ANNUAL REVIEW OF
BIOPHYSICS AND
BIOMOLECULAR STRUCTURE

EDITORIAL COMMITTEE (1992)

ANNUAL REVIEW OF BIOPHYSICS AND BIOMOLECULAR STRUCTURE

VOLUME 21, 1992

DONALD M. ENGELMAN, *Editor*
Yale University

CHARLES R. CANTOR, *Associate Editor*
Lawrence Berkeley Laboratory, University of California, Berkeley

THOMAS D. POLLARD, *Associate Editor*
The Johns Hopkins University School of Medicine

ANNUAL REVIEWS INC. 4139 EL CAMINO WAY P.O. BOX 10139 PALO ALTO, CALIFORNIA 94303-0897

R ANNUAL REVIEWS INC.
Palo Alto, California, USA

International Standard Serial Number: 1056-8700
International Standard Book Number: 0-8243-1821-8
Library of Congress Catalog Card Number: 79-188446

Annual Review and publication titles are registered trademarks of Annual Reviews
Inc.

∞ The paper used in this publication meets the minimum requirements of American National Standard for Information Sciences—Permanence of Paper for Printed
Library Materials, ANSI Z39.48-1984.

Annual Reviews Inc. and the Editors of its publications assume no responsibility
for the statements expressed by the contributors to this *Review*.

TYPESET BY BPCC-AUP GLASGOW LTD., SCOTLAND
PRINTED AND BOUND IN THE UNITED STATES OF AMERICA

PREFACE

Over the past decade, the *Annual Review of Biophysics* has sought to formulate a vision of biophysics that emphasizes the solution of significant biological problems using approaches based on the methods and concepts of the physical sciences. Initially, we reformulated the name of the *Review* to emphasize the use of physical chemistry (i.e. the *Annual Review of Biophysics and Biophysical Chemistry*). We recently reviewed the actual content of the *Review* over this decade, and noted that structural biology, a field of great current interest, is heavily represented. We therefore considered whether a new name might be appropriate.

But the name "Structural Biology" seemed imprecise in that it, in an ideal view, includes many scales of characterization of biological structure, ranging from gross morphological observation through the levels of light and electron microscopy to the finest details of molecular architecture. The particular focus of our interest in this publication resides in the properties of biomolecules. Consequently, while recognizing the dislocations that a change of name might produce, the Editors have decided to rename the series as the *Annual Review of Biophysics and Biomolecular Structure*.

DONALD M. ENGELMAN
EDITOR

CONTENTS

SOME RELATED ARTICLES IN OTHER *ANNUAL REVIEWS*

From the *Annual Review of Biochemistry*, Volume 61 (1992):

Enzymes and Molecular Mechanisms of Genetic Recombination, S. C. West

Prokaryotic DNA Replication, K. J. Marians

Telomerases, E. H. Blackburn

Transcription Factors: Structural Families and Principles of DNA Recognition, C. O. Pabo and R. T. Sauer

Catalytic Antibodies, S. J. Benkovic

Constrained Peptides: Models of Bioactive Peptides and Protein Substructures, J. Rizo and L. M. Gierasch

Mass Spectrometry of Peptides and Proteins, K. Biemann

Control of Nonmuscle Myosins by Phosphorylation, J. L. Tan, S. Ravid, and J. A. Spudich

Neuronal $Ca^{2+}/Calmodulin$-Dependent Protein Kinases, P. I. Hanson and H. Schulman

Proton Transfer in Reaction Centers from Photosynthetic Bacteria, M. Y. Okamura and G. Feher

Zinc Proteins: Enzymes, Storage Proteins, Transcription Factors, and Replication Proteins, J. Coleman

Small Catalytic RNAs, R. H. Symons

From the *Annual Review of Cell Biology*, Volume 7 (1991):

Structures of Bacterial Photosynthetic Reaction Centers, J. Deisenhofer and H. Michel

Microtubule Dynamics: Mechanism, Regulation and Function, V. Gelfand and A. D. Bershadsky

Molecular Mechanisms of Axon Growth and Guidance, J. L. Bixby and W. A. Harris

Signal Transduction in the Visual System of Drosophila, D. P. Smith, M. A. Stamnes, and C. S. Zuker

Structure and Biological Role of Vitronectin, K. T. Preissner

Microfilament Structure and Function in the Cortical Cytoskeleton, A. Bretscher

Biochemical Mechanisms of Constitutive and Regulated Pre-mRNA Splicing, M. R. Green

Analyses of the Cytoskeleton in Saccharomyces cerevisiae, F. Solomon

From the *Annual Review of Microbiology*, Volume 46 (1992):

Treatment of the Picornavirus Common Cold by Inhibitors of Viral Uncoating and Attachment, M. A. McKinlay, D. C. Pevear, and M. G. Rossmann

From the *Annual Review of Physical Chemistry*, Volume 42 (1991):

Vibrational and Vibronic Relaxation of Large Polyatomic Molecules in Liquids, T. Elsaesser and W. Kaiser

High-Resolution Zero Kinetic Energy (ZEKE) Photoelectron Spectroscopy of Molecular Systems, K. Müller-Dethlefs and E. W. Schlag

Structures and Transitions in Lipid Monolayers at the Air-Water Interface, H. M. McConnell

Simulated Annealing in Crystallography, A. T. Brünger

Generation of High-Resolution Protein Structures in Solution from Multidimensional NMR, T. L. James and V. J. Basus

Vibrational Energy Relaxation and Structural Dynamics of Heme Proteins, R. J. D. Miller

From the *Annual Review of Physiology*, Volume 54 (1992):

Charge Movement and the Nature of Signal Transduction in Skeletal Muscle Excitation-Contraction Coupling, E. Rios, G. Pizarro, and E. Stefani

Mechanotransduction, A. S. French

Role of cGMP and Ca^{2+} in Vertebrate Photoreceptor Excitation and Adaptation, U. B. Kaupp and K.-W. Koch

Transmembrane Receptors and Intracellular Pathways That Control Cell Proliferation, J. Pouysségur and K. Seuwen

Adaptations to High Hydrostatic Pressure, G. N. Somero

Structural Elements Involved in Specific K^+ Channel Functions, L. Y. Jan and Y. N. Jan

Application of Localized In Vivo NMR to Whole Organ Physiology in the Animal, A. Koretsky and D. S. Williams

NMR Spectroscopy of Cells, B. S. Szwergold

Nuclear Magnetic Resonance and Its Application to Physiological Problems, R. J. Gillies

Solving Solution Structures of Physiologically Relevant Proteins by NMR Spectroscopy, N. E. MacKenzie, P. R. Gooley, and L. A. Hardaway

The Utilization of Magnetic Resonance Imaging in Physiology, J. R. Alger and J. A. Frank

From the *Annual Review of Plant Physiology and Plant Molecular Biology*, Volume 42 (1991):

Plant Lipoxygenase: Structure and Function, J. N. Siedow

Thionins, H. Bohlmann and K. Apel

Chlorophyll Fluorescence and Photosynthesis: The Basics, G. H. Krause and E. Weis

The Roles of Heat Shock Proteins in Plants, E. Vierling

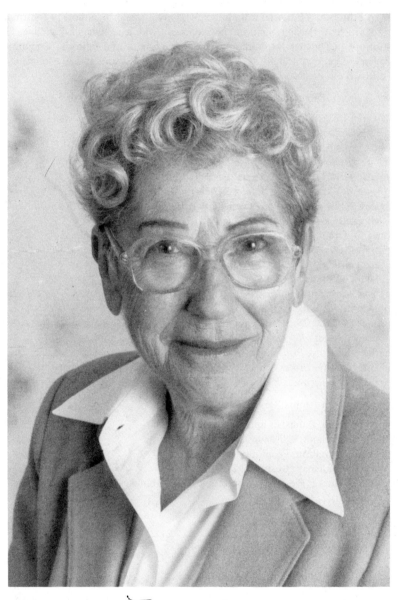

Mildred Cohn

Annu. Rev. Biophys. Biomol. Struct. 1992. 21:1–24

ATOMIC AND NUCLEAR PROBES OF ENZYME SYSTEMS

M. Cohn

Department of Biophysics and Biochemistry, University of Pennsylvania, School of Medicine, Philadelphia, Pennsylvania 19104–6089

KEY WORDS: autobiographical sketch

CONTENTS

PERSPECTIVES AND OVERVIEW

It is deeply gratifying to have been invited by the Editors to present my reminiscences and reflections on science and participation in research. I feel particularly honored when I note who my illustrious predecessors have been. Unlike some *Annual Reviews,* which present a prefatory chapter every year, the *Annual Review of Biophysics* has only done so sporadically. Perhaps a partial explanation is the difficulty the Editors have had identifying biophysicists—the prefatory editorial remarks in many volumes deal with the question of defining the field of biophysics. I, however, am comfortable with the term *biophysics* because I have been familiar with hybrid fields of science for more than fifty years; the term "chemical physics" was introduced in the early 1930s when I was a graduate student. My PhD mentor, Harold Urey, founded the *Journal of Chemical Physics* and was its first editor. In the first issue of January, 1933, he editorialized:

1

1056–8700/92/0610–0001$02.00

At present the boundary between the sciences of physics and chemistry has been completely bridged. Men who must be classified as physicists on the basis of training and of relations to departments or institutes of physics are working on the traditional problems of chemistry; and others who must be regarded as chemists on similar grounds are working in fields which must be regarded as physics. These men, regardless of training and affiliations, have a broad knowledge of both sciences and their work is admired and respected by their coworkers in both sciences. The methods of investigation used are, to a large extent, not those of classical chemistry and the field is not of primary interest to the main body of physicists, nor is it in the traditional field of physics.

In 1947, the term "chemical physics" was used by Francis Crick in his application to the Medical Research Council for a research student's grant (39):

The particular field which excites my interest is the division between the living and the non-living, as typified by, say, proteins, viruses, bacteria and the structure of chromosomes. The eventual goal, which is somewhat remote, is the description of these activities in terms of their structure, i.e., the spatial distribution of their constituent atoms, in so far as this may prove possible. This might be called the *chemical physics of biology*.

Of course, the name that caught on was molecular biology and the first two prefatory chapters published in the *Annual Review of Biophysics* have the term "molecular biology" in their titles. Many areas in biology can benefit from a chemical physics approach, and any combination of the terms physics, chemistry, and biology can be used for its description. For my own work, I prefer the designation *biophysical chemistry*.

In this chapter, I present some of my background, the progress of my career, and then some of my research work as an independent scientist. To have a career as a scientist was my choice, but the particular fields in which I have been working since 1937 are quite accidental. I was born and grew up in New York City and was educated in its public schools. In high school, biology, a required course, did not appeal to me, but I did very well in mathematics. I elected to study two years of chemistry, which was taught by an excellent teacher, and I tentatively considered majoring in chemistry at college. There were no scientists in my family, although both sides had a long rabbinical tradition, the most common form of intellectual and scholarly pursuit in the Jewish communities of eastern Europe. My mother and father had independently emigrated from the same Russian town about 1906—my father had come alone to avoid being ordained as a rabbi and to avoid military service in the Czarist army. He was a man of advanced ideas, a militant atheist, with strong convictions on many political and moral issues and with an inordinate respect for learning and scholarship. When my only brother decided to become a lawyer, my father was sorely disappointed; he had hoped to have his son get a PhD in philosophy. As for me, he indoctrinated me with the belief that I could achieve anything I chose to—of course, not without difficulty since I was female and a Jew. He was a realist. My mother was more conventional in her attitudes and had modest goals for my future.

In my first years at Hunter College (the family took for granted that I would attend Hunter, the free city college for women), I was excited by many of the subjects I was exposed to. Nevertheless, I decided in my sophomore year to major in chemistry and minor in physics (no major in physics was available). With the arrogance of youth at the age of 15, I had concluded that I could study the humanities and social sciences on my own, but for the physical sciences, I needed formal instruction. My fascination with science was sufficiently strong to withstand erosion by inferior education. Although Hunter had excellent instruction in the humanities and social sciences, the attitude of the college towards science education was epitomized by the chemistry department chairman who declared that it was not ladylike for women to be chemists; his sole purpose was to prepare us to be chemistry teachers. My persistence was rewarded in my senior year with a good course in physical chemistry and an inspiring course on introduction to modern physics. For the first time, I appreciated the general principles in chemistry and the excitement of current developments in physics. The year was 1931, and I was determined to go on to graduate school to learn more in both areas. My father encouraged me, but my mother tried to persuade me to become a school teacher. I turned down an offer of a career in merchandising made by the buyer in the electrical goods department at Macy's, where I had been working as a salesgirl on Saturdays and school holidays for two years, an opportunity most of my classmates would have jumped at in that jobless period.

My father's business failed in the Great Depression, and the family could not finance my graduate studies. Although I had an excellent academic record, my applications for scholarships or other forms of financial support to some 20 graduate schools were unsuccessful. By living at home, I could attend Columbia University and pay for one year's tuition, about $300, from savings I had accumulated from summer jobs. Columbia would not accept my application for a teaching assistantship since in 1931 only men were permitted to be assistants in Columbia College, an all male school. I eked out financial solvency that year by babysitting.

That first year at Columbia was a revelation to me as well as a traumatic experience. I was introduced to thermodynamics, classical mechanics, and molecular spectroscopy. I resented the fact that my undergraduate education had not given me a broad view of what chemistry was all about. Urey and Hammett shared the thermodynamics course, and Urey taught molecular spectroscopy; the latter course opened up the field of chemical physics and quantum chemistry for me. I found Urey enthusiastic and inspiring and decided to try to do research with him as my mentor should I have the opportunity to become a PhD candidate. The prospect of at last doing research had sustained me in my efforts to attend graduate school, so I was disappointed to learn that first-year graduate students were limited to course work. At the end of the year, I was granted a master's degree; no thesis was required.

Since I had no funds, I had to leave Columbia and try to find a job, no easy task in 1932. Fortunately in my senior year at college, I had passed a federal civil service examination for Junior Chemist and as my year at Columbia ended, I was offered a job at the NACA (National Advisory Committee for Aeronautics) laboratory in Langley Field, Virginia. I accepted with alacrity. Initially I was assigned to do computational work, tedious and boring, but I managed to be transferred to a research position in the engine division where the goal was to develop a fuel-injection, spark-ignition, airplane engine that operated on the Diesel cycle. I had a most supportive superior, a physicist named A. M. Rothrock, who not only taught me the workings of an engine but found time to study Tolman's *Statistical Mechanics* with me. I became quite interested in the phenomenon of combustion in engines and was shocked to learn that so little was understood of the basic physics and chemistry of flame propagation. I asked one of my engineer colleagues, "How can you do research on engine design when you don't even understand what's going on inside?" He answered, "If we had to wait for you chemists to explain the combustion process, we still wouldn't have an engine." If I learned nothing else on this first job, I developed a healthy respect for applied research and realized that in seeking a solution to a practical problem, one must tackle it on all levels.

After two years, I had published two reports; I served as senior author on the second. With the help of the best support staff I have ever encountered in my scientific career, I designed and they constructed a combustion apparatus capable of withstanding 2000 psi. Kinetics of combustion could be measured with millisecond time resolution as a function of (*a*) air pressure, (*b*) delay time (in 10^{-3} s) between fuel injection and spark ignition, and (*c*) air/fuel ratio. After two years, I had reached the top salary of my rank, junior scientific aide, and I was informed that I would never be promoted. The director of the agency did not approve of women in research. I was the only one among seventy men, an unenviable position for a naive 20-year old almost 60 years ago. Faced with a dead end in my position, I decided to return to graduate school. My studies were financed by my savings from my $1300–1750 annual salary.

I had become interested in the rate of vaporization of the injected fuel in relation to its efficacy of utilization, a problem suitable for a PhD in chemical engineering. It might be more feasible financially, I reasoned, to take a leave of absence, complete the requisite courses as a candidate for the PhD in chemical engineering, and return to do the experimental work for my thesis at the NACA. A leave of absence was duly granted and I returned to my parents' home in New York.

GRADUATE STUDIES

In an interview with the chairman of the chemical engineering department at Columbia, I was informed that women had never been admitted to the graduate program and that no change in policy was in the offing. So I returned to my first love, physical chemistry. I sought out Professor Urey to ask if he would accept me as a graduate student. His first response was, "You don't want to be my graduate student, I don't pay attention to my graduate students." This did not worry me unduly because my experience at the NACA had given me considerable self-confidence in my ability to do research independently. When I told him that I wanted to have his mentorship notwithstanding, he agreed to accept me and sent me to his friend Professor I. I. Rabi for guidance on the physics courses I should take. After a semester of additional course work including quantum chemistry and advanced physics lab, I passed my qualifying exams and became an official candidate for the PhD.

Both chemistry and physics were in ferment at that time and Columbia shared in the excitement. Urey was separating stable isotopes; down the hall Hammett was laying the foundations of physical organic chemistry; in the next building Rabi was determining nuclear magnetic moments with his molecular beams; and in the summer of 1936, I audited a splendid course given by Fermi on artificial radioactivity. Urey introduced a seminar series in the chemistry department in chemical physics; he thought the existing one in physical chemistry didn't suffice. Instead of having a journal club, we studied current developments in depth, including low temperature phenomena, absolute reaction rate theory, separation of stable isotopes, production of artificial radioactivity, etc. Urey was well qualified to lead such a seminar because he had been a postdoctoral fellow in the Bohr Institute and had coauthored with Ruark the definitive text at that time on *Atoms, Molecules and Quanta*.

Urey was a man of broad interests, encouraging the use of isotopes to solve biological problems, even suggesting some uses himself. He was also interested in geochemistry, in the origin and distribution of the elements, a field that became his chief interest many years later. Of all the great scientists I've known, he had the fastest mind. I learned to prepare myself carefully for a discussion with him; otherwise I would be on point 2 when he was already at point 5. He also never forgot his humble beginnings and always fought for the underdog—in particular, he seemed to be the only professor in the department who was concerned about the welfare of the graduate students. Towards the end of my graduate student days when he surmised that I was in need of funds he said, "Ever since I've gotten the Nobel Prize, I've wanted to help my students. Why don't you let me lend you some money and someday when you have a job, you can pay me back." I did not avail myself of his well-meant offer, but I never forgot his generosity.

At that time, Urey was separating the stable isotopes by taking advantage of the deviation from the value of 1.000 for the equilibrium constant of isotopic exchange reactions, e.g. $H_2^{18}O + C^{16}O_2 \rightleftharpoons H_2^{16}O + C^{16}O^{18}O$ ($K_{eq} = 1.047$ at $0°C$). In a two-phase system, the reactants could be brought to equilibrium many times, and enrichment of the same isotope would occur in one component and loss in the other. I was assigned the problem of separating ^{12}C and ^{13}C. The first three months were spent calculating equilibrium constants of possible exchange reactions as described by Urey & Greiff (64) by using spectroscopic data to evaluate the ratios of partition functions of the appropriate ^{12}C and ^{13}C compounds. The goal was to find a suitable reaction with a large fractionation factor at a reasonable temperature. This was my first realization that a nuclear property such as mass could affect molecular and chemical properties of molecules, and furthermore, that one could take advantage of the small difference in properties to achieve a practical result. The next three months were devoted to learning to blow glass and repeating an experiment of a postdoctoral fellow on determining the equilibrium constant of the H_2O-CO_2 oxygen exchange reaction. The theoretical and experimental approaches that I was indoctrinated with in the first six months in Urey's lab have guided me throughout my scientific career.

After I wasted a year and failed to separate ^{12}C and ^{13}C, partly because the newly constructed mass spectrometer was nonfunctional, Urey suggested that I study exchange reactions of $H_2^{18}O$ with organic compounds, in particular, acetone in the vapor state. The concentration of ^{18}O could hopefully be measured using the density difference between $H_2^{16}O$ and $H_2^{18}O$. This method would obviate the necessity of an operating mass spectrometer. Initial experiments were analyzed using density methods, but eventually the mass spectrometer became operational.

Urey had succeeded in enriching the ^{18}O concentration of H_2O from the natural abundance of 0.2% to 2.0%, and I was in the unique position of having access to the only source of enriched ^{18}O and water de-enriched in

$H_2{}^{18}O$. I soon found that the acetone-water exchange did occur slowly in the vapor phase but that the acid or base-catalyzed reaction in solution proceeded at a reasonable rate at 25°C. I reported to Urey that I thought it would be more interesting to study the reaction in solution, whereupon he said, "I understand something about the solid state and something about the gaseous state but the liquid state is a complete mystery to me and I do not like experiments where I have no theory to guide me. If you feel strongly about studying the reaction in solution, why don't you talk to Professor Hammett. He knows all about what goes on in solution." And so I did. My thesis became a typical research problem in physical organic chemistry rather than in chemical physics, except for the analytical methodology (22).

Urey developed an interest in the mechanism of the reaction once I presented the experimental results to him. In fact, since he could not find me a job (as he sadly put it, "Nobody wants you"), he offered me a postdoctoral position to extend the use of ^{18}O to determine the mechanisms of organic reactions that I had selected. In 1937, the economy was still in a depression and jobs were scarce. Most of the PhD graduates took industrial positions. The big companies (du Pont, Standard Oil, etc) would send recruiters to the Columbia chemistry department every spring and the notices would appear on the bulletin board, "Mr. _____ of _____ Company will interview all prospective PhDs of this year—Male, Christian." I was out on two counts.

My luck held, however, and I was offered another postdoctoral position. Vincent du Vigneaud, then Professor of Biochemistry at George Washington University Medical School, wanted to introduce isotopic tracers into his research program on sulfur-amino acid metabolism and was looking for a qualified postdoctoral fellow. He approached Schoenheimer and Rittenberg at Columbia College of Physicians and Surgeons, who were pioneers in the application of isotopic tracers to intermediary metabolism. They had close ties to Urey who supplied them with isotopes such as ^{15}N; Rittenberg had preceded me as a graduate student in Urey's lab by a few years. They recommended me to du Vigneaud. Urey and I discussed the offer, and Urey thought it would be better for me to go to another laboratory rather than stay at Columbia. I had been infected by the enthusiasm of Rittenberg and Schoenheimer for applying isotopic tracers to biological problems and the prospects seemed legion in this newly opened field. I accepted the offer and I have never regretted the decision. I began my wanderings using chemical physics in biology, a most rewarding experience, far more rewarding I daresay than chemical physics per se, even if a career in the latter would ever have materialized for me.

POSTDOCTORAL YEARS

My first task in du Vigneaud's laboratory was to set up a procedure for measuring the deuterium content of organic compounds. In Urey's lab, I had already assembled an apparatus for measuring density of water to 1 ppm for the determination of D_2O or $H_2^{18}O$ concentration, the "falling drop" method (4), which I then duplicated at George Washington. Rittenberg graciously allowed me to spend some time in his laboratory to learn how to convert the hydrogen of organic compounds to water for isotopic analysis.

In du Vigneaud's laboratory, I found myself in a new world where metabolic pathways and molecular structure were viewed from the vantage of organic chemistry. The organization of research as a team effort was also unfamiliar to me; each member of the team contributed his or her expertise to the master plan designed by the professor. As the only group member with a background in physics and physical chemistry, I was called upon to repair galvanometers, modify telephone circuits, and other tasks quite beyond me. I did later build an electrophoresis apparatus at 10,000 volts for the lab and eventually constructed a mass spectrometer. I also had to learn how to feed rats by stomach tube.

After about nine months at George Washington Medical School, I moved with du Vigneaud to Cornell Medical College in New York City. Again luck was with me because I had just married a theoretical physicist, Henry Primakoff, who was also offered a job in New York City; we had estimated the probability that we both would have jobs in the same city to be close to zero.

In one of the early isotopic tracer experiments, du Vigneaud found that, contrary to reports in the literature, young rats did not grow when homocysteine (deuterated) was substituted for methionine in the diet. The opinion within the conservative elements in the biochemical community who distrusted this newfangled tracer technique ascribed the difficulty to the deuterium, which, of course, du Vigneaud demonstrated was not the case. By carefully comparing the pure amino acid, pure vitamin diet being fed to rats in his experiments with the diet of Rose, whose animals did grow, he noted a difference—Rose used tiki tiki as the source of the vitamin B complex. In a brilliant flash of intuition, du Vigneaud said, "transmethylation from N-methyl of choline, a component of tiki tiki, to S-methyl of homocysteine to form methionine."

I spent most of the next seven years participating in studies of transmethylation. Unlike other group members, I was generally not involved in synthetic work such as the syntheses of 10 of the amino acids used in the rat diets, which were not available commercially. Du Vigneaud did ask me to synthesize deuterated methyl alcohol to be used as a source of the labeled methyl group in the synthesis of deuteromethyl methionine. I remembered that Professor Zanetti in the Columbia chemistry department had synthesized CD_3OD. He generously permitted me to use his laboratory with its homemade compressor to reduce CO with deuterium gas at 10,000 pounds pressure at 300°C with an unknown duPont catalyst. I managed to produce about 100 grams of CD_3OD in a month. Labeled methionine was synthesized, and the group showed that the deutero methyl group of methionine was indeed the source of the methyl groups of choline and creatine (27). The universality of transmethylation from methionine is currently known to be much greater than we realized at the time.

In my opinion, the most elegant tracer experiment done in du Vigneaud's lab used doubly labeled methionine to study this compound's conversion to cystine in the rat. Kilmer synthesized methionine with ^{13}C in the β and γ-positions (^{14}C was not yet available) and with ^{34}S. None of the carbon and all of the ^{34}S was transferred from fed methionine to cystine isolated from the hair (28). I also worked on the peptide hormones from the posterior pituitary, determining their isoelectric points in an apparatus I devised (17). Occasionally I could do an experiment outside the group effort. Because of his interest in insulin, du Vigneaud approved of my attempt to determine the valence states of the metal in paramagnetic cobalt and nickel insulin by comparing their magnetic susceptibilities with that of the diamagnetic zinc insulin. I had been inspired by Pauling's work on the magnetic susceptibility of various forms of hemoglobin (53). Unfortunately, even the sensitive Gouy balance that I used in the Columbia physics department gave equivocal results because of the large contribution of the diamagnetic susceptibility of the protein to the measured value. Some ten years later, I went back to magnetochemistry because electron paramagnetic resonance had been discovered and the diamagnetism of components other than the paramagnetic metal ion in the system no longer interfered.

The World War II years were spent in du Vigneaud's laboratory. The young men of draft age and du Vigneaud devoted their time to war work, but du Vigneaud thought that I and the draft-exempt men should continue to do basic research to maintain a minimum continuity until the war was over. By 1946, I felt that I had been initiated in the bioorganic approach and appreciated the high standards that could be achieved in this work, but that I had served my apprenticeship in this type of biochemistry long enough. When my husband was offered a position in the physics department at Washington University, I urged him to accept it, which he did. Our choice of academic institutions was limited because all state universities and many private ones had nepotism rules forbidding a husband and wife from holding jobs in the same institution. du Vigneaud, who had been reluctant to have me leave as long as I remained in New York, then helped me obtain a research associateship in the biochemistry department of Washington University Medical School, newly chaired by Carl Cori. We left New York with our two children and never returned.

What a warm welcome I received in St. Louis. On my first appearance at the laboratory, Gerty Cori, who was awarded the Nobel prize jointly with her husband the following year, greeted me with "I understand you are more fortunate than I; you have a daughter and a son; I have only a son." I had two objectives for my future research, one was to work independently, an ardent wish after almost nine years as a member of a team, and the other was to use isotopes not merely as tracers of metabolic pathways in intact animals but for insight into the mechanism of enzyme-catalyzed reactions in isolated systems. In discussions with Carl Cori, who generously endorsed both objectives, I suggested two possible projects for the elucidation of mechanisms: one, a comparison of rates of hydrogen, deuterium, and tritium in appropriate enzyme reactions and two, the use of ^{18}O to determine the position of bond cleavage in various enzymatic reactions of phosphate compounds. I had wished to extend the approach in my PhD thesis into the biochemical arena for some time—hence my interest in the second proposal. Cori preferred this project because of his great interest in the reactions of phosphate intermediates in glycolysis and glycogenolysis. When I informed him that it would be necessary to construct a mass spectrometer (none were available commercially at that time), he assured me that he was prepared to finance it and also make technical help available to me. I also set up a facility for measuring radioactive isotopes for the department—in 1946 both radioactive isotopes and measuring instruments began to be commercially available.

Cori's laboratory, the center of enzymology in the U.S. at that time, was an ideal environment for any young scientist interested in enzymology, and especially for me because Gerty Cori took me under her wing to teach me enzymology. The Coris had gathered a group of highly talented young scientists. Their faculty included Earl Sutherland, Sidney Velick, Oliver Lampen, and John Taylor. The postdoctoral fellows included Graham Webster, Ed Krebs, Victor Najjar, Arthur Kornberg, and visitors came from abroad, including Lindberg from Sweden, the Walaas's from Norway, Helen Porter from England, Shlomo Hestrin from Israel, Baranowski from Poland, de Duve from Belgium, Posternak from Switzerland, and many others. Daily discussions at lunch in the departmental library were lively. Conversations ranged over a broad spectrum of subjects and were not necessarily scientific but always consisted of challenging questions and an intolerance for sloppy thinking. The more formal weekly seminars were stimulating and covered all aspects of biochemistry. Cori himself covered progress in photosynthesis annually and Velick often brought us up to date on progress in X-ray studies of hemoglobin. I remember one year when Cori decided he wanted to know, and thought all of us should know, the current state of elementary particle physics, and he invited Henry Primakoff to present a seminar on the subject.

I had set up a system for radioactivity measurements and I collaborated with Gerty Cori in the first use of ^{32}P and ^{14}C in the Cori laboratory. Doudoroff, Barker & Hassid (25) in a landmark paper had postulated that a covalent enzyme-glucose intermediate existed on the basis of an exchange between the phosphate group of glucose-1-phosphate and inorganic phosphate (^{32}P) catalyzed by sucrose phosphorylase in the absence of acceptor. This finding led many enzymologists to generalize the existence of such covalent intermediates to all group-transfer enzymatic reactions. We showed that neither muscle nor potato phosphorylase in the absence of acceptor catalyzed any such exchange reaction between either inorganic phosphate (^{32}P) or glucose (^{14}C) with glucose-1-phosphate (10). Another collaborative experiment with Sutherland, Posternak, and Cori on the mechanism of the phosphoglucomutase reaction involved the equilibration of $^{32}P,^{14}C$-labeled glucose-1-phosphate with the obligatory cofactor glucose 1,6 diphosphate (62). The equilibration of both isotopes eliminated several mechanisms and was consistent only with the mechanism proposed by Leloir and coworkers (41) whereby the glucose-1,6 diphosphate transfers a phosphoryl group to glucose-1- or glucose-6-phosphate.

INDEPENDENT RESEARCH ACTIVITIES 1946–1985

A common thread that characterized many of my research efforts is the strategy of revealing in an enzyme system what reaction has taken place or its rate, not by isolation of intermediates, but indirectly by observation of the transfer of a labeled atom or a spectroscopic line shape. This strategy was resorted to only when a direct approach was ineffective. An example was elaborated in 1951 in the use of ^{18}O as a probe of enzymatic reactions (6):

> If inorganic phosphate labeled with ^{18}O is taken up in organic linkage by the formation of a carbon-oxygen linkage, as in the phosphorylase reactions, the oxygen bridging the carbon and phosphorus is thus labeled with O^{18}. Should the organic phosphate now be cleaved by the rupture of the phosphorus-oxygen bond, the organic moiety remaining would contain O^{18}. Furthermore, should inorganic phosphate be formed in such a reaction, it would be diluted with normal oxygen. This leads (a) to the possibility of identifying phosphorylated intermediates which are too unstable or too low in concentration to be isolated as such, by establishing the presence of O^{18} in the depho-

sphorylated product; and (b) to the possibility of detecting reactions otherwise unobservable by following the O^{18} content of the inorganic phosphate.

Nuclear magnetic resonance (NMR), which I began to use in 1958, lends itself particularly to this strategy as exemplified in (a) deducing structural features of the binding sites of kinases when various substrates are bound from the effect of Mn(II) on the proton relaxation rates of water in the enzyme-metal-substrate complex; (b) determining distances at the active site of enzyme-substrate complexes from the effect of paramagnetic Mn(II) on the relaxation rates of nuclei in the substrates; (c) evaluating the reaction rates of the central complexes in kinase reactions from the line width of the ^{31}P resonances, a static measurement to define a dynamic parameter; (d) estimating the distance between substrate and an amino acid residue of the enzyme on the basis of the nuclear Overhauser effect (NOE) between the two in proton NMR. Electron paramagnetic resonance (EPR) can also yield structural information on the immobilization of bound Mn(II) and the asymmetry of the Mn(II) complex from the distribution of spectral lines; distance information can be obtained between two paramagnetic species on the same molecule using the intensity loss of the spectral lines.

Oxygen-18 as a Probe

Although my ultimate goal was to understand the structural basis of both substrate and enzyme that explained enzyme catalysis, I realized that first one had to define the reactions, the bond cleaved, and the structures of the substrates and the intermediates. Forty-five years ago it was not even known which bond was cleaved in enzyme-catalyzed reactions of organic phosphates. Oxygen-18 could answer that question. I compared the nonenzymatic and enzymatic hydrolytic reactions of glucose-1-phosphate in $H_2^{18}O$. The same substrate, glucose-1-phosphate labeled with ^{18}O, was converted to glycogen and sucrose catalyzed by glycogen and sucrose phosphorylases, respectively (5). In acid hydrolysis, the C-O bond was ruptured, but in enzymatic hydrolyses (whether catalyzed by acid or alkaline phosphatases) the P-O bond was cleaved. However, in the phosphorylase reactions, the C-O bond of glucose-1-phosphate was cleaved, thus indicating that the phosphorylase enzymes are glucosyl-transfering enzymes, but the phosphatases are phosphoryl-transfering enzymes. The same pattern was observed in many other enzyme-catalyzed reactions of organic phosphates. In those reactions where Pi is taken up to form organic phosphate, the C-O bond is involved, e.g. reaction catalyzed by glyceraldehyde-3-phosphate dehydrogenase (GAPDH). In contrast, when an organic phosphate transfers phosphate to water or another acceptor, then the P-O bond is involved. Thus, 1,3 diphosphoglyceric acid, like glucose-1-phosphate, has its P-O bond cleaved when its carboxyphosphate moiety transfers its phosphoryl group to ADP to yield ATP in the 3-phosphoglycerate kinase reaction. However, its C-O bond is cleaved when it transfers its acyl group to GAPDH to yield acyl-enzyme. This aspect of the ^{18}O work demonstrating a universal feature of all enzymatic phosphoryl transfer reactions was summarized in 1959 (8). Furthermore, I found that reactions of ATP involving transfer of the adenyl group rather than the γ-phosphoryl group showed cleavage of the P-O bond of the α-phosphate of ATP. This finding emphasized the similarity of adenyl transfer reactions (pyrophosphorylases) with phosphoryl transfer reactions (kinases) rather than with reactions catalyzed by phosphorylases.

Upon the urging of my colleague, Graham Webster, I embarked in 1950 on an investigation of oxidative phosphorylation with ^{18}O-labeled Pi with the hope of throwing some light on the unknown mechanism of phosphorylation coupled with electron transport. At that time, by analogy with glycolysis, an organic phosphate intermediate between the initial Pi and the final ATP was postulated but never identified. The result of experiments with rat liver mitochondria was unexpected; in the phosphorylation accompanying electron transport, ^{18}O-labeled Pi lost not 25% of its ^{18}O but 90%, indicating that inorganic phosphate had undergone a phosphorus-oxygen cleavage reaction about eight times during the formation of one ATP molecule (7). This phenomenon did not occur in substrate-level phosphorylation.

Further work on the phosphate-water exchange associated with oxidative phosphorylation, some done in collaboration with postdoctoral fellows George Drysdale (12, 26) and Nobutomo Itada (35) only succeeded in proving that the mechanism could not be the same as substrate-level phosphorylation in glycolysis, in which a -C-O-P intermediate forms. Only after Mitchell in 1961 pointed out that oxidative phosphorylation occurred without an organic phosphate intermediate did Boyer and his coworkers, after many years of work, unravel the complex phosphate-water exchanges involved in oxidative phosphorylation and delineate the detailed alternate-site mechanistic implications (2).

Many years later in the late 1970s, I became involved with phosphate-^{18}O again quite accidentally. In connection with some work on the GTPase activity of the elongation factor, EF-Tu, I decided to use isotopic oxygen for mechanistic studies. Because I had given away my mass spectrometer more than 10 years earlier and I was now focused on ^{31}P-NMR, I decided to use $H_2{}^{17}O$ to follow the phosphate-water exchange reaction by NMR. As I anticipated, the quadrupolar ^{17}O so broadened the ^{31}P resonance spectrum of Pi that the ^{31}P peak decreased in intensity as the ^{17}O in water substituted for the ^{16}O in phosphate as the exchange reaction proceeded.

To share my excitement over this observation, I showed the spectra to two of my postdoctoral fellows, George Reed and Jacques Reuben. One of them said, "The resonance has structure," and the other said, "Maybe it's an isotope effect," whereupon I looked at the label of the water I had used in the experiment and learned that it contained not only 11% ^{17}O but about 60% ^{18}O. This serendipitous observation proved to be an isotope effect; preparation of Pi containing approximately 50% ^{18}O, 50% ^{16}O recorded at 145.8 MHz was resolved into 5 lines separated by about 0.02 ppm ranging from $P^{16}O_4$ to $P^{18}O_4$ and all intermediate species in the expected distribution (13). Further NMR experiments indicated how this distribution of ^{18}O phosphate species could be used to gain insight into enzyme mechanisms as also demonstrated by Boyer and collaborators using mass spectrometric methods (33). Preparations of ATP labeled with ^{18}O in various positions (14) showed that the chemical shift resulting from a bridge ^{18}O differed from that of a nonbridge ^{18}O. Several investigators used this effect to specify the stereochemical pathway of many enzymatic phosphate reactions.

The observation of the ^{18}O effect on ^{31}P-NMR gave me pleasure far exceeding its scientific importance because I felt I had come full circle. Forty-five years had passed since as a graduate student I had calculated equilibrium constants of isotopic exchange reactions from the isotopic mass effect on energy levels in molecular spectra, and now I observed the isotopic mass effect of oxygen-18 on the nuclear energy levels of ^{31}P in the nuclear magnetic resonance spectrum of ^{31}P. In NMR spectroscopy, the phenomenon could also be applied to study chemical reactions.

Electron Paramagnetic Resonance

At the same time that I was pursuing the intractable problem of the synthesis of ATP coupled to electron transport, I turned to what I hoped was a more tractable area of research, the mechanism of reactions utilizing ATP, the phosphoryl transferring enzymes, the kinases, and the adenyl transferring enzymes. One characteristic of all enzymatic reactions with ATP as substrate is the requirement of a divalent metal ion. The investigation of the role of the divalent metal ion appealed to me for three reasons: (a) the simplicity of a single atomic species; (b) the possibility that the site of bond cleavage at the α or β-P of ATP was determined by the structure of the metal chelate of ATP involved in the reaction; and (c) the fact that the paramagnetic Mn(II) could always substitute, although Mg(II) was the activator in most cases.

I had learned about EPR, an active field of research in the physics and chemistry departments of Washington University, in 1953, and I speculated that Mn complexes of ATP and Mn-ATP-enzyme complexes should be good candidates for study. Although Jack Townsend, who had built one of the most sensitive EPR instruments available, and I succeeded in observing free Mn(II) concentrations of 100 μM to 1 mM, we did not observe any complex (21). The quantitation of free Mn(II) concentration permitted the determination of association constants of the Mn complexes but yielded no information on the structure of these complexes. More than a decade later at the University of Pennsylvania with a postdoctoral fellow, George Reed, we succeeded in observing the complex EPR spectra of Mn(II) protein complexes (55) and of ternary and quaternary complexes composed of enzyme and substrates (56). The observation was made possible by the theoretical understanding of the dependence of the spectral intensity and distribution of transitions on the immobilization of Mn(II) in the complex and the asymmetry of the complex. The information gathered on the structure of these complexes and their relation to enzyme mechanism in the extension of Mn(II) EPR is discussed below in connection with the experiments on the effect of Mn(II) on the proton relaxation rate of water in the same complexes.

NMR Spectroscopy

While I was on sabbatical in 1955 in Kreb's laboratory at Oxford, it occurred to me that perhaps I could get at the structure of metal-ATP-enzyme complexes by using ^{1}H and ^{31}P-NMR. When I returned to St. Louis early in 1956, I found that the home-built NMR spectrometer in the chemistry department was limited to protons. Consequently, I wrote to Varian in Palo Alto explaining my problem and asking if I could use their instruments. Their reply was most enthusiastic and they suggested I come immediately. At this time, I had three children aged 6 to 13 and it was not easy for me to be absent from home for an extended period. A couple of years later, the whole family planned to spend the summer in Palo Alto because Henry was invited to be a visiting professor at Stanford for the summer quarter. When I then wrote to Varian, I received a cool reception; in the two years that had elapsed, the organic chemists had discovered NMR and the applications laboratory at Varian was very busy indeed. Nevertheless, they agreed to allow me access.

During the summer of 1958, the 60-MHz NMR spectrometer at Varian was available to me for only two days in spite of my introduction by Felix Bloch. One day was made available for proton spectra and, about six weeks later, one day for ^{31}P spectra. Nevertheless, the time sufficed to demonstrate feasibility—the adenine and ribose protons were resolved; the α-, β-, and γ-P of ATP were well resolved; Mg(II) chelation caused a considerable shift in the β-peak; and stoichiometric amounts of Mn(II) made all three peaks disappear.

The next fall, I learned that the nearest suitable spectrometer was in the chemistry department of the University of Illinois. Through friends at Urbana, the NMR spectrometer was made available to me on weekends, and I availed myself of this opportunity about four or five times. Fortunately, I could dispense with this long commute because NIH invited Sam Weissman, an outstanding EPR and NMR spectroscopist in the chemistry department of Washington University, to apply for a grant for a Varian DP60 spectrometer. He, in turn, invited me to participate in the application with the understanding that I would have time on the instrument.

The instrument duly arrived, and Tom Hughes, a physics graduate student, was given responsibility for its operation. After several months, it was operating smoothly and Tom obtained with a single scan in a 5 mm tube a high resolution spectrum of 0.5 M ATP with the ^{31}P-^{31}P couplings well resolved. Low resolution spectra in 12 mm nonspinning tubes could be obtained with 90 mM solutions. We published two papers, one on the pH dependence of the resonances of ADP and ATP (15) and the second on the metal nucleotides—the effects of the diamagnetic divalent ions Mg, Ca, and Zn and of the paramagnetic ions Mn, Cu, and Co (16). All three diamagnetic metal ions caused similar changes in the chemical shifts in the ^{31}P peaks of ADP and ATP, primarily in the β-P of ATP; no significant changes occurred in any of the proton peaks with the exception of a shift of 0.2 ppm in the H–8 peak of adenine induced by Zn(II). Low concentrations of both Mn(II) and Co(II) broadened all three ^{31}P peaks of ATP, but Cu(II) broadened only the β- and γ-peaks because Cu(II) could form only square coplanar complexes but Mn(II) and Co(II) could form octahedral complexes. I submitted the results of the metal ion effects on the ^{31}P-NMR of ATP as a communication to the *Journal of the American Chemical Society* early in 1960; it was rejected. It was subsequently published in the *Journal of Biological Chemistry* and eventually became a "citation classic." I attempted and failed to see any effect of hexokinase on the ^{31}P-NMR spectrum of MgATP; as I found out many years later, the effect was too small to observe at the ratio of hexokinase to MgATP that I had used.

In 1960, Henry accepted a position as Donner Professor of physics at the University of Pennsylvania. I joined the Johnson Foundation/Biophysics Department, which was under the direction of Britton Chance, and continued my research program there. This move could not have come at a more auspicious moment in my career. Not only was Britton Chance interested in energy transduction and in my work on oxidative phophorylation and ATP-utilizing reactions, but he was a master of spectroscopy and most supportive of my efforts to explore magnetic resonance spectroscopy. He not only gave me access to his excellent shop but introduced me to a talented undergraduate electrical engineering student, Jack Leigh.

I realized that the high concentrations needed for NMR spectroscopy of substrates or enzymes made this study impractical to pursue. However, one component of the enzymatic reaction system, namely water, was not limited in concentration, and because the effect of 1 M Mn(II) on the proton relaxation rates (T_1 and T_2) of water is about a factor of 10,000, and the value in complexes depends on the number of water molecules in the first coordination sphere of the metal ion that exchanges with solvent water, the measurement of relaxation rates promised to have sufficient sensitivity to yield information on the number of water molecules in Mn(II) complexes. Fortunately, when I arrived in Philadelphia, I found that Jack Leigh had constructed a pulsed NMR spectrometer to measure relaxation rates of water by the spin echo technique. The only magnet available was from an EPR instrument. For purposes of temperature control, I used the Varian ^{31}P probe (24.3 MHz), which I had persuaded the chemistry department to purchase as an accessory to their 60 MHz NMR spectrometer.

The first measurements on MnADP and MnATP were a surprise; the proton relaxation rate (T_1) of water (PRR) due to Mn(II) was enhanced, rather than de-enhanced, by a factor of about 1.5 in the presence of nucleotide. Furthermore, upon addition of the enzyme creatine kinase, enhancement increased to about 10 in the ternary enzyme-metal nucleotide complex. With the enzyme enolase, maximum enhancement was observed with the binary Mn-enzyme complex and was reduced in the ternary Mn-enzyme-substrate complex (19). Because the number of water ligands to Mn(II) must decrease in a complex, the enhancement could only be explained by an increase in the correlation time for the interaction between the electron spin and the nuclear spin, sufficient to more than overcome the decreased number of water ligands. Again, we were lucky; unbeknownst to us at the time, the proton relaxation rate (PRR) enhancement for protein complexes is near maximum at 25 MHz. A similar PRR enhancement had been observed (31) on the binding of Mn(II) to nucleic acids, the first example of PRR enhancement of water on binding of paramagnetic ions to a macromolecule. Early experiments carried out by Al Mildvan on serum albumin (44) and pyruvate kinase (45) and Bill O'Sullivan on creatine kinase (52) yielded an enhancement parameter characteristic of each metal complex that could be used to determine its binding constant. Two classes of enzymes were distinguished, in which the metal ion was bound either to the nucleotide only (creatine kinase) or was bound directly to the enzyme (pyruvate kinase). Extensions of these measurements to many metal-enzyme-substrate complexes have been reviewed (29, 47).

Delving further into the phenomenon through measurements of PRR enhancement as a function of frequency and temperature, Jacques Reuben (58) revealed that in Mn(II) enzyme complexes, the relevant correlation time was the electron spin relaxation time of Mn(II) rather than the rotational correlation time of the complex. Simultaneously, George Reed (56) obtained EPR spectra of the Mn complexes that, as judged by line widths and positions and symmetry considerations, complemented the information from PRR enhancement. Since the Mn(II)-H_2O distance was known, the number of water protons in the first Mn(II) coordination sphere exchangeable with solvent water protons could be calculated. The measurements were extended to several kinases (9) and the following generalization emerged: as each successive substrate was bound to the enzyme, the apparent number of water molecules, n, in the first coordination sphere of Mn(II) progressively decreased. For example with arginine kinase investigated by Buttlaire (3), n equals 2 for the ternary E-MnADP complex, n equals 1 for the quaternary E-MnADP-L-arginine, and n equals ~ 0.4 for the transition state analog E-MnADP-nitrate-L-arginine.

Two possible explanations of this phenomenon were presented: as more subsites of the active site of enzymes become occupied, either the Mn(II) water ligands are replaced by protein or substrate ligands, or the number of water ligands remains constant but the changed active-site conformation leads to a decreased rate of exchange between water in the first coordination sphere of Mn(II) with solvent water or a combination of both. In either case, the active site becomes less and less accessible to solvent water. A similar phenomenon has been observed with X-ray crystallography of hexokinase and its substrate complexes (1). Subsequently, Reed and his coworkers (57) resolved the ambiguity of the PRR results for the creatine kinase complexes and other enzyme complexes by establishing the complete ligand assignment of Mn(II) in the complexes by observing the [17]O superhyperfine coupling in elegant Mn(II) EPR experiments using [17]O-labeled substrates and/or water.

In the years between 1966 and 1974, we attempted to exploit every technically feasible aspect of magnetic resonance for structure and function of enzymes that we could think of, in addition to EPR and water PRR of Mn(II) complexes. General narrowing of proton resonances of proteins in solution by magic angle spinning did not occur; we observed only narrowing of the aromatic protons of high molecular weight poly-γ-glutamate and the methyl group of the silicone rubber gasket of the sample cell (18).

Al Mildvan and Jack Leigh succeeded in quantitating the distance between Mn(II) and ^{19}F at the active site of pyruvate kinase in its fluorokinase reaction using the electron spin-nuclear spin interaction, i.e. the paramagnetic effect on T_1 and T_2 of ^{19}F-NMR (46). Tom James used internuclear double resonance techniques (INDOR) and NOE to implicate the lysyl residue at the active site of creatine kinase as the binding site of formate, a proven analog of the γ-phosphoryl group of ATP (38).

Two graduate students, June Taylor and Jack Leigh, and I (64) succeeded in estimating the distance between the nitroxide-free radical bound covalently to the S-H group of creatine kinase and Mn(II), Co(II), or Ni(II) on the enzyme-bound metal nucleotide by observing the effect of the electron spin-electron spin interaction in the EPR spectrum of the nitroxide-free radical. Leigh (40) developed a quantitative theory of the effect.

With the goal of mapping the three-dimensional configuration at the creatine kinase active site, Leigh & McLaughlin (43) encountered difficulties in determining distances between paramagnetic probes, Mn(II) and the nitroxide free radical covalently bound to creatine kinase, and the bound substrate nuclei in creatine kinase-substrate complexes. Their efforts to evaluate T_1 and T_2 of the relevant bound substrate nuclei were hampered in solutions containing excess substrate over enzyme by insufficiently rapid exchange between free and bound substrates and by the presence of a mixture of complexes.

To characterize the enzyme-substrate complexes, we therefore decided to do experiments in which more than 90% of the substrates were in the bound form with stoichiometric amounts of enzyme. Experiments with Mg(II), the normal activator, carried out on four kinase enzymes by Nageswara Rao (9), a visiting scientist, yielded a surprising result. Regardless of the equilibrium constant of the overall reaction measured in the presence of catalytic amounts of enzyme, for example in the 3-phosphoglycerate kinase reaction with an equilibrium constant of $\sim 3 \times 10^{-4}$, the equilibrium constant of the central complexes determined by ^{31}P-NMR is always close to 1 (49). Thus the free energy change of the chemical transformation on the surface of the enzymes is close to zero; the significant free energy changes are involved in the binding of substrate to enzyme and/or the dissociation of products. This remarkable feature of enzyme catalysis appears to be fairly general for many enzyme reactions. Furthermore in the NMR experiments, the interconversion rates of the central complexes at equilibrium can be determined from analysis of the line shapes of the ^{31}P resonances of the exchanging nuclei (48).

In certain respects, the results of ^{31}P NMR of enzyme-bound substrates were somewhat disappointing. When the nucleotides or their Mg chelates bind to kinases, very little change in ^{31}P chemical shifts is observed except for the β-P of ADP, which incidentally indicates that the electronic environment of the β-P of MgADP when bound to kinases is different from that of MgATP (20). Upon binding to adenylate kinase, the molecular symmetry of the inhibitor diadenosine pentatophosphate breaks down, accompanied by significant changes in chemical shift indicating that the two ADP substrate molecules are in very different environments when enzyme-bound (50). Upon binding of phosphoenolpyruvate (PEP) to pyruvate kinase, progressive chemical shift changes are observed downfield by 1.1 ppm in E.PEP, 3.2 ppm in E.Mg.PEP, and 4.5 ppm in Mg.E.MgADP.PEP (51). Even in those cases in which significant changes were observed, the results were uninterpretable in terms of structural parameters because of the lack of a satisfactory theory of ^{31}P chemical shifts.

The ^{31}P chemical shifts of phosphates are not greatly perturbed by binding because the four oxygen atoms shield the phosphorus. However, if an oxygen is substituted by a sulfur, large changes occur (30). A study of the metal ion dependence of the ^{31}P-NMR of ATP phosphorothioate analogs by Eileen Jaffe, a graduate student (36), indicated that Mg(II) chelates via oxygen and Cd(II) via sulfur with ATPβS as would be anticipated for hard and soft metals, respectively. Hence, the the β-γ bidentate chelate of Mg and Cd with the same diastereomer of ATPβS yields opposite stereochemical configurations in the chelate, as occurs in ATPαS in α-β or α-β-γ chelates. For the first time, a NMR result suggested an enzyme experiment to determine how the Mg(II) was chelated to ATP in various enzyme reactions, the question that motivated my original interest in NMR. The rationale was the following: if MgATPβS (R) and CdATPβS (S) are preferred substrates in a particular enzymatic reaction, such reversal indicates unequivocally that the metal is chelated to the β phosphate in a rate-determining step in the reaction. In the hexokinase reaction (37), the ratio of V_{Max}, V_S/V_R, increased monontonically for ATPβS from 0.0017 with Mg(II) through a series of metal ions to 37 for Cd(II); on the other hand, the V_S/V_R for ATPαS of ∼20 varied little with metal ion. The study concluded that the β,γ bidentate ATP is the substrate, as supported by prior results with substitution-inert Co(III) metal complexes (23). This approach, extended to other kinase reactions, emphasized that the structure of the MgATP chelates differs even when all the enzymes catalyze the phosphoryl group transfer reaction.

A discussion of the many systems that have been investigated with paramagnetic and nuclear probes is beyond the scope of this chapter. However, some important studies of tRNA include: water PRR of Mn(II) binding in collaboration with A. Danchin and M. Grunberg-Manago (11);

nitroxide spin labeling of ^{1}H-NMR relaxation carried out by Walter Daniel (24); NMR of ^{19}F-substituted tRNA in collaboration with Horowitz et al (34). Ed Wilson and colleagues investigated EF-Tu, water PRR of Mn(II) complexes, and nitroxide-labeled Tu (66, 67). In addition, the stoichiometric equilibrium of methionyl tRNA synthetase was investigated using ^{31}P-NMR in collaboration with Fayat, Blanquet, and Nageswara Rao (32), as was mechanistic aspects of the synthetase reaction with the thio analog of ATP in collaboration with Linda Smith (61) and Ed Rossomando (59).

The technology, particularly of NMR, has advanced spectacularly over the past 30 years. With the introduction of high field superconducting magnets and Fourier transform spectroscopy, the barrier of NMR insensitivity encountered in the late 1950s necessitating the use of concentrations inapplicable to enzyme systems has largely been overcome. In addition, the introduction of 2D and 3D techniques and of higher resolution has made possible the reliable determination of interatomic distances in proteins in solution complementary to X-ray crystallographic data.

New approaches in enzymology, arising from introduction of molecular biological techniques, in particular site-directed mutagenesis, have obviated the use in many cases of indirect methods of studying structure-function relations. The focus of enzymatic studies has also shifted towards the phenomenon of regulation. In the 1980s, I had the tool to answer the question, does the thermodynamics, i.e. magnitude, of the free energy of ATP hydrolysis determine the calcium gradient established in the sarcoplasmic reticulum by the Mg-Ca ATPase as suggested by Tanford (63)? Lerman (42), a visiting scientist, had observed that the free energy of hydrolysis of ATPβS to ADPβS is more exergonic than the hydrolysis of ATP by approximately 2.5 kcal/mol. A collaborative study with Pintado and Scarpa (54) showed that the magnitude of the Ca(II) gradient accompanying nucleotide triphosphate hydrolysis was invariant with substrate ATP or ATPβS (R or S) and was consequently independent of the free energy of hydrolysis in the sarcoplasmic reticulum system.

I became intrigued with calcium regulation of enzymes via calmodulin. A postdoctoral fellow, Steve Seeholzer, used ^{1}H-NMR to investigate one aspect of this regulatory process, what changes in structural and dynamic properties occurred in each component upon complexing of calmodulin and its ligand, melittin, an analog of the binding domain for calmodulin on myosin light chain kinase (60). Perdeuterated calmodulin was prepared by expressing the calmodulin gene in *Escherichia coli* in collaboration with Anthony Means and John Putkey, who had cloned the chicken gene for calmodulin, and Henry Crespi, who grew the *E. coli* in D_2O and deuterated medium. The calmodulin, >99% deuterated, simplified observation of conformational changes in the spectrum of the mellitin and exchange rates in the NH region of calmodulin. The work was followed up by Joshua Wand and his collaborators using 2D techniques to make proton resonance assignments and determine conformational changes quantitatively.

CONCLUDING REMARKS

My formal career was somewhat unusual inasmuch as I held the rank of research associate for 21 years before becoming an associate professor. However, because 12 of those years were in Cori's department in St. Louis, I did independent research, and in the last 6 years, I was an Established Investigator of the American Heart Association. In spite of the obvious disadvantages of my status, it held a number of positive features. I had no teaching or administrative duties; I was able to stay home if a child was seriously ill and could spend two months vacationing with my family every summer. Furthermore, I was not competing on the academic ladder, so I could choose technically difficult, long-range problems because there was no pressure to publish quickly. After one year at the University of Pennsylvania, I was promoted to full professorship and shortly thereafter awarded a Career Investigatorship of the American Heart Association, an enlightened organization with a policy of supporting people rather than projects. Again I could devote almost all my time to research. Britton Chance not only made his excellent technical support staff available to me but encouraged and supported me in developing a group of my own.

In retrospect, the most important aspect of my career is that it's been fun—the joy of predicted results materializing, the even more rewarding experience of serendipitously discovering an entirely unexpected phenomenon, and the special gratification of having the results applied to medical problems. And I have been so lucky, always finding myself in a stimulating milieu, interacting with first-class minds, first my mentors, then my colleagues, and finally my postdoctoral fellows and students. My greatest piece of luck was marrying Henry Primakoff, an excellent scientist who treated me as an intellectual equal and always assumed that I should pursue a scientific career and behaved accordingly.

Literature Cited

1. Bennett, W. S. Jr., Steitz, T. 1978. *Proc. Natl. Acad. Sci. USA* 75: 4848–52
2. Boyer, P. D. 1989. *FASEB J.* 3: 2164–78
3. Buttlaire, D. H., Cohn, M. 1974. *J. Biol. Chem.* 249: 5741–48
4. Cohn, M. 1946. *Preparation and Measurement of Isotopic Tracers*, ed. D. Wright Wilson, pp. 51–59. Ann Arbor, MI: Edwards. 108 pp.
5. Cohn, M. 1949. *J. Biol. Chem.* 180: 771–81
6. Cohn, M. 1951. *Phosphorus Metabolism*,

ed. M. D. McElroy, B. Glass, 1: 374–76. Baltimore: The Johns Hopkins Press. 762 pp.
7. Cohn, M. 1953. *J. Biol. Chem.* 201: 735–50
8. Cohn, M. 1959. *J. Cell. Comp. Physiol.* 54(Suppl. 1): 17–32
9. Cohn, M. 1984. *Current Topics in Cellular Regulation*, ed. M. deLuca, pp. 1–13. New York: Academic
10. Cohn, M., Cori, G. T. 1948. *J. Biol. Chem.* 175: 89–93
11. Cohn, M., Danchin, A., Grunberg-Manago, M. 1969. *J. Mol. Biol.* 39: 199–217
12. Cohn, M., Drysdale, G. R. 1955. *J. Biol. Chem.* 216: 831–46
13. Cohn, M., Hu., A. 1978. *Proc. Natl. Acad. Sci. USA* 75: 200–3
14. Cohn, M., Hu., A. 1980. *J. Am. Chem. Soc.* 102: 913–16
15. Cohn, M., Hughes, T. R. 1960. *J. Biol. Chem.* 235: 3250–53
16. Cohn, M., Hughes, T. R. 1962. *J. Biol. Chem.* 237: 176–81
17. Cohn, M., Irving, G. W. Jr., du Vigneaud, V. 1941. *J. Biol. Chem.* 137: 635–42
18. Cohn, M., Kowalsky, A., Leigh, J. S. Jr., Maricic, S. 1967. See Ref. 30a, pp. 45–48
19. Cohn, M., Leigh, J. S. Jr. 1962. *Nature* 193: 1037–40
20. Cohn, M., Nageswara Rao, B. D. 1978. *Frontiers in Physico-Chemical Biology*, ed. B. Pullman, pp. 191–211. New York: Academic. 503 pp.
21. Cohn, M., Townsend, J. 1954. *Nature* 173: 1090–93
22. Cohn, M., Urey, H. C. 1938. *J. Am. Chem. Soc.* 60: 679–87
23. Cornelius, R. D., Cleland, W. W. 1978. *Biochemistry* 17: 3279–85
24. Daniel, W. E. Jr., Cohn, M. 1975. *Proc. Natl. Acad. Sci.. USA* 72: 2582–86
25. Doudoroff, M., Barker, H. A., Hassid, W. Z. 1947. *J. Biol. Chem.* 168: 725–36
26. Drysdale, G. R., Cohn, M. 1958. *J. Biol. Chem.* 233: 1574–77
27. du Vigneaud, V., Cohn, M., Chandler, J. P., Schenck, J. R., Simmonds, S. 1941. *J. Biol. Chem.* 140: 625–41
28. du Vigneaud, V., Kilmer, G. W., Rachele, J. R., Cohn, M. 1944. *J. Biol. Chem.* 155: 645–51
29. Dwek, R. A. 1973. *Nuclear Magnetic Resonance in Biochemistry*, pp. 213–84. Oxford: Clarendon. 390 pp.
30. Eckstein, F., Goody, R. S. 1976. *Biochemistry* 15: 1685–91
30a. Ehrenberg, A., Malmstrom, B. G., Vanngard, T., eds. 1967. *Magnetic Resonance in Biological Systems*. Oxford:

Pergamon. 431 pp.
31. Eisinger, J., Shulman, R. G., Blumberg, W. E. 1961. *Nature* 192: 963–64
32. Fayat, G., Blanquet, S., Nageswara Rao, B. D., Cohn, M. 1980. *J. Biol. Chem.* 255: 8164–69
33. Hackney, D. D., Sleep, J. A., Rosen, G., Hutton, R. L., Boyer, P. D. 1979. *NMR in Biochemistry*, ed. S. Opella, P. Lu, pp. 285–300. New York: Marcel Dekker. 434 pp.
34. Horowitz, J., Ofengand, J., Daniel, W. E. Jr., Cohn, M. 1977. *J. Biol. Chem.* 252: 4418–20
35. Itada, N., Cohn, M. 1963. *J. Biol. Chem.* 238: 4026–31
36. Jaffe, E. K., Cohn, M. 1978. *Biochemistry* 17: 652–57
37. Jaffe, E. K., Cohn, M. 1979. *J. Biol. Chem.* 254: 10839–45
38. James, T. L., Cohn, M. 1974. *J. Biol. Chem.* 249: 2599–2603
39. Judson, H. F. 1979. *The Eighth Day of Creation*, pp. 109–10. New York: Simon and Schuster. 636 pp.
40. Leigh, J. S. 1969. *J. Chem. Phys.* 52: 2608–12
41. Leloir, L. F., Trucco, R. E., Cardini, C. E., Paladini, A., Caputto, R. 1948. *Arch. Biochem.* 19: 339–40
42. Lerman, C. L., Cohn, M. 1980. *J. Biol. Chem.* 255: 8756–60
43. McLaughlin, A., Leigh, J. S. Jr., Cohn, M. 1976. *J. Biol. Chem.* 251: 2777–87
44. Mildvan, A. S., Cohn, M. 1963. *Biochemistry* 2: 910–11
45. Mildvan, A. S., Cohn, M. 1965. *J. Biol. Chem.* 240: 238–45
46. Mildvan, A. S., Cohn, M., Leigh, J. S. Jr. 1967. See Ref. 30a, pp. 113–17
47. Mildvan, A. S., Cohn, M. 1970. *Adv. Enzymol.* 33: 1–70
48. Nageswara Rao, B. D., Buttlaire, D. H., Cohn, M. 1976. *J. Biol. Chem.* 251: 6981–86
49. Nageswara Rao, B. D., Cohn, M. 1977. *Proc. Natl. Acad. Sci. USA* 74: 5355–57
50. Nageswara Rao, B. D., Cohn, M., Scopes, R. K. 1978. *J. Biol. Chem.* 253: 8056–60
51. Nageswara Rao, B. D., Kayne, F., Cohn, M. 1979. *J. Biol. Chem.* 254: 2689–96
52. O'Sullivan, W. J., Cohn, M. 1966. *J. Biol. Chem.* 241: 3116–25
53. Pauling, L., Coryell, C. D. 1936. *Proc. Natl. Acad. Sci. USA* 22: 210–14
54. Pintado, E., Scarpa, A., Cohn, M. 1982. *J. Biol. Chem.* 257: 11346–52
55. Reed, G. H., Cohn, M. 1970. *J. Biol. Chem.* 245: 662–64
56. Reed, G. H., Cohn, M. 1972. *J. Biol. Chem.* 247: 3073–81

57. Reed, G. R., Leyh, T. 1980. *Biochemistry* 19: 5472–80
58. Reuben, J., Cohn, M. 1970. *J. Biol. Chem.* 245: 6539–46
59. Rossomando, E. F., Smith, L. T., Cohn, M. 1979. *Biochemistry* 18: 5670–74
60. Seeholzer, S. H., Cohn, M., Putkey, J. A., Means, A. R., Crespi, H. L. 1986. *Proc. Natl. Acad. Sci. USA* 83: 3634–38
61. Smith, L. T., Cohn, M. 1981. *Biochemistry* 20: 385–91
62. Sutherland, E. W., Cohn, M., Posternak, T., Cori, C. F. 1949. *J. Biol. Chem.* 180: 1285–95
63. Tanford, C. 1981. *J. Gen. Physiol.* 77: 223–29
64. Taylor. J. S., Leigh, J. S. Jr., Cohn, M. 1969. *Proc. Natl. Acad. Sci. USA* 64: 219–26
65. Urey, H. C., Greiff, L. J. 1935. *J. Am. Chem. Soc.* 57: 321–27
66. Wilson, G. E. Jr., Cohn, M. 1977. *J. Biol. Chem.* 252: 2004–9
67. Wilson, G. E., Cohn, M., Miller, D. L. 1978. *J. Biol. Chem.* 253: 5764–68

Annu. Rev. Biophys. Biomol. Struct. 1992. 21:25–47

SOLID-STATE NMR APPROACHES FOR STUDYING MEMBRANE PROTEIN STRUCTURE

Steven O. Smith and Olve B. Peersen

Department of Molecular Biophysics and Biochemistry, Yale University, New Haven, Connecticut 06511

KEY WORDS: rotational resonance, REDOR, magic angle spinning, peptides, dipolar interactions

CONTENTS

PERSPECTIVES AND OVERVIEW

The proteins that span the cell membrane perform an array of functions ranging from signal transduction to ion transport. In the past few years, gene sequencing of membrane proteins has yielded an abundance of amino acid sequence data that in turn has generated structural models for many of these proteins (13, 14, 52, 61). Unfortunately, high resolution structures of integral membrane proteins in phospholipid bilayers have been notoriously difficult to obtain using either X-ray diffraction or solution NMR methods. It has generally been a challenge to grow well-ordered crystals of large hydrophobic molecules for diffraction studies, while solution NMR

25

1056–8700/92/0610–0025$02.00

approaches for determining protein structure rely on rapid isotropic molecular motion and are often not suitable for membrane systems in which proteins have restricted motions and exhibit broad NMR resonances. Lysolipids and detergents have been used to solubilize hydrophobic proteins and increase mobility for solution studies, but have the drawback of forming micellar rather than bilayer structures (5, 21, 55). In comparison, solid-state NMR spectroscopy has become an effective approach for studying membrane proteins, such as gramicidins (45, 78), rhodopsins (71), and phage-coat proteins (49, 50). Solid-state NMR approaches have the potential for obtaining accurate internuclear distances and orientations that can be translated into molecular structure, and recent advances in magic angle spinning (MAS) methods for measuring both homonuclear and heteronuclear dipolar couplings have begun to tap this potential. Currently, using specific ^{13}C and ^{15}N isotopic labels, distances in the range of 2–7 Å can be measured within ~ 0.5 Å, and the relative orientations between peptide planes can be measured to better than $10°$. This review covers several solid-state NMR methods that have emerged in the past few years for the analysis of membrane proteins, and the studies discussed serve to outline the strengths and limitations of the approaches.

SOLID-STATE NMR METHODS

The NMR spectrum, in both solution and the solid-state, results from interactions of the observed nuclear spins with a large external magnetic field and many small local internal fields. These interactions are described by the nuclear spin Hamiltonian ($\mathscr{H}$).

$$\mathscr{H} = \mathscr{H}_Z + \mathscr{H}_{RF} + \mathscr{H}_{CS} + \mathscr{H}_D + \mathscr{H}_J \qquad 1.$$

One must have an idea of the physical basis for each term of the spin Hamiltonian and its size before discussing the methods for extracting structural information from the NMR spectrum. In depth discussions can be found in several reviews (6, 40, 49, 71, 89). The Zeeman ($\mathscr{H}_Z$) and radio-frequency Hamiltonians ($\mathscr{H}_{RF}$) describe the interaction of nuclear spins with the external magnetic field and with local internal fields created by radio-frequency pulses in the NMR probe, respectively. The RF fields are about 10^3 times smaller than the field generated by the external magnet and stimulate transitions between NMR energy levels. The chemical-shift term ($\mathscr{H}_{CS}$) describes the shielding of a nuclear spin from the external field by surrounding electrons. The distribution of electrons around a nucleus is usually not uniform, and consequently the effective shielding is often anisotropic. The size of the chemical-shift anisotropy (CSA) increases with the asymmetry and number of occupied outer electron orbitals and is typically on the order of 1–20 kHz. $\mathcal{H}_D$ describes through-space dipolar interactions, while $\mathcal{H}_J$ describes indirect through-bond dipolar interactions (or J couplings) that are mediated via electrons. The direct dipole-dipole coupling (D) ranges from 0–50 kHz depending on the gyromagnetic ratio (γ) of each of the coupled spins, their through-space separation, and Plank's constant (h), where $D = h\gamma_1\gamma_2r^{-3}$. The J couplings are generally much smaller (0–200 Hz), but play an important role in solution NMR in which the larger direct dipolar interactions are averaged and only contribute to the NMR spectrum through relaxation effects. Finally, an additional term $\mathcal{H}_Q$ dominates the NMR spectra of quadrupolar nuclei, such as ^2H and ^{14}N. Deuterium NMR has been used extensively to study the dynamics of membrane lipids and proteins (12, 17, 65, 68, 70, 79) but is not covered in this review.

Solid-state and solution NMR differ in the molecular motions that are effective in averaging these nuclear spin interactions. In solution, rapid isotropic rotational motion of proteins leads to averaging of dipolar interactions to zero and chemical shifts to an isotropic value, resulting in narrow resonances with small splittings due to J couplings that are not averaged. In contrast, for molecules that have restricted or anisotropic motion, these spin interactions lead to broad NMR resonances. The broad NMR lineshapes contain a wealth of structural information because both the chemical-shift anisotropy and dipolar interactions depend directly on molecular structure and orientation with respect to the external magnetic field. This information is lost in solution studies. The challenge in solid-state NMR is to counter problems of resolution and sensitivity in order to extract structural details from the NMR spectrum.

One can improve both resolution and sensitivity in solid-state NMR studies in several ways. The first is by specific isotopic labeling. In protein studies, ^{13}C and ^{15}N enrichment is often used to great advantage to enhance the signals from single sites over natural-abundance backgrounds. A second approach is to orient or align samples relative to the external magnetic field, increasing both resolution and sensitivity as broadening resulting from differences in molecular orientation is greatly reduced. The macroscopic orientation of lipid bilayers has been accomplished by coating glass slides with phospholipid multilayers (30, 41, 67) or by the use of strong magnetic fields (62, 66, 72). Finally, narrow linewidths approaching those in solution can be obtained through magic angle spinning (MAS) (1, 37, 63). In MAS, the sample is physically rotated at high speeds in the magnetic field in order to average the nuclear-spin interactions. Structural studies of membrane proteins usually rely on isotopic labeling in combination with either macroscopic orientation of the sample or MAS. High resolution ^{1}H NMR studies, analogous to those in solution, are severely limited in solids because of strong proton-proton dipolar interactions.

Figure 1 illustrates the distinctive ^{13}C lineshapes for the carboxyl and α-carbon resonances of free glycine. These lineshapes arise from the random orientation of glycine molecules in a polycrystalline sample and are representative of the broad NMR resonances (or powder patterns) mentioned above. A single molecule or crystallite in the sample contributes a narrow Lorentzian component to the overall lineshape at a frequency dependent on its orientation with respect to the external magnetic field. In Figure 1 (top), the powder pattern lineshapes represent the sum of all of the molecular orientations in the sample and result solely from anisotropy in the

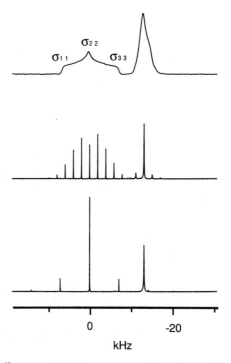

Figure 1   Solid-state ^{13}C NMR spectra of glycine illustrating the broad NMR resonances in static samples (*top*) and the effects of magic angle spinning at 2.0 kHz (*middle*) and 7.2 kHz (*bottom*). The principal values of the chemical-shift tensor are shown for the ^{13}C carboxyl resonance and correspond to the down-field inflection point (σ_{11}), the maximum (σ_{22}), and the up-field inflection point (σ_{33}). MAS collapses the broad lineshapes into sharp centerbands at the isotropic chemical shifts (σ_{iso}) and rotational sidebands spaced at the spinning frequency. The frequency scale is centered on the carboxyl centerband.

chemical-shift interaction because dipolar interactions between ^{13}C and ^{1}H spins have been eliminated by proton decoupling. The glycine CSA is ~ 15 kHz for the carboxyl resonance and ~ 5 kHz for the methylene resonance at a magnetic field strength of 9.4 T (100.6 MHz ^{13}C frequency). In Figure 1 (middle and bottom), the CSA has been averaged by spinning the sample at an angle θ of 54.7° relative to the external magnetic field. This is the "magic angle." Both the chemical shift ($\mathscr{H}_{CS}$) and dipolar ($\mathscr{H}_{D}$) Hamiltonians have terms that contain factors of $(3\cos^2\theta - 1)$, and at the magic angle, these terms vanish. The spinning speed of the sample has a pronounced effect on the appearance of the spectrum. Spinning at a rotational frequency that is much less than the frequency width of the CSA results in each broad lineshape breaking up into a centerband at the isotropic chemical shift and into sets of spinning sidebands spaced at the rotational frequency. One can see this effect in Figure 1 (middle), where the spinning speed is 2.0 kHz. The relative intensities of the spinning sidebands can be used to determine the CSA while providing a substantial gain in signal-to-noise over the powder pattern (27). Faster spinning collapses the line intensity into the centerband, thereby increasing sensitivity but removing information about the CSA.

The standard solid-state cross-polarization (CP) pulse sequence used for observing dilute S spins, such as ^{13}C and ^{15}N, is shown in Figure 2 (top). The 90° pulse on the ^{1}H spins and simultaneous spin-locking pulses on the ^{1}H and S spins transfer the much larger polarization of the ^{1}H spins to the S spins, thereby increasing sensitivity (57, 63). The use of ^{1}H CP also allows for a faster pulse repetition rate governed by the shorter proton T_1. Proton irradiation is generally used during the acquisition period to eliminate heteronuclear dipolar coupling.

ORIENTATION-DEPENDENT APPROACHES

Diffraction and NMR methods differ greatly in how the data specify the three-dimensional structure of a protein. Diffraction data define the coordinates of atoms in a crystal lattice, while NMR methods yield relative distances and orientations between nuclei. Solution NMR structures are derived mainly from short (< 5 Å) ^{1}H $\cdots$ ^{1}H distance constraints, estimated from nuclear Overhauser effects (NOEs), and are refined using torsion-angle data calculated from J couplings (6, 16, 89). In solids, direct dipolar interactions and the chemical-shift anisotropy are exploited to obtain both distance and orientation information that constrain structural models. One solid-state NMR approach, developed by Opella, Cross, and coworkers focuses on the determination of torsion angles in the polypeptide backbone of a protein as a way to generate protein structures solely from orientation

Cross Polarization

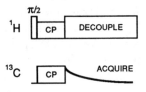

Rotational Resonance

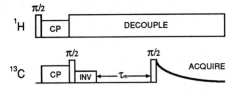

REDOR

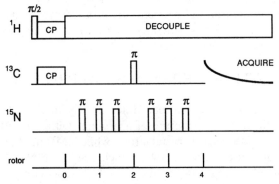

Figure 2   Solid-state NMR pulse sequences used for orientation and distance measurements. The standard cross-polarization sequence (*top*) enhances dilute spin signals by transferring the larger proton polarization to the dilute spins. The pulse sequence used in rotational resonance experiments (*middle*) adds a flip-back pulse followed by a selective inversion and a time delay to allow for magnetization exchange. The pulse sequence for REDOR experiments (*bottom*) requires at least three RF channels. A ^{13}C spectrum is collected with and without the ^{15}N pulse train, and the difference between them is used to determine the dipolar coupling. This figure illustrates a four-cycle REDOR experiment.

constraints (9, 10, 50). The following two sections briefly describe the theory for this orientation-dependent approach and several applications to membrane systems.

Theory

The α-carbons of adjacent amino acids in a polypeptide chain are joined by the amide C-N bonds. The six atoms that form this peptide linkage lie roughly in a plane, and the relative orientation of adjacent planes is defined by the ϕ and ψ torsion angles (Figure 3). The secondary structure of the peptide backbone can be determined by sequentially establishing the orientation of each peptide plane relative to a common axis, the z-axis of the external magnetic field. Measurements of both the dipolar and chemical shift interactions are necessary to limit the number of possible orientations and define the peptide structure (9, 45, 50, 77).

The orientation dependence of the dipolar interaction has the form:

$$\Delta v = D (3 \cos^2 \theta - 1), \qquad\qquad 2.$$

where Δv is the observed dipolar splitting, D is the dipolar coupling constant, and θ is the angle between the internuclear vector connecting the spins and the external magnetic field. The dipolar interactions point along the bond axes and are axially symmetric. The observed dipolar splitting ranges from 0 to $2D$ for bonds aligned at the magic angle and parallel to the z-axis of the magnetic field, respectively. One of the problems in

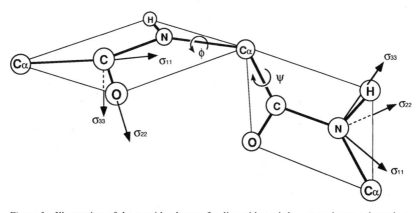

Figure 3   Illustration of the peptide planes of a dipeptide and the approximate orientations of the amide ^{15}N and carbonyl ^{13}C chemical-shift tensors with respect to the molecular frame (22). The ϕ and ψ angles define the orientation of the planar peptide linkages and are determined by measuring the N-C and N-H bond orientations, as well as the orientation of the ^{15}N and ^{13}C shift tensors.

determining peptide plane orientations is that the experimental Δv specifies two or four different values for θ depending on the size of D relative to Δv (9). Consequently, several bond orientations need to be measured to arrive at a unique solution for the peptide-plane orientation. The ^{15}N-^{1}H and ^{15}N-^{13}C bond orientations are the most readily measured dipolar interactions because they involve spin $\frac{1}{2}$ nuclei, but ^{14}N quadrupole and dipole splittings can also be measured and used as orientation constraints (49, 81, 82).

Additional constraints for peptide-plane orientations are derived from the amide ^{15}N and carbonyl ^{13}C chemical-shift tensors. The orientation dependence of the chemical-shift interaction has the form:

$$\sigma = \sigma_{11}\cos^2\alpha\sin^2\beta + \sigma_{22}\sin^2\alpha\cos^2\beta + \sigma_{33}\cos^2\beta, \qquad 3.$$

where σ is the observed chemical shift; σ_{11}, σ_{22}, and σ_{33} are the principal components of the chemical shift tensor; and α and β are the Euler angles relating the principal axis system (PAS) of the chemical-shift tensor to the lab frame (73). It is important to realize that although the dipolar interaction points along the internuclear axis and is related to the magnetic field axis by a single rotation about an angle θ, the orientation (or PAS) of the chemical-shift tensor must be determined relative to a molecular axis and relative to the magnetic field axis. The standard approach for establishing the orientation of a chemical-shift tensor relative to a molecular axis system has been through NMR studies of single crystals in which the molecular axis orientation can be determined independently using X-ray methods (18, 34, 53). More recently, however, other approaches have been developed that make use of the axial orientation of dipolar interactions as a convenient frame of reference (22, 23, 47, 48).

Structural Studies of Membrane Proteins

The orientation-dependent approach has been applied extensively to gramicidin, a channel-forming protein whose small size (15 amino acids) facilitates specific isotopic labeling and reconstitution into lipid bilayers. The secondary structure of larger proteins can be studied using these approaches as well, depending on the ability to incorporate labels in regions of interest. Bacterial phage-coat proteins (~ 50 amino acids) and bacteriorhodopsin (256 amino acids) have been studied using the orientation dependence of the chemical-shift interaction. In these cases, the orientation-dependent approach is turned upside-down, and the strategy is to compare the NMR data to spectral simulations generated using standard secondary structures.

GRAMICIDIN A   Gramicidin A is a small hydrophobic peptide composed of 15 alternating L and D amino acids (86a). The peptide dimerizes in membranes and forms channels that conduct monovalent cations. One motivation for studying the structure of gramicidin using NMR methods is the substantial differences between two crystal structures of the peptide (33, 87) and the bilayer structure that has been proposed on the basis of circular dichroism measurements (83–85).

Cross has undertaken a series of elegant orientation-dependent solid-state NMR studies to address the structure of gramicidin in membranes (41, 45, 46, 78). Figure 4 illustrates the data obtained from ^{15}N- and ^{13}C-labeled gramicidin oriented in lipid bilayers that are used to determine the ϕ and ψ torsion angles for the alanine residue at position 3 in the gramicidin sequence. The measurements are of the Gly2-Ala3 and Ala3-Leu4 peptide bonds and yield the dipolar splittings (Δv) of the amide ^{15}N resonances resulting from the directly bonded carbonyl carbons. The top spectra show the ^{15}N resonances of oriented gramicidin that is singly labeled at the amide nitrogens of Ala3 (left) and Leu4 (right), and the bottom spectra illustrate the dipolar splitting of the ^{15}N by ^{13}C when the peptide bonds are doubly labeled. The observed dipolar splittings are 670 Hz for the ^{13}C-

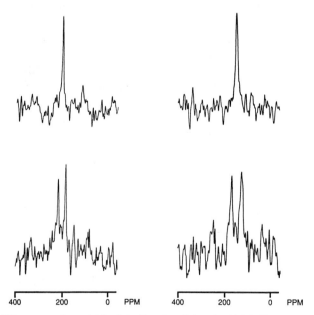

Figure 4 ^{15}N spectra of gramicidin A in dimyristoylphosphatidylcholine (DMPC) bilayers. The top spectra are of gramicidin singly labeled with ^{15}N at the amides of Ala3 (*left*) and Leu4 (*right*), and the bottom spectra illustrate the dipolar splitting observed when the peptide bonds are doubly labeled with ^{13}C. The spectra result from ~12,000 acquisitions collected at a ^{15}N frequency of 20.3 MHz. Reproduced from Ref. 78 with permission.

Gly2-^{15}N-Ala3 bond and 820 Hz for the ^{13}C-Ala3-^{15}N-Leu4 bond. An accurate bond length is the only additional information needed to calculate the angle θ. A 1.34-Å C-N bond length taken from the crystal structure of alanylalanine translates into a dipolar coupling constant (D) of 1.26 kHz, and using Equation 2, these data define four possible orientations for each C-N bond because D is larger than the observed splittings (78).

To further limit the number of possible structures, independent constraints on the peptide plane orientations are obtained from the ^{15}N-^{1}H dipolar couplings and the ^{15}N chemical-shift tensor. The ^{15}N-^{1}H dipolar couplings are determined using separated local field experiments (11, 31, 42, 43, 77, 78) and yield only two possible orientations for each N-H bond because the ^{15}N-^{1}H dipolar coupling constant is smaller than the observed splittings. Since the orientation of the ^{15}N chemical shift tensor relative to the molecular frame has been established in model compounds (22, 23, 43, 47, 48, 77), the observed ^{15}N chemical shifts provide a way to discriminate between several of the orientations of the N-H and N-C bonds suggested by the observed dipolar couplings. Together, these data along with several geometric constraints define two possible sets of torsion angles for the Ala3 position with errors in the ϕ and ψ angles of $\pm 6°$ and $\pm 5°$, respectively (Figure 5).

The two structures defined by the Ala3 torsion angles are right-handed β-type helices. The difference in the structures lies in the orientation of the Ala3-Leu4 linkage where the carbonyl group points towards the channel axis in the left structure ($\psi = 153°$) and away from it in the right structure ($\psi = 122°$). The left structure is the favored model because it is thought that the selectivity of cations over anions by gramicidin arises from the partial negative charges of the backbone carbonyls, which may solvate the cations that have been stripped of water upon entering the channel.

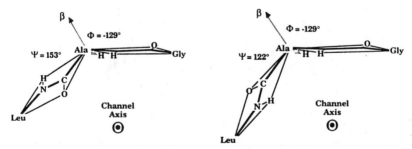

Figure 5 Two possible structures for the peptide planes at Ala3 in gramicidin A. Both correspond to right-handed β-type helices but differ in the orientation of the Ala3 carbonyl group, which points toward the gramicidin channel axis (*left*) or away from it (*right*). Reproduced from Ref. 78 with permission.

PHAGE-COAT PROTEINS The filamentous bacteriophages are simple structures consisting of a strand of DNA protected by a surrounding coat of protein. This outer protein shell is composed of a few specialized cell-attachment proteins and several thousand copies of a coat protein (88). The coat proteins are generally small (~ 50 amino acids) and have a C-terminal stretch of 20–25 hydrophobic amino acids that is α-helical (64, 75). They are assembled into the virus shell in a process that first involves incorporation into the membrane of the host cell.

Opella and coworkers have extensively studied the structure and dynamics of phage-coat proteins in oriented fibers (11) and in membrane bilayers (69). Solution NMR studies of the phage Pf1 coat protein show that the sequence contains two α-helical segments, a short helix from residues 6 to 13 and a longer hydrophobic helix from residues 19 to 42. Based on these data, ^{15}N chemical shift measurements of oriented Pf1 coat protein have provided a picture of the orientation of these two helical segments in phospholipid bilayers. The ^{15}N chemical shift tensor of the amide bond is nearly axially symmetric ($\sigma_{11} = \sigma_{22} \neq \sigma_{33}$), resulting in a ^{15}N frequency close to σ_{33} when the amide N-H bond is nearly parallel to the z-axis of the magnetic field, and in a frequency near σ_{11} when the N-H bond is perpendicular to the applied field (see Equation 3 and Figure 3). In an α-helix, the N-H bond is nearly parallel to the helix axis. Consequently, if the two helical segments are retained in bilayers, only a single measurement of the ^{15}N chemical shift from one amino acid in each helix is needed to define the helix orientation. Measurement of the ^{15}N resonance of Glu9 in the N-terminal segment argues that this helix is oriented parallel to the membrane plane, and ^{15}N labeling of Tyr25 and Tyr40 show that the second helix lies perpendicular to the bilayer plane (69). These data have led to a model that uses the short N-terminal helix as an initiation site for phage assembly (44).

BACTERIORHODOPSIN Structural studies of bacteriorhodopsin based on the orientation dependence of the chemical-shift tensor have shown that the orientation-dependent approach can be extended to large membrane proteins. Many different structural studies have focused on bacteriorhodopsin since the pioneering electron diffraction work of Henderson & Unwin (25), which suggested that the protein spans the membrane in seven transmembrane α-helices. Jap & Glaeser (29) later challenged this original model and proposed that up to four β-strands might cross the membrane. In an attempt to resolve this issue, Griffin and coworkers compared the chemical shift spectrum of bacteriorhodopsin ^{13}C-labeled at the backbone carbonyl of all 36 leucine residues with simulations based on models that had various secondary structures (36).

The NMR approach used for these studies differs from the work described on gramicidin and phage-coat proteins in that the protein is not macroscopically oriented relative to the external magnetic field. This observation has two important consequences. First, a broad NMR resonance is observed for the leucine carbonyls rather than the sharp lines characteristic of oriented samples. Second, because the protein undergoes rapid rotational diffusion about an axis perpendicular to the membrane plane, the chemical shift tensors of the carbonyls are averaged, but the extent of averaging depends on their orientation relative to the diffusion axis. That is, the rapid rotational diffusion imparts an orientation dependence to each molecule in an otherwise unoriented sample because the motion of the protein is highly anisotropic. In the case of bacteriorhodopsin, most of the leucine residues (34 of 36) are in the predicted transmembrane region of the protein and have an easily calculated orientation relative to the axis of diffusion.

The experimental spectrum obtained from ^{13}C-leucine-bacteriorhodopsin was compared with spectra calculated from structures where the leucine carbonyls are incorporated into transmembrane helices and β-strands. The orientation of the carbonyl chemical-shift tensor relative to a molecular axis is taken from model compound studies, in this case glycylglycine (74) (see Figure 3). Such comparisons showed that either of two structures could fit the experimental data equally well; one structure consisted entirely of α_I-helices oriented at 20° to the membrane plane, and a second structure had a combination of 60% α_{II}-helices (32) oriented perpendicular to the membrane plane and 40% antiparallel β-sheets tilted at 10–20°. The recent high resolution structure of the protein by Henderson and coworkers has confirmed the original model with seven α-helical transmembrane segments, of which four are significantly tilted (24).

DISTANCE-DEPENDENT APPROACHES

The second class of methods used to determine protein structure by solid-state NMR rely on an accurate determination of weak dipolar couplings between nuclear spins. A set of distances determined from the dipolar couplings serve to constrain the structure, analogous to the use of $^1H \cdots {}^1H$ distance constraints from NOE data in solution NMR. Because ^1H studies in membranes are hampered by the strongly coupled proton spins, alternative approaches have been developed that measure $^{13}C \cdots {}^{15}N$ and $^{13}C \cdots {}^{13}C$ distances. The difficulty in these measurements is that the weak couplings are virtually impossible to observe in the broad NMR powder spectra, while they are averaged to zero in magic angle spinning spectra. The problem is readily illustrated in the splittings of the sharp ^{15}N res-

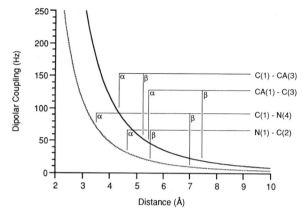

Figure 6 Plot of the r^{-3} distance dependence of the dipolar interaction for $^{13}C \cdots {}^{13}C$ homonuclear couplings (*solid line*) and $^{13}C \cdots {}^{15}N$ heteronuclear couplings (*stippled line*). Also indicated are the approximate distances between backbone atoms in α-helix and β-sheet secondary structures (C, carbonyl carbons; CA, α-carbons; N, amide nitrogens). For both the REDOR ($^{13}C \cdots {}^{15}N$) and RR ($^{13}C \cdots {}^{13}C$) experiments, the lower limit for measuring dipolar couplings is about 30 Hz.

onances for the ^{15}N-^{13}C pairs in gramicidin A (Figure 4, bottom). These labeled sites are 1.34 Å apart and yield relatively large splittings of 670 and 820 Hz. For longer distances (4–5 Å) these splittings would decrease dramatically and fall below the narrow linewidths exhibited by oriented samples, making accurate measurements difficult at best. Figure 6 plots the r^{-3} distance dependence of the $^{13}C \cdots {}^{13}C$ and $^{15}N \cdots {}^{13}C$ dipolar couplings and shows graphically how they decrease with increasing distance.

The following sections discuss two approaches, rotational echo double-resonance (REDOR) and rotational resonance (RR) NMR, that circumvent these difficulties. Both methods use magic angle spinning (MAS) to narrow the NMR lines. As a result, the small dipolar couplings are not directly observed as splittings in the NMR spectrum, but calculated from intensity changes in observed resonances.

REDOR NMR

Rotational echo double-resonance (REDOR) NMR methods are used to measure weak heteronuclear dipolar couplings such as those between ^{13}C, ^{15}N, and ^{31}P (19, 51). The approach relies on the dephasing of magnetization of the observed spin (typically ^{13}C) through coupling to a second spin (such as ^{15}N). The dipolar coupling between these two spins is determined by the difference between two NMR spectra. The first spectrum is obtained using a standard cross polarization pulse sequence with a π pulse on the observed nucleus (e.g. ^{13}C) in the middle of an evolution period (Figure 2, bottom). During this period, the observed magnetization evolves under the influence of the chemical shift interaction and a heteronuclear dipolar interaction. The π pulse refocuses both interactions, leading to a signal S during the acquisition period. The second spectrum is obtained with an additional train of π pulses on the dipole-coupled spin (e.g. ^{15}N) (20). These pulses affect the observed signal by interfering with the dipolar interaction during the evolution period. The magnetization is not completely refocused and the signal intensity drops by an amount ΔS. For weak dipolar coupling, the change in signal intensity is related to the distance between the coupled spins by the equation

$$\Delta S/S = K D^2 N_c^2 v_r^{-2} \qquad\qquad 4.$$

where N_c is the number of rotor cycles during the evolution period, v_r is the spinning speed, D is the dipolar coupling constant, and K is a dimensionless constant equal to 1.066. The REDOR experiment is generally done at slow spinning speeds and over several rotor cycles so as to increase the size of the difference signal.

The basic REDOR experiment is incredibly versatile and has been extended by Schaefer and coworkers to include two-dimensional versions and experiments involving three or more S spins (19). The two-dimensional experiments yield ΔS directly as function of the evolution time in the second dimension; however, the sensitivity is reduced compared to the one-dimensional experiment. Rotational echo triple-resonance (RETRO) experiments are a more promising approach to edit natural-abundance background signals by selecting unique spin triplets. A third rare spin, such as ^2H, ^{19}F, or ^{31}P, is used to distinguish the signal arising from a specific ^{13}C-^{15}N pair from that of the natural-abundance background (28).

EMERIMICIN NONAPEPTIDES   The ability to accurately measure weak $^{13}C \cdots {}^{15}N$ couplings provides a way to determine the secondary structure of a polypeptide chain. Schaefer and coworkers have illustrated the potential of this method on microcrystals of a hydrophobic fragment of the antibiotic emerimicin (38). The peptide was specifically labeled with ^{13}C at the backbone carbonyl of Aib2 (Aib = aminoisobutyric acid or 2-methylalanine) and with ^{15}N at the amide nitrogen of Gly6. These labels are across one turn of an α-helix, 4.13 Å apart in the X-ray crystal structure of the peptide (39). Figure 7 shows the ^{13}C NMR spectrum (bottom) of the peptide without ^{15}N dephasing pulses, and the difference spectrum (top) obtained by subtracting a spectrum collected with the dephasing

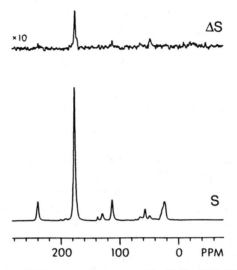

Figure 7 ^{13}C REDOR NMR spectra of microcrystalline [1-^{13}C-Aib2, ^{15}N-Gly6] emerimicin nonapeptide. The full signal S (*bottom*) was obtained without ^{15}N pulses, and the REDOR difference spectrum ΔS (*top*) is the result of subtracting a spectrum collected with ^{15}N π pulses. The sample contained 120 mg of peptide spinning at 3205 Hz, and 162,000 acquisitions were collected with an 8-cycle REDOR evolution time. Reproduced from Ref. 38 with permission.

pulses. The intensities of the carbonyl resonance in these spectra yield the values for ΔS and S, and a $\Delta S/S$ ratio of 0.0267.

To translate the ΔS and S measurements into an internuclear distance, one must first consider the natural-abundance ^{13}C (1.10%) and ^{15}N (0.37%) backgrounds. The full S signal has a 7% contribution from the natural-abundance ^{13}C of the peptide carbonyls that must be subtracted in order to obtain the intensity solely from the specific ^{13}C label at Aib2. The ΔS signal has contributions both from ^{13}C-labeled Aib2 coupled to natural-abundance ^{15}N and from ^{15}N-labeled Gly6 coupled to natural-abundance ^{13}C. The largest contributions to the ΔS signal arise from dipolar couplings to natural-abundance carbons and nitrogens that are separated by one or two bonds from the labeled positions. The one- and two-bond distances are estimated to be 1.33 and 2.46 Å, which correspond to couplings of 1.26 kHz and 200 Hz, respectively. Despite the sizeable contribution of the natural-abundance dipolar couplings to the ΔS signal when the coupling being measured is weak, Schaefer and coworkers find that the couplings can be estimated or measured very accurately and that the error in the final distance determination is on the order of a few tenths of an Ångstrom. In the case of the emerimicin peptide, the natural-abundance contribution to ΔS was estimated at more than 50% of the signal, leaving a residual $\Delta S/S$ of 0.0129 arising from the two labeled sites. Using Equation 4, with an eight-cycle evolution period and a spinning speed of 3205 Hz, the $\Delta S/S$ measurement translates into a $^{13}C \cdots ^{15}N$ coupling of 44.1 Hz, corresponding to an internuclear distance of 4.07 Å. This value is in good agreement with the 4.13-Å distance determined in the X-ray crystal structure of the peptide and is consistent with other α-helical structures.

Rotational Resonance NMR

Rotational-resonance (RR) NMR methods have been developed for measuring weak homonuclear dipolar couplings between two spins that have different chemical shifts. In the REDOR experiment, the dipolar coupling is generally observed as intensity changes resulting from dephasing of the dipole-coupled resonances. In RR, these changes result from an exchange of magnetization between two spins, and an analysis of the exchange rate is used to determine the coupling. In most cases, the rate of spin diffusion between dilute spins is slow (4, 26, 76, 86). However, the rate is greatly enhanced when the spinning speed (v_r) of the sample matches the frequency separation (Δv) between the two spins, or more generally when $\Delta v = nv_r$, where $n = 1, 2, 3$, etc (1a, 1b, 7, 60). The rate enhancement can be related to internuclear distance by theoretical simulations (35).

Figure 2 shows the RR pulse sequence. It consists of a standard cross polarization sequence immediately followed by a ^{13}C flip-back pulse and selective inversion of one of the two resonances being studied. After a variable mixing time for magnetization exchange (τ_m), the NMR signal is acquired. If the two rotationally coupled resonances are also close in space and coupled by a dipolar interaction, their intensities will vary as a function of the mixing time due to a transfer of magnetization. When spinning at the $n = 1$ rotational resonance condition, the initial rate of magnetization transfer is dominated by the strength of the dipolar coupling. As the value of n increases, the rate of transfer decreases and contributions from the orientations of the chemical-shift tensors become more pronounced, making interpretation of the transfer rate more difficult. Consequently, the $n = 1$ experiments are the most important. Theoretical simulations of strongly coupled sites also predict line-shape effects and oscillations in the transfer curves that result from the relative orientations of the exchanging sites (35).

ALAMETHICIN UNDECAPEPTIDES   To test the limits of the rotational resonance approach, a series of peptides were synthesized bearing pairs of ^{13}C groups separated by various distances (54, 56; O. Peersen, S. Yoshimura, H. Hojo, S. Aimoto & S. Smith, submitted). The peptide has the sequence Boc-L-Ala-Aib-Ala-Aib-Ala-Glu(OBzl)-Ala-Aib-Ala-Aib-Ala-OMe and has been used as a model for the N terminus of alamethicin, a small membrane channel-forming peptide. The crystal structure of the undecapeptide has been solved to 0.9-Å resolution by Jung and coworkers using crystals grown from dichloromethane solutions (3) and in our laboratory using crystals grown from methanol (S. O. Smith, unpublished results). In both crystals, the peptide forms a canonical α-helix, and the rms difference in backbone atom positions is 0.11 Å. The ^{13}C labels have been placed on pairs of backbone carbonyl and alanine methyl carbons in the first five residues of the peptide such that the distances between them serve as markers of a helical structure. Figure 8 illustrates rotational resonance transfer at $n = 1$ in crystals of the peptide in which the ^{13}C labels are 3.7, 4.8, and 6.8 Å apart. In the top spectrum, the ^{13}C-labeled carbonyl line (175 ppm) has been selectively inverted while spinning at rotational resonance with the ^{13}C-labeled methyl resonance (20 ppm), but exchange has not yet taken place. The subsequent spectra are difference

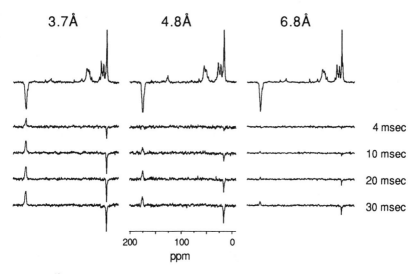

Figure 8 ^{13}C rotational resonance NMR spectra of three microcrystalline alamethicin undecapeptides at $n = 1$. Each peptide bears two ^{13}C labels, one label at a backbone carbonyl and a second label at an alanine methyl, separated by the indicated distances. The top spectrum corresponds to zero mixing time, and the subsequent spectra are the differences obtained by subtraction of the zero-time spectrum from those with mixing times of 4, 10, 20, and 30 ms. Each ^{13}C-labeled peptide has been diluted 10-fold with unlabeled peptide. Crystallization for these peptides was done by evaporation of methanol, and the distances are calculated from the crystal structure obtained from methanol (S. O. Smith, unpublished results). The spectra are from 1024 acquisitions of 10-mg labeled peptide spinning at 8 kHz.

spectra obtained by subtraction of this zero mixing time spectrum from those obtained using 4-, 10-, 20-, and 30-ms mixing times, clearly illustrating a positive increase in the carbonyl signal coupled to a reduction of the methyl signal. Furthermore, the exchange is limited to the two rotationally coupled lines, with little or no transfer to the natural-abundance α-carbons (50 ppm) or Aib methyl groups (25 ppm). Figure 9 summarizes the $n = 1$ data and shows the normalized transfer curves for all five ^{13}C-labeled peptides. For this study, the ^{13}C-labeled peptides were diluted 1:10 with unlabeled peptide, resulting in a natural-abundance contribution to the spectrum equivalent to that of a 10-kilodalton (kDa) protein.

The transfer curve shows the largest transfer of magnetization between labels at the carbonyl of Aib4 and the methyl of Ala5, which are only 3.7 Å apart in the X-ray structure. In this case, the transfer is rapid enough to illustrate the oscillations that occur with strong dipolar couplings and to show that they are being damped out within 30 ms. The next two transfer curves correspond to ^{13}C pairs that directly test the secondary

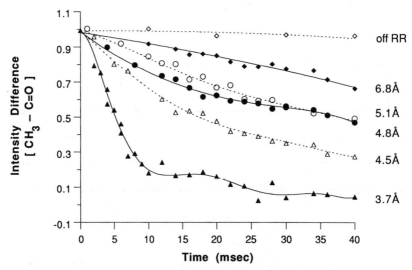

Figure 9 Normalized magnetization transfer curves for five microcrystalline alamethicin undecapeptides showing the correlation between internuclear distance and the rate of magnetization transfer. The curves are obtained by summing the intensities of the two ^{13}C resonances (after natural-abundance subtraction) as a function of mixing time and normalizing to an initial value of 1.0. The off-rotational resonance data are from the 6.8-Å sample spinning at 8500 Hz, 541 Hz faster than the $n = 1$ condition. The line fits illustrate the trend of the data and are not theoretical simulations of transfer (35). The estimated error in the normalized curves is 0.05 or less for all of the peptides.

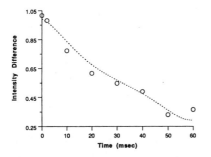
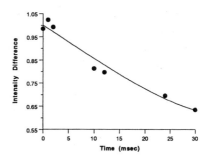

Figure 10 Normalized magnetization transfer curves for alamethicin peptide-dipal-mitoylphosphatidylcholine (DPPC) complexes using the 5.1-Å peptide at $n = 1$ (*left*) and the 4.8-Å peptide at $n = 2$ (*right*). The solid lines correspond to the crystal data for each peptide, and the large dots are the data from 10 mg of peptide reconstituted into DPPC at a molar ratio of 1:10 (58).

structure of the peptide. Both pairs use one label at the Ala5 methyl group and a second label at either the carbonyl of Ala1, yielding a 4.8-Å distance along the helix axis or at the carbonyl of Aib$_2$, yielding a 4.5-Å distance diagonally across the face of the helix. In these cases, the oscillations in the transfer curves are no longer observed. The last two peptides incorporate ^{13}C labels that have larger separations in a helical geometry. The longest distance, 6.8 Å, tests the limit of the rotational resonance method. As shown in Figures 8 and 9, appreciable transfer takes place at this distance, and it is easily resolved from the off rotational resonance case, in which no transfer takes place.

The structure of the peptide when bound to a membrane has been addressed by reconstituting ^{13}C-labeled peptides into lipid bilayers (58) and repeating the NMR experiments on these complexes. For these studies, the NMR experiments were done at $-40°C$ in order to reduce peptide motion and improve signal intensity. Figure 10 shows a comparison of the transfer rates in the crystals and in the lipid for the 4.8-Å and 5.1-Å peptides, where the labels are one turn apart and across the helix from each other, respectively. The close correlation with the crystal data strongly suggests that the helical conformation is maintained upon reconstitution into membranes, and demonstrates that rotational resonance can be used to investigate the local secondary structure of membrane proteins.

BACTERIORHODOPSIN   Rotational resonance NMR methods have also been shown to be effective in larger membrane proteins. In a rotational resonance study of bacteriorhodopsin, Griffin and coworkers incorporated two specific ^{13}C labels into the retinal chromophore of the protein, one label at the C_{18} position on the ionone ring and the other at position C_8 of the polyene chain (8). In order to remove the large natural-abundance background in these studies, the intensities of the ^{13}C labels were obtained from difference spectra between bacteriorhodopsin regenerated with ^{13}C-labeled retinal and with unlabeled retinal. The distance between the labels depends on the conformation about the C_6-C_7 bond. Model compound studies showed that in the s-*cis* conformation the labels are ~3.1 Å apart, while the distance is closer to 4.2 Å in the s-*trans* conformation. In the protein, the magnetization transfer rates agreed well with a separation of 4.2 Å, arguing that the retinal has an s-*trans* geometry. These studies set the stage for distance measurements between the retinal and amino acid residues in the retinal binding site.

CONCLUSIONS

Relatively few structural studies have yet been undertaken on membrane peptides and proteins using solid-state NMR approaches. Nevertheless, these studies illustrate that solid-state NMR approaches are well suited to address specific structural questions in membranes. The methods used have several features in common that roughly define the range of problems that are accessible. First, there is the need for specific isotopic labels. Specific labels have the advantage of highlighting regions of interest, but the disadvantage of limiting the scope of an investigation. Often, however, the focus is on a few residues that are known from biochemical and molecular biological experiments to be critical in protein function or struc-ture. Second, solid-state NMR approaches have the potential for yielding accurate distances and orientations. Short-range distance measurements are possible and can be exploited in membrane systems where proteins generally have regular secondary structures that span the membrane, such as helices of 20–25 hydrophobic amino acids (14). In this case, distances between residues four amino acids apart in the sequence can establish helical periodicity as has been shown in the emerimicin and alamethicin peptides. Several labeling schemes and predicted dipolar couplings for characterizing α-helix and β-sheet structures are shown in Figure 6. The 4- to 7-Å range for distance measurements also opens the way for determining interhelical distances and characterizing helix-helix interactions. The side chains of adjacent helices pack together in a space of 4–6 Å, and specific side chain-side chain and side chain-backbone interactions are in part responsible for the tertiary fold of membrane proteins.

What are the prospects for solid-state NMR on membrane proteins? Currently, the systems most accessible to these methods are peptides that can be synthesized directly and larger proteins in which a bound ligand or cofactor has been selectively labeled. The future lies in the further development of both NMR and biochemical methods for targeting specific sites in larger proteins. There are several additional approaches for determining dipolar couplings in solids that have not yet been applied to membrane systems (15, 80). Also, two-dimensional and spectral editing versions of the REDOR and RR experiments are envisioned that will select unique sites in proteins that contain several isotopic labels. Protein-engineering techniques provide ways to tailor unique sites in large proteins (59), to recombine protein or peptide fragments (2, 58), and to create novel protein chimeras (M. Lemmon, B. J. Bormann, J. Flanagan, J. Hunt, D. Engelman, et al., submitted). These approaches should greatly facilitate the targeting of specific protein groups. In summary, the limited number of solid-state NMR studies to date on membrane proteins and peptides have shown that these techniques can be effective in determining protein distances and orientations, and have illustrated the potential for addressing larger and more varied problems.

Literature Cited

1. Andrew, E. R., Bradbury, A., Eades, R. G. 1958. *Nature* 182: 1659
1a. Andrew, E. R. Bradbury, A., Eades, R. G., Wynn, V. T. 1963. *Phys. Lett.* 4: 99–100
1b. Andrew, E. R., Clough, S., Farnell, L. F., Glenhill, T. D., Roberts, I. 1966. *Phys. Lett.* 21: 505–6
2. Bibi, E., Kaback, H. R. 1990. *Proc. Natl. Acad. Sci. USA* 87: 4325–29
3. Bosch, R., Jung, G., Schmitt, H., Winter, W. 1985. *Biopolymers* 24: 961–78
4. Bronniman, C. E., Szeverenyi, N. M., Maciel, G. E. 1983. *J. Chem. Phys.* 79: 3694–3700
5. Brown, L. R., Wüthrich, K. 1981. *Biochim. Biophys. Acta* 647: 95–111
6. Clore, M. G., Gronenborn, A. M. 1991. *Annu. Rev. Biophys. Biophys. Chem.* 20: 29–63
7. Colombo, M. G., Meier, B. H., Ernst, R. R. 1988. *Chem. Phys. Lett.* 146: 189–96
8. Creuzet, F., McDermott, A., Gebhard, R., van der Hoef, K., Spijker-Assink, et al. 1991. *Science* 251: 783–86
9. Cross, T. A. 1986. *Biophys. J.* 49: 124–26
10. Cross, T. A., Opella, S. J. 1983. *J. Am. Chem. Soc.* 105: 306–8
11. Cross, T. A., Opella, S. J. 1985. *J. Mol. Biol.* 182: 367–81
12. Davis, J. H. 1983. *Biochim. Biophys. Acta* 737: 117–71
13. Eisenberg, D. 1984. *Annu. Rev. Biochem.* 53: 595–623
14. Engelman, D. M., Steitz, T. A., Goldman, A. 1986. *Annu. Rev. Biophys. Biophys. Chem.* 15: 321–53
15. Engelsberg, M., Yannoni, C. S. 1990. *J. Magn. Reson.* 88: 393–400
16. Ernst, R. R., Bodenhausen, G., Wokaun, A. 1987. *Principles of Nuclear Magnetic Resonance in One and Two Dimensions.* New York: Oxford Univ. Press
17. Griffin, R. G., Beshah, K., Ebelhäuser, R., Huang, T. H., Olejniczak, et al. 1988. In *Deuterium NMR Studies of Dynamics in Solids*, ed. G. J. Long, F. Grandjean, pp. 81–105. New York: Kluwer Academic
18. Griffin, R. G., Ellett, J. D. Jr., Mehring, M., Bullitt, J. G., Waugh, J. S. 1972. *J. Chem. Phys.* 57: 2147–55
19. Gullion, T., Schaefer, J. 1989. In *Advances in Magnetic Resonance*, ed. W. S. Warren, 13: 57–83. New York: Academic
20. Gullion, T., Schaefer, J. 1991. *J. Magn. Reson.* 92: 439–42

21. Hagen, D. S., Weiner, J. H., Sykes, B. D. 1979. *Biochemistry* 18: 2007–12
22. Hartzell, C. J., Pratum, T. K., Drobny, G. 1987. *J. Chem. Phys.* 87: 4324–31
23. Hartzell, C. J., Whitfield, M., Oas, T. G., Drobny, G. P. 1987. *J. Am. Chem. Soc.* 109: 5966–69
24. Henderson, R., Baldwin, J. M., Ceska, T. A., Zemlin, F., Beckmann, E., et al. 1990. *J. Mol. Biol.* 213: 899–929
25. Henderson, R., Unwin, P. N. T. 1975. *Nature* 257: 28–32
26. Henrichs, P. M., Linder, M., Hewitt, J. M. 1986. *J. Chem. Phys.* 85: 7077–86
27. Herzfeld, J., Berger, A. E. 1980. *J. Chem. Phys.* 73: 6021–30
28. Holl, S. M., McKay, R. A., Gullion, T., Schaefer, J. 1990. *J. Magn. Reson.* 89: 620–26
29. Jap, B. K., Maestre, M. F., Hayward, S. B., Glaeser, R. M. 1983. *Biophys. J.* 43: 81–89
30. Jarrell, H. C., Jovall, P. A., Giziewicz, P. A., Turner, L. A., Smith, I. C. P. 1987. *Biochemistry* 26: 1805–11
31. Kolbert, A. C., Levitt, M. H., Griffin, R. G. 1989. *J. Magn. Reson.* 85: 42–49
32. Krimm, S., Dwivedi, A. M. 1982. *Science* 216: 407–8
33. Langs, D. A. 1988. *Science* 241: 188–91
34. Lauterbur, P. 1958. *Phys. Rev. Lett.* 1: 343–44
35. Levitt, M. H., Raleigh, D. P., Creuzet, F., Griffin, R. G. 1990. *J. Chem. Phys.* 92: 6347–64
36. Lewis, B. A., Harbison, G. S., Herzfeld, J., Griffin, R. G. 1985. *Biochemistry* 24: 4671–79
37. Lowe, I. J. 1959. *Phys. Rev. Lett.* 2: 285–87
38. Marshall, G. R., Beusen, D. D., Kociolek, K., Redlinski, A. S., Leplawy, et al. 1990. *J. Am. Chem. Soc.* 112: 963–66
39. Marshall, G. R., Hodgkin, E. E., Langs, D. A., Smith, G. D., Zabrocki, J., et al. 1990. *Proc. Natl. Acad. Sci. USA* 87: 487–91
40. Mehring, M. 1983. *Principles of High Resolution NMR in Solids*. Berlin: Springer-Verlag. 2nd ed.
41. Moll, F. III, Cross, T. A. 1990. *Biophys. J.* 57: 351–62
42. Munowitz, M., Aue, W. P., Griffin, R. G. 1982. *J. Chem. Phys.* 77: 1686–89
43. Munowitz, M. G., Griffin, R. G., Bodenhausen, G., Huang, T. H. 1981. *J. Am. Chem. Soc.* 103: 2529–33
44. Nambudripad, R., Stark, W., Opella, S. J., Makowski, L. 1991. *Science* 252: 1305–8
45. Nicholson, L. K., Cross, T. A. 1989. *Biochemistry* 28: 9379–85
46. Nicholson, L. K., Teng, Q., Cross, T. A.
1991. *J. Mol. Biol.* 218: 621–37
47. Oas, T. G., Hartzell, C. J., Dahlquist, F. W., Drobny, G. P. 1987. *J. Am. Chem. Soc.* 109: 5962–66
48. Oas, T. G., Hartzell, C. J., McMahon, T. J., Drobny, G. P., Dahlquist, F. W. 1987. *J. Am. Chem. Soc.* 109: 5956–62
49. Opella, S. J. 1982. *Annu. Rev. Phys. Chem.* 33: 533–62
50. Opella, S. J., Stewart, P. L., Valentine, K. G. 1987. *Q. Rev. Biophys.* 19: 7–49
51. Pan, Y., Gullion, T., Schaefer, J. 1990. *J. Magn. Reson.* 90: 330–40
52. Paul, C., Rosenbusch, J. P. 1985. *EMBO J.* 4: 1593–97
53. Pausak, S., Pines, A., Waugh, J. S. 1973. *J. Chem. Phys.* 59: 591–95
54. Peersen, O. B., Aimoto, S., Smith, S. O. 1991. *Biophys. J.* 59: 300a (Abstr.)
55. Peersen, O. B., Pratt, E. A., Truong, H. T. N., Ho, C., Rule, G. S. 1990. *Biochemistry* 29: 3256–62
56. Peersen, O., Yoshimura, S., Hojo, H., Aimoto, S., Smith, S. 1991. In *Peptide Chemistry* 1990, ed. Y. Shimonishi, pp. 399–404. Osaka: Protein Research Foundation
57. Pines, A., Gibby, M. G., Waugh, J. S. 1973. *J. Chem. Phys.* 59: 569–90
58. Popot, J.-L., Gerchman, S. E., Engelman, D. M. 1987. *J. Mol. Biol.* 198: 655–76
59. Püttner, I. B., Kaback, H. R. 1988. *Proc. Natl. Acad. Sci. USA* 85: 1467–71
60. Raleigh, D. P., Levitt, M. H., Griffin, R. G. 1988. *Chem. Phys. Lett.* 146: 71–76
61. Rees, D. C., DeAntonio, L., Eisenberg, D. 1989. *Science* 245: 510–13
62. Sanders, C. R. I., Prestegard, J. H. 1990. *Biophys. J.* 58: 447–60
63. Schaefer, J., Stejskal, E. O. 1976. *J. Am. Chem. Phys.* 98: 1031–32
64. Schiksnis, R. A., Bogusky, M. J., Tsang, P., Opella, S. J. 1987. *Biochemistry* 26: 1373–81
65. Seelig, J. 1977. *Q. Rev. Biophys.* 10: 353–418
66. Seelig, J., Borle, F., Cross, T. A. 1985. *Biochim. Biophys. Acta* 814: 195–98
67. Seelig, J., Gally, H. U. 1976. *Biochemistry* 15: 5199–5204
68. Seelig, J., Seelig, A. 1980. *Q. Rev. Biophys.* 13: 19–61
69. Shon, K. J., Kim, Y., Colnago, L. A., Opella, S. J. 1991. *Science* 252: 1303–5
70. Smith, R. L., Oldfield, E. 1984. *Science* 225: 280–88
71. Smith, S. O., Griffin, R. G. 1988. *Annu. Rev. Phys. Chem.* 39: 511–35
72. Speyer, J. B., Sripada, P. K., Gupta, S. K. D., Shipley, G. G., Griffin, R. G. 1987. *Biophys. J.* 51: 687–91
73. Spiess, H. W. 1978. In *NMR: Basic Prin-*

ciples and Progress, ed. P. Diehl, E. Fluck, R. Kosfeld, 15: 55–214. New York: Spring-Verlag
74. Stark, R. E., Jelinski, L. W., Ruben, D. J., Torchia, D. A., Griffin, R. G. 1983. *J. Magn. Reson.* 55: 266–73
75. Stark, W., Glucksman, M. J., Makowski, L. 1988. *J. Mol. Biol.* 199: 171–82
76. Suter, D., Ernst, R. R. 1985. *Phys. Rev. Ser. B* 32: 5608–27
77. Teng, Q., Cross, T. A. 1989. *J. Magn. Reson.* 85: 439–47
78. Teng, Q., Nicholson, L. K., Cross, T. A. 1991. *J. Mol. Biol.* 218: 607–19
79. Torchia, D. A. 1984. *Annu. Rev. Biophys. Bioeng.* 13: 125–44
80. Tycko, R., Dabbagh, G. 1990. *Chem. Phys. Lett.* 173: 461–65
81. Tycko, R., Opella, S. J. 1987. *J. Chem. Phys.* 86: 1761–74
82. Tycko, R., Stewart, P. L., Opella, S. J. 1986. *J. Am. Chem. Soc.* 108: 5419–25
83. Urry, D. W. 1971. *Proc. Natl. Acad. Sci. USA* 68: 672–76
84. Urry, D. W., Goodall, M. C., Glickson, J. D., Mayers, D. F. 1971. *Proc. Natl. Acad. Sci. USA* 68: 1907–11
85. Urry, D. W., Walker, J. T., Trapane, T. L. 1982. *J. Membr. Biol.* 69: 225–31
86. VanderHart, D. L. 1987. *J. Magn. Reson.* 72: 13–47
86a. Wallace, B. A. 1990. *Annu. Rev. Biophys. Biophys. Chem.* 19: 127–57
87. Wallace, B. A., Ravikumar, K. 1988. *Science* 241: 182–87
88. Webster, R. E., Lopez, J. 1985. In *Structure and Assembly of the Class I Filamentous Bacteriophage*, ed. S. Casjens, pp. 235–67. Boston: Jones and Bartlett
89. Wüthrich, K. 1986. *NMR of Proteins and Nucleic Acids*. New York: Wiley-Interscience

Annu. Rev. Biophys. Biomol. Struct. 1992. 21:49–76

STRUCTURE AND FUNCTION OF ACTIN

Wolfgang Kabsch and Joël Vandekerckhove

Max-Planck-Institut für medizinische Forschung, Abteilung Biophysik, Jahnstrasse 29, W–6900 Heidelberg, Germany and Laboratory of Physiological Chemistry, State University of Ghent, K.L. Ledeganckstraat 35, B–9000 Gent, Belgium

KEY WORDS: cytoskeleton, actin-binding proteins, microfilaments, ATPase, ATP binding

CONTENTS

PERSPECTIVES AND OVERVIEW

Actin is one of the most abundant proteins in eukaryotic cells. In 1942, Straub (103) isolated it as a water soluble component of muscle acetone powder. At increased ionic strength, G-actin molecules polymerize into filaments, known as F-actin. This process is reversible and is the basis of most purification procedures (109). F-actin is the main component of the

49

1056–8700/92/0610–0049$02.00

thin filaments in sarcomeres of muscle cells. Muscle sarcomeres use ATP hydrolysis to produce mechanical force by sliding the thin actin filament past thick myosin filaments (45, 46). Actin was later also found in non-muscle cells (38) in which its organization has been visualized using indirect immunofluorescence microscopy (62). The next important step came with the elucidation of the amino acid sequence, which provided a solid basis for all further actin research (28). This advancement allowed researchers to locate chemical and enzymatic modifications in the amino acid sequence and to correlate these changes with alterations in the properties of the molecule. Comparative sequence analysis revealed the highly conserved nature of the molecule throughout evolution. Unexpectedly, investigators found that actin isoforms were more closely related within the tissue in which they were expressed than between species (120).

Actin research originally focused on the molecular basis of muscular contraction (for review, see 98). The discovery of actin-based motile systems and their transient character in nonmuscle cells led to intensive studies on actin organization and its control system. In the early 1980s, the basic principles of actin polymerization were elucidated (see 33, 56), and the first actin-binding proteins (ABPs) were characterized and classified according to their in vivo and in vitro activities (21). The discovery of many additional classes of actin-binding proteins, often with overlapping functions, dampened the initial optimism that actin organization in cells might be explained in terms of a few simple interactions with actin-binding proteins. The inventory of discovered proteins still grows steadily, reaching toward a level of nearly unmanageable complexity. Such complexity might well reflect the need of the cell to provide sufficient redundancy for maintaining crucial cellular functions. For instance, several actin regulatory proteins that were conserved throughout various species and thought to be essential for actin organization can be deleted by mutagenesis, often without noticeable effect on the cell performance in the laboratory (81).

Structural studies on actin have recently advanced to atomic detail (51). A combination of X-ray crystallographic results with fiber diffraction data has further led to an atomic model of filamentous actin (43). Advances in cryoelectron microscopy have provided important new information about the structure of F-actin and the location of the binding sites for myosin and tropomyosin (72). Furthermore, these cryoelectron microscopic image reconstructions are in excellent agreement with the atomic model of the actin filament. Forthcoming three-dimensional structures will show actin complexed with different ABPs at atomic detail. This is expected to lead to a recognition of the underlying principles of the molecular mechanism of muscle contraction and various types of actin-based cell motility. Although these structures are not at hand yet, already a large body of implicit structural information is available at the sequence level, such as information derived from cross-linking experiments, chemical and proteolytic modifications, and inhibition studies with mimetic peptides and antibodies. We discuss these data in the framework of the primary and tertiary structure of actin.

For recent introductory reviews on actin and actin binding proteins, we refer to papers by Korn (56), Weeds (130), Stossel et al (102), Pollard & Cooper (89), Vandekerckhove (117), Pollard (88), Holmes & Kabsch (42), Janmey (47), Carlier (17), Noegel & Schleicher (81), and Hartwig & Kwiatkowski (37).

STRUCTURE OF ACTIN

Actin can exist either as a monomeric molecule, G-actin, or as a filamentous polymer, F-actin. The former is obtained in low salt buffers while the latter is spontaneously formed upon addition of physiological concentrations of salt. Actin consists of a single polypeptide chain of about 375 residues whose amino acid sequence and biochemical properties are highly conserved throughout evolution. It binds one molecule of ATP or ADP and has a single high affinity and several low affinity binding sites for divalent cations, believed to be Mg^{2+} in the cell. The Mg^{2+} can be replaced by Ca^{2+}, which somewhat affects the kinetic properties of actin. The tightly bound cation is directly associated with the phosphates of the nucleotide (115). In the presence of Ca^{2+}, nucleotide exchange is relatively slow, and monomeric actin is a slow ATPase. Replacement of Ca^{2+} by Mg^{2+} and EGTA leads to a much faster dissociation of the bound nucleotide.

Judging from the assembly properties of isolated actin, most of the monomeric actin in cells must exist as a complex with associated proteins that reversibly inhibit its polymerization. This role was attributed to profilin, one of the first actin-binding proteins to be discovered (19). More recently, thymosin β_4, a 43-amino acid-long polypeptide present in several tissues at high concentrations was recognized as an important actin regulatory polypeptide (94).

The assembly of ATP-actin into filaments is initiated by an unfavorable nucleation step and propagated by the addition of subunits to the two ends of the growing filament at different rates. The ends of the filament are referred to as "barbed" and "pointed" according to the polarity of the arrowhead-like structure generated on binding myosin subfragment 1 (S1) or heavy meromyosin. ATP-actin binds faster to the barbed end than to the pointed end. After incorporation of an actin molecule into a filament, bound ATP is hydrolyzed to ADP. This behavior leads to the phenomenon of treadmilling (97). Formation of F-actin stimulates the actin ATPase. However, the release of phosphate proceeds more slowly than the formation of the filament so that the growing filament has a cap of ATP-actin at its barbed end, while monomers containing ADP and phosphate transiently accumulate in the rest of the filament (17a). The mature filament, however, contains only ADP-actin. ADP-actin may also be induced to form polymers in vitro by raising the salt concentration. Janmey et al (48) recently proposed that such ADP-F-actin polymers may be different in structure from normal F-actin. However, their results are in conflict with the observation that the dynamic elasticity and viscosity of filaments assembled from ATP-actin or ADP-actin are the same (T. D. Pollard, I. Goldberg & W. Schwarz, personal communication). A physiological role of the putative ADP-F-actin has yet to be established.

Actin is present in cells in a variety of supramolecular structures. In striated muscle, it forms the stably organized thin filaments of the sarcomere. In nonmuscle cells, however, organization of actin can be transiently modified in response to extra- or intracellular stimuli. These structures are variations on the theme of filament organization: networks of individual filaments in the cortical cytoplasm; bundled filaments, called stress fibers in interphase fibroblasts; short actin bundles in microvilli and stereocilia; filament bundles ending in focal contacts; filaments running parallel with the membrane at the membrane-cytoskeletal interface. Initially, F-actin stability and the isoelectric point of the isoforms were thought to be correlated. The most stable structures could generally be associated with the low pI actins (e.g. the muscle actins). Later studies showed that the primary cause of actin organization was its interaction with ABPs.

Crystal Structure of Actin in Complex with DNase I

The strong tendency of G-actin to polymerize interferes with the formation of crystals. Although three-dimensional crystals of G-actin can be grown from 4–14% polyethylene glycol 6000 (85), these crystals have never been studied using X-ray diffraction. A more successful approach is based upon the idea that actin may crystallize as a complex with an actin-binding protein that keeps actin in its monomeric form. So far, crystals suitable for X-ray diffraction studies have been obtained as complexes with profilin (18, 96), deoxyribonuclease I (DNase I) (63, 67, 106), and recently with the segment I domain of gelsolin (H. G. Mannherz, personal communication). At present, the only structure known at atomic detail has been obtained from the analysis of crystals of rabbit skeletal muscle actin in complex with bovine pancreatic DNase I—in both the ATP and ADP forms (51)—at resolutions of 2.8 Å and 3.0 Å, respectively. Both structures are very similar.

In agreement with earlier results at low resolution (50, 104), actin consists of a small and a large domain with one molecule of ATP or ADP residing in the cleft between the two domains (Figure 1). The overall dimensions of the molecule are approximately $55 \times 55 \times 35$ Å. It is now known that the two domains are not very different in size. The small domain contains both the amino- and carboxy-terminus of actin and is built from residues 1–144 and 338–375. The large domain is made up of residues 145–337. The atomic structure revealed that each domain can be further subdivided into two subdomains. The small domain consists of subdomain 1 (residues 1–32, 70–144, and 338–375) and subdomain 2 (residues 33–69). The large domain comprises subdomain 3 (residues 145–180 and 270–337) and subdomain 4 (residues 181–269). The course of the

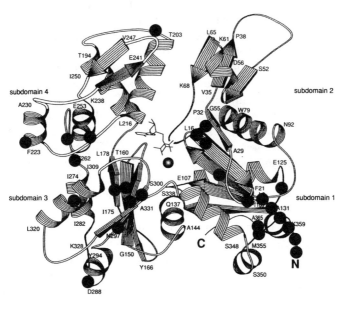

	1	2	3	4	5	6	10	16	17	76	103	129	153	162	176	201	225	260	267	272	279	287	297	299	358	365
α	D	E	D	E	T	T	C	L	V	I	T	V	L	N	M	V	N	T	I	A	Y	I	N	M	T	A
β	-	D	D	D	I	A	V	M	C	V	V	T	M	T	L	T	Q	A	L	C	F	V	T	L	S	S
γ	-	E	E	E					I																	

Figure 1 Schematic representation of the structure of actin (51). ATP and Ca^{2+} are located between the small (*right*) and large (*left*) domain. Solid circles indicate the position of amino acid differences between mammalian cytoplasmic actins and rabbit skeletal muscle actin (120). The first residue is absent in the cytoplasmic actins.

polypeptide chain is very similar in subdomains 1 and 3, where it forms a five-stranded β-sheet consisting of a β-meander and a right-handed $\beta\alpha\beta$ unit flanked by several α-helices. Quantitatively, 75 pairs of corresponding residues have been identified that can be superimposed by an approximate two-fold rotation with a root-mean-square difference of 2.8 Å. A similar chain fold is found in hexokinase (4) and in the 44-kilodalton (kDa) ATPase fragment of the heat-shock protein HSC70 (31, 32)—see below. Subdomains 1 and 3 may have evolved by gene duplication, and subdomains 2 and 4 may have been subsequently inserted into subdomains 1 and 3, respectively.

Actin appears to be a rather flexible molecule. The polypeptide chain crosses over from the small into the large domain at residue 140 and comes back at residue 338. The α-carbon atoms of these two residues are only 4 Å apart, suggesting the possibility of a hinge at that region. The relative orientation of the domains is fixed, however, by the adenine nucleotide and the associated divalent cation found at the strategic position between the small and the large domain. The nucleotide and the metal are involved in numerous interactions with both domains, thereby contributing to the stability of the actin molecule. Indeed, as indicated by the temperature factors of the refined model, those parts in the molecule involved in nucleotide binding are significantly less mobile than other regions in the structure (Figure 2). Actin denatures rapidly after removal of the nucleotide and the tightly bound metal. Bertazzon et al (10) used differential scanning microcalorimetry to study thermal unfolding of actin. They concluded that denaturation cannot be described by a single transition between the native and the unfolded state. The melting curve, which has a maximum at 57°C for G-actin, is broad and can be explained by two independent two-state transitions suggesting the existence of domains of different thermal stability. For F-actin, the melting temperature is 67°C. A state of G-actin similar to that of the heat-denatured form is obtained by removing the tightly bound Ca^{2+} with EGTA. As judged using circular dichroism spectra, both forms retain 60% of the α-helical content of the native G actin, and the completely unfolded state cannot be reached by further heating to 95°C. A complete unfolding can be obtained in 5 M guanidinium chloride or 8 M urea.

During the unfolding of actin caused by removal of the actin-bound adenine nucleotide, several intermediate states can be distinguished by the number of exposed thiols (23, 24) using the reagent 2,4-dinitrophenylcysteinyldisulfide ([¹⁴C]DNPSSC) for radioactive labeling (30). These states may be identical to those observed during thermal denaturation as described above. Rabbit skeletal muscle actin contains five cysteine residues, at positions 10, 217, 257, 285, and 374 (28). The initial

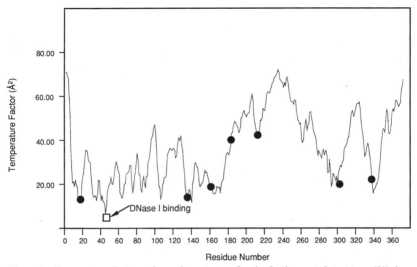

Figure 2   Temperature factors of α-carbon atoms of actin. In the crystal structure (51), low temperature factors are found in regions of the molecule that are in contact with DNase I or that interact with the nucleotide and its associated divalent metal (*filled circles*).

state of ATP-G-actin is characterized by the exposure of a single thiol group, Cys374. Exchange of ATP for ADP also uncovers Cys10. The transition between the two states is reversible: addition of ATP or of excess divalent metal ions restores the initial state. Drewes & Faulstich (24) conclude that, after the exchange of ATP for ADP, the ADP-G-actin slowly but reversibly undergoes conformational transition to the state in which Cys10 is exposed. Removal of the nucleotide irreversibly leads to a third state characterized by the exposure of Cys257 in addition to Cys374 and Cys10 (23). Actin in this state is still able to polymerize. Unfolding proceeds by uncovering Cys217 and finally Cys285. Exposure of cysteine residues has also been estimated using the reagent 7-dimethylamino-4-methyl-(N-maleimidyl)coumarin (DACM) (64). Liu et al (64) found that Cys285 was completely inaccessible to DACM and that Cys10, 217, and 374 were much less reactive than Cys257. These results are different from those obtained by using [^{14}C]DNPSSC, indicating that the reactivity of the cysteine residues strongly depends upon their environment and the thiol reagent used. [^{14}C]DNPSSC is probably more suitable for estimating solvent exposure of cysteine residues in a protein because this reagent is very selective for thiol groups and largely independent of the hydrophobicity of the environment (23).

In the crystal structure of the actin: DNase I complex in both the ADP and ATP form, the calculated exposed area (52) of Cys10, 217, 257, and 285 is between 0 and 6 Å^2. Hence the average number of water molecules in contact with the cysteine residues is between 0 and 0.6. Cys374 is not present in the crystal structure because, in order to grow crystals, the last three residues in the actin sequence are removed by mild trypsin treatment after complex formation with DNase I. However, model building has yielded an estimate of the coordinates of the missing residues. In this model, Cys374 becomes well exposed to solvent. In the search for isomorphous heavy-atom derivatives during the X-ray analysis, investigators found that only Cys10 reacts with methylmercuriacetate. Larger compounds such as *p*-chloromercuribenzoate did not bind at all. Cys217 and 257 are close neighbors in subdomain 4; the distance between the two sulfur atoms is approximately 3.8 Å. The absence of exposed cysteine residues indicates that the crystal structure corresponds to the native state as defined by Drewes & Faulstich (24).

Actin contains one nucleotide ATP (or ADP) located in the cleft between the small and large domains together with a Ca^{2+} ion bound to the phosphate moiety (Figures 1 and 3) (see Figure 4 in 51). The adenine base is in the anti conformation with respect to the ribose, which assumes a 2'-endo pucker. The 2'- and 3'-hydroxyl groups of the ribose participate in hydrogen bonds with one of the oxygen atoms of the carboxylate groups

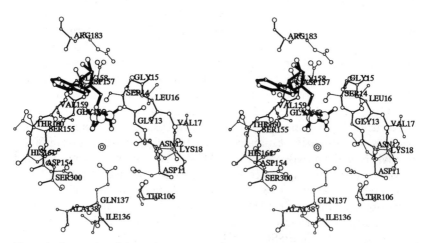

Figure 3   Stereo plot of the environment of Ca^{2+} and ATP in actin (51). The calcium ion is in the center of the picture. The atoms belonging to ATP are connected by thick lines. An approximate two-fold axis (vertical in the figure) passes through the calcium ion and relates the two phosphate-binding loops and associated β-sheets. Published with permission, © 1990, Macmillan Magazines Ltd. (51).

of Glu214 and Asp157, respectively. The adenine binds into a hydrophobic pocket between subdomains 3 and 4. The floor of this pocket comprises one turn of a 3_{10} helix 302–308. The glycine residue at position 302, which is hydrogen-bonded to the α-phosphate group, is essential for nucleotide binding because there is no space for a side chain between this residue and the ribose-phosphate moiety. The back of the pocket is formed by the side chain of Tyr306. The rest of the pocket consists of the hydrophobic parts of Glu214, Lys213, and Lys336. Glu214 is held in place by a hydrogen bond to the ribose 2′OH and a salt bridge to Arg210, while Lys213 forms a hydrogen bond to the carbonyl group of Gly182.

In the case of ATP, the β-phosphate is bound by the β-bend formed by residues Ser14, Gly15, and Leu16, and the γ-phosphate is bound by the β-bend formed by Asp157, Gly158, Val159 (Figure 3). These two phosphate-binding loops are equivalent with respect to the approximate two-fold rotation relating subdomains 1 and 3. In each case, the amide groups of the β-bends are orientated so as to hydrogen-bond the phosphate oxygens. In the case of ADP, only the β-phosphate is bonded, and Lys18 forms a bidentate complex with the α- and β-phosphate oxygens; in the ATP form, Lys18 interacts with the main-chain carbonyl and side-chain carboxyl of Asp11.

The position of the Ca^{2+} ion with respect to the phosphate groups is in agreement with biochemical evidence that the tightly bound divalent metal ion interacts with the β- and γ-phosphates of ATP and shows a high specificity for the Λ isomer (115). The divalent cation is at the center of a hydrophilic pocket formed by the di- or triphosphate moiety of the nucleotide and residues Asp11, Asp154, Lys18, and Gln137. The ion is shielded from the bulk solvent, which may explain its tight binding.

DNase I Binding

Deoxyribonuclease I (DNase I) from bovine pancreas is an endonuclease of molecular weight 30,400 that degrades double-stranded DNA through hydrolysis of the P-O3′ bond to yield 5′-oligonucleotides. DNase I consists of a single polypeptide chain of 260 amino acid residues with a carbohydrate side chain attached to Asn18. The atomic structure of the protein has been determined through X-ray analysis of single crystals at 2-Å resolution (83, 105). Although the physiological significance of the interaction is still obscure, DNase I forms a stable 1 : 1 complex with actin from many different sources. The interaction inhibits DNase I activity (61) as well as the ability of actin to polymerize (41, 66). The only exceptions known so far are actin from *Entamoeba histolytica* (70) and from *Tetrahymena thermophila* (40), which do not bind DNase I. These actins are the only known examples of sequences that differ in the DNase I binding region.

Knowledge of the atomic structure of DNase I has been extremely useful for solving the structure of the actin: DNase I complex (51). DNase I binds to actin at two regions. The area of these contacts is 1849 Å^2, found by subtracting the solvent-accessible area of the complex from the sum of the accessible area of actin and DNase I computed separately (52). The binding energy between the two proteins comes from hydrogen bonds as well as from electrostatic and hydrophobic interactions. The minor contact region involves residues Thr203 and Glu207 in subdomain 4 and Glu13 and His44 in DNase I. The major contact is found in subdomain 2, involving residues Arg39-Gly46 and Lys61-Ile64. Lys61 forms a salt bridge with Glu69 in DNase I, whereas residues Gly42, Val43, and Met44 are attached as an additional parallel strand of the six-stranded β-sheet in DNase I with partners Tyr65, Val66, and Val67 (see Figure 2 in 51).

The tight binding leads to a deviation in the α-carbon positions of residues 65–67 by as much as 1.8 Å from their original locations in the native DNase I structure. Except for this region, the native structure of DNase I does not significantly change by forming the complex with actin. Because the hydrophobic residues in the loop 40–49 would become much more exposed to solvent without DNase I and because the DNase I structure is locally disturbed by the binding to actin, it is reasonable to expect that the actin structure, as found in the complex with DNase I, differs also from the native G-actin conformation. However, the structural similarity between actin and the ATPase domain of the heat-shock protein HSC70 (32) leads one to believe that these changes are likely to be of a local nature, probably involving the loop 40–49 in subdomain 2, and do not affect all of the actin structure. The loop His40-Gln49 has no counterpart in HSC70, but the three strands of the β-sheet and the α-helix connecting the second with the third strand in subdomain 2 of actin do not differ much from the equivalent residues in HSC70. The environment of the phosphate groups is essentially identical: the relative orientation of domains 1 and 2 is the same in both proteins. As described below, the similarity between actin and HSC70 includes all four subdomains as well as the bound nucleotide, and therefore it seems reasonable to assume that the structure of actin determined in complex with DNAse I is very like the structure of G-actin.

X-ray analysis of crystals of actin in its complex with profilin (96) and with the segment I domain of gelsolin (see below) is in progress and is expected to provide an undistorted structure of subdomain 2 because the contact region between these two proteins and actin is different from the DNase I binding sites.

Comparison with Other Structures

The structural similarity between actin and hexokinase and the 44-kDa ATPase fragment of the bovine heat-shock cognate protein HSC70 is striking (31). This discovery was rather unexpected, as these proteins share almost no sequence homology.

The similarity between actin and HSC70 extends over 241 pairs of equivalent amino acid residues in the two structures whose α-carbon positions can be superimposed with a root-mean-square difference in distance of 2.3 Å (32). Among the equivalent residues, only 39 are identical and another 56 are conservative substitutions. Subdomains 1, 2, 3, and 4 of actin roughly correspond to HSC70 domains IA, IB, IIA, and IIB as defined by Flaherty et al (31). The structural differences between the two molecules mainly occur in loop regions of actin known to be involved in interactions with other monomers in the actin filament or with actin binding proteins. The similarity also includes the conformations of the adenine nucleotides and their environments in both proteins. Despite the absence of significant global sequence similarity between actin, hexokinase, and HSC70, a characteristic sequence fingerprint,

$$(I/L/V)X(I/L/V/C)DXG(T/S/G)(T/S/G)XX(R/K/C),$$

of the adenine nucleotide β-phosphate-binding pocket has been derived that, in addition, identifies members of the glycerol kinase family likely to have similar structures in their nucleotide-binding domains (32).

The structure of hexokinase b (4) can be matched with the actin structure by moving the large and small domains of hexokinase with respect to each other, such that the β-sheets of the large and small (residues 63–188) domains in hexokinase coincide with the equivalent β-sheets of actin. The resulting movement consists of a rotation of 37° and a small translational component along the rotation axis of 2.5 Å. This rotation is greater than necessary to superimpose hexokinase b onto hexokinase a (99), suggesting that even hexokinase a is not completely closed. In analogy with hexokinase, the domains of actin may open up to enable nucleotide and divalent cation exchange. After rotation of the domains, the structures of hexokinase b and actin become quite similar, and include also the β-sheets of subdomains 2 and 4. Also, these three proteins may share a similar mechanism of ATP hydrolysis with His161 as a candidate proton acceptor for the ATPase reaction in actin (32). To be effective as a base, this histidine would need to be part of a charge-relay system.

Structure of the Actin Filament

The actin filament can be described as a left-handed helix, the genetic helix, with a rise per monomer of 27.5 Å and a rotation angle of $-166.2°$ around the filament axis. Because the rotation per monomer is close to 180°, the structure has the appearance of two right-handed long-pitch helices that slowly twist around each other. F-actin can be orientated in capillary tubes (91), and the resulting gel gives X-ray fiber patterns that diffract to better than 8 Å. The observed fiber diagram has been explained in terms of a unique rigid-body transformation of the actin monomer with respect to the filament (43). The transformed coordinates from the crystal structure (51) then lead to an atomic model of the filament as shown in Figure 4. The maximum diameter of the filament is between 90 and 95 Å. The large domain is located near the central axis of the filament, and the small domain is at a large radius from the filament axis. In the middle of the fiber, the density is low. The N-terminus of actin is well exposed at a large radius. Extensive interactions occur between molecules along the long-pitch actin helix, involving residues 322–325 with residues 243–245; 286–289 with 202–204; and 166–169 and 375 with 41–45. Contacts along the left-handed genetic helix occur between residues 110–112 and 195–197. A trimeric contact may exist involving the loop 264–273 that fits between two molecules of the opposing strand (43). This loop may be rebuilt as an antiparallel β-sheet with residues Phe266-Ile-Gly-Met in the β-bend, thereby forming a hydrophobic plug that fits into the pocket consisting of residues 63–64 and 40–45 in one molecule and residues 166, 169, 171, 173, 285, and 289 in an adjacent one along the long-pitch helix.

The atomic model of the actin filament is in agreement with many biochemical observations (43) as well as with electron micrograph image reconstructions (14a, 71, 72). Moreover, these and other results imply the polarity of the filament: the barbed end in the model must be at the bottom in Figure 4.

Some changes between monomeric and F-actin are to be expected that, perhaps, might consist of slightly different orientations of the four sub-domains. Therefore, the subdomains were allowed to move independently in a new refinement against the fiber diffraction data. A marked improvement in the fit to the fiber diagram was obtained with small shifts (1–2 Å), except for subdomain 2, which moved about 6 Å.

The number of interacting residues found in the model indicates that the interactions between monomers in the long-pitch helix are stronger than along the genetic helix. This view is supported by the findings of Aebi et al (2) and Erickson (29) as well as by earlier results obtained from image reconstructions of negatively stained Mg-paracrystals of F-actin (82). Furthermore, recent cryoelectron microscopic work on F-actin and F-actin decorated with myosin S1 embedded in vitreous ice (72) now shows a stronger connectivity along the long-pitch helix as compared with previous results (71, 114).

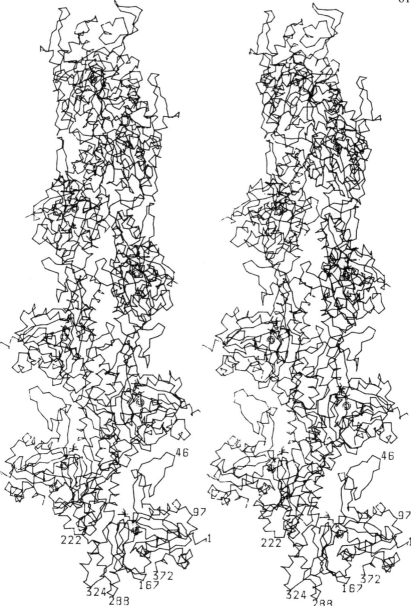

Figure 4 Atomic model of F-actin as a stereo pair (43). The barbed end of the filament is at the bottom. α-Carbon positions of eight monomers, ADP, and Ca²⁺ are shown. A few amino acid sequence numbers are given for the actin monomer at the bottom. Strong contacts are made along the long-pitch helices. Published with permission, © 1990, Macmillan Magazines Ltd. (43).

The new results (72) provide important details about the shape of F-actin and the location of the binding sites of myosin and tropomyosin. Furthermore, the atomic model of the filament, when reduced to comparable resolution, agrees well with the cryoelectron microscopic pictures (42). Milligan et al (72) were also able to localize the C terminus by labeling Cys374 with an undecagold derivative. The radius of 27 Å they obtained is in good agreement with the value obtained by Holmes et al (43). The structure obtained for S1-decorated actin shows additional important detail (e.g. the second myosin binding site) that could not be seen in the earlier results (71). Moreover, it bears a welcome family resemblance to the original reconstructions of decorated actin (76).

Electron micrographs of single actin filaments taken with negative staining show considerable variability in the pitch of the long-pitch two-start helix and the radius of the filament. These two phenomena have been studied by Egelman et al (25) as "cumulative angular disorder" and by Millonig et al (73) as the "lateral slipping" model. However, these effects seem much less pronounced in vitreous ice (see Figure 11c in 101; 72).

Actin Isoforms

In two-dimensional (2D) gels of total cellular extracts, actin migrates as slightly different spots with constant molecular weights (42 kDa) and, depending on the tissue and/or the species, with very similar pI values (around 5.4) (34). Amino acid sequence analysis of skeletal muscle actin (28) and other isoforms of actin (122) confirmed the conserved length (374–375 residues) and explained the pI differences in terms of the number and nature of the acidic residues present in the extreme N termini (121). Warm-blooded vertebrates all contain six isoforms of actin expressed solely in a tissue-specific way independent of the species: two striated-muscle actins (cardiac and skeletal muscle), two smooth-muscle actins (vascular and visceral), and two nonmuscle actins (β and γ) in all nonmuscle cells. The muscle actins are typically found in chordates. Early subphyla have only one type. Later, because of consecutive gene duplication (one from Chondrichthyes to Amphibia and one from Amphibia to Reptilia), the ancestral actin branched into four types: two striated- and two smooth-muscle actins (123). The cytoplasmic actins are evolutionarily older and found in all cells of lower eukaryotes, invertebrates, and in nonmuscle cells of vertebrates.

The positions of the amino acid exchanges that distinguish skeletal muscle from nonmuscle vertebrate actins are mapped in the atomic structure (Figure 1). Most exchanges occur in three-dimensional clusters. The most important cluster is found in the right-hand lower corner of subdomain 1 and contains positions 1, 2, 3, 4, 5, 6, 103, 129, 357, and 364.

Another cluster is present in the central β-sheet of subdomain 3 with substitutions at residues 153, 162, 176, and 298. The third cluster is less pronounced and is located at the interdomain region of subdomains 3 and 4 comprising residues 225, 259, 266, and 271. Interestingly, subdomains 2 and 4 are conserved.

In considering the actin-actin contact sites (43), one should note that, except for the I287V and the T201V substitutions, which are part of or adjacent to contact sites 286–288 and 202–204, respectively, none of the substitutions are part of the strong interactions along the long-pitch helix. Two other exchanges, I267L and A272C, are in the loop 264–273, which is supposed to form the hypothetical trimeric contact with the opposite strand. The conserved nature of the presumed actin-actin contacts also applies for all other actin isoforms sequenced so far, suggesting that they may all exhibit similar, if not identical, polymerization properties. Several lines of experimental evidence support this assumption: (a) polymerization rates, critical monomer concentrations, and relative viscosities are nearly identical for a large number of actins; (b) copolymerization studies showed that most actins displayed very similar polymerization properties (for reviews, see e.g. 19a, 55); (c) a mutation, G245D, in a human fibroblast β-actin (119) resulted in a poorly polymerizing protein (53) because this mutation disturbs the most conserved actin-actin binding region, 243–245.

Most of the substitutions located in subdomain 1 coincide with the presumed binding sites of a variety of actin binding proteins (see below). Variations in this region may therefore be considered as structural adaptations to match the contacts with the different associated proteins. For instance, the differences in the activation of myosin Mg^{2+}-ATPase by sarcomeric and smooth-muscle actins can be explained by amino acid exchanges in the N terminus and in residues 17 and 89, which are all located within the presumed myosin S1 binding site (80). This observation suggests that the differences between the isoforms of actin serve to accomodate interactions with associated proteins rather than to vary polymerization properties.

FUNCTION OF ACTIN

Actin has no important enzymatic activity, although it is a slow ATPase. However, it does inhibit DNase I and activate the myosin ATPase. Various other enzymes interact with actin (for review, see 102).

Perhaps even more important is actin's structural and dynamic role as a major component of the cytoskeleton in the cell. Both properties depend on its capacity to assemble and disassemble a variety of filamentous structures. Together with the other components of the cytoskeleton, it may help to organize cellular processes in space as well as in time.

In addition to its structural role, actin is also an important element in cellular motility processes. Actin filaments activate the myosin-Mg^{2+}-ATPase activity, and movement of myosin along acting filaments produces force for muscle contraction and other less specialized types of cell movements (20). Moreover, amoeboid movements that are responsible for the motility of or in individual cells, such as locomotion and cell ruffling, are important in biological processes such as embryonic development, wound healing, and tumor invasion. Although much new information was recently obtained (113), the molecular mechanisms of this process are still poorly understood.

All motility processes involving actin are controlled by the interaction in the G- or the F-form with various actin-binding proteins. These proteins are generally classified according to their effects on actin organization in vivo and in vitro: ABPs that bind monomeric actin and hinder polymerization (e.g. the profilins); ABPs able to cap one of the ends of the filament (e.g. cap Z36); ABPs that sever filaments and bind to the barbed ends (e.g. gelsolin); ABPs that bind laterally along the filaments (e.g. tropomyosin); ABPs that can move along the filaments (e.g. myosins); and ABPs that connect the filaments with each other and form networks or bundles (e.g. α-actinin, synapsin, villin) (37, 89, 102, 117). Comparison of their primary structures allows a similar classification. In addition, it was also possible to recognize smaller entities as either actin-binding domains or regulatory domains, linking the actin-binding activities with cellular signals. These domains could be isolated through limited proteolytic cleavage or generated as recombinant fragments, and their individual actin-binding properties could be studied.

The three-dimensional structure of actin (51) and the derived atomic model of the filament (43) obtained recently now allow the location of some of the ABP binding sites in the structure. In the following sections, we discuss some of the best-characterized ABPs and their interactions with actin.

Tropomyosin

Skeletal muscle tropomyosin is a two-chain parallel coiled-coil α-helical structure of length about 400 Å that follows the long-pitch actin helix at a filament radius of 37–38 Å (12, 72) thereby interacting with 7 actin molecules. The amino acid sequence of α-tropomyosin from rabbit skeletal muscle consists of 284 residues. It contains 14 pseudorepeats of acidic, basic, and hydrophobic residues, which is consistent with the knob-into-hole packing expected for a coiled-coil structure and equivalent interaction with the 7 actin monomers. Each actin molecule interacts with 2 chains of tropomyosin of about $39\frac{1}{2}$ residues. This observation agrees well with the pseudorepeat of 19 2/3 found in the sequence (100). Tropomyosin is part of the regulatory system that controls actin-myosin interaction in muscle. There is good evidence in vitro and in live muscle that tropomyosin shifts its position on the actin filament when relaxed muscle is activated to contract. This shift may result in a physical blocking or unblocking of the interaction site with myosin (86), but the mechanism is likely to involve more subtle structural changes that activate the myosin independently of its affinity for actin.

Comparison of the atomic model of the helical actin filament (43) with Figures 4a,b of Milligan et al (72) suggests that, in the presence of S1 and Ca^{2+}, tropomyosin runs along the interface between subdomains 3 and 4 with contacts around Lys215 and Pro307. Figure 5 shows the trace of tropomyosin on actin, which corresponds to the on state. This assignment is consistent with the fact that modifications of Lys238 impair tropomyosin binding (27) and that the same residue is shielded in the F-actin-tropomyosin complex (110). The α-helix Asp222-Ser233 could well be also part of this contact. This is in agreement with the observation that eight amino acids in the region 222–233 of the sequence of *Tetrahymena* actin (22, 39), which does not bind muscle tropomyosin (40), differ from the same region of the rabbit muscle sequence. Also, the region Cys217-Leu236 in actin must have an actin-specific function, because it is replaced by the short stretch Ser275-Thr278 in HSC70 (32).

Modification of Arg28, Arg95, and Arg147 with dione derivatives reportedly results in total loss of tropomyosin binding (49). Furthermore, reactivities of Lys326, Lys328, Lys336, and Arg95 were strongly reduced in the F-actin-tropomyosin complex (110). Figure 5 makes clear that the reactivities of Lys326 and 328 are reduced when tropomyosin occupies the on-state; but the other biochemical data can be explained only if one assumes that actin has a second binding site of tropomyosin that includes residues Arg28, 95, 147, and Lys336. If tropomyosin occupies this second site, the filament should be in the off-state because it overlaps with the S1 strong binding site (see Figure 5). The two binding regions of tropomyosin as shown in Figure 5 are approximately parallel to each other at a distance of 37–38 Å from the filament axis and can be superimposed by a rotation of $\approx 50°$ around the filament axis.

On the other hand, it has also been reported that the peptide containing residues 355–375 interacts with tropomyosin (75), a result that is difficult to explain by the simple model shown in Figure 5.

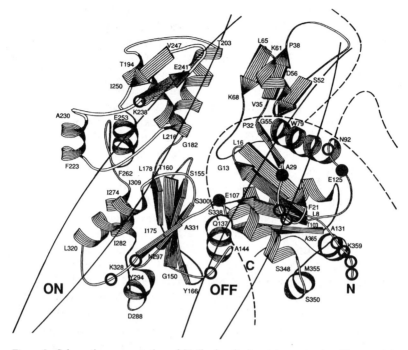

Figure 5 Schematic representation of S1 (*broken line*) and tropomyosin with respect to an actin molecule in the filament as derived from cryoelectron microscopic pictures, biochemical information, and the atomic model of the actin filament. The on position of tropomyosin is assumed in the presence of Ca^{2+} and S1 in the rigor state. The off position of tropomyosin, which overlaps with the strong binding site of S1 on actin, is drawn in agreement with biochemical data and model-building studies. Residues in actin known to be involved in the binding of S1 and of tropomyosin are marked by a solid circle. Open circles show residues that interact with either tropomyosin or S1.

Myosin

Myosin consists of two identical heavy chains with two light chains attached to the globular head of each heavy chain. The cyclic interaction between the thick myosin filament and the thin actin filament with concomitant ATP hydrolysis leads to the production of mechanical force in muscle (for review see 20, 35, 57, 79, 126).

Comparison of the atomic model of the actin helix (43) with Figures 4c,d of Milligan et al (72) shows that S1 in the rigor state mainly binds to the outer face of subdomain 1 as outlined by the broken line in Figure 5.

This is in agreement with the positions of known myosin-binding residues of actin comprising Asp1, Glu2, Asp3, Glu4, Asp24, Asp25, Arg28, Glu93, Arg95, and Lys336 (see discussion in 43, 51). Moreover, the reconstruction shows that the rigor myosin binding site spans two subunits. Above the major site of interaction is an additional thin bridge of density extending between the main body of S1 and the top of the outer domain in the adjacent long-pitch actin monomer (Figure 5). Inspection of the atomic structure suggests that residues Glu93 and Arg95 may take part in this interaction. The idea of two distinct myosin binding sites on actin may be of significance for theories of muscle contraction (see Figure 6 in 36). On the myosin side of the complex, the use of peptide mimetics showed that residues within the region 690–725 of S1 are involved in binding to actin (54). Cross-linking experiments (131) suggest that a second possible binding site may be located at the junction between the 50-kDa and 20-kDa fragments of S1.

By comparing actin decorated with S1(A1) or with S1(A2) (S1 containing A1 or A2 light chains), researchers could locate the extra density missing from the A2 light chain that corresponds to the 41 N-terminal residues in the A1 light chain (72). The N-terminal region of the A1 light chain is known from cross-linking results to bind to residues 360–364 in actin (107). The extra density is found on the undersurface of the actin monomer, which is consistent with the position of residues 360–364 in the atomic model of the actin filament.

The main actin-S1 contact appears to be effectively blocked by tropomyosin in its off position (Figure 5). The second, more tenuous actin-S1 contact, which is near the α-helix Trp79-Asn92, may not be affected by tropomyosin, because S1 density interacting in this region comes from a different direction. It is therefore tempting to speculate that this is the contact involved in the so-called weak binding state of myosin. Thus, the transition between weak and strong binding states, which represents the power stroke in the contraction mechanism, appears to be regulated by the switching of tropomyosin between its on and off position. X-ray analysis of crystals of S1 (93) and of tropomyosin (87), now in progress, will lead to a better understanding of actin-myosin interactions and their regulation.

Caldesmon

Caldesmon is an F-actin and Ca^{2+}-calmodulin binding protein regulating the actomyosin interactions in smooth muscle and nonmuscle cells (for review see 68). The caldesmon family forms a group of elongated molecules with sizes varying between 87 and 130 kDa that are believed to lie along the actin filament covering about 7–10 actin protomers (124). Limited proteolysis of caldesmon has been used to locate its functional domains

(111). The F-actin binding site is located in a globular head close to the Ca^{2+} calmodulin binding site in the C-terminal 10-kDa fragment of the molecule (7). This region was narrowed down to a calmodulin binding region, residues 629–666, flanked on either side by F-actin binding sites: a high affinity site located between Leu597 and Ala628, and a low affinity site located between residues Arg711 and Pro736 that is important for inhibition of actomyosin ATPase activity (125). Again, caldesmon can be cross-linked to the N terminus of actin (8) as for many other ABPs. The caldesmon amino acid sequences that are supposed to be involved in actin binding are 483–508, 597–629, and 711–756 (see Figure 5 in 125; 16).

The Cofilin Family

Cofilin belongs to a family of widely distributed and structurally related ABPs with apparent molecular mass of 21 kDa. These proteins form a 1: 1 complex both with monomeric actin and with F-actin protomers resulting in a depolymerization. Proteins similar in function are actin-depoly- merizing factor (ADF) from chick embryonic brain, destrin from mam- malian brain, depactin from echinodermatous oocytes, and actophorin from *Acanthamoeba*. The sequences of several members of this family were recently published (1, 69, 77) and show a high degree of structural homology, suggesting that they may have similar actin-binding activities.

Potential actin binding sites have been mapped either on the basis of sequence homology with other ABPs or by cross-linking and peptide- inhibition experiments. A dodecapeptide, WAPECAPLKSKM, has been found in the cofilin sequence (residues 104–115) that binds specifically via one or both of its lysine residues to the N-terminal region 1–12 of actin, and inhibits actin polymerization (132). Matsuzaki et al (69) also reported that the heptapeptide, DAIKKKL, which occurs in the cofilin sequence, competes with cofilin for actin binding.

Profilin

Profilins are small actin-binding proteins expressed in high concentrations in the cytoplasm of nonmuscle cells. Actin forms a 1: 1 complex with profilin, and this complex does not assemble into filaments. Profilin is believed to act as an actin monomer buffer. The complex can be dissociated by phosphatidyl inositol 4-monophosphate (PIP) and phosphatidyl inosi- tol 4,5-bisphosphate (PIP$_2$), resulting in profilin binding to poly- phosphoinositide integrated in micelles and polymerization-competent actin (59, 60). The complex of actin and profilin from *Acanthamoeba castellanii* can be cross-linked between Glu364 of actin and Lys115 of profilin (118), which is consistent with the finding that profilin binds to the barbed end of actin filaments. This binding site coincides with the

S1(A1) light chain binding site on actin. X-ray analysis of crystals of profilin (65) and of the actin: profilin complex (96) is in progress. In both cases, crystallographic work turned out to be quite difficult: progress towards a solution of the profilin structure has been delayed by the lack of suitable heavy-atom derivatives, although the crystals are of good quality. In the case of the actin: profilin complex, the crystals displayed extensive polymorphism with considerable variation in the length of the c-axis. In addition, the b-axis shows a superlattice at low pH that causes dissociation of profilin (96). The crystals were obtained from high salt in the presence of EDTA, which is likely to remove the essential divalent cation. Under these conditions, one might expect that the two domains of actin could swing apart as in hexokinase, thereby explaining the large changes in cell constants observed. Despite these difficulties, a low resolution electron density map of the crystalline complex between G-actin and profilin has been published (96). The structure shows actin to have two domains with the nucleotide sitting at the top of the cleft between the two domains. Furthermore, Schutt et al (96) emphasize the importance of the packing of the actin monomers observed in the crystal that results in a zig-zag shaped actin helix, the "ribbon structure," with a rise per monomer of 36 Å along the two-fold screw-axis b and a twist per monomer of 180°. These authors speculate that the ribbon structure is related by a simple transformation to the normal actin helix, which has a rise of 27.5 Å and a twist of 166°. The atomic model (43) and recent cryoelectron microscopic image reconstructions (72) of the actin helix indicate that similar actin-actin contacts are probably not involved in the ribbon structure.

α-Actinin and Related Proteins

α-Actinin is an F-actin cross-linking protein found in both muscle and nonmuscle cells at points where actin filaments are anchored to a variety of intracellular structures (e.g. the attachment of the actin cytoskeleton to the cell membrane or the anchorage of thin filaments to the Z-disc). In nonmuscle cells, most of the α-actinin is in the cytoplasm, often in association with thin filaments. α-Actinin is a rod-shaped molecule, 300–400 Å in length, consisting of two subunits oriented in an antiparallel manner, explaining the bivalent affinity for F-actin. The α-actinin subunit consists of an N-terminal 27-kDa actin-binding globular domain, followed by a rod-like region consisting of four internal repeats of 122 amino acids, homologous to repeated sequences in spectrin and dystrophin, and a C-terminal region containing two EF hand-like Ca^{2+}-binding motifs. The latter domain is responsible for the Ca^{2+} sensitivity of α-actinin and is probably nonfunctional in muscle α-actinin (for a review, see 13).

Cross-linking experiments suggest that the N-terminal 27-kDa domain binds actin at two sites involving residues 1–12 and 86–119 or 123 of actin, respectively (74). A region for actin binding has been narrowed down to a linear sequence containing only 27 residues that is homologous to other α-actinins, *Dictyostelium* ABP-120, human filamin, *Drosophila* β spectrin, and human and chick dystrophin (15). This finding suggests that these proteins may share common F-actin binding properties.

Myosin and α-actinin can be cross-linked to similar, if not identical, side chains in actin (11, 74). This is in accordance with the observation that tropomyosin can inhibit the interactions of both α-actinin and myosin with F-actin (84). However, a comparison of the sequences in the α-actinin and myosin interfaces has so far not revealed any similarity.

Gelsolin

Gelsolin is a Ca^{2+}-dependent actin binding protein of 82 kDa, found in blood plasma and in many types of cells in vertebrate tissues. It severs actin filaments, caps their fast-growing ends, and also accelerates polymerization by forming a stable nucleating complex with two actin monomers. Cytoplasmic and secreted gelsolins are identical except for the plasma extension sequence (58). The homology between the cytoplasmic forms of human and pig gelsolins is 98%, consisting of 704 out of 730 identical amino acid residues and 11 conservative substitutions (129). Extensive homologies to gelsolin throughout their lengths have also been found for severin (5), fragmin (3), villin (6, 9), gCap39 (133), Mbh1 (92), and adseverin (95), indicating a close evolutionary relation between these proteins (129). This family of actin-severing proteins has apparently evolved from an ancestral sequence of 120 to 130 amino acid residues that are repeated three times in the case of severin, fragmin (3), gCap39, and Mbh1, and six times for gelsolin (129), villin, and probably also adseverin. The strong tandem repeat in the N- and C-terminal halves (58) suggests that gelsolin and villin have evolved by gene triplication of the ancestral motif followed by gene duplication (129). In gelsolin, these six repeating segments are connected by proteolytically sensitive regions between segments 1 and 2 and segments 3 and 4. Each of the three proteolytic fragments, segment 1, segment 4–6, and segment 2–3, bind to actin. Human plasma gelsolin as well as several deletion mutants lacking some of the segments have been expressed in high yield and soluble form in *Escherichia coli*, and the actin binding properties of these mutants have been subsequently explored (90, 127, 128). The deletion mutant consisting of segment 1 (residues 1–150) binds one actin monomer with high affinity independent of calcium. Cross-linking experiments have shown that segment 1 binds to the acidic residues in the N-terminal region 1–18 of actin

(108). Regions in the segment 1 mutant involved in the binding have been identified using several smaller mutants truncated at either the N- or C-terminal ends (128). Apparently, the regions close to the N and C termini of segment 1 are essential for binding to actin. Furthermore, the complex between segment 1 and actin contains an additional Ca^{2+}-binding site (128). The mutant consisting of segments 2–3 (residues 151–406) binds stoichiometrically to F-actin subunits in a calcium-independent way, but in the intact gelsolin molecule, this interaction with actin is calcium sensitive. This binding involves residues 305–326 (44) in gelsolin and 1–18 in actin (108). The mutant consisting of segments 4–6 (residues 407–755) binds a single actin monomer only in the presence of calcium. Candidate residues for cross-linking are Lys359, Glu361, Asp363, Glu364, Lys373, and Phe375 (108) in actin and residues 660–738 in gelsolin (14). Based on these observations and the structure of actin, a schematic model for the interaction of gelsolin with actin has been proposed (26, 90).

Recently, crystals of the complex between actin and the segment 1 mutant of gelsolin (128) were obtained (H. G. Mannherz, personal communication) that are suitable for X-ray analysis. A native data set at 3-Å resolution of good quality has been collected (P. McLaughlin, personal communication), and it appears likely that the structure of this complex will be known by the time this volume is published. The new structure will undoubtedly contribute to the understanding of the capping and severing mechanism. In addition, it will show the undisturbed structure of subdomain 2 of actin since the binding of gelsolin does not interfere with the binding of DNase I to actin.

CONCLUDING REMARKS

The N-terminal residues 1–4, the C-terminal residues 357–375, and residues located around Glu100 show a frequent participation in interactions with ABPs. This information was generally obtained by chemical cross-linking studies. These regions all map at the surface in the lower right-hand corner of subdomain 1 (see Figure 1). The cross-linking success rate of the actin N terminus is particularly striking, as explained by its high flexibility and the fact that it contains numerous cross-linkable side chains. Indeed, the α-carbon backbone of residues 1 to 5 is 15 Å long, and in addition, a distance of 13 Å connects the α-carbon atoms of the Glu and Lys residues cross-linked via a zero-length isopeptide linkage. This means that in the fully extended configuration, residues that are up to 28 Å apart could be cross-linked in the complexes of actin with actin-binding proteins. Consequently, the cross-linking results must be interpreted cautiously.

Our reservations about these cross-linking results seem to be supported by the absence of any sequence homology between the segments that are supposed to interact with the actin N terminus. The picture that does arise suggests that several ABPs interact with subdomain 1, probably via different motifs or three-dimensional entities. Due to the high flexibility and reactivity of the N terminus, isopeptide connections form most frequently with this region.

Interestingly, subdomain 1 is not only a target for several G-actin binding proteins (profilins, cofilin), but also for severing and capping ABPs (fragmin, gelsolin, actolinkin) and for F-actin binding proteins (myosin S1 and α-actinin). This observation came somewhat as a surprise, as one would have expected that ABPs that exert different actin-organizing properties would bind at a greater number of different locations on the actin molecule. It seems that these proteins bind to the same region but probably in different orientations, and some may additionally interact with other sites either in the same [gelsolin (44)] or the neighboring (myosin S1) actin protomer. In this respect, it is also interesting to recall that this subdomain is characterized by a high frequency of isoactin-specific amino acid exchanges, suggesting that substitutions in this area may modulate interactions of actin isoforms with ABPs.

In analogy with small sequence motifs, defining specific protein signals (such as nuclear or ER-targeting) one could also analyze the ABP-sequences for the presence of small motifs of linear sequences that could function as actin-recognition signals. A hexapeptide motif, LKHAET, was found in actobindin, tropomyosin, thymosin β_4, myosin heavy chain, and *Dictyostelium* α-actinin. This motif, of which Leu1, Lys2, and Glu5 are absolutely conserved, interacts with the N-terminal residues 1–3 and residue Glu100 of actin (116). Its actin-binding properties have meanwhile also been demonstrated by direct peptide synthesis (K. Vancompernolle, M. Goethals & J. Vandekerckhove, unpublished results). A second motif, LXDYLXG, appears in *Acanthamoeba* profilin, yeast profilin, fragmin, severin, villin, and gelsolin. This stretch interacts with the helix 359–365 located in the actin C terminus (118). Deletion mutagenesis on truncated severin confirmed its participation in actin capping (26). Interestingly, a similar motif, but lacking the conserved last glycine residue, was also noticed in the actin sequence 185–191. This observation supported the notion that actin and actin-binding proteins might use common themes (112). A third motif is found in cofilin, actophorin, and tropomyosin. It is a basic hexapeptide, DAIKKK, which probably interacts with the acidic residues in subdomain 1. Also in this case, actin-binding has been confirmed by the use of a synthetic peptide (132).

Although identification of such motifs may be helpful in understanding actin-ABP interactions, not all motifs may consist of easily recognizable linear segments. For instance, the adenine nucleotide β-phosphate binding motif present in actin, HSC70, and hexokinase (32) has been recognized only after the crystal structures have been solved.

In the case of actin, a synthesis of X-ray crystallography, X-ray fiber diffraction, and electron microscopy yields a consistent near atomic picture of the structure of the actin filament. It is now possible to place functional amino acid sequences of actin-interacting molecules identified by biochemical methods into a three-dimensional context. Forthcoming X-ray structures of actin-ABP complexes combined with protein chemical information will, hopefully, lead to a recognition of the underlying principles of actin organization and its control system in the cell.

ACKNOWLEDGMENTS

We would like to thank Drs. Goody and Holmes for discussions and critically reading the manuscript. J.V. is supported by grants from the Belgian National Fund for Scientific Research.

Literature Cited

1. Adams, M. E., Minamide, L. S., Duester, G., Bamburg, J. R. 1990. *Biochemistry* 29: 7414–20
2. Aebi, U., Millonig, R., Salvo, H., Engel, A. 1986. *Ann. N. Y. Acad. Sci.* 483: 100–19
3. Ampe, C., Vandekerckhove, J. 1987. *EMBO J.* 6: 4149–57
4. Anderson, C. A., Stenkamp, R. E., Steitz, T. A. 1978. *J. Mol. Biol.* 123: 15–33
5. André, E., Lottspeich, F., Schleicher, M., Noegel, A. 1988. *J. Biol. Chem.* 263: 722–28
6. Arpin, M., Pringault, E., Finidori, J., Garcia, A., Jeltsch, J.-M., et al. 1988. *J. Cell Biol.* 107: 1759–66
7. Bartegi, A., Fattoum, A., Derancourt, J., Kassab, R. 1990. *J. Biol. Chem.* 265: 15231–38
8. Bartegi, A., Fattoum, A., Kassab, R. 1990. *J. Biol. Chem.* 265: 2231–37
9. Bazari, W. L., Matsudaira, P., Wallek, M., Smeal, T., Jakes, R., Ahmed, Y. 1988. *Proc. Natl. Acad. Sci. USA* 85: 4986–90
10. Bertazzon, A., Tian, G. H., Lamblin, A., Tsong, T. Y. 1990. *Biochemistry* 29: 291–98
11. Bertrand, R., Chaussepied, P., Kassab, R., Boyer, M., Roustan, C., Benyamin, Y. 1988. *Biochemis. ·y* 27: 5728–36
12. Bivin, D. B., Stone, D. B., Schneider, D. K., Mendelson, R. A. 1991. *Biophys. J.* 59: 880–88
13. Blanchard, A., Ohanian, V., Critchley, D. 1989. *J. Muscle Res. Cell Motil.* 10: 280–89
14. Boyer, M., Feinberg, J., Hue, H. K., Capony, J. P., Benyamin, Y., Roustan, C. 1987. *Biochem. J.* 248: 359–64
14a. Bremer, A., Millonig, R. C., Sütterlin, R., Engel, A., Pollard, T. D., Aebi, U. 1991. *J. Cell Biol.* In press
15. Bresnick, A. R., Warren, V., Coondeelis, J. 1990. *J. Biol. Chem.* 265: 9236–40
16. Bryan, J., Imai, M., Lee, R., Moore, P., Cook, R. G., Lin, W.-C. 1989. *J. Biol. Chem.* 264: 13873–79
17. Carlier, M.-F. 1991. *Curr. Opin. Cell Biol.* 3: 12–17
17a. Carlier, M.-F. 1991. *J. Biol. Chem.* 266: 1–4
18. Carlsson, L., Nystroem, L.-E., Lindberg, U., Kannan, K. K., Cid-Dresdner, H., et al. 1976. *J. Mol. Biol.* 105: 353–66
19. Carlsson, L., Nystroem, L.-E., Sundkvist, I., Markey, F., Lindberg, U. 1977. *J. Mol. Biol.* 115: 465–83
19a. Clarke, M., Spudich, J. A. 1977. *Annu. Rev. Biochem.* 46: 797–822

20. Cooke, R. 1990. *Curr. Opin. Cell Biol.* 2: 62–66
21. Craig, S. W., Pollard, T. D. 1982. *Trends Biochem. Sci.* 7: 88–91
22. Cupples, C. G., Pearlman, R. E. 1986. *Proc. Natl. Acad. Sci. USA* 83: 5160–64
23. Drewes, G. 1991. Dissertation. Univ. Heidelberg
24. Drewes, G., Faulstich, H. 1991. *J. Biol. Chem.* 266: 5508–13
25. Egelman, E. H., Francis, N., DeRosier, D. 1982. *Nature* 298: 131–35
26. Eichinger, L., Noegel, A. A., Schleicher, M. 1991. *J. Cell Biol.* 112: 665–76
27. El-Saleh, S. C., Thieret, R., Johnson, P., Potter, J. D. 1984. *J. Biol. Chem.* 259: 11014–21
28. Elzinga, M., Collins, J. H., Kuehl, W. M., Adelstein, R. S. 1973. *Proc. Natl. Acad. Sci. USA* 70: 2687–91
29. Erickson, H. P. 1989. *J. Mol. Biol.* 206: 465–70
30. Faulstich, H., Merkler, I., Blackholm, H., Stournaras, C. 1984. *Biochemistry* 23: 1608–12
31. Flaherty, K. M., DeLuca-Flaherty, C., McKay, D. 1990. *Nature* 347: 623–28
32. Flaherty, K. M., McKay, D., Kabsch, W., Holmes, K. C. 1991. *Proc. Natl. Acad. Sci. USA* 88: 5041–45
33. Frieden, C. 1985. *Annu. Rev. Biophys. Biophys. Chem.* 14: 189–210
34. Garrels, J. I., Gibson, W. 1976. *Cell* 9: 793–805
35. Geeves, M. A. 1991. *Biochem. J.* 274: 1–14
36. Goody, R. S., Holmes, K. C. 1983. *Biochim. Biophys. Acta* 726: 13–39
37. Hartwig, J. H., Kwiatkowski, D. J. 1991. *Curr. Opin. Cell Biol.* 3: 87–97
38. Hatano, S., Oosawa, F. 1966. *Biochim. Biophys. Acta* 127: 488–98
39. Hirono, M., Endoh, H., Okada, N., Numata, O., Watanabe, Y. 1987. *J. Mol. Biol.* 194: 181–92
40. Hirono, M., Tanaka, R., Watanabe, Y. 1990. *J. Biochem.* 107: 32–36
41. Hitchcock, S. E. 1980. *J. Biol. Chem.* 255: 5668–73
42. Holmes, K. C., Kabsch, W. 1991. *Curr. Opin. Struct. Biol.* 1: 270–80
43. Holmes, K. C., Popp, D., Gebhard, W., Kabsch, W. 1990. *Nature* 347: 44–49
44. Houmeida, A., Hanin, V., Feinberg, J., Benyamin, Y., Roustan, C. 1991. *Biochem. J.* 274: 753–57
45. Huxley, A. F., Niedergerke, R. 1954. *Nature* 173: 971–73
46. Huxley, H. E., Hanson, J. 1954. *Nature* 173: 973–76
47. Janmey, P. A. 1991. *Curr. Opin. Cell Biol.* 3: 4–11
48. Janmey, P. A., Hvidt, S., Oster, G., Lamb, J., Stossel, T., Hartwig, J. 1990. *Nature* 347: 95–99
49. Johnson, P., Blazyk, J. M. 1978. *Biochem. Biophys. Res. Commun.* 82: 1013–18
50. Kabsch, W., Mannherz, H. G., Suck, D. 1985. *EMBO J.* 4: 2113–18
51. Kabsch, W., Mannherz, H. G., Suck, D., Pai, E. F., Holmes, K. C. 1990. *Nature* 347: 37–44
52. Kabsch, W., Sander, C. 1983. *Biopolymers* 22: 2577–2637
53. Kakunaga, T., Leavitt, J., Hamada, H., Hirakawa, T. 1983. In *Genes and Proteins in Oncogenesis*, pp. 351–67. New York: Academic
54. Kean, A. M., Trayer, I. P., Levine, B. A., Zeugner, C., Ruegg, J. C. 1990. *Nature* 344: 265–68
55. Korn, E. D. 1978. *Proc. Natl. Acad. Sci. USA* 75: 588–99
56. Korn, E. D. 1982. *Physiol. Rev.* 62: 672–737
57. Korn, E. D., Hammer, J. A. 1988. *Annu. Rev. Biophys. Biophys. Chem.* 17: 23–45
58. Kwiatkowski, D. J., Stossel, T. P., Orkin, S. H., Mole, J. E., Harvey, R. C., et al. 1986. *Nature* 323: 455–58
59. Lassing, I., Lindberg, U. 1985. *Nature* 314: 472–74
60. Lassing, I., Lindberg, U. 1988. *J. Cell. Biochem.* 37: 255–67
61. Lazarides, E., Lindberg, U. 1974. *Proc. Natl. Acad. Sci. USA* 71: 4742–46
62. Lazarides, E., Weber, K. 1974. *Proc. Natl. Acad. Sci. USA* 71: 2268–72
63. Lindberg, U. 1966. *J. Biol. Chem.* 241: 1246–48
64. Liu, D. F., Wang, D., Stracher, A. 1990. *Biochem. J.* 266: 453–59
65. Magnus, K. A., Lattman, E. E., Sato, M., Pollard, T. D. 1986. *J. Biol. Chem.* 261: 13360–61
66. Mannherz, H. G., Barrington-Leigh, J., Leberman, R., Pfrang, H. 1975. *FEBS Lett.* 60: 34–38
67. Mannherz, H. G., Kabsch, W., Leberman, R. 1977. *FEBS Lett.* 73: 141–43
68. Marston, S., Lehman, W., Moody, C., Pritchard, K., Smith, C. 1988. *Calcium and Calcium Binding Proteins*, ed. C. Gerdy, R. Gilles, L. Bolis, pp. 69–81. Heidelberg: Springer Verlag
69. Matsuzaki, F., Matsumoto, S., Yahara, I., Yonezawa, N., Nishida, E., Sakai, H. 1988. *J. Biol. Chem.* 263: 11564–68
70. Meza, I., Sabanero, M., Cazares, F., Bryan, J. 1983. *J. Biol. Chem.* 258: 3936–41

71. Milligan, R. A., Flicker, P. F. 1987. *J. Cell Biol.* 105: 29–39
72. Milligan, R. A., Whittaker, M., Safer, D. 1990. *Nature* 348: 217–21
73. Millonig, R., Sutterlin, R., Engel, A., Pollard, T. D., Aebi, U. 1989. The "lateral slipping" model of F-actin filaments. In *Cytoskeletal and Extracellular Proteins, Springer Series in Biophysics*, ed. U. Aebi, A. Engel, 3: 51–53. Berlin: Springer-Verlag
74. Mimura, N., Asano, A. 1987. *J. Biol. Chem.* 262: 4717–23
75. Moir, A., Levine, B. 1986. *J. Inorg. Biochem.* 27: 1–8
76. Moore, P. B., Huxley, H. E., DeRosier, D. 1970. *J. Mol. Biol.* 50: 279–95
77. Moriyama, K., Nishida, E., Yonezawa, N., Sakai, H., Matsumoto, S., et al. 1990. *J. Biol. Chem.* 265: 5768–73
78. Deleted in proof
79. Mornet, D., Bonet, A., Audemard, E., Bonicel, J. 1989. *J. Muscle Res. Cell Motil.* 10: 10–24
80. Mossakowska, M., Strzelecka-Golaszewska, H. 1985. *Eur. J. Biochem.* 153: 373–81
81. Noegel, A. A., Schleicher, M. 1991. *Curr. Opin. Cell Biol.* 3: 18–26
82. O'Brien, E. J., Couch, J., Johnson, G. R. P., Morris, E. P. 1983. In *Actin: Its Structure and Function in Muscle and Non-Muscle Cells*, ed. dos Remedios, Barden, pp. 3–16. London: Academic
83. Oefner, C., Suck, D. 1986. *J. Mol. Biol.* 192: 605–32
84. Ohtaki, T., Tsukita, S., Mimura, N., Tsukita, S., Asano, A. 1985. *Eur. J. Biochem.* 153: 609–20
85. Oriol, C., Dubord, C., Landon, F. 1977. *FEBS Lett.* 73: 89–91
86. Parry, D. A. D., Squire, J. M. 1973. *J. Mol. Biol.* 75: 33–55
87. Phillips, G. N., Fillers, J. P., Cohen, C. 1986. *J. Mol. Biol.* 192: 111–31
88. Pollard, T. D. 1990. *Curr. Opin. Cell Biol.* 2: 33–40
89. Pollard, T. D., Cooper, J. A. 1986. *Annu. Rev. Biochem.* 55: 987–1035
90. Pope, B., Way, M., Weeds, A. C. 1991. *FEBS Lett.* 280: 70–74
91. Popp, D., Lednev, V. V., Jahn, W. 1987. *J. Mol. Biol.* 197: 679–84
92. Prendergast, G. C., Ziff, E. B. 1991. *EMBO J.* 10: 757–66
93. Rayment, I., Winkelmann, D. A. 1984. *Proc. Natl. Acad. Sci. USA* 81: 4378–80
94. Safer, D., Elzinga, M., Nachmias, V. T. 1991. *J. Biol. Chem.* 266: 4029–52
95. Sakurai, T., Kurokawa, H., Nonomura, Y. 1991. *J. Biol. Chem.* 266: 4581–85
96. Schutt, C. E., Lindberg, U., Myslik, J., Strauss, N. 1989. *J. Mol. Biol.* 209: 735–46
97. Selve, N., Wegner, A. 1986. *J. Mol. Biol.* 187: 627–31
98. Squire, J. 1981. *The Structural Basis of Muscular Contraction.* New York: Plenum
99. Steitz, T. A., Shoham, M., Bennett, W. S. 1981. *Philos. Trans. R. Soc. London Ser. B* 293: 43–52
100. Stewart, M., McLachlan, A. D. 1975. *Nature* 257: 331–33
101. Stokes, D. L., DeRosier, D. J. 1987. *J. Cell Biol.* 104: 1005–17
102. Stossel, T. P., Chaponnier, C., Ezzell, R. M., Hartwig, J. H., Janmey, P. A., et al. 1985. *Annu. Rev. Cell Biol.* 1: 353–402
103. Straub, F. B. 1942. *Stud. Univ. Szeged* 2: 3–15
104. Suck, D., Kabsch, W., Mannherz, H. G. 1981. *Proc. Natl. Acad. Sci. USA* 78: 4319–23
105. Suck, D., Oefner, C., Kabsch, W. 1984. *EMBO J.* 3: 2423–30
106. Sugino, H., Sakabe, N., Sakabe, K., Hatano, S., Oosawa, F., et al. 1979. *J. Biochem.* 86: 257–60
107. Sutoh, K. 1982. *Biochemistry* 21: 3654–61
108. Sutoh, K., Yin, H. L. 1989. *Biochemistry* 28: 5269–75
109. Szent-Gyorgyi, A. 1951. In *Chemistry of Muscular Contraction*, p. 10. New York: Academic. 2nd ed.
110. Szilagyi, L., Lu, R. C. 1982. *Biochim. Biophys. Acta* 709: 204–11
111. Szpacenko, A., Dabrowska, R. 1986. *FEBS Lett.* 202: 182–86
112. Tellam, R. L., Morton, D. J., Clarke, F. M. 1989. *TIBS* 14: 130–33
113. Theriot, J. A., Mitchison, T. J. 1991. *Nature* 352: 126–31
114. Trinick, J., Cooper, J., Seymour, J., Egelman, E. H. 1986. *J. Microsc.* 141: 349–60
115. Valentin-Ranc, C., Carlier, M.-F. 1989. *J. Biol. Chem.* 264: 20871–80
116. Vancompernolle, K., Bubb, M. R., Vandekerckhove, J., Korn, E. D. 1991. *J. Biol. Chem.* 266: 15427–31
117. Vandekerckhove, J. 1990. *Curr. Opin. Cell Biol.* 2: 41–50
118. Vandekerckhove, J. S., Kaiser, D. A., Pollard, T. D. 1989. *J. Cell Biol.* 109: 619–26
119. Vandekerckhove, J., Leavitt, J., Kakunaga, T., Weber, K. 1980. *Cell* 22: 893–99
120. Vandekerckhove, J., Weber, K. 1978. *Eur. J. Biochem.* 90: 451–62

121. Vandekerckhove, J., Weber, K. 1978. *J. Mol. Biol.* 126: 783–802
122. Vandekerckhove, J., Weber, K. 1979. *Differentiation* 14: 123–33
123. Vandekerckhove, J., Weber, K. 1984. *J. Mol. Biol.* 179: 391–413
124. Velaz, L., Hemric, M. E., Benson, C. E., Chalovich, J. M. 1989. *J. Biol. Chem.* 264: 9602–10
125. Wang, C.-L., Wang, L. W. C., Xu, S., Lu, R. C., Saavedra-Alanis, V., Bryan, J. 1991. *J. Biol. Chem.* 266: 9166–72
126. Warrick, H. M., Spudich, J. A. 1987. *Annu. Rev. Cell Biol.* 3: 379–421
127. Way, M., Gooch, J., Pope, B., Weeds, A. G. 1989. *J. Cell Biol.* 109: 593–605
128. Way, M., Pope, B., Gooch, J., Hawkins, M., Weeds, A. C. 1990. *EMBO J.* 9: 4103–9
129. Way, M., Weeds, A. G. 1988. *J. Mol. Biol.* 203: 1127–33
130. Weeds, A. 1982. *Nature* 296: 811–15
131. Yamamoto, K. 1989. *Biochemistry* 28: 5573–77
132. Yonezawa, N., Nishida, E., Iida, K., Kumagai, H., Yahara, I., Sakai, H. 1991. *J. Biol. Chem.* 266: 10485–89
133. Yu, F.-X., Johnston, P. A., Sudhof, T. C., Yin, H. L. 1990. *Science* 250: 1413–15

Annu. Rev. Biophys. Biomol. Struct. 1992. 21:77–93

APPROACHING ATOMIC RESOLUTION IN CRYSTALLOGRAPHY OF RIBOSOMES

Ada Yonath

Department of Structural Biology, Weizmann Institute, Rehovot, Israel, and Max-Planck-Research-Unit for Ribosomal Structure, Hamburg, Germany

KEY WORDS: image reconstruction, neutron diffraction, organo-metallic clusters, undecagold cluster, cryobiocrystallography

CONTENTS

77

1056–8700/92/0610–0077$02.00

PERSPECTIVES AND OVERVIEW

The translation of the genetic code into proteins is facilitated by a universal cellular organelle, the ribosome. The fundamental significance of the ribosome triggered intensive studies that led to important advancements: the determination of the primary sequences of many ribosomal components; sound propositions for the secondary structures of the rRNA chains; suggestions for spatial proximities between several ribosomal components; an insight into aspects in evolution; elaborate genetic manipulations; approximations of the size and the shape of the ribosome; and a fairly detailed description of the overall process of protein biosynthesis. At the same time these studies showed that a reliable molecular model of the ribosome is a prerequisite for the determination of the mechanism of protein biosynthesis.

The ribosome is an assembly of proteins and RNA chains. A typical bacterial ribosome contains some 56 different proteins and three RNA chains weighing a total of 2.3 million daltons. This assembly is unstable, flexible, and possesses no internal symmetry, and therefore is considered a rather complicated object for crystallographic analysis. Even its crystallization was believed to be a formidable task. However, natural in vivo organizations of eukaryotic ribosomes in periodic structures were detected in organisms exposed to stressful conditions, such as suboptimal temperatures, wrong diet, or lack of oxygen (for review see 42). The existence of these ordered formations stimulated extensive attempts to grow three-dimensional crystals of prokaryotic ribosomes. These were chosen because they are well characterized biochemically and may provide systems for in vitro crystallization, independent of in vivo events, environmental influences, and physiological factors that might be difficult or impossible to control and to reproduce.

As a result, natural and mutated 70S ribosomes and their small (30S) and large (50S) subunits were crystallized. Quality crystals were also obtained from chemically modified (with heavy atom clusters) particles and from complexes, which mimicked defined functional states in protein biosynthesis (Table 1). To facilitate subsequent crystallographic analysis, novel procedures for data collection and for derivatization have been established and low resolution images have been reconstructed.

This chapter describes the initial, intermediate, and current states of the structural studies of ribosomes. The crystallographic work with both X-rays and neutrons is addressed and the results obtained through image reconstructions from ordered arrays are compared with those derived from investigations of single particles. The review highlights the influence of structural results on subsequent functional studies and the contribu-

Table 1   Characterized three-dimensional crystals of ribosomal particles

Source[a]	Grown form	Cell dimensions (Å)	Resolution (Å)[b]
70S T.t.	MPD[c]	524 × 524 × 306; P4₁2₁2	approx. 20
70S T.t. +			
m-RNA & t-RNA[d]	MPD	524 × 524 × 306; P4₁2₁2	approx. 15
30S T.t.	MPD	407 × 407 × 170; P42₁2	7.3
50S H.m.	PEG[c]	210 × 300 × 581; C222₁	3.0
50S T.t.	AS[c]	495 × 495 × 196; P4₁2₁2	8.7
50S B.st.[e]	A[c]	360 × 680 × 920; P2₁2₁2	approx. 18
50S B.st.[e,f]	PEG	308 × 562 × 395; 114°; C2	approx. 11

  [a] B.st., *Bacillus stearothermophilus*; T.t., *Thermus thermophilus*; H.m., *Haloarcula marismortui*.
  [b] Represents the highest resolution for which sharp diffraction spots could be consistently observed. In many instances, we could not collect useful crystallographic data to this resolution.
  [c] MPD, PEG, A, AS = crystals grown by vapor diffusion in hanging drops from solutions containing methyl-pentane-diol (MPD), polyethyleneglycol (PEG), ammonium sulphate (AS), or low molecular weight alcohols (A).
  [d] A complex including 70S ribosomes, two equivalents of PhetRNA^Phe and an oligomer of 35 ± 5 uridines, serving as mRNA.
  [e] Same form and parameters for crystals of large ribosomal subunits of a mutant (missing protein BL11) of the same source and for modified particles with an undecagold-cluster.
  [f] Same form and parameters for crystals of a complex of 50S subunits, one tRNA molecule and a segment (18–20 mers) of a nascent polypeptide chain.

tion of biochemical experiments to the progress of the crystallographic work.

THE INITIAL STAGES: OBTAINING CRYSTALS

Choosing Halophilic and Thermophilic Prokaryotic Ribosomes

The key for obtaining diffracting crystals was the choice of the appropriate organism. The initial targets for crystallization were the ribosomes from *Escherichia coli* as they are fully characterized biochemically. Because these ribosomes are rather sensitive and unstable, only small two-dimensional arrays (24) or micro three-dimensional crystals (41) could be grown from them. Consequent extensive screening efforts showed that the most suitable sources for crystallizable ribosomes are extreme halophilic and thermophilic bacteria, probably because these ribosomes are rather stable.

The 50S subunits of the moderate thermophile, *Bacillus stearothermophilus*, were the first ribosomal particles to be crystallized (47). Although the initially grown micro-crystals were not suitable for crystallographic analysis, they played a crucial role in the progress of ribosomal crystallography because their diffraction patterns contained features to 3.5-Å resolution, with spacings compatible with those obtained from gels of prokaryotic ribosomes (20). Seven crystal forms of 50S subunits, one of 30S subunits, and one of whole 70S ribosomes were grown from these bacteria under a variety of conditions (43). Among them, the two forms suitable for medium-resolution studies (Table 1) (30) may provide unique information, because they could be specifically derivatized, using mutagenesis, with a multi heavy-atom cluster (see below) (39).

The ribosomes of the archaebacterium, *Haloarcula marismortui* (previously called *Halobacterium marismortui* or *Halobacterium* of the Dead Sea), maintain their integrity, stability, and biological functioning under high salt concentrations, conditions that usually cause denaturation of proteins and dissociation of protein assemblies with nucleic acids. Therefore these ribosomes provide a system suitable for crystallization under most favorable conditions. Furthermore, the determination of their structure should not only illuminate the process of protein biosynthesis, but also may reveal some factors governing the formation of assemblies of nucleic acid with protein. Five crystal forms of 50S subunits and one of the 30S subunits from this bacterium were grown; one of them diffracts to the highest resolution obtained so far, 3 Å (Figure 1, Table 1) (26, 37a).

The ribosomes of the extreme thermophile *Thermus thermophilus* are currently being characterized biochemically in several laboratories because of the growing interest in thermal stability of biological macromolecules. The 70S ribosomes of this bacterium were crystallized in two similar, however not identical, forms (35, 36, 43). Diffracting crystals were also obtained from 30S (44) and 50S subunits (37) as well as from complexes of 70S ribosomes with mRNA and tRNA (14). Thus, structural analysis of the crystalline ribosomal particles from this bacterium (Table 1) should provide information concerning conformational changes correlated with selected steps in the process of protein biosynthesis.

Several common properties have been observed in crystallization of prokaryotic ribosomal particles, regardless of their source. Functional activity is a prerequisite for crystal growth, but not every active preparation yields high quality crystals. Thus, it seems that the requirements for crystallization are more severe than those for biological activity, and extreme care in growing the cells and in the preparation of the ribosomes is necessary for obtaining crystallizable particles. It was found that the basic factors governing the quality of crystals are related more to the quality of the ribosomal particles than to choice of the crystallizing agent (49); however, the exact conditions for the growth of quality crystals must still be refined for each preparation. In all cases, the crystallized material retains its integrity and biological activity for long periods, in contrast to the short lifetime of isolated ribosomes.

Several Aspects of Nucleation and Crystal Growth

As ribosomes are large enough to be seen using electron microscopy, some steps in the nucleation and in the growth of ribosome crystals could be directly observed (45). It was observed that under proper crystallization conditions, the process of crystal growth starts within the first few hours by nonspecific aggregation, which is likely to inhibit the natural tendency of ribosomes to disintegrate. These amorphous aggregates undergo rearrangements toward the formation of nuclei of different morphologies, including star-shaped crystallites and various helical arrangements. These organizations may explain the extreme sensitivity of the crystallization process to small changes in external conditions and the commonly observed high mosaicity. Thus, it is not surprising that several different crystal forms were developed under similar conditions, and that small variations in the growth media introduced large differences in the crystallographic constants (e.g. the presence of 0.2 M KCl caused a change of 65 Å in the length of one axis of the crystals of 70S ribosomes from *T. thermophilous*) (36, 43).

In general, Mg^{2+} plays an essential role in maintaining the integrity of ribosomes. Our studies showed that it is also most crucial for their crystallization. For example, in spontaneous crystallization of several crystal types, the lower the Mg^{2+} concentration is, the thicker the crystals are. Interestingly, the upper critical value of Mg^{2+} permitted for the growth of three-dimensional crystals of 50S from *B. stearothermophilus* is the lowest needed for obtaining two-dimensional arrays (1).

The optimal conditions for the crystallization of halophilic ribosomes were established according to the complementary effects of mono and divalent ions. Mild variations in the delicate equilibrium of these ions enabled the development of a sophisticated seeding procedure (26, 49). Subsequent studies led to the establishment of a procedure that allows the crystallization of the halophilic ribosomes at the lowest concentrations of salts essential to maintain their integrity and the collection of diffraction data from crystals soaked in solutions mimicking their physiological environment.

Minute quantities of additives, such as metal ions with a high coordination of organic materials with a low surface tension, dramatically influenced the appearance or the quality or the morphology of several crystal types, in accord with observations obtained for isolated proteins (28). In particular, the addition of 1 mM Cd^{2+} to the growth media of 50S subunits from *H. marismortui* resulted in crystals diffracting to 3-Å resolution, with reasonable mosaicity and superb mechanical stability (37a).

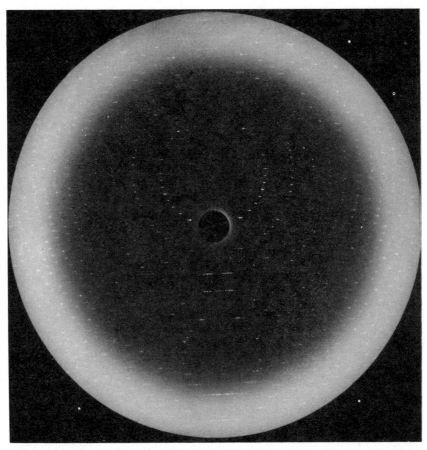

Figure 1   Rotation photograph of a crystal of 50S ribosomal subunits from *H. marismortui* grown by vapor diffusion in Linbro dishes coupled with individual seeding at 19°C from 6–8 µl of: 5 mg/ml 50S subunits, 1.2 M potassium chloride, 0.5 M ammonium chloride, 0.005 M magnesium chloride, 0.001 M cadmium chloride, and 5–6% polyethyleneglycol (6000), at pH 5.6 equilibrated with 1 ml reservoir of 1.7 M KCl and all the other components of the drop. The crystal was kept in 3 M potassium chloride, 0.5 M ammonium chloride, 0.005 M magnesium chloride, 0.001 M cadmium chloride, and 8% polyethyleneglycol (6000) at pH 5.6. Before cooling, it was soaked for 15 minutes in a solution containing the above storage components and 18% ethyleneglycol. The pattern was obtained at 90 K at Station F1/CHESS, operating at about 5.3 Gev and 50–80 mA. The crystal to film distance was 220 mm, the diameter of the collimator = 0.1 mm; wave length = 0.9091 Å.

INTERMEDIATE RESULTS: RECONSTRUCTED MODELS AT LOW RESOLUTION

Electron Microscopy of Sectioned Three-Dimensional Crystals

Some of the naturally occurring eukaryotic periodic organizations (see Perspectives and Overview) enabled image reconstruction studies that yielded low resolution information about the interactions between the particles, the outer contour of the ribosome, and the inner distribution of its components (for review, see 42). Similar procedures were employed for the analysis of the initially obtained three-dimensional crystals from prokaryotic sources. These were too small for X-ray or neutron crystallography, but too thick for direct investigation using electron microscopy. Therefore, positively stained thin sections of cross-linked and embedded crystals were investigated. Such analysis is limited by the inherent lower resolution induced by the embedding process, by the uncertainty regarding the exact sectioning direction, and by the unknown factors governing the stain distribution within the particle. However, despite these shortcomings, useful information could be extracted concerning the packing of the crystals of the 70S ribosome from *E. coli* (41) and the stain-distribution within the 50S subunits from *B. stearothermophilus*. The latter was obtained through three-dimensional reconstructions using four different crystal forms at a very low resolution, 60–90 Å. The resulting models, built of two domains of unevenly distributed density (25), were strikingly similar to models obtained a few years later at significantly higher resolution, 28 Å, from two-dimensional arrays (Figure 2) grown under different crystallization conditions and exposed to radically different experimental treatments (46).

Image Reconstruction from Two-Dimensional Arrays

Investigations of negatively stained isolated ribosomes using electron microscopy, coupled with immunology, performed in many laboratories, led to the estimation of the sizes and the shapes of the ribosomal particles and to suggestions for possible locations of several ribosomal components (for review, see 15, 17). Two-dimensional ordered arrays differ fundamentally from single particles in their suitability for image reconstruction in three dimensions. Based on diffraction data, rather than on averaging of selected particles, the reconstruction is inherently more objective. In addition, the particles in the two-dimensional arrays are held by lattice forces, which may reduce structural deformations caused by the contacts of the particles with the flat microscopical grids.

The growth of the first two-dimensional arrays of bacterial ribosomal particles was reported over a decade ago (24). A few years later these

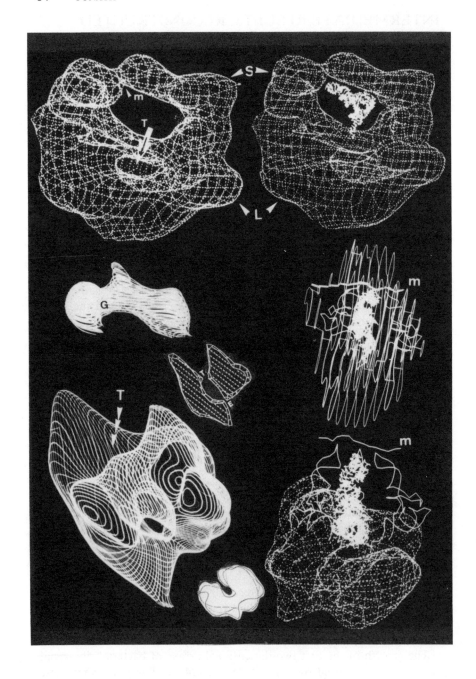

alcohol-grown arrays of ribosomal subunits from *E. coli* reached a size marginally suitable for image reconstruction (8, 31). The initial two-dimensional arrays of 50S subunits from *B. stearothermophilus* were also obtained from alcohols by employing essentially the same crystallization conditions used for the growth of three-dimensional crystals of these particles (47) while increasing the relative Mg^{2+} concentrations (1). The second-generation arrays, obtained a few years later, were grown within less than 1 min, directly on electron microscopy grids using salt-alcohol mixtures. Tilt series of two-dimensional arrays of 70S ribosomes and 50S subunits of *B. stearothermophilus*, negatively stained with gold thioglucose, led to reconstructed images at 47 and 28 Å, respectively (Figure 2) (2, 46). These showed several key features, associated mainly with internal vacant spaces or partially filled hollows, that were not detected earlier. The significant similarities in the overall shapes and in several specific features of corresponding regions in several reconstructed models allowed the assessment of their reliability, the location of the 50S subunit within the 70S ribosome, the extraction of an approximate model for associated 30S subunits, and the tentative assignment of biological functions to several structural features (Figure 2) (43, 50). However, an accurate determination of the shape and the size of the ribosome, as well as a detailed assignment of its functional sites, still awaits higher resolution data.

Figure 2 Computer-graphic displays of models obtained by three-dimensional reconstructions of 70S ribosomes (at 47-Å resolution) and 50S ribosomal subunits (at 28-Å resolution) of *B. stearothermophilus*, from tilt series of negatively stained (with gold-thioglucose) two-dimensional arrays, viewed using electron microcopy. S and L mark the small and the large subunits, respectively. T shows the entrance to the tunnel and E its exit. G marks the groove in the small subunit, presumed to be the path of m, the mRNA.

(*Top left*) The 70S ribosome, shown as a net.

(*Bottom left*) The 50S subunit, shown in fine lines. Inserts: (*upper right corner*) a slice of 20-Å thickness of this subunit; (*bottom right corner*) the reconstructed stain density from positively stained thin sections of three-dimensional micro crystals from the same source.

(*Middle left*) The shape of the 30S subunit as obtained by subtracting the density of the 50S subunit from that of the 70S ribosome.

(*Top right*) A tRNA molecule, positioned by model building in the intersubunit free space in the 70S ribosome (*top left*).

(*Middle right*) A perpendicular view of the model shown in top right. The ribosome is outlined by vertical lines. Fitted into the intersubunit space of the ribosome by model building are the backbones of a chain of 28 nucleotides in an arbitrary conformation, and of two molecules of tRNA. The third tRNA shown in the middle is highlighted by including all its atoms (as in top right).

(*Bottom right*) The 50S subunit in the same orientation as it is in the ribosome shown in the middle right panel, together with the components included by model building. The outline of the whole ribosome was removed for clarity.

POSSIBLE FUNCTIONAL RELEVANCES IN THE RECONSTRUCTED MODELS

Approximate Shapes of the Ribosomal Subunits Within the Assembled 70S Ribosome

Based on common structural elements, the reconstructed model of the isolated 50S subunit was fitted into that of the 70S ribosome. The overall agreement in the shapes of the reconstructed isolated 50S subunit and the part of the ribosome it was assigned to is quite striking. The few slight differences, detected mainly in two regions, one of which is close to the subunit interface, may reflect conformational changes occurring upon the association of the subunits, or resulting from the differences in the resolutions of the two reconstructions (5).

The approximate shape of the associated 30S subunit was deduced by subtracting the part assigned as the 50S subunit from the model of the whole ribosome (Figure 2). There is a significant similarity in the volumes and in the overall shapes of isolated (for review, see 15, 17) and bound 30S subunits, but the isolated particles appear somewhat wider than those extracted from the assembled ribosome. Flattening of isolated 30S particles on the microscopic grids may account for these differences. Such deformations are virtually eliminated in the two-dimensional arrays used for the reconstruction of the assembled ribosomes, because in these arrays, most of the contacts of the ribosomes with the electron microscopical grids are through the 50S subunits. Alternatively, the differences could result from conformational changes of the 30S subunits upon their incorporation into the ribosome.

Tentative Assignments for the Path of the Nascent Proteins and for the Site for the Biosynthetic Reaction

A prominent feature in the reconstructed models of both 70S ribosomes and 50S subunits is a tunnel spanning the 50S subunit of about 100 Å in length and up to 25 Å in diameter (Figure 2) (46). A tunnel within the large ribosomal subunit was predicted more than two decades ago, when it was shown that the ribosome masks the latest synthesized segments of nascent chains (27). This tunnel may be the path of the newly synthesized proteins because it leads from the intersubunit space, which was presumed to be the peptidyl transferase site (see below), to a location that may be compatible with that suggested as the site for the emerging nascent polypeptide by immuno electron microscopy experiments (4). A similar feature was also apparent in image-reconstructed 80S eukaryotic ribosomes (29) and in neutron diffraction maps of 50S subunits of *H. maris-mortui* (10). The current resolution does not permit an accurate determination of the diameter of the tunnel. However, the tunnel seems spacious enough to impose no restrictions to the sequence of the growing peptides and may accommodate amino acids to which bulky groups, such as biotin, have been bound (23). In recent immuno electron microscopy experiments, the N-termini of nascent chains were detected in two locations: one close to the subunit interface, where the end of short polypeptides were detected, and the second at the other end of the particle (34), where the N-termini of longer chains were found. Further studies indicated that ribosomes protect natural proteins more efficiently than artificial homopolymers (21) and that the latter may choose a path slightly different from that chosen by naturally occurring proteins (16).

Thus, it seems that the amino termini of natural proteins have a common feature that guides nascent chains into the tunnel. Homopolypeptides lacking this feature may miss the entrance to the tunnel. Thus, the differences in the migration of short and long chains of polyphenylalanine and polylysine (16) may be correlated with a mechanism in which newly formed peptides that hit the correct exit path continue to grow and migrate normally out of the ribosome, whereas those that miss the tunnel adhere to the surface of the ribosome and cause early termination of the biosynthetic pathway. This hypothesis may explain why only 40–60% of most ribosomal preparations are found to be active in the synthesis of relatively long polypeptides, although almost all well-prepared ribosomes bind mRNA and tRNA (14, 32). In fact under some conditions, short nascent homopolypeptides adhere to ribosomes of *E. coli* (13). Furthermore, complexes of short chains of polyphenylalanine or polylysine with 50S subunits from *B. stearothermophilus* and *H. marismortui* were crystallized (43).

The small and large ribosomal subunits are well separated in most reconstructions of whole ribosomes, regardless of the source of the ribosome, the staining material, and the computational treatments (2, 11, 29, 38, 50). An empty space, comprising about 20% of the volume of the ribosome, located at the interphase between the two ribosomal subunits was clearly resolved in reconstructed images of 70S ribosomes from *B. stearothermophilus* (Figure 2) (50). This space may provide the flexibility, dynamics, and the mobility needed for the process of protein biosynthesis. Volume calculations showed that it is large enough to accommodate up to three tRNA molecules together with other factors participating in this process. Therefore it was tentatively assigned as the site of protein biosynthesis.

Regions rich in rRNA were detected through preferential staining of the two-dimensional arrays, in several locations on the walls of the free space, one of them in the vicinity of a groove in the 30S subunit (50). In accord with biochemical evidence and modeling experiments (7), this groove was tentatively assigned as the path of the mRNA chain. In a model-building experiment, a molecule of tRNA was placed in the inter-subunit space with its anticodon close to the tentative mRNA binding site and its CCA-terminus positioned so that the peptidyl group could extend into the tunnel (Figure 2) (43, 50). In this orientation, the tRNA interacts at many sites with the walls of the intersubunit space. These interactions may account for noncognate affinity of the tRNA to the ribosome and provide a mechanism for communication between the path of the nascent chain and the decoding region.

Crystallizable Complexes Mimicking Defined Functional States

The characteristic low resolution of all crystals of whole ribosomes obtained so far may be related to the inherent conformational het-erogeneity of their preparations. Reassembled ribosomes from purified 50S and 30S subunits, which are expected to be fairly homogenous, yielded crystals containing solely the 50S subunits (14), showing that the inter-particle interactions in the crystals of the 50S subunits are stronger than the affinity between the large and small subunits in 70S particles kept for long periods without having the opportunity to participate in protein biosynthesis. This experiment highlights the readiness of the large riboso-mal subunits to crystallize, a property also reflected by the large number of crystal forms obtained from these particles (26, 30, 37, 37a, 42, 43, 47, 48). It also is in accord with observations made on two-dimensional arrays of 80S ribosomes, which showed that these arrays could be depleted of the small subunits and still maintain their packing integrity (22).

To minimize the flexibility of the ribosomes and to increase the hom-ogeneity of the crystallized material, complexes were prepared that mim-icked defined stages in protein biosynthesis. A model complex of 70S ribosomes from *T. thermophilus* with two equivalents of phetRNA^{phe} and a chain of about 35 uridyl residues was first crystallized. The repro-ducibility of the growth of crystals and their internal order dramatically improved (Table 1) (14). To assess the individual contributions of the different components to the stability of this complex, 70S ribosomes were cocrystallized together with a chain of 35 uridines. Only poorly shaped crystals were occasionally grown, indicating the larger contribution of the tRNA molecule to the stability of this system.

CURRENT CRYSTALLOGRAPHIC ANALYSIS

X-Ray Data Collection with Synchrotron Radiation at Cryotemperature

The diffracting power of crystalline ribosomal particles is so weak that synchrotron radiation is required for virtually all the crystallographic studies. At ambient temperatures, the radiation damage of the ribosomal crystals is so rapid that all reflections beyond approximately 15–18 Å decay within a few minutes, a period shorter than the time required to obtain a single useful X-ray pattern. This severe decay led to under-estimation of the real resolution, to occasional assignment of wrong unit cell constants, and to unsuccessful attempts to collect complete diffraction data sets. Only the pioneering introduction of a procedure for crys-tallography at cryogenic temperature enabled productive studies. Thus, shock-frozen, irradiated crystals measured surrounded by a nitrogen stream at about 90 K did not show radiation damage over long periods, enabling the collection of complete diffraction data sets from individual crystals (18).

All ribosomal crystals could be measured at cryotemperature, although a thorough search to establish individual freezing conditions for each crystal form was essential. This work revealed that the resolution limits and the mosaicity obtained at cryotemperatures from ribosomal crystals equaled those obtained at ambient temperature. However, as there is practically no time limit for irradiation at cryotemperature, the reflections with the highest resolution, which are usually the weakest, could be detected. Comparisons of diffraction data collected at intervals of 0.5, 2, and 153 days from the same crystal showed no significant differences in the intensities or in the cell parameters.

Attempts at Phasing

Fourier summation, the operation leading from diffraction patterns to electron density maps, requires information about the direction, ampli-tude, and phase of each reflection. The directions and amplitudes can be measured, whereas the phases have to be determined indirectly. The most common method for extracting phases in crystallography of macro-molecules is multiple isomorphous replacement (MIR). This method involves the introduction of electron-dense atoms to the crystalline lattice at distinct locations, causing measurable changes in the diffraction pattern, while keeping the crystal isomorphous with that of the native molecule. For proteins of average size, useful isomorphous derivatives are obtained using one or a few heavy-metal atoms. Because of the large size of the ribosome, compact clusters of a proportionally larger number of heavy atoms should be used for its derivatization.

To maximize the extent of derivatization, sophisticated synthetic procedures were developed. An undecagold cluster, consisting of a compact core of eleven gold atoms linked directly to one another (19), was prepared as a monofunctional reagent, specific for sulfhydryl groups (39). As the core of the undecagold cluster is about 8.2 Å in diameter, it can be treated as a single scatterer at low to medium resolution. At this resolution, the structural ambiguities in the location of the reactive moiety on the cluster are negligible. To enhance the accessibility of this bulky cluster, its functional arm was extended with aliphatic chains of varying lengths. A spacer of about 10 Å was needed for efficient binding of the cluster to ribosomal particles, isolated ribosomal components, or modified tRNA molecules. The yield and the specificity of cluster binding to the ribosomal particles was optimized by minimizing the number of exposed sulfhydryl moieties. In this way, the 70S ribosome and the 30S subunits of *T. thermophilus* (43) were fully derivatized without impairing their integrity and their ability to crystallize.

However, direct binding of the cluster to intact ribosomal particles cannot be fully controlled. Therefore, whenever applicable, the cluster was bound to free sulfhydryl moieties of isolated ribosomal components. These were, in turn, reconstituted into core particles. In this way, modified 50S subunits were formed by the binding of the gold cluster to isolated protein BL11 and the incorporation of the cluster-bound protein into cores of mutated ribosomes from *B. stearothermophilus* lacking this protein (39). X-ray diffraction data, of a quality comparable to that of native crystals, were collected from crystals of the modified particles, and the resulting difference Patterson maps included features that could be interpreted as the bound cluster.

Selected proteins can be removed quantitatively from eubacterial ribosomes through mutagenesis (9) or stepwise addition of salts (3). The significant resistance of the halophilic ribosomes to mutations dictates almost exclusively in vitro selective detachment of ribosomal proteins, but at the same time, the high salinity required for the integrity of halophilic ribosomes does not allow substantial alterations. However, treatment with dioxane enabled quantitative removal of several proteins from ribosomes of *H. marismortui*, all of which could be reconstituted quantitatively into core particle. One of the removed proteins, HL11, quantitatively binds reagents specific to sulfhydryls. However, in contrast to protein BL11 from *B. stearothermophilus*, which was reconstituted into core particles even when a group as large as the gold cluster was bound to it, the modified halophilic protein HL11 reconstitutes only when its sulfhydryl group is free. Even binding of small organic compounds to the sulfhydryl of the isolated protein prevented its association with core particles. Using this property, we could prepare halophilic 50S core particles quantitatively depleted of protein HL11. These were crystallized under the same conditions as that used for native 50S subunits, indicating that the removal of this protein did not cause conformational changes of the 50S subunit.

Obvious carriers for indirect derivatization are tRNA and mRNA. Conditions for stoichiometric binding of tRNA to several ribosomal particles were determined, and complexes that contain tRNA molecules have been crystallized (12, 14, 43). For the derivatization of these complexes, the gold cluster was chemically attached to the X base (at position 47) of tRNAphe from *E. coli*. The modified tRNA molecule could be charged with its cognate amino acid and attached to 70S ribosomes and to 30S ribosomal subunits, in the presence or absence of mRNA, under the same conditions and with the same stoichiometry as native tRNA (S. Weinstein, F. Franceschi, C. Glotz, T. Boeck, M. Laschever & A. Yonath, unpublished data).

A different approach for phasing at low resolution is the use of the reconstructed models in several variations of the molecular replacement method. These procedures are based on the positioning of approximate models of the studied object in the crystallographic unit cells. Such attempts may yield valuable intermediate information concerning mainly the packing of the crystals. To facilitate these studies, crystallographic data for 70S ribosomes from *T. thermophilus* and for 50S subunits from *H. marismortui* and *T. thermophilus* were used together with the models of these particles from *B. stearothermophilus* (see Intermediate Results, above), assuming that prokaryotic ribosomes are of similar structures at low resolution.

Parallel studies have been performed using single crystal neutron diffraction accompanied by contrast variation. This method has already provided useful phasing information, as well as hints about the internal distribution of different components for large cellular assemblies (e.g. 33; reviewed in 10). Neutron diffraction data to 30-Å resolution were collected from crystals of 50S ribosomal subunits from *H. marismortui*. Phased using direct methods, these data led to a relatively clean map, which contained several compact features with a shape similar to that obtained by image reconstruction of the large subunit from *B. stearothermophilus* (10).

CONCLUDING REMARKS

This article demonstrates that crystallographic studies on intact ribosomal particles are feasible, despite the facts that a straightforward application of conventional macromolecular crystallographic techniques was not adequate and considerable effort had to be invested in developing conceptual and experimental procedures. Of special significance are the development of innovative procedures for crystallization and seeding, the introduction of cryotemperature techniques, and the sophisticated extension of existing evaluation techniques. Also, the combination of metalo-organic biochemistry, genetic manipulations, and functional studies enabled specific labeling of the crystals of the ribosomal particles and of their complexes, without introducing major changes in their crystallizability, integrity, or biological activity. In addition, the interplay with other diffraction methods, such as neutron crystallography and three-dimensional image reconstructions from two-dimensional arrays investigated using electron microscopy led to the elucidation of medium-resolution models, to the tentative assignments of several functional sites, and to the design of subsequent functional and structural experiments.

ACKNOWLEDGMENTS

All stages of the studies presented here were carried out in active collaboration under the inspiration and guidance of the late Prof. H. G. Wittmann. This work was performed at the Weizmann Institute of Science in Israel, the Max-Planck-Research-Unit at DESY in Hamburg, the Max-Planck-Institute for Molecular Genetics in Berlin, the EMBL Laboratory in Heidelberg, the ILL neutron diffraction facility in Grenoble, and the following synchrotron facilities: EMBL/DESY, Hamburg; CHESS, Cornell University; SSRL, Stanford University; SRS, Daresbury, UK; and KEK, Japan. Support was provided by the National Institute of Health (NIH GM 34360), the Federal Ministry for Research and Technology (BMFT 05 180 MP BO), the USA-Israel Binational Foundation (BSF 85-00381), the France-Israel Binational Foundation (NCRD-334190), the Kimmelman Center for Macromolecular Assembly at the Weizmann Institute, and the Minerva and Heinemann Foundations (4694 81). The author holds the Martin S. Kimmel Professorial chair.

Literature Cited

1. Arad, T., Leonard, K. R., Wittmann, H. G., Yonath, A. 1984. *EMBO J.* 3: 127
2. Arad, T., Piefke, J., Weinstein, S., Gewitz, H. S., Yonath, A., Wittmann, H. G. 1988. *Biochimie* 69: 1001
3. Atsmon, A., Spitnik-Elson, P., Elson, D. 1969. *J. Mol. Biol.* 45: 125
4. Barnebeu, C., Lake, J. A. 1982. *Proc. Natl. Acad. Sci. USA* 79: 3111
5. Berkovitch-Yellin, Z., Wittmann, H. G., Yonath, A. 1990. *Acta Crystallogr.* B46: 637
6. Deleted in proof
7. Brimacombe, R., Atmadja, J., Stiege, W., Schueler, D. 1988. *J. Mol. Biol.* 199: 115
8. Clark, W., Leonard, K., Lake, J. 1982. *Science* 216: 999
9. Dabbs, E. 1987. *Mol. Genet. Life Sci. Adv.* 6: 61

10. Eisenstein, M., Sharon, R., Berkovitch-Yellin, Z., Gewitz, H.-S., Weinstein, S., et al. 1991. *Biochemie* In press
11. Frank, J., Verschoor, A., Radamaacher, M., Wagenknecht, T. 1990. See Ref. 17, pp. 107
12. Gewitz, H. S., Glotz, C., Piefke, J., Yonath, A., Wittmann, H. G. 1988. *Biochimie* 70: 645
13. Gilbert, W. 1963. *Cold Spring Harbor Symp. Quant. Biol.* 28: 287
14. Hansen, H., Volkmann, N., Piefke, J., Glotz, C., Weinstein, S., et al. 1990. *Biochim. Biophys. Acta* 1050: 1
15. Hardesty, B., Kramer, G., eds. 1986. *Structure, Function and Genetics of Ribosomes.* Heidelberg/New York: Springer Verlag
16. Hardesty, B., Picking W. D., Odom O. W. 1990. *Biochim. Biophys. Acta* 1050: 197
17. Hill, E. W., Dahlberg, A., Garrett, R. A., Moore, P. B., Schlesinger, D., Warner, J. R., eds. 1990. *The Ribosomes: Structure, Function and Evolution.* Washington, DC: Am. Soc. Microbiol.
18. Hope, H., Frolow, F., von Böhlen, K., Makowski, I., Kratky, C., et al. 1989. *Acta Crystallogr.* B45: 190
19. Jahn, W. 1989. *Z. Naturforsch.* 44b: 1313
20. Klug, A., Holmes, K. C., Finch, J. T. 1961. *J. Mol. Biol.* 3: 87
21. Kolb V. A., Kommer A., Spirin A. S. 1990. *FEBS Workshop on Translation, Leiden,* p. 84a
22. Kuhlbrandt, W., Unwin, P. N. T. 1982. *J. Mol. Biol.* 156: 611
23. Kurzchalia, S. V., Wiedmann, M., Breter, H., Zimmermann, W., Bauschke, E., Rapoport, T. A. 1988. *Eur. J. Biochem.* 172: 663
24. Lake, J. 1980. In *Ribosomes Structure, Function and Genetics.* ed. G. Chambliss, G. R. Craven, J. Davies, K. Davies, J. Kahan, N. Nomura, p. 207. Baltimore: Univ. Park Press
25. Leonard, K. R., Arad, T., Tesche, B., Erdmann, V. A., Wittmann, H. G., Yonath, A. 1982. In *Electron Microscopy* 1982, 3: 9. Hamburg: Offizin Paul Hartung
26. Makowski, I., Frolow, F., Saper, M. A., Wittmann, H. G., Yonath, A. 1987. *J. Mol. Biol.* 193: 819
27. Malkin, L. I., Rich, A. 1967. *J. Mol. Biol.* 26: 329
28. McPhearson, A., Koszelak, S., Axelrod, H., Day, J., Williams, R. 1986. *J. Biol. Chem.* 261: 1969
29. Milligan, R. A., Unwin, P. N. T. 1986. *Nature* 319: 693
30. Müssig, J., Makowski, I., von Böhlen, K., Hansen, H., Bartels, K. S., et al. 1989. *J. Mol. Biol.* 205: 619
31. Oakes, M., Henderson, E., Scheiman, A., Clark, M., Lake, J. 1986. See Ref. 15, pp. 47–67
32. Rheinberger, H.-J., Nierhaus, K. H. 1990. *Eur. J. Biochem.* 193: 643
33. Roth, M., Lewit-Bentley, A., Michel, H., Deisenhofer, J., Huber, R., Oesterheld, D. 1989. *Nature* 340: 659
34. Ryabova, L. A., Selivanova, O. M., Baranov, V. I., Vasiliev, V. D., Spirin, A. S. 1988. *FEBS Lett.* 226: 255
35. Trakhanov, S. D., Yusupov, M. M., Agalarov, S. C., Garber, M. B., Ryazantsev, S. N., et al. 1987. *FEBS Lett.* 220: 319
36. Trakhanov, S. D., Yusupov, M. M., Shirokov, V. A., Garber, M. B., Mitschler, A., et al. 1989. *J. Mol. Biol.* 209: 327
37. Volkmann, N., Hottentrager, S., Hansen, H., Zayzsev-Bashan, A., Sharon, R., et al. 1990. *J. Mol. Biol.* 216: 239
37a. von Böhlen, K., Makowski, I., Hansen, H. A. S., Bartels, H., Berkovitch-Yellin, Z., et al. 1991. *J. Mol. Biol.* In press
38. Wagenknecht, T., Carazo, J. M., Radermacher, M., Frank, J. 1989. *Biophys. J.* 55: 455
39. Weinstein, S., Jahn, W., Wittmann, H. G., Yonath, A. 1989. *J. Biol. Chem.* 264: 19138
40. Deleted in proof
41. Wittmann, H. G., Müssig, J., Gewitz, H. S., Piefke, J., Rheinberger, H. J., Yonath, A. 1982. *FEBS Lett.* 146: 217
42. Yonath, A. 1984. *TIBS* 9: 227
43. Yonath, A., Bennett, W., Weinstein, S., Wittmann, H. G. 1990. See Ref. 17, p. 134
44. Yonath, A., Glotz, C., Gewitz, H. S., Bartels, K., von Böhlen, K., et al. 1988. *J. Mol. Biol.* 203: 831
45. Yonath, A., Khavitch, G., Tesche, B., Müssig, J., Lorenz, S., et al. 1982. *Biochem. Int.* 5: 629
46. Yonath, A., Leonard, K. R., Wittmann, H. G. 1987. *Science* 236: 813
47. Yonath, A., Müssig, J., Tesche, B., Lorenz, S., Erdmann, V. A., Wittmann, H. G. 1980. *Biochem. Int.* 1: 428
48. Yonath, A., Saper, M. A., Makowski, I., Müssig, J., Piefke, J., et al. 1986. *J. Mol. Biol.* 187: 633
49. Yonath, A., Wittmann, H. G. 1988. *Methods Enzymol.* 164: 95
50. Yonath, A., Wittmann, H. G. 1989. *TIBS* 14: 329

Annu. Rev. Biophys. Biomol. Struct. 1992. 21:95–118

THE MECHANISM OF α-HELIX FORMATION BY PEPTIDES

J. Martin Scholtz and Robert L. Baldwin

Department of Biochemistry, Stanford University Medical School, Stanford, California 94305–5307

KEY WORDS: α-helix propensities, side-chain interactions in peptides, α-helix stability

CONTENTS

95

1056–8700/92/0610–0095$02.00

PERSPECTIVES AND SCOPE

The systematic study of helix formation by peptides of defined length and sequence is less than 10 years old. The field began with an effort to understand helix formation in water by an apparently exceptional short peptide, the 13-residue C-peptide from the N terminus of ribonuclease A (RNase A). At that time, other short peptides, with fewer than 20 residues, generally failed to show observable helix formation, and host-guest studies indicated that all short peptides should not show any measurable helix formation if they obey the same rules as random-sequence copolymers. One explanation for the contradiction was that the C-peptide helix might be stabilized by specific side-chain interactions because these should have little effect on helix stability in random sequence copolymers. Amino acid substitution experiments in C-peptide confirmed this explanation and demonstrated that specific side-chain interactions, such as ion-pair and charge-helix dipole interactions, can stabilize short helices in water.

Unexpectedly, however, substitution experiments sometimes revealed large changes in helicity, both in C-peptide and other peptide systems. Moreover, investigators found that they could design short peptide sequences that show good α-helix formation in water, first by using ion-pair interactions to stabilize the helix and later by making use of the unexpectedly strong helix-forming tendency of alanine. These results brought into question the accepted values of helix propensities of the different amino acids, and also raised questions about limitations on the validity of the Zimm-Bragg model of α-helix formation.

The field of peptide helix formation is now at an exciting but speculative stage. Many basic questions are unanswered, but the tools needed to answer these questions are now available. The long-range goal is to understand the mechanism of α-helix formation in water to help elucidate the mechanism of protein folding. A specific goal is to predict the helicity of any arbitrary peptide sequence and further to predict the pattern of helicity residue by residue.

The scope of our review is limited to studies of the past 10 years on α-helix formation in water by peptides of defined length and sequence. We summarize earlier work as background. Insistence on water as the solvent follows from the aim of elucidating the folding mechanisms of water-soluble proteins because they are unfolded by organic solvents. Peptides whose sequences are derived from proteins were the first systems studied. The direction of the field changed when it became possible to study helices formed by sequences of de novo design. This development allowed the isolation and analysis of individual factors in helix formation. Our review closes by considering the implications of peptide helix studies for the mechanism of protein folding.

HISTORY

A Thermodynamic Model of α-Helix Formation

In 1955, four years after Pauling and coworkers (56) proposed the α-helix as a basic structural motif in proteins, Schellman (68) estimated the stability of the α-helix in water, based on a model still debated today. His model preceded by a few years the 1959 paper by Kauzmann (29) on the hydrophobic interaction. The hydrophobic interaction does not appear in Schellman's model, which assumes that the α-helix is stabilized by the peptide hydrogen bond and destabilized by the loss in backbone conformational entropy. Thus, the free energy change per residue for helix formation was first separated into an enthalpy and an entropy term. In modern usage, *residue* means an α-carbon flanked on both sides by peptide linkages (see below):

$$\Delta G^\circ_{res} = \Delta H^\circ_{res} - T\Delta S^\circ_{res}. \qquad\qquad 1.$$

The term ΔH°_{res}, estimated to be -1.5 kcal/mol from data on the dimerization of urea in water (67), was identified with the enthalpy of peptide hydrogen-bond formation in water. The entropy change per residue for helix formation, ΔS°_{res}, was taken to be $-R\ln j$, where j is the number of equivalent torsional conformations of the peptide backbone, per residue, in the random coil form. If j is about 10, ΔS°_{res} is about -4.6 eu and $T\Delta S^\circ_{res}$ is about -1.4 kcal/mol at 25°C. Thus, Schellman (68) concluded that an isolated α-helix should be marginally stable in water.

His formulation of the problem showed the importance of answering the following questions. (*a*) What is the enthalpy of peptide hydrogen-bond formation in water, and what is the value of ΔH°_{res}? (*b*) What is the actual value of j, and how much do side chains contribute to ΔH°_{res}? (*c*) How does the hydrophobic interaction affect the values of ΔH°_{res} and ΔS°_{res}? Given the basic nature of this problem, it is surprising that firm answers to these questions were not obtained long ago. The difficulties resulted chiefly from using polypeptides to study helix formation in water. The use of short peptides with defined sequences allows one to bypass some of these difficulties.

The standard free energy change of forming a helix with n residues is a linear function of ΔH°_{res} and ΔS°_{res}, but it is not proportional to n. One of the two end effects (68) is taken into account by using the modern definition of a residue (see above). The ϕ,φ backbone angles are unconstrained by helix formation in each of the two end amino acids of an unblocked peptide. These two end amino acids are not, however, counted as residues unless the N and C termini have blocking groups that create two additional peptide units. The second end effect is that the first four NH groups of an unblocked peptide do not form hydrogen bonds in an α-helix, and neither do the four CO groups at the C terminus. Therefore, we must subtract an enthalpy term corresponding to four peptide hydrogen bonds, but the counting system is based on residues (n), not amino acids ($n+2$). The net result is that the term $2\Delta H^{\circ}_{res}$ needs to be subtracted. Thus, the standard free energy of helix formation by an unblocked peptide, using the modern definition of a residue, is:

$$\Delta G^{\circ}_{helix} = (n-2)\Delta H^{\circ}_{res} - nT\Delta S^{\circ}_{res} \qquad 2.$$

The end effects make formation of a short helix difficult and cause helix stability to depend strongly on chain length. Note that when acetyl and amide blocking groups are present at the N and C termini, they form peptide bonds, contribute two additional peptide units, and increase n, the number of residues, by 2.

Statistical Mechanical Models of α-Helix Formation

Several similar theories of α-helix formation based on statistical mechanics appeared in 1958 and afterwards, and Schellman's model was used to treat the problem with statistical thermodynamics (69). These theories are presented and discussed in the book by Poland & Scheraga (58); the textbook by Cantor & Schimmel (11) gives a clear introduction to the subject. In statistical mechanics treatments, helix formation is a two-step process: helix nucleation can occur at random locations, and helix propagation can take place only after a helical nucleus has been formed. Thus, the process of forming an α-helix is quite different from those biophysical processes that occur in a definite sequence of steps at defined sites, and with unique intermediates. Often with a short peptide, one cannot drive α-helix formation to completion in the conditions available. Because the only possible unique product is the complete helix, the products of the reaction comprise a broad distribution of partly helical molecules with frayed ends. This behavior is predicted by helix-coil theory and is confirmed by current experiments. One basic consequence is that the two-state model (random coil ⇌ complete helix) is normally a poor approximation to use in treating problems of α-helix formation.

Current practice is to report the parameters of the Zimm-Bragg theory (91, 92) even if another, similar, theory has been used to evaluate the experimental data. These parameters are σ, the helix nucleation parameter, and s, the helix propagation parameter. In the Zimm-Bragg theory, the first helical residue (i), which initiates a helix, is given statistical weight σs

and the second helical residue $(i+1)$ is given statistical weight s. The original Zimm-Bragg theory (92) defined the chain length as the number of peptide units that, in the notation used here, is $n+1$ for an unblocked peptide.

The basic assumption made in applying the Zimm-Bragg model to helix formation by a peptide containing different amino acids is that a single value of s can be used for each type of residue: each value of s is independent of neighboring amino acids and also of the amino acid's position in the helix. The nucleation parameter σ is usually thought to depend on the conformational properties of the peptide backbone in the random coil conformation; thus σ should have similar values for residues with similar ϕ,φ maps (excluding glycine and proline). The intrinsic helix-forming tendency of a residue, or its helix propensity, is assumed to be measured by its value of s, the helix propagation parameter.

The assumption that s is independent of neighboring amino acids is an oversimplification for charged amino acids, which form specific ion-pair interactions with each other and which interact nonspecifically through coulombic interactions. Likewise, the s value of a charged residue depends on its position in the helix through the charge-helix dipole interaction. Several workers have studied the problem of taking account of specific charge interactions while retaining the Zimm-Bragg formalism, which is reviewed briefly below. Nonspecific interactions of an uncharged residue with neighboring side chains may also be significant: this problem is being studied (S. Padmanabhan & R. L. Baldwin, unpublished data).

In the Lifson-Roig model (34) of α-helix formation, a residue is counted as helical or nonhelical according to its ϕ,φ values, in contrast to the Zimm-Bragg model in which it is helical if its peptide NH group is hydrogen bonded. Qian & Schellman (60) discuss the difference between the two models, and also current usage of terms such as residue, in a forthcoming article. The Lifson-Roig theory is particularly useful in studies of helix formation by short peptides because it gives positional information on helix formation: the helicity of each residue can be predicted, once values have been assigned to the nucleation (v) and propagation (w) parameters for each type of residue. Although the v and w parameters of the Lifson-Roig theory differ from the σ and s parameters of the Zimm-Bragg theory, σ and s may be computed readily from v and w by using relations derived by Qian & Schellman (60).

Tests of Helix-Coil Theory and Values for Parameters

In 1959, Zimm et al (93) tested the Zimm-Bragg theory by fitting the helix-coil transitions of a set of polypeptides with different average chain lengths

(26–1500 residues). The peptides were polymers of γ-benzyl-L-glutamate, which does not ionize, and the solvent system was a mixture of a helix-breaker, dichloroacetic acid, and a helix-former, ethylene dichloride. The thermal transition curves for the entire set of polypeptides were fitted satisfactorily by three parameters: σ (assumed independent of temperature), s (at 25°C), and ΔH° (assumed independent of temperature). The value they obtained for s was 2×10^{-4}.

The dependence of s on temperature is written as:

$$-RT\ln s = \Delta H^\circ - T\Delta S^\circ, \qquad\qquad 3.$$

where ΔH° and ΔS° are temperature independent. The enthalpy change ΔH° can be identified with ΔH°_{res} in Equation 1, which is measured using calorimetry. Later, the value of ΔH° found by Zimm et al (93) was confirmed using calorimetry (1). The transition curve of the infinite-chain polypeptide gives directly the temperature at which $s = 1$ as the temperature midpoint (T_m) of the unfolding transition, and the shape of the transition curve depends in a simple way on σ and ΔH°. The van't Hoff enthalpy change, ΔH°_{vH}, calculated for a two-state reaction (helix $\rightleftharpoons$ coil) of an infinite-chain polypeptide is given by (2):

$$\Delta H^\circ_{vH} = \Delta H^\circ / \sigma^{1/2}, \qquad\qquad 4.$$

where ΔH° is the calorimetrically determined enthalpy change per residue, which appears in Equation 3. The ratio $\Delta H^\circ_{vH}/\Delta H^\circ$ gives the size of the cooperative unit, or the average number of residues in a helical segment at T_m. If $\sigma = 10^{-4}$, the cooperative unit is 100 residues.

The helix-coil transition of γ-benzyl-L-glutamate is inverted in the solvent system studied by Zimm et al (93): the helix is formed at high temperatures. This unusual behavior results from preferential binding by the peptide of one of the two solvent components, and from a change in preferential binding on helix formation (6).

The agreement between helix-coil theory and experiment was excellent in this first studied system (93), which employed a nonionizing amino acid and an organic solvent system. Little further work has been done on testing the theory in systems of this kind, although other properties of the helix-coil transition, such as hydrodynamic properties, have been studied extensively.

The next problem was to study α-helix formation in water. The basic difficulty was that helix-forming amino acids such as Ala and Met yield polypeptides that are not water-soluble, whereas amino acids whose polypeptides are water-soluble, such as Ser, Thr, Asn, Gln, Asp, His, and Arg, do not form the α-helix in water. Only Glu and Lys show helix formation in water, and then only under special conditions. The uncharged amino acid forms the helix and the ionized form does not, but the uncharged helix aggregates. Zimm & Rice (94) analyzed theoretically the problem of removing charge effects by extrapolation in 1960. They obtained a solution that proved to be quite general (see 49) and widely applicable, and the extrapolations were experimentally feasible. The value of ΔH° (Equation 3) for both Glu and Lys was found to be close to -1 kcal/mol residue (for review, see 59). Rialdi & Hermans (61) measured ΔH° for α-helix formation by Glu with calorimetry and confirmed the value found using the Zimm-Rice method. A value of $\sigma = 0.0025$ was found both for Glu and Lys (59).

Host-Guest Studies

Scheraga and coworkers have used the host-guest method (13, 79, 85, 88) to obtain values of s for all 20 amino acids in the genetic code. Random copolymers of two amino acids are made using the Leuchs synthesis: the host residue is hydroxybutyl- or hydroxypropyl-L-glutamine (HBLG or HPLG) (35), and the guest residue is any of the 20 amino acids. The copolymer is water-soluble and nonionizing unless the guest residue ionizes. Helix-coil transition curves are analyzed using a theory for random-sequence copolymers. A basic assumption of the host-guest method is that the copolymer sequences are truly random. Deviations from randomness seriously affect the shape of the transition curve. For this reason, extracting the value of σ for the guest residue is difficult, and the temperature dependence of s should also be regarded with caution.

The host-guest values of s at 20°C for all 20 amino acids have been determined (88). They show several striking properties. Most values of s cluster closely around 1 ($\pm 20\%$). A value of $s = 1$ means that an amino acid is neither a strong helix-former nor a helix-breaker, but rather is helix-indifferent. The host-guest values for s in water differ strikingly from observations of helix formation by polypeptides in nonpolar solvents, which indicate that β-branched amino acids are helix-breakers (7): Ile shows one of the highest s values found by the host-guest method. The nonionized form of an acidic or basic amino acid always has a higher s value than the ionized form: this is particularly evident for Glu. The temperature dependences of s found using the host-guest method are striking chiefly because of their variability from one amino acid to the next.

Serious contradictions arise between the host-guest values of s and the results of experiments on helix formation with short peptides. These contradictions are discussed in the section below on helix formation by peptides of de novo design.

HELIX FORMATION BY SEQUENCES FROM PROTEINS

Early Studies

In 1968–1971, peptide sequences from helical regions of three proteins were studied. Epand & Scheraga (16) found no significant helix formation at 25°C in peptides from myoglobin, and Taniuchi & Anfinsen (81) reported similar results for staphylococcal nuclease. On the other hand, Brown & Klee (10 and references therein) did find evidence from circular dichroism (CD) studies that the C-peptide (residues 1–13) and the S-peptide (residues 1–20) of ribonuclease A (RNase A) show partial helix formation at low temperatures. Residues 3–13 form a helix in native RNase A, when helical residues are counted as ones that have helical hydrogen bonds. The CD-detected structure in C-peptide corresponds to only about 25% helix at 0°C; it undergoes thermal unfolding so that its helicity is small at 25°C. Brown & Klee found using sedimentation equilibrium that C-peptide is monomeric in conditions in which helical structure is detected. When they used guanidium chloride (GuHCl) to induce helix unfolding, they obtained puzzling CD spectra.

The problem of whether or not C-peptide forms an α-helix in water was reinvestigated by Bierzynski et al (5) in 1982, following a report, using NMR, that structure can be detected in S-peptide (8) at 10°C. Their NMR results showed that residues at well-separated positions participate in structure formation, and the structure undergoes cooperative thermal unfolding. Their CD spectra were consistent with α-helix formation.

pH Dependence of Helix Formation by C Peptide

Helix formation by C-peptide contradicts the host-guest values of s, which predict that no short peptide should show measurable α-helix formation in water (5). The authors used an approximate form of the Zimm-Bragg equation that is not suitable for values of s close to 1; however, a later calculation (75) using the full equation reached a similar conclusion. The stability of the C-peptide helix was found to depend strongly on pH: helix content follows a bell-shaped curve with a maximum near pH 5 (5). At least two ionized groups, one with a pK_a near 3.5 and one with a pK_a near 6.5, are needed for maximum helical stability of C-peptide (5); this observation suggested that specific side-chain interactions stabilize the C-peptide helix and that they explain the contradiction with the host-guest results. A $Glu9^- \cdots His12^+$ ion pair was suggested. The helix content and thermal stability of the C-peptide helix change in parallel as the pH varies, and later studies showed the same parallelism in amino acid substitution experiments.

Helix Stop in S Peptide

The average length of α-helices in proteins is about 11 residues, whereas the average length of a helical segment in a synthetic polypeptide, containing a single type of amino acid, is estimated to be 30–100 residues at T_m (see Equation 4). Thus, proteins have helix termination signals of some kind. Rico and coworkers (63) and, independently, Kim & Baldwin (31) used NMR to study the localization of the helix in S-peptide. Both groups concluded that the helix stops near Met13, and consequently that the helix is localized in S-peptide in a way that resembles helix localization in RNase A.

These investigations provided the first good evidence that studies of α-helix formation in peptides might yield useful information about the mechanism of protein folding. Because helix localization in S-peptide can be explained by helix propensities only if the differences between the s values of different amino acids are large, either some specific side-chain interaction acts as a helix stop signal in S-peptide or else the host-guest values of s are not applicable to helix formation in S-peptide.

In later studies, a trifluoroethanol (TFE)-H_2O solvent system was used to find out if the helix propagates to the end of S-peptide in the presence of TFE (50); in another study, Asp14, Ser15, and Ser16 were each replaced by Ala (42). Neither study found helix propagation to the C terminus of S-peptide. By providing a fixed nucleus to initiate the helix in S-peptide, Pease et al (57) succeeded in increasing substantially its helix content, and in demonstrating that the helix can be detected four to five residues beyond Met13.

Charge-Helix Dipole Interactions

Chemical synthesis of C-peptide analogs and pH titration of their helix contents (75) showed that $Glu2^-$ and $His12^+$ are the two ionized groups needed for maximal stability of the C-peptide helix. Chemical modification studies (62) pointed earlier to the involvement of $Glu2^-$. Substitution studies confirmed that $Glu2^-$ and $His12^+$, which are far apart in the helix, act independently of each other. Each might interact with the helix dipole because they are close to ends of the helix.

The possibility that charge-helix dipole interactions might affect the stability of the C-peptide helix was tested by Shoemaker et al (76), who used chemical synthesis to vary the charge on the N-terminal residue from $+2$ to -1. They found substantial changes in helix content, and NaCl screening experiments indicated that a charge-helix dipole interaction was responsible. Important experiments from this same period by Ooi and coworkers on the charge-helix dipole interaction are discussed below under peptides of de novo design.

A later study (18) compared the effects on helix stability of the α-NH$_3^+$ group and the α-COO$^-$ group, and asked if the increase in helix stability found by removing the charge (either with a chemical blocking group or by pH titration) resulted from a charge-helix dipole interaction or from hydrogen bonding. A $-$OCH$_3$ group, which cannot hydrogen bond to a peptide CO group, was used to block the α-COO$^-$ group; the same increase in helix stability was found as with a $-$NH$_2$ blocking group, which can hydrogen bond. The results fit the helix dipole model and showed that hydrogen bonding is not involved. If all charge-helix dipole interactions involved hydrogen bonding of the charged side chain to a free peptide NH or CO group, helix-destabilizing interactions should not occur.

The term "charge-helix dipole" interaction may be misleading. The interaction occurs chiefly between the charged group and partial charges on non-hydrogen-bonded groups at either end of the helix (four free NH groups at the N terminus and four free CO groups at the C terminus). Tidor & Karplus (82) recently analyzed the interaction with free energy perturbation calculations for the case of a His $\rightarrow$ Arg mutation near the C terminus of a protein helix, and Åquist et al (3) made the same point using electrostatic theory.

Phe8 $\cdots$ His12$^+$ Interaction in C Peptide

The demonstration (75) that His12$^+$ is one of two charged residues that stabilize the C-peptide helix provoked interest in the mechanism by which His$^+$ acts because: (a) His12$^+$ is close to the C terminus of the helix and might stabilize it by interacting with the helix dipole; (b) in the X-ray structure of RNase A, the rings of Phe8 and His12 are close together and might interact; (c) in host-guest studies (88), His$^+$ has a lower s value (i.e. is more helix-breaking) than His^0, and His12$^+$ has to overcome this intrinsic effect of a low helix propensity to stabilize the C-peptide helix. Substitution experiments, combined with pH titration of helix stability, resolved the puzzle (74). They showed that: (a) the helix-stabilizing effect results from a Phe $\cdots$ His interaction; (b) it is specific for an $i,i+4$ spacing of Phe and His, and (c) the interaction is specific for His$^+$ and vanishes when His12$^+$ is titrated to give His^0. The results also confirmed the earlier puzzling observation that the helix-stabilizing effect of His12$^+$ cannot be screened using NaCl, in contrast to the charge-helix dipole interactions studied earlier.

A current study of the Phe8 $\cdots$ His12$^+$ interaction (R. Fairman, K. M. Armstrong & R. L. Baldwin, unpublished results) shows that the above properties are almost unchanged when the Phe-His residues are transferred into an alanine-based peptide with a simple sequence. This study also suggests that His$^+$ stabilizes the helix by interacting with the helix dipole, since the helix-stabilizing effect of the Phe-His pair is observed when His is close to the C terminus of the peptide, but not when it is in the center of the peptide.

A molecular dynamics simulation of the C-peptide helix by Tirado-Rives & Jorgensen (83) does not show an interaction between Phe8 and His12$^+$ but does show His12$^+$ in a favorable conformation for interacting with the helix dipole.

Glu2$^-$ $\cdots$ Arg10$^+$ Interaction in C Peptide

The problem posed by identifying Glu2$^-$ as one of the two charged residues that stabilize the C-peptide helix (75) is similar to the problem posed by His12$^+$: does Glu2$^-$ exert its effect by interacting with the helix dipole (since Glu2$^-$ is close to the N terminus of the helix) or by an ion-pair interaction with Arg10$^+$, which can be seen in the X-ray structure of RNase A? The Glu2$^-$ $\cdots$ Arg10$^+$ interaction produces a small kink in the RNase A helix near the N terminus. This kinked conformation was detected using NMR in solution in a study by Osterhout et al (53), who observed an unusual nuclear Overhauser effect (NOE) that is absent if the helix is straight. They also observed a second helical conformation of C-peptide, a straight, extended helix.

The putative helix-stabilizing effect of Arg10$^+$ cannot be demonstrated directly using pH titration because the pK$_a$ of arginine is too high. Substitution experiments (19) gave complex results, probably because the helix straightens out and becomes extended when Ala is substituted for Arg10. By combining substitution experiments with NaCl titrations, however, Fairman et al (19) demonstrated the helix-stabilizing effect of Arg10$^+$. When the substitution X $\rightarrow$ Ala is made and NaCl titrations of helix stability are performed, the curves of helicity versus [NaCl] are nearly parallel for the two peptides with X or with Ala if residue X does not affect helix stability by an electrostatic interaction. If X does interact, and the interaction can be screened with NaCl, then the two curves are nonparallel, and the extent of the deviation from parallelism measures the strength of the interaction.

A molecular-dynamics simulation of the C-peptide helix (83) shows the Glu2$^-$ $\cdots$ Arg10$^+$ ion-pair interaction, but it is a solvent-separated ion pair rather than the contact ion pair seen in the X-ray structure of RNase A.

Studies of Helix Propensities in C Peptide

Initially, investigators conducted substitution experiments in C-peptide (45, 77) to find out if the replacement of a single noninteracting residue can measurably affect the helicity of C-peptide, and to compare the results with expectations based on the host-guest values of s. The results showed that single amino acid substitutions do affect C-peptide helicity, although substitutions made at the N- or C-terminal residue show little effect (77), and the behavior of Ala $\rightarrow$ Gly (77) or Ala $\rightarrow$ Ser (45) substitutions fit expectation based on earlier host-guest studies. A later study of Ala $\rightarrow$ Pro substitutions (78) showed that insertion of a proline residue effectively terminates the C-peptide helix.

Substitution experiments to analyze the Phe8 $\cdots$ His12$^+$ (74) and Glu2$^-$ $\cdots$ Arg10$^+$ (19) interactions sometimes revealed surprisingly large changes in peptide helicity in control experiments, in which the substitution should not have affected any known specific interaction. Later, the explanation for these surprising results was sought through substitution experiments in peptides with simple sequences.

To study systematically the effects of helix propensities on substitution experiments in C-peptide, Fairman et al (17) made the same substitution (Ala $\rightarrow$ X) at each of three positions in C-peptide (Ala4,5,6) using five different amino acids as X (Glu, His, Phe, Lys, and Arg). They made pH titrations of helicity to aid in sorting out charge interactions and to obtain data on the uncharged forms of Glu and His as well as on their charged forms. The surprising result of this study is that position 5 has a general position effect. Replacement of Ala5 by any of the other five amino acids generally results in a higher helix content in the substituted peptide than when Ala4 or Ala6 is replaced. The reason for this position effect is not known.

The Nascent Helix

NMR study of an immunogenic peptide, corresponding to one helix (residues 69–87) of myohemerythrin, by Dyson et al (15) revealed that residues in the C-terminal half of the peptide have backbone ϕ,φ angles that correspond to the α-helical conformation, although medium-range NOEs characteristic of the helix could not be detected, nor could the helix be observed using CD. Upon addition of TFE, the C-terminal half of the peptide became helical. Consequently, its conformation in aqueous solution was deduced to be a precursor to the helix, and was termed the nascent helix (15). The observation that antibodies made against peptides often cross-react with intact proteins has increased interest in the analysis of peptide conformations in aqueous solution. Dyson et al (14) also found that a single β-turn can be populated sufficiently in a short peptide in water for its conformation to be analyzed using NMR and for the sequence requirements for its formation to be determined. Wright et al (89) reviewed peptide conformations in water and their analysis using NMR, as well as their implications for the initiation of protein folding.

HELIX FORMATION IN PEPTIDES OF DE NOVO DESIGN

Introduction

The studies of α-helix formation in peptides derived from RNase A identified specific side-chain and charge-dipole interactions that affect the stability of the α-helix. The C- and S-peptide derivatives of RNase A, are not, however, ideal systems for these studies. To isolate and study specific interactions and to measure intrinsic helix-forming tendencies of all of the amino acids, a simple model peptide system is desired. Several independent investigations of α-helix formation in short peptides of de novo design have been made using different model peptides as hosts and different design strategies.

The ideal host peptide should show monomolecular α-helix formation, and its transition from helix to coil must be reversible. An ideal host peptide should, if possible, contain only neutral residues so as to avoid complications from charge-dipole and charge-charge interactions. The stability of the peptide host should derive exclusively from the properties of the polypeptide backbone itself; interactions between side-chain residues should be avoided.

Marqusee & Baldwin (41) described the first de novo-designed α-helical peptide system. It has some of the desirable properties necessary for a simple α-helical host. The peptides in this system mostly contain Ala, with Glu and Lys inserted for solubility. The N- and C-terminal residues are blocked with acetyl and carboxamide, respectively, to eliminate unfavorable charge-dipole effects. The peptides contain oppositely charged residues spaced either $i,i+3$ or $i,i+4$; stabilizing side-chain interactions have been observed for the $i,i+4$ spacing but not for the $i,i+3$ spacing. These peptides, which exhibit ~75% helical structure, demonstrate that simple peptides can be designed and characterized and that specific interactions between side chains can be observed.

This initial success in designing a simple, α-helical peptide led to the design of other helical peptides. Lyu et al (37) synthesized two peptides that contain primarily Glu and Lys; they found modest α-helical structure in solution. These peptides do not contain many Ala residues; rather, the helical structure results solely from ion-pair formation between appropriately spaced Glu and Lys residues (see section below on helix-stabilizing side-chain interactions). Wang et al (87) reported recently that a 285-residue peptide from the smooth muscle protein caldesmon apparently forms a single long helix and contains numerous pairs of Glu-Lys residues spaced $i, i+4$.

Bradley et al (9) took a contrasting design approach in their studies of another set of monomeric α-helical peptides. They intentionally incorporated many different types of residues to facilitate the NMR assignments. They used NMR to find evidence for an unequal distribution of α-helical structure throughout the chain.

Marqusee et al (43) provided the first direct demonstration of the high helix-forming tendency of alanine. Peptides that contain only Ala, plus either Glu or Lys for solubility, show substantial α-helix formation in water. Because no stabilizing side-chain interactions occur in these peptides, the helical structure results exclusively from the high helix propensity of alanine. Another example of the high helix-forming tendency of alanine is provided by a completely neutral, water-soluble peptide, containing Ala and Gln residues, which exhibits α-helix formation in water (72). This completely neutral peptide, devoid of stabilizing side-chain interactions, meets almost all criteria for an ideal host peptide. With this neutral host, the effects of single charged residues on helix stability, as well as the interactions between charged side chains, can be studied in isolation.

Several attempts have been successful at designing peptides whose α-helical structure in water is stabilized either by covalent or noncovalent interactions between side chains. Felix et al (20) and Madison et al (40) described analogs of human growth hormone-releasing factor (GRF) that contain a covalent linkage between Asp8 and Lys12 in the helical portion of GRF. These covalently cross-linked analogs show enhanced α-helical structure in solution as well as increased biological activity. Ösapay & Taylor (52) employed the same design strategy in their design of an amphiphilic α-helical peptide containing three pairs of covalently linked Glu-Lys residues. The peptide containing cross-linked Glu-Lys pairs did not, however, show substantially greater α-helical structure than the control peptide with Glu-Lys ion pairs. A recent report by Jackson et al (28) describes the use of single disulfide bond-bridging residues i and $i+8$ to stabilize α-helical structure in peptides as short as eight amino acids. They demonstrate that a D and L pair of isomers of a cysteine homolog, when oxidized to form an intramolecular disulfide bond, can stabilize the α-helicity of the resulting peptide.

Peptide-metal complexes have also been used to stabilize α-helices. Ghadiri and coworkers have designed peptides that contain two histidines, which can serve as exchange-labile ligands for various transition metals (23) or can form an exchange-inert complex with Ru(III) (24). In the latter case, a 17-residue peptide-metal complex exhibits about 80% α-helical structure in water at 21°C. Ruan et al (66) reported a similar approach to metal-stabilized peptide helices. In their design, which employs an unnatural amino acid with an aminodiacetic acid side chain, a substantial increase in peptide helicity could be observed in the presence of any of several transition metals.

Helix Propensities Studied in Substitution Experiments

The remarkable success in designing and characterizing short peptides that exhibit substantial α-helix formation in water has prompted a renewed interest in determining the helix-forming tendencies of all the amino acids. Several different approaches have been used, and different host peptides employed, and the results are all qualitatively similar. They show large differences between helix propensities for the various amino acids, larger than those found from host-guest studies (88). The α-helix propensities determined in different systems are, however, quantitatively different; these differences are discussed below. Some of the experiments yield helix propensities measured by values of s; others yield only the change in helix content compared with the host peptide.

Padmanabhan et al (55) provided the relative helix-forming tendencies of the nonpolar amino acids. Marqusee et al (43) describe the host peptide for these studies; X gives the position of an amino acid substitution:

Ac-Y-K-A-A-X-A-K-A-A-X-A-K-A-A-X-A-K-(NH$_2$).

The reference peptide is devoid of stabilizing side-chain interactions and thus the α-helical structure is stabilized solely by the intrinsic helix-forming tendencies of the constituent amino acids. Of the nonpolar residues studied, Ala, Leu, Ile, Phe, and Val, only Leu shows α-helix formation comparable to Ala. The results do not correlate with the s values determined in host-guest studies (88).

A direct demonstration of the disparity between the s values determined in host-guest studies (88) and those determined in short, alanine-based peptides came from the work of Chakrabartty et al (12). By studying the position-dependent effect of a single Ala $\rightarrow$ Gly substitution in an Ala-Lys host peptide used earlier (43, 55), and by analyzing the results with the Lifson-Roig theory (34), they found a large ratio of the s values for Ala : Gly, approximately 100. This ratio is in striking contrast to the host-guest ratio of s for Ala : Gly, which is only 1.8 (88). The effect of an amino acid substitution on helix content depends strongly on its position only if the ratio of s values is large. The effect arises from fraying of the ends of the helix.

Merutka et al (44, 46) provided a comprehensive investigation of the helix-forming tendencies of all the amino acids. The host peptide for their substitution experiments,

Ac-Y-E-A-A-A-K-E-A-X-A-K-E-A-A-A-K-A-(NH$_2$),

is the $i,i+4$ E,K peptide designed by Marqusee & Baldwin (41) and contains three $i,i+4$ stabilizing ion pairs between Glu and Lys residues. They substituted, in turn, each of the 20 residues for the central residue, X, in this 17-residue peptide and determined the helix content of each peptide using CD. Their results show that a single substitution, even in a host peptide that has stabilizing side-chain interactions, can dramatically affect the observed helicity of a short, monomeric peptide.

Another study of the helix propensities of several neutral amino acids was reported by Lyu et al (36). The host peptide employed in these studies,

Suc-Y-S-E-E-E-E-K-K-K-K-X-X-X-E-E-E-E-K-K-K-K-(NH$_2$),

is based on the earlier peptide described by Lyu et al (37); it contains eight Glu and eight Lys residues appropriately spaced to form eight possible ion pairs. The three central residues, X, were used as substitution sites, and the helical content of each peptide was determined by CD. In addition to using CD to measure the average α-helical content of each peptide, Lyu et al (36, 39) used NMR methods to localize the helical structure within the peptide chain. They find evidence for a nonuniform distribution of helical structure within the peptide; the residues at the ends of the chains are much less helical than those in the middle.

A related study of the helix-forming tendencies of the amino acids has been reported by O'Neil & DeGrado (51), who made single substitutions of all 20 amino acids at a surface-exposed position in a dimeric coiled-coil peptide. Although the coiled-coil is not a monomeric α-helix, O'Neil & DeGrado have selected a substitution site that is solvent-exposed and is not in direct contact with the dimerization surface of the coiled-coil. They determined the effect of the guest residue on the stability of the coiled-coil dimer helix using both urea denaturation and the dependence of helix formation on peptide concentration, and then fitted the results to a two-state reaction between helical dimer and random coil monomers in order to calculate free energy changes. Their results are qualitatively similar to the other substitution results discussed above, but not to the host-guest (88) results. They can also be correlated quantitatively with the data obtained by Lyu et al (36), but not with the host-guest results (88), the Chou-Fasman Pα scales, nor with the results of Chakrabartty et al (12) for Ala → Gly.

Padmanabhan & Baldwin (54) and Lyu et al (38) further investigated the effect of side-chain conformational freedom on α-helical stability. As proposed much earlier by Blout (7), nonpolar β-branched amino acids are helix-breaking, whereas nonpolar straight-chain amino acids are helix-forming. This result indicates that conformational freedom of a side chain is a major factor in determining its helix-stabilizing tendency. This effect can be analyzed, and even predicted, by free energy simulations. Yun et al (90) conducted a study of this kind for the substitution Ala → Pro in an alanine helix.

The contradiction between host-guest values of s and the results found from substitution experiments in short peptides may result from a helix-stabilizing hydrophobic interaction between the host residues, as suggested by Marqusee et al (43). The host residue, either hydroxypropyl- or hydroxybutyl-L-glutamine (HPLG or HBLG) forms a helix in water that, according to Lotan et al (35), is stabilized by hydrophobic interactions among the long alkyl chains of the host. The net effect is that the intrinsic helix-forming tendency of the guest is masked by the guest's perturbing effect on the stability of the host.

Thermodynamics of α-Helix Formation

All short peptide helices studied thus far, except template-initiated helices and ones stabilized by covalent cross-links, show similar thermally induced unfolding. This observation suggests that helix formation is enthalpically driven. The enthalpy change of helix formation should have two components. The temperature-independent component should reflect formation of peptide hydrogen bond and van der Waals contacts, whereas hydrophobic interactions should be reflected in the temperature-dependent portion of $\Delta H°$.

Scholtz et al (70) have measured the enthalpy of helix formation using differential scanning calorimetry (DSC). The peptide they studied,

Ac-Y-(A-E-A-A-K-A)$_8$-F-(NH$_2$),

has 50 residues and blocked N and C termini and is well-suited to studies of the thermodynamics of the helix-coil transition associated with the polypeptide backbone itself.

The value of $\Delta H°$ for helix formation is about -1 kcal/mol residue. The breadth of the thermal transition precludes determining the change in heat capacity, ΔC_p, accurately, but ΔC_p does not appear to be large. Analysis of the thermal unfolding curves for the 50-residue peptide, as monitored by either CD or DSC, reveals a van't Hoff enthalpy change for helix formation (ΔH_{vH}) of -11.2 kcal/mol of peptide, whereas the calorimetric enthalpy change is approximately -1 kcal/mol residue or about -50 kcal/mol peptide. It will be important to determine the enthalpy change of helix formation for other peptides to test the generality of this result and also to measure ΔC_p for the transition. The value of $\Delta H°$ found for an alanine-based helix is close to the values found using the Zimm-

Rice method for poly-L-glutamate and poly-L-lysine (for review, see 59) and to the value found calorimetrically for poly-L-glutamate (61). Ben-Naim (4) recently proposed that, considering only the polypeptide backbone, a value for $\Delta H°$ of about -1 kcal/mol residue should be expected for the formation of a solvent-exposed α-helix in water. He suggests that the ability of the peptide CO group to form more than one hydrogen bond is a key factor in determining the value of $\Delta H°$.

Application of Helix-Coil Transition Theory

A fundamental problem in the study of α-helix formation in water, either by short peptides or by polypeptides, is to determine the applicability of helix-coil transition theory. In testing the applicability of the Zimm-Bragg and Lifson-Roig theories, one must avoid side-chain interactions as much as possible and be aware of possible limitations of the simple model in which the helix propensity of each type of amino acid residue is described by a single value of s, independent of neighboring amino acids and of position in the helix.

Scholtz et al (71) took the same approach used by Zimm et al (93) to test the Zimm-Bragg theory for helix formation by poly-γ-benzyl-L-glutamate in a mixed organic solvent. They studied helix formation in water by a series of simple, repeating-sequence, alanine-based peptides of varying chain lengths, using the thermally induced helix-coil transition monitored by CD. The generic formula is

$$Ac\text{-}Y\text{-}(A\text{-}E\text{-}A\text{-}A\text{-}K\text{-}A)_k\text{-}F\text{-}(NH_2) \quad k = 2\text{–}8.$$

They fitted the helix-coil transition curves with three parameters from helix-coil theory (σ, s at $0°C$, and $\Delta H°$), but they also needed to express the values of $[\theta]_{222}$, the mean residue ellipticity (222 nm) of the complete helix and random coil, as functions both of temperature and of chain length. Lack of definite values for these spectroscopic parameters limited the accuracy of the results. Nevertheless, the results were encouraging. They found a value for $\Delta H°$ (-0.95 kcal/mol residue) in good agreement with the value measured calorimetrically (70), and the value determined for σ of 0.003 agreed satisfactorily with the earlier determinations on poly-L-glutamate and poly-L-lysine ($\sigma = 0.0025$) (for review, see 59).

A second determination of σ for a series of peptides of defined sequence and length in water has been done (C. A. Rohl, J. M. Scholtz, E. J. York, J. M. Stewart & R. L. Baldwin, in preparation). This study, which probes α-helix formation by using amide proton exchange and NMR, determined a value for σ of 0.0019 for the series of peptides:

Ac-(A-A-K-A-A)$_k$-Y-(NH$_2$) $k = 1$–10.

The agreement between these two independent determinations of σ, using two different probes to monitor α-helix formation, suggests that σ may be relatively independent of side-chain type, although further work in this area is needed to resolve this issue.

Studies of Helix-Stabilizing Side-Chain Interactions

Marqusee & Baldwin (41) reported the first observation of ion-pair formation in designed peptides. They used pH and NaCl titrations to investigate the effects of spacing and orientation of putative ion pairs and found evidence for $i,i+4$ but not for $i,i+3$ ion pairs. They also found greater helix stabilization by Glu$^-$ $\cdots$ Lys$^+$ than by Lys$^+$ $\cdots$ Glu$^-$ ion pairs. Lyu et al's (37) pH titration of the initial host peptide, which contains eight possible Glu$^-$ $\cdots$ Lys$^+$ ion pairs, shows that the helix becomes unstable when the Lys$^+$ residues are titrated to Lys^0 at pH 12, but not when the Glu$^-$ residues are titrated to Glu^0 at pH 2. This result suggests that singly charged Glu^0 $\cdots$ Lys$^+$ hydrogen bonds may contribute to α-helix stability, as suggested by Marqusee & Baldwin (41).

Merutka & Stellwagen (47, 48) studied the relative effectiveness of several different ion pairs in stabilizing an alanine-based α-helix. They studied Glu-Lys, Glu-Orn, and Glu-Arg ion pairs as well as ion pairs of Asp with each of these three basic residues. Their results indicate that $i,i+4$ ion pairs of all these types can stabilize α-helix formation; differences in helix content were attributed chiefly to the different intrinsic helix-forming tendencies of the various charged residues. The length dependence of helicity was also investigated for the most helical sequences of the peptides studied (48), the $i,i+4$ Glu-Arg peptide. These authors found that increasing the length of the peptide to 27 residues gives a peptide that appears to be completely α-helical under optimal helix-forming conditions.

The problem of quantitating specific side-chain interactions in α-helices is only beginning to be solved. A hierarchical nesting approach has been put forward recently by Robert (64) for incorporating side-chain interactions into the Zimm-Bragg model. He uses existing data in the literature to show how side-chain interactions can be evaluated. Earlier, Vasquez & Scheraga (84) had also proposed a formalism for including side-chain interactions in the Zimm-Bragg model. Gans et al (22) propose a related formalism and use it to evaluate data in the literature. They show that a single set of parameters cannot reproduce the different results found using various host peptides. Their conclusion suggests that the problem of context dependence is a major unsolved problem: how does the apparent s

value of a residue depend on neighboring amino acids, and what are the reasons for these dependencies?

Gans et al (22) use their formalism to calculate the energetic contribution of $i,i+4$ E,K ion pairs to α-helix stability. The two peptides that are compared are:

Suc-Y-S-E-E-E-E-K-K-K-K-E-E-E-E-K-K-K-K-(NH$_2$)   E$_4$K$_4$ and

Suc-Y-S-E-E-K-K-E-E-K-K-E-E-K-K-E-E-K-K-(NH$_2$)   E$_2$K$_2$.

By comparing the helix contents of two peptides that differ only in the spacing of eight possible ion pairs, such that one peptide, E$_4$K$_4$, can form stabilizing ion pairs and the other, E$_2$K$_2$, cannot, Gans et al calculate that ion-pair formation contributes 0.50 kcal/mol to the stability of the α-helix in these peptides. The entire helical structure of E$_4$K$_4$ results from ion-pair formation; E$_2$K$_2$ shows no α-helical structure in water at neutral pH.

Finkelstein and coworkers (21) recently described a computational approach for estimating the helix contents of a wide range of α-helical peptides. They use the Zimm-Bragg formalism with many additional parameters for specific and nonspecific interactions between side chains and the helix macrodipole. They contend that the s values determined from host-guest studies (88) are sufficient to describe the observed α-helix formation by short peptides, provided one includes the energetic contributions to helix formation from side-chain interactions, interactions with the helix macrodipole, and context- and position-dependent adjustments to the intrinsic helix-forming tendencies of the amino acids. Their complex function requires numerous experimental parameters, several of which are not known precisely.

The other major way that a charged side chain can affect the stability of an α-helical peptide, apart from specific ion-pair formation, is the electrostatic interaction between a charged side chain and the helix macrodipole (25, 26, 86). Ooi and coworkers (27, 80) performed a classic set of experiments, which illustrate the properties of the charge-helix dipole interaction and its importance for α-helix stability. They made double-block copolymers of known block lengths, first of Glu and Ala (27) and later of Lys and Ala (80), with 20 residues in each block. In the first block copolymer of each set, the block of ionizing residues was at the N terminus of the alanine block, and in the second block copolymer it was at the C terminus. Stabilization of the alanine helix was observed whenever a block of oppositely charged residues was close to one pole of the helix macrodipole, and helix destabilization was observed if the block of charged residues was of the same sign as the nearby pole of the helix dipole.

Literature Cited

1. Ackermann, T., Neumann, E. 1967. *Biopolymers* 5: 649–62
2. Applequist, J. 1963. *J. Chem. Phys.* 38: 934–41
3. Åquist, J., Luecke, H., Quiocho, F. A., Warshel, A. 1991. *Proc. Natl. Acad. Sci. USA* 88: 2026–30
4. Ben-Naim, A. 1991. *J. Phys. Chem.* 95: 1437–44
5. Bierzynski, A., Kim, P. S., Baldwin, R. L. 1982. *Proc. Natl. Acad. Sci. USA* 79: 2470–74
6. Bixon, M., Lifson, S. 1966. *Biopolymers* 4: 815–21
7. Blout, E. R. 1962. See Ref. 76a, pp. 275–79
8. Blum, A. D., Smallcombe, S. H., Baldwin, R. L. 1978. *J. Mol. Biol.* 118: 305–16
9. Bradley, E. K., Thomason, J. F., Cohen, F. E., Kosen, P. A., Kuntz, I. D. 1990. *J. Mol. Biol.* 215: 607–22
10. Brown, J. E., Klee, W. A. 1971. *Biochemistry* 10: 470–76
11. Cantor, C. R., Schimmel, P. R. 1980. *Biophysical Chemistry*, Vol. 3. New York: Freeman
12. Chakrabartty, A., Schellman, J. A., Baldwin, R. L. 1991. *Nature (London)* 351: 586–88
13. Chou, P. Y., Wells, M., Fasman, G. D. 1972. *Biochemistry* 11: 3028–43
14. Dyson, H. J., Rance, M., Houghten, R. A., Lerner, R. A., Wright, P. E. 1988. *J. Mol. Biol.* 201: 161–200
15. Dyson, H. J., Rance, M., Houghten, R. A., Wright, P. E., Lerner, R. A. 1988. *J. Mol. Biol.* 201: 201–17
16. Epand, R. M., Scheraga, H. A. 1968. *Biochemistry* 7: 2864–2872
17. Fairman, R., Armstrong, K. M., Shoemaker, K. R., York, E. J., Stewart, J. M., Baldwin, R. L. 1991. *J. Mol. Biol.* 221: 1395–1401
18. Fairman, R., Shoemaker, K. R., York, E. J., Stewart, J. M., Baldwin, R. L. 1989. *Proteins Struct. Funct. Genet.* 5: 1–7
19. Fairman, R., Shoemaker, K. R., York, E. J., Stewart, J. M., Baldwin, R. L. 1990. *Biophys. Chem.* 37: 107–19
20. Felix, A. M., Heimer, E. P., Wang, C.-T., Lambros, T. J., Fournier, A., et al. 1988. *Int. J. Pept. Protein Res.* 32: 441–54
21. Finkelstein, A. V., Badretdinov, A. Y., Ptitsyn, O. B. 1991. *Proteins Struct. Funct. Genet.* 10: 287–99
22. Gans, P. J., Lyu, P. C., Manning, M. C., Woody, R. W., Kallenbach, N. R. 1991. *Biopolymers.* Submitted
23. Ghadiri, M. R., Choi, C. 1990. *J. Am. Chem. Soc.* 112: 1630–32
24. Ghadiri, M. R., Fernholz, A. K. 1990. *J. Am. Chem. Soc.* 112: 9633–35
25. Hol, W. G. J. 1985. *Prog. Biophys. Mol. Biol.* 45: 149–95
26. Hol, W. G. J., van Duijnen, P. T., Berendsen, H. J. C. 1978. *Nature (London)* 273: 443–46
27. Ihara, S., Ooi, T., Takahashi, S. 1982. *Biopolymers* 21: 131–45
28. Jackson, D. Y., King, D. S., Chmielewski, J., Singh, S., Schultz, P. G. 1991. *J. Am. Chem. Soc.* Submitted
29. Kauzmann, W. 1959. *Adv. Protein Chem.* 14: 1–63
30. Kemp, D. S., Boyd, J. G., Muendel, C. C. 1991. *Nature (London)* 352: 451–54
31. Kim, P. S., Baldwin, R. L. 1984. *Nature (London)* 307: 329–33
32. Kirkwood, J. G. 1943. In *Proteins, Amino Acids and Peptides*, ed. E. J. Cohn, J. T. Edsall, pp. 276–303. New York: Reinhold
33. Lesk, A. M. 1991. *Nature (London)* 352: 379–80
34. Lifson, S., Roig, A. 1961. *J. Chem. Phys.* 34: 1963–74
35. Lotan, N., Yaron, A., Berger, A. 1966. *Biopolymers* 4: 365–68
36. Lyu, P. C., Liff, M. I., Marky, L. A., Kallenbach, N. R. 1990. *Science* 250: 669–73
37. Lyu, P. C., Marky, L. A., Kallenbach, N. R. 1989. *J. Am. Chem. Soc.* 111: 2733–34
38. Lyu, P. C., Sherman, J. C., Chen, A., Kallenbach, N. R. 1991. *Proc. Natl. Acad. Sci. USA* 88: 5317–20
39. Lyu, P. C., Wang, P. C., Liff, M. I., Kallenbach, N. R. 1991. *J. Am. Chem. Soc.* 113: 1014–19
40. Madison, V. S., Fry, D. C., Greeley, D. N., Toome, V., Wegrzynski, B. B., et al. 1990. In *Proceedings of the 11th American Peptide Symposium*, ed. J. E. Rivier, G. R. Marshall, pp. 575–77. Leiden, the Netherlands: ESCOM
41. Marqusee, S., Baldwin, R. L. 1987. *Proc. Natl. Acad. Sci. USA* 84: 8898–8902
42. Marqusee, S., Baldwin, R. L. 1990. In *The Protein Folding Problem*, ed. J. King, L. Gierasch, pp. 85–94. Washington, DC: Am. Assoc. Adv. Sci
43. Marqusee, S., Robbins, V. H., Baldwin, R. L. 1989. *Proc. Natl. Acad. Sci. USA* 86: 5286–90
44. Merutka, G., Lipton, W., Shalongo, W., Park, S.-H., Stellwagen, E. 1990. *Biochemistry* 29: 7511–15
45. Merutka, G., Stellwagen, E. 1989. *Biochemistry* 28: 352–57

46. Merutka, G., Stellwagen, E. 1990. *Biochemistry* 29: 894–98
47. Merutka, G., Stellwagen, E. 1991. *Biochemistry* 30: 1591–94
48. Merutka, G., Stellwagen, E. 1991. *Biochemistry* 30: 4245–48
49. Nagasawa, M., Holtzer, A. 1964. *J. Am. Chem. Soc.* 86: 538–43
50. Nelson, J. W., Kallenbach, N. R. 1986. *Proteins Struct. Funct. Genet.* 1: 211–17
51. O'Neil, K. T., DeGrado, W. F. 1990. *Science* 250: 646–51
52. Ösapay, G., Taylor, J. W. 1990. *J. Am. Chem. Soc.* 112: 6046–51
53. Osterhout, J. J., Baldwin, R. L., York, E. J., Stewart, J. M., Dyson, H. J., Wright, P. E. 1989. *Biochemistry* 28: 7059–64
54. Padmanabhan, S., Baldwin, R. L. 1991. *J. Mol. Biol.* 219: 135–37
55. Padmanabhan, S., Marqusee, S., Ridgeway, T., Laue, T. M., Baldwin, R. L. 1990. *Nature (London)* 344: 268–70
56. Pauling, L., Corey, R. B., Branson, H. R. 1951. *Proc. Natl. Acad. Sci. USA* 37: 205–11
57. Pease, J. H. B., Storrs, R. W., Wemmer, D. E. 1990. *Proc. Natl. Acad. Sci. USA* 87: 5643–5647
58. Poland, D., Scheraga, H. A. 1970. *Theory of Helix-Coil Transitions in Biopolymers.* New York: Academic
59. Ptitsyn, O. B. 1972. *Pure Appl. Chem.* 31: 227–44
60. Qian, H., Schellman, J. A. 1992. *J. Phys. Chem.* Submitted
61. Rialdi, G., Hermans, J. Jr. 1966. *J. Am. Chem. Soc.* 88: 5719–20
62. Rico, M., Gallego, E., Santor, J., Bermejo, F. J., Nieto, J. L., Herranz, J. 1984. *Biochem. Biophys. Res. Commun.* 123: 757–63
63. Rico, M., Nieto, J. L., Santor, J., Bermejo, F. J., Herranz, J., Gallego, E. 1983. *FEBS Lett.* 162: 314–19
64. Robert, C. H. 1990. *Biopolymers* 30: 335–47
65. Deleted in proof
66. Ruan, F., Chen, Y., Hopkins, P. B. 1990. *J. Am. Chem. Soc.* 112: 9403–4
67. Schellman, J. A. 1955. *C. R. Trav. Lab. Carlsberg Ser. Chim.* 29: 223–29
68. Schellman, J. A. 1955. *C. R. Trav. Lab. Carlsberg Ser. Chim.* 29: 230–59
69. Schellman, J. A. 1958. *J. Phys. Chem.* 62: 1485–94
70. Scholtz, J. M., Marqusee, S., Baldwin, R. L., York, E. J., Stewart, J. M., et al. 1991. *Proc. Natl. Acad. Sci. USA* 88: 2854–58
71. Scholtz, J. M., Qian, H., York, E. J., Stewart, J. M., Baldwin, R. L. 1991. *Biopolymers.* In press
72. Scholtz, J. M., York, E. J., Stewart, J. M., Baldwin, R. L. 1991. *J. Am. Chem. Soc.* 113: 5102–4
73. Shoemaker, K. R., Fairman, R., Kim, P. S., York, E. J., Stewart, J. M., Baldwin, R. L. 1987. *Cold Spring Harbor Symp. Quant. Biol.* 52: 391–98
74. Shoemaker, K. R., Fairman, R., Schultz, D. A., Robertson, A. D., York, E. J., et al. 1990. *Biopolymers* 29: 1–11
75. Shoemaker, K. R., Kim, P. S., Brems, D. N., Marqusee, S., York, E. J., et al. 1985. *Proc. Natl. Acad. Sci. USA* 82: 2349–53
76. Shoemaker, K. R., Kim, P. S., York, E. J., Stewart, J. M., Baldwin, R. L. 1987. *Nature* 326: 563–67
76a. Stahmann, M. A., ed. 1962. *Polyamino Acids, Polypeptides and Proteins.* Madison: Univ. Wis. Press
77. Strehlow, K. G., Baldwin, R. L. 1989. *Biochemistry* 28: 2130–33
78. Strehlow, K. G., Robertson, A. D., Baldwin, R. L. 1991. *Biochemistry* 30: 5810–14
79. Sueki, M., Lee, S., Powers, S. P., Denton, J. B., Konishi, Y., Scheraga, H. A. 1984. *Macromolecules* 17: 148–55
80. Takahashi, S., Kim, E.-H., Hibino, T., Ooi, T. 1989. *Biopolymers* 28: 995–1009
81. Taniuchi, H., Anfinsen, C. B. 1969. *J. Biol. Chem.* 244: 3864–75
82. Tidor, B., Karplus, M. 1991. *Biochemistry* 30: 3217–28
83. Tirado-Rives, J., Jorgensen, W. L. 1991. *Biochemistry* 30: 3864–71
84. Vasquez, M., Scheraga, H. A. 1988. *Biopolymers* 27: 41–58
85. Von Dreele, P. H., Lotan, N., Ananthanarayanan, V. S., Andreatta, R. H., Poland, D., Scheraga, H. A. 1971. *Macromolecules* 4: 408–17
86. Wada, A. 1976. *Adv. Biophys.* 9: 1–63
87. Wang, C.-L., Chalovich, J. M., Graceffa, P., Lu, R. C., Mabuchi, K., Stafford, W. F. 1991. *J. Biol. Chem.* 266: 13958–63
88. Wójcik, J., Altmann, K.-H., Scheraga, H. A. 1990. *Biopolymers* 30: 121–34
89. Wright, P. E., Dyson, H. J., Lerner, R. A. 1988. *Biochemistry* 27: 7167–75
90. Yun, R. H., Anderson, A., Hermans, J. 1991. *Proteins Struct. Funct. Genet.* 10: 219–28
91. Zimm, B. H. 1962. See Ref 76a, pp. 229–33
92. Zimm, B. H., Bragg, J. K. 1959. *J. Chem. Phys.* 31: 526–35
93. Zimm, B. H., Doty, P., Iso, K. 1959. *Proc. Natl. Acad. Sci. USA* 45: 1601–7
94. Zimm, B. H., Rice, S. A. 1960. *Mol. Phys.* 3: 391–407

Annu. Rev. Biophys. Biomol. Struct. 1992. 21:119–43

RUBISCO: Structure and Mechanism

Gunter Schneider, Ylva Lindqvist, and Carl-Ivar Brändén

Department of Molecular Biology, Swedish University of Agricultural Sciences, Biomedical Center, Box 590, S-751 24 Uppsala, Sweden

KEY WORDS: ribulose-1,5-bisphosphate carboxylase, X-ray crystallography, photosynthesis, photorespiration, protein engineering

CONTENTS

PERSPECTIVES AND OVERVIEW

Solar energy that is captured and converted to chemical energy during photosynthesis sustains almost all lifeforms on earth. Most of this energy is stored by converting CO_2 to polymerized sugar molecules from which most nonphotosynthetic organisms ultimately obtain the energy needed to drive their cellular reactions. The initial step in this photosynthetic fixation of CO_2, the carboxylation of ribulose-1,5-bisphosphate (RuBP), is

119

1056–8700/92/0610–0119$02.00

catalyzed by the enzyme ribulose-1,5-bisphosphate carboxylase oxygenase (Rubisco). This enzyme is responsible for the annual net fixation of 10^{11} tons of CO_2 from the atmosphere to the biosphere. This amount can be compared to our annual net consumption of crude oil, which is about 3×10^9 tons.

Rubisco is perhaps the most abundant protein on earth; it is certainly the most abundant enzyme: up to 50% of leaf proteins in plants are Rubisco. This large amount does not result primarily from the enormous task the enzyme has to carry out, but rather reflects the catalytic inefficiency of Rubisco as a catalyst, which is manifested by a turnover number of $3 \, s^{-1}$.

Not only is the enzyme slow, it also catalyzes a competing oxygenase reaction that leads to loss of energy by photorespiration. In this reaction, O_2 instead of CO_2 is added to RuBP, yielding phosphoglycolate as one of the oxidation products. Phosphoglycolate is metabolized in the glycolate pathway, which eventually produces CO_2 and energy in the form of heat. The net efficiency of photosynthesis is reduced by up to 50% by this photorespiratory pathway, which also severely affects a plant's water-use efficiency and nitrogen budget.

For these reasons, genetic redesign of Rubisco with the aim of constructing transgenic plants with improved photosynthetic efficiency and thereby increased agricultural productivity has attracted a lot of interest. Detailed kinetic studies of the catalytic reactions of Rubisco have been carried out during the past two decades and are summarized in several excellent reviews (10, 47, 48, 79, 96). This review describes recent advances in our knowledge of the molecular details of the enzyme's function that have emerged from genetic and X-ray structural studies.

PHYSIOLOGICAL AND GENETIC ASPECTS

Photosynthesis and Photorespiration

Rubisco is one of the key enzymes in the carbon metabolism of plants. The enzyme catalyzes the initial step in CO_2 fixation, the carboxylation of RuBP, yielding two molecules of phosphoglycerate. RuBP, the initial CO_2 acceptor, is regenerated in the Calvin cycle, and the fixed carbon is incorporated into carbohydrates such as sucrose and starch. The oxygenation of RuBP results in the formation of one molecule of phosphoglycerate, which can be metabolized in the Calvin cycle, and one molecule of phosphoglycolate. To salvage some of the carbon of phosphoglycolate, C-3 plants have developed the glycolate pathway, in which some of the phosphoglycolate is converted to phosphoglycerate. This rescue pathway consumes considerable amounts of energy, however, and 50% of the carbon is still lost as CO_2.

Carboxylation and oxygenation of RuBP occur at the same catalytic site of Rubisco; both gaseous substrates compete for the second substrate, RuBP. Therefore, the ratio of carboxylation towards oxygenation is influenced by the relative concentrations of CO_2 and O_2. Higher CO_2 concentrations result in more efficient photosynthesis with faster production of biomass (52). The present efforts to increase the concentration of atmospheric CO_2 might result in higher agricultural yields on a global scale. A doubling of atmospheric CO_2 concentration is expected to increase agricultural yields by approximately 33% (72).

Rubisco activity is highly regulated in vivo. A wealth of experimental data has accumulated showing that regulation operates at transcriptional as well as translational and posttranslational levels. Andrews & Lorimer (10) and Gutteridge & Gatenby (48) recently summarized the complicated patterns of Rubisco regulation.

Synthesis and Assembly

Rubisco from higher plants and most photosynthetic microorganisms is built up of two types of subunits, large (L chain, $M = 52,000–55,000$) and small (S chain, $M = 13,000$). The holoenzyme is a complex of eight L and eight S subunits (L_8S_8 Rubisco) forming a molecule with 422 symmetry (13). The only well-established exceptions from this quaternary structure are the enzymes found in the photosynthetic bacteria *Rhodospirillum rubrum* (121, 138) and *Rhodobacter sphaeroides* (44). These organisms contain a simpler type of Rubisco that consists of only two large subunits (L_2 Rubisco). Interestingly, *R. sphaeroides* also expresses an L_8S_8 Rubisco (44).

The genes for the L_8S_8 Rubisco molecule from higher plants are present in two different genomes. The gene for the L subunit is part of the chloroplast genome, whereas the S subunits are coded by the nuclear genome. Each chloroplast DNA molecule has only one gene for the L subunit. Even though each chloroplast contains several DNA molecules and each cell contains hundreds of chloroplasts, a nonhybrid plant will have only one unique sequence for all L subunit proteins. In contrast, a family of genes on the nuclear genome codes for the S subunits. These genes are strongly homologous. For example in *Arabidopsis thaliana*, four genes have been identified that show more than 90% sequence identity in their gene products (75). The S-subunit genes are differentially expressed in different cell types, but specific functional roles for individual genes have not been demonstrated (31, 102). Amino acid sequences are known for about 20 different L chains from various species and 35 different S chains, mostly deduced from the corresponding genes or cDNA sequences.

S subunits are translated as preproteins that contain an extra peptide of about 50 residues at the amino end of the polypeptide chain. This peptide directs the S subunit into the chloroplast, where it is cleaved off after passage of the preprotein through the membranes (29).

Assembly of the L subunits with mature S subunits inside the chloroplast is mediated by a chaperone protein, Rubisco binding protein (16, 101, 117). This protein, which is present in large amounts in plants, belongs to the chaperonin family, one member of which is the classic chaperone protein GroEL from *Escherichia coli* (43). The Rubisco binding protein and GroEL show about 50% amino acid sequence identity (56). The chaperonin protein is believed to prevent improper aggregation of L subunits by protecting exposed hydrophobic surfaces during the last stages of the folding or assembly process (34, 45).

The gene for the *R. rubrum* L subunit has been cloned and expressed in *E. coli* (104, 130). Functional L_2 molecules are obtained in high yield (111), and this system has been extensively used for site-directed mutagenesis experiments to probe the function of critical residues in the active site (50, 51, 53, 55, 77, 78, 100, 107, 131, 132, 142). In contrast, expression in *E. coli* of Rubisco L- and S-subunit genes from higher plants yield insoluble aggregates with no catalytic activity (40, 42). The subunits do not assemble into functional L_8S_8 molecules, presumably because of lack of proper chaperone proteins. However, L and S subunits from cyanobacteria obtained by coexpression in *E. coli* of the corresponding genes assemble into catalytically competent L_8S_8 molecules. In these cyanobacteria, the genes for Rubisco L and S subunits are on the same operon, and apparently assembly does not require cyanobacterial chaperone proteins. This is the system of choice for making and analyzing mutations in the S subunit (28, 38, 41, 46, 70, 139).

CHEMICAL MECHANISM

Activation—the Ternary Complex of Enzyme, CO_2, and $Mg(II)$

A common feature of all Rubisco molecules analyzed so far is a chemical modification step necessary to convert the enzyme from its inactive to its active form. The activation process consists of the formation of a carbamate group by reaction of a CO_2 molecule with the ε-amino group of a lysine residue at the active site (80, 87). This activator CO_2 molecule is separate from the CO_2 molecule that becomes incorporated into RuBP during catalysis (81, 95). Formation of the carbamate is followed by rapid binding of Mg(II), resulting in the active ternary complex—enzyme, CO_2, and Mg(II) (81, 84).

In the ternary complex, the Mg(II) ion can be replaced by several different metal ions such as Mn(II), Fe(II), Ca(II), Cu(II), Co(II), and Ni(II). However, the degree of catalytic activity depends both on the type of metal and the type of Rubisco. In L_2 Rubisco, catalytic activity has been observed upon replacement of Mg(II) by Fe(II), Ca(II), and Cu(II) (26, 27, 106, 113, 116, 133). In the L_8S_8 enzyme, activity has been observed with Mg(II), Ni(II), Co(II), Fe(II), Mn(II), and Cu(II) (19, 20, 26, 27, 146, 147). A very interesting observation is that the metal bound at the activator site can influence partitioning between carboxylation and oxygenation. Rubisco molecules from *R. rubrum* activated with Co(II) (26, 116) and from spinach activated with Cu(II) (19) are active as oxygenases, but lack carboxylase activity. This indicates an intimate involvement of the metal ion in at least one catalytic event: the addition of the gaseous substrate, CO_2 or O_2, respectively, to RuBP.

Formation of the carbamylated ternary complex is accompanied by changes in the chemical properties of the enzyme. Carbamylation affects the reactivity and nucleophilicity of certain lysine residues at the active site, reflected by different chemical labeling patterns observed in experiments with affinity labels (39, 57) or group-specific reagents (54). Also, the affinities for the substrate RuBP (66) and other phosphorylated compounds (68, 94) are influenced by the carbamylation state of the enzyme.

Overall Carboxylation Reaction

This review focuses on the carboxylation reaction of Rubisco, which is far better understood than the oxygenation reaction. Carboxylation of RuBP is a complicated reaction that involves a series of events and several intermediates. A preliminary mechanism for the carboxylation reaction, which has subsequently been modified, was first proposed by Calvin (21). The overall reaction can be divided into a number of individual steps (Figure 1). This overall scheme is supported by many isotope-labeling experiments. Lorimer (79) provides an excellent summary of these data. The first step in this mechanism is the enolization of RuBP, resulting in the 2,3 enediol(ate). Carboxylation at the nucleophilic center at C-2 creates a six-carbon intermediate 2-carboxy-3-keto-arabinitol 1,5 bisphosphate (3-keto-CABP), which undergoes hydration to the gem diol form. Deprotonation of the gem diol at O-3 of the six-carbon intermediate initiates carbon-carbon cleavage that results in one molecule of 3-P-glycerate and the C-2 carbanion form of another 3-P-glycerate molecule. The carbanion is then stereospecifically protonated at C-2, yielding the second 3-P-glycerate molecule. The release of products completes the catalytic cycle.

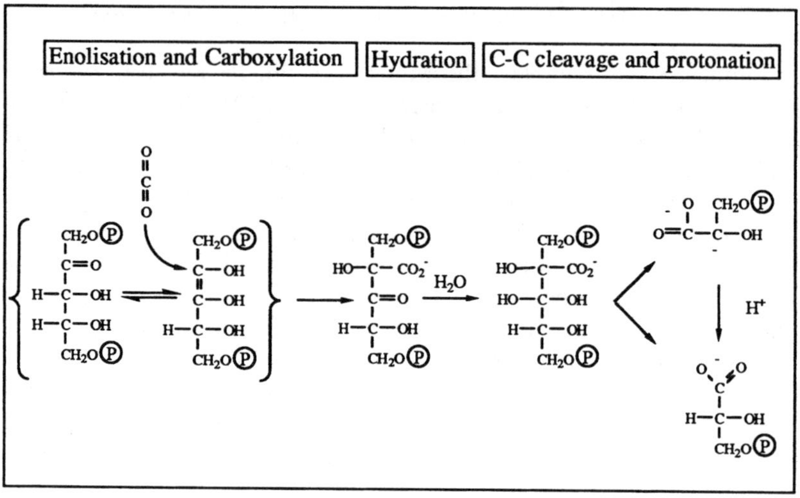

Figure 1 Mechanism of the carboxylation reaction.

Partial Reactions and Reaction Intermediates

ENOLIZATION OF RuBP: THE 2,3 ENEDIOL(ATE)   Enolization of bound RuBP is considered to be the very first step in the catalytic cycle. In fact, this step is common to both the carboxylation and oxygenation reactions. Enolization, which is initiated by abstraction of the C-3 proton of the substrate, leads to formation of the 2,3 enediol(ate) of RuBP as the first intermediate during turnover. This partial reaction, the exchange of the proton at C-3 of RuBP, can be followed by the wash in of solvent ^{3}H into C-3 of RuBP and the wash out of [3-^{3}H]RuBP into the solvent (119, 136).

CARBOXYLATION: 3-keto-CABP   At the stage of the 2,3 enediol(ate), the reaction proceeds either towards carboxylation or oxygenation. In both reactions, the gaseous substrates, CO_2 or O_2, respectively, react with the C-2 carbon atom of RuBP. Electrophilic attack of CO_2 on the C-2 carbon atom yields the six-carbon intermediate, 3-keto-CABP. After acid quenching of the carboxylation reaction, the intermediate can be trapped by borohydride reduction to the corresponding 2' carboxypentitol bisphosphate (120). The borohydride reduction of the intermediate occurs only in free solution, not when bound to the enzyme. This probably results from the fact that the six-carbon intermediate exists on the enzyme predominantly as the hydrated C-3 gem diol, which cannot be reduced by borohydride (83).

One of the unique features of the carboxylation reaction is that the intermediate 3-keto-CABP can be isolated and is surprisingly stable (83, 110). By acid quenching of the reaction, sacrificing large amounts of enzyme, the intermediate can be isolated and stored at $-80°C$ for months. At room temperature, 3-keto-CABP is reasonably stable: it decarboxylates with a half-time of approximately 1 h (83).

HYDRATION AND CARBON-CARBON BOND CLEAVAGE: THE GEM DIOL   On the enzyme, the intermediate 3-keto-CABP exists predominantly in the gem diol form, resulting from the addition of a water or hydroxide molecule to the C-3 carbon atom. The O-3 oxygen of RuBP is completely retained during carboxylation (82, 135). Thus, the hydration step is either kinetically reversible and/or stereospecific. Abstraction of a proton from the gem diol initiates carbon-carbon bond cleavage between C-2 and C-3, yielding one molecule of 3-phospho-glycerate and the C-2 carbanion of 3-phospho-glycerate.

The isolated 3-keto-CABP can be added back to the enzyme and is then hydrolyzed to products. However, Rubisco catalyzes the hydrolysis of 3-keto-CABP at rates that are only 3% of the maximal rate of carboxylation. This discrepancy between rates of carboxylation and hydrolysis led Cleland (30) to question the kinetic competence of 3-keto-CABP as a true reaction intermediate. He suggests a modified mechanism in which the carboxylation and the hydration steps occur in a concerted reaction, resulting in the gem diol. Therefore, in his proposal, 3-keto-CABP is not a true reaction intermediate. However, other effects might cause the observed discrepancy in reaction rates (see below), and in our opinion, the experimental evidence for 3-keto-CABP as a reaction intermediate (summarized in 10) is compelling.

The availability of the six-carbon intermediate provides another partial reaction for probing the functional defects of site-directed mutants. Mutant Rubiscos deficient in the overall carboxylation reaction might be able to catalyze the hydrolysis of the six-carbon intermediate to products. One can thus distinguish between mutants deficient in the enolization reaction, verified by the wash in or wash out experiments, or mutants deficient in one of the subsequent steps of catalysis.

PROTONATION: THE C-2 CARBANION   The carbon-carbon bond cleavage of the gem diol results in the formation of one molecule of 3-phosphoglycerate and one molecule of the C-2 carbanion of 3-phosphoglycerate. However, no firm experimental evidence for the existence of the C-2 carbanion as an intermediate has been obtained so far. Stereochemical considerations (10) suggest that the enzymic base donating the proton to the C-2 carbanion is different from the groups involved in proton-proton transfer during the earlier enolization-carboxylation steps of catalysis.

THREE-DIMENSIONAL STRUCTURE

The Overall Structure of Rubisco as Revealed by Protein Crystallography

Because of the central role of Rubisco in the carbon cycle, several groups are engaged in crystallographic studies of this enzyme from various sources. Crystallographic studies of Rubisco were first reported for the enzyme from tobacco (12, 13). These low resolution studies indicated that the molecule was a two-layered structure with 422 symmetry. The studies also showed a central channel running through the molecule. However, the crystals used were not sufficiently well ordered to allow structure determination to high resolution. Subsequently, preliminary crystallographic data were reported for the homodimeric enzyme from R. $rubrum$ (25, 63, 122, 123) and for the L_8S_8 molecule from tobacco (14, 137), spinach (1, 3, 15), potato (65), $Alcaligenes\ eutrophus$ (18, 109), $Chromatium$ $vinosum$ (103), and $Synecococcus$ (105).

Following the initial reports, the structure of the nonactivated $R.\ rubrum$ enzyme was solved to 2.9-Å resolution (125). This study revealed the two-domain structure of the L subunit, with one smaller N-terminal domain and a larger C-terminal domain folded as an eight-stranded parallel α/β barrel, and also located the active site in the subunit interface at the C-terminal end of the β strands in the α/β barrel. The model of the non-activated enzyme from $R.\ rubrum$ has now been refined to 1.7-Å resolution (126). The structures of several different complexes of Rubisco from $R.$ $rubrum$ have also been reported (89–92).

Chapman et al (22, 23) reported preliminary descriptions of the non-activated L_8S_8 enzyme from tobacco at 3.0-Å and 2.6-Å resolution. Andersson et al (2) described the active site of Rubisco based on the structure of nonactivated $R.\ rubrum$ enzyme and activated spinach Rubisco complexed with 2-carboxy arabinitol 1,5 bisphosphate (CABP), an analog of the six-carbon intermediate. Knight et al (73) described the fold of the small subunit that in the work by Chapman et al (23) had not been correctly determined. Knight et al (74) provided a complete description of the spinach Rubisco structure refined at 2.4-Å resolution.

THE L SUBUNIT   The catalytic activity of Rubisco resides on the L subunit, the structure of which is very similar in L_2 and L_8S_8 Rubisco (124) despite the low amino acid sequence identity, 28%. The L subunit consists of two clearly separated domains (Figure 2). The N-terminal domain, residues 1–150,[1] is folded into a central mixed five-stranded β-sheet with two α-helices

---

[1] All sequence numbering is based on the amino acid sequence of Rubisco from spinach. In the case of the L subunits, this is the unified numbering system as suggested in Schneider et al (124).

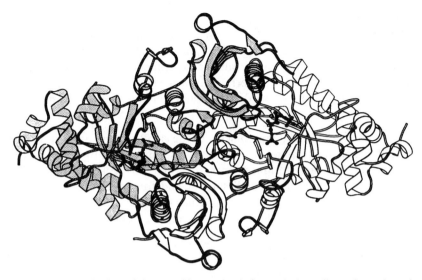

Figure 2 Schematic view of the L₂ Rubisco molecule from *Rhodospirillum rubrum*. One of the two L subunits is shown in gray. Bound substrate, ribulose bisphosphate, is included.

on one side of the sheet. The larger C-terminal α/β barrel domain consists of amino acids 151–475. This structural motif has been observed in many functionally nonrelated enzymes with completely different amino acid sequences (36).

Eight consecutive $\beta\alpha$ units are folded such that the β-strands form the core of a barrel surrounded on the outside by the eight α-helices. The active site is located at the carboxyl side of the β-strands; several of the last residues in the β-strands, or the first residues in the loops between the strands and helices, are involved in catalysis.

THE L₂ DIMER: THE MINIMAL FUNCTIONAL UNIT   The L₂ dimer has the shape of a distorted ellipsoid with dimensions $45 \times 70 \times 105$ Å and tight interactions between the subunits. The core of the molecule is made up of the C-terminal domains from both subunits. The contacts at the interface between these domains involve interactions of the loops between the carboxyl ends of the β strands and the α-helices from the α/β barrels across the local two-fold axis of the molecule.

The second contact area between the subunits involves the active site at the carboxy terminii of the β strands in the α/β barrel of the C-terminal domain. This side of the barrel is partly covered by the N-terminal domain of the other subunit, and residues from both domains contribute to the formation of the active site. This interaction area includes an intricate network of charges and hydrogen bonds involving conserved sidechains. Replacing one of these, Lys175, with an aspartate sidechain (78) disrupts the balance of charges, and the repulsion prevents dimerization. In addition, site-directed double mutant experiments have shown that the active site is located at the interface between subunits (77). Thus, because of this subunit packing, the dimer of large subunits is the minimal functional unit.

THE S SUBUNIT   The 123 amino acids of the small subunit are arranged in a four-stranded anti-parallel β-sheet covered on one side by two α-helices. The amino-terminal residues form an arm of irregular structure that extends to a neighboring small subunit and forms the interaction area between small subunits that form S_4 clusters. Structure determination of the spinach enzyme revealed deviations from the published sequence (93).

THE L_8S_8 MOLECULE   The L_8S_8 molecule is shaped like a cube with rounded edges and sides of approximately 110 Å each. The fundamental unit of the L_8 part of the molecule is the L_2 dimer. Each small subunit binds in a deep crevice formed between the tips of two adjacent elongated L_2 dimers at each end of the L_8S_8 molecule. Four faces of the cube-shaped molecule are thus formed from pairs of adjacent L_2 dimers, whereas the remaining two faces are formed by the S_4 clusters.

The interaction areas between the small and the large subunits are quite extensive in L_8S_8 Rubisco and involve several regions of residues that are conserved in all small subunits. Some of these have been probed in the *Anabena eutrophus* enzyme with mutations (38) that give subunits that do not assemble with the L subunits to form functional L_8S_8 molecules. One of these mutations (Glu13-Val) disrupts a network of ion-pair interactions and would bury an unbalanced positive charge, thus preventing assembly. Another mutant (Pro73-His) would result in burying a polar side chain in an otherwise very hydrophobic environment. Thus, it is not surprising that this mutant does not form a stable holoenzyme.

The surface of the L_2 dimer in the spinach L_8S_8 enzyme is somewhat less hydrophobic than expected (74) for a molecular entity involved in subunit interactions. Its surface is more like that of a monomer or a fully assembled oligomer, perhaps indicating an intermediate role for the dimer in the assembly process. This observation is also true for the $(L_2)_4$ core of large subunits. Nevertheless, researchers have been unable to isolate L subunits from plant Rubisco without concomittant aggregation and/or precipitation (67, 69, 118, 145), probably because of the exposure of highly hydrophobic patches on the surface of the L subunits upon release of S subunits. In contrast, in Rubisco from cyanobacteria in which the subunits can be easily separated to give isolated S subunits and stable $(L_2)_4$ cores

(5, 6, 11, 61, 62, 67, 140), several of these conserved hydrophobic residues are changed to polar or even charged side chains. The $(L_2)_4$ core Rubisco binds small subunits and reassembles to form a species indistinguishable from the native, undissociated enzyme. This phenomenon has been explored by constructing Rubisco hybrids with $(L_2)_4$ from one species and S subunits from another species (7, 9, 61, 144). The general conclusion from these experiments is that the hybrids show the character of the parent $(L_2)_4$ rather than the parent small subunit. In particular, they exhibit the same carboxylase/oxygenase ratio as the parent $(L_2)_4$.

Structural Differences Between the L_2- and L_8S_8-Type Rubisco: a Function of the Small Subunit

The small subunits profoundly influence the catalytic properties of L_8S_8 Rubisco (5, 6, 61, 62, 67, 140). The L_8 core of the enzyme retains a small intrinsic activity in the absence of small subunits (4). Structural studies (2, 22, 74) have shown that the small subunits do not contribute any residues to the active site. Thus, the dramatic effect of the small subunits on catalytic activity must be exerted by inducing long-range effects in the active site through interactions remote from the active site. Schneider et al (124) discussed how this might be accomplished, showing that the position of helix 8 with respect to the rest of the α/β barrel is different in the L_2 versus the L_8S_8 type of Rubisco. These structural differences extend to loop 8, which forms one of the phosphate binding sites in the active site, and to helix 7 and loop 7, which are also part of the active site and contain a strictly conserved serine residue involved in inhibitor, substrate, and product binding (2, 89, 90, 92). These structural differences could be the basis for the higher catalytic efficiencies of the L_8S_8 enzymes compared to *R. rubrum* Rubisco. The difference in structure is caused by the binding of small subunits that form extensive interactions with α-helix 8 and parts of loop 8. The position adopted by α-helix 8 in the *R. rubrum* enzyme would be sterically hindered in the L_8S_8 enzyme because of overlap with the small subunit. This conformational difference is also reflected in the C-terminal region of the L chain, which forms a helical extension to the α/β barrel. An intrinsic difference between the *R. rubrum* and the plant enzyme in this part of the structure is that the L_2 enzyme has two additional α-helices.

The C-terminal residues (459–466) of Rubisco from *R. rubrum* show a remote sequence homology to residues 13–20 of the small subunit of L_8S_8 Rubisco. A possible function of these residues as a substitute for the small subunit in L_2 Rubisco was tested by truncation of the polypeptide chain at position 458 (115) or 460 (98). The truncated chains form a mutant protein with almost undisturbed activities, showing that these residues are not essential for proper function. Truncation at positions 431 or 423 (115), which removes helices αG, αH, αI, and αJ, leads to insoluble protein aggregates because of the exposure of a hydrophobic patch at the surface of the mutant protein. Curiously, truncation at position 441 leads to the formation of an L_8 Rubisco, different in packing from the $(L_2)_4$ core of the higher plant enzymes. Disruption of the hydrophobic patch by site-directed mutagenesis prevents the formation of the L_8 particles (115).

Another species difference involves the N-terminal residues. The first α-helix in the *R. rubrum* enzyme is absent in the spinach enzyme. In the bacterial enzyme, this α-helix covers one side of the N-terminal β-sheet, which is thus more exposed in the spinach enzyme where the corresponding residues have the conformation of an extended chain. Differences in the N-terminal region might be of interest with regard to catalysis. Removal of the eight first residues in spinach (60) and wheat (49) Rubisco does not affect catalytic activity, whereas removal of six additional residues drastically reduces catalytic activity. The crystal structure of the spinach enzyme (74) shows that the side chain Phe13 is buried between the small subunit and the large subunit, causing extensive interactions. The dramatic effect on activity following removal of residues 8–14 in the large subunit indicates that the interactions in this area are important to maintain a catalytically competent enzyme.

The Active Site

The active site of Rubisco is located at the interface between the C-terminal domain of one subunit and the N-terminal domain of the second subunit (2, 22, 125). As in all α/β barrel enzymes known so far, the active site is found at the carboxy ends of the β-strands of the barrel. Residues in the loops from the β-strands to the α-helices of the barrel contain most of the conserved amino acid side chains essential for substrate binding and catalysis.

Loop 1 contains the sequence Lys175-Pro176-Lys177, which is conserved in all Rubisco molecules. In all Rubisco structures determined at sufficiently high resolution, the proline peptide bond is in the *cis*-conformation.

Lys175 has been identified as an active-site residue through affinity labeling (58), crystallography (2, 23, 89, 125), and site-directed mutagenesis (55). The side chain of Lys177 also points into the active site and interacts with the side chains of Glu60 and Glu204. Both lysine residues are part of a complicated network of charges and hydrogen bonds, involving residues Glu60, Lys175, Lys177, Asp203, and Glu204. The disruption of this delicate balance of charges by site-directed mutagenesis severely affects tertiary and quaternary structure. Substitution of Asp203 with Asn induces local and global conformational changes (E. Söderlind, G. Schneider & S.

Gutteridge, unpublished results), whereas the replacement of Lys175 with an aspartic acid side chain prevents the formation of dimers (78).

Loop 2 also contains several conserved amino acid residues, Lys201, Asp203, and Glu204. These three amino acids form the activator site. The side chain of Lys201 becomes carbamylated during activation, and the carbamate, together with the side chains of Asp203 and Glu204, forms the metal-binding site (2, 91, 92).

Loops 3 and 4 are involved in subunit-subunit interactions, but do not contribute any residues directly involved in catalysis or substrate binding. In the enzyme from *R. rubrum*, Asp245 forms a bifurcate hydrogen bond to the main-chain nitrogen atoms of residues 113 and 114 at the N-terminal end of helix αC in the N-terminal domain of the second subunit (126).

Loop 5 contains two conserved histidine residues, His294 and His298. His294 is close to the bound substrate and inhibitor and has been implicated in catalysis (2, 74, 92). The function of His298 has been probed using site-directed mutagenesis. Substitution of this side chain by Ala produces a mutant enzyme with 40% activity (107), demonstrating that this residue is not essential for catalytic activity. A conserved arginine residue, Arg295, within this loop is involved in the binding of one of the phosphate groups of CABP (2, 90) or RuBP (92).

Loop 6 is a flexible loop that is disordered in the crystals of nonactivated Rubisco from *R. rubrum* (125, 126). In those structures, where this loop is ordered, it has been observed in both an open and a closed conformation (2, 32, 74). The closed conformation is found in complexes of the activated enzyme with the inhibitor CABP bound at the active site (2, 32). A conserved lysine residue, Lys334, resides on this loop.

Loop 7 contains a conserved serine residue involved in the binding of product (89), inhibitor CABP (2, 90), and substrate RuBP (92). Loop 8 forms a short, glycine-rich helix that is part of the second phosphate binding site.

Two regions from the N-terminal domain of the second subunit are close to the active site and are in fact involved in substrate binding. One region comprises residues 58–78. This peptide segment contains the highly conserved sequence 58–65. The side chain of Glu60 at the end of helix αC is involved in a subunit-subunit interaction across the active site. Residues 66–76 form a loop that is disordered in nonactivated Rubisco from *R. rubrum* (125, 126). In the quaternary complex of Rubisco from spinach and tobacco (2, 32, 74), this loop partly covers the active site, and some of its residues are in van der Waals contact to the substrate.

The second region from the N-terminal domain that contributes to the active site consists of residues 122–130. This loop contains the conserved residue Asn123. In the activated complex of Rubisco from *R. rubrum* (91), this side chain is part of the coordination sphere of the metal ion. Upon binding of the substrate RuBP, this ligand is replaced by oxygen atoms from the substrate, and Asn123 interacts with the C-4 hydroxyl group of RuBP (92). This interaction is conserved in the quaternary complex with CABP (2, 74). Electron paramagnetic resonance (EPR) measurements with Cu(II)-substituted Rubisco are in agreement with these observations. In the ternary complex, enzyme-CO_2-Cu(II), the EPR spectra show a nitrogen hyperfine splitting and suggest a nitrogen ligand close to the metal ion (134). Upon addition of substrate or inhibitor, this hyperfine structure disappears, indicating coordination of Cu(II) only to oxygen atoms in the quaternary complex.

Binding of Phosphorylated Compounds to Rubisco

The structure of two complexes of phosphorylated sugar compounds with nonactivated Rubisco have been determined (89, 90). The binding of the product, phosphoglycerate (PGA), revealed the location of the active site and one of the phosphate binding sites. The phosphate group is bound close to loops 5 and 6 with residues Arg295, His327, and main-chain nitrogen atoms of residues 328 and 329 interacting with the phosphate group. Furthermore, the side chain of Ser379 from loop 7 forms a hydrogen bond to the bridging oxygen atom of the phosphate group. The carboxyl group of PGA interacts with the side chain of Lys201. This side chain is changed to a negatively charged carbamate during activation and changes its character from an anion-binding site to a metal-binding center.

Nonactivated Rubisco binds the inhibitor CABP across the active site, with one of the phosphate groups bound at the binding site close to loops 5 and 6 described above. The second phosphate binding site is located on the other side of the barrel, close to loop 8. The phosphate group interacts with the main chain nitrogen of conserved residue 403, which is located at the N-terminal end of a very short helix. Other interactions with the enzyme are through hydrogen bonds and salt bridges with Lys175, Lys334, and Asn123.

The crystal structure analysis of the quaternary complex of spinach Rubisco with bound inhibitor CABP (2, 74) provided the first evidence of the binding of substrate analogs to the active site of the activated enzyme. Studies of the activated complex of tobacco Rubisco with CABP (32) confirmed these results and demonstrated the high similarity of the active sites of the two L_8S_8 enzymes. A schematic view of the interactions of the analog with the active site of Rubisco is shown in Figure 3. The reaction intermediate analog binds in an extended conformation at the active site. The two phosphate groups bind at the two phosphate sites of the α/β barrel. The P1 phosphate interacts with the main-chain nitrogens of residues 403

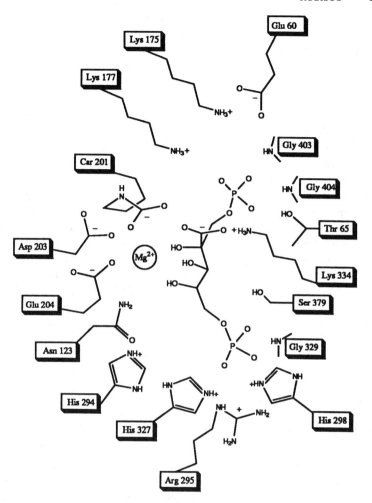

Figure 3 Schematic view of the inhibitor CABP bound at the active site of spinach Rubisco.

and 404 of the short helix in loop 8 as well as with the main-chain nitrogen of residue 381 of loop 7. A hydrogen bond to the side chain of Thr65 and two salt links, involving Lys175 and Lys334, also contribute to the interactions at that phosphate-binding site (74). The P2 phosphate-binding site is formed by residues Arg295, His327, and Ser379. One of the oxygen atoms of the 2-carboxyl group that simulates the substrate CO_2 after the carboxylation event is a ligand to the Mg(II) ion. The second oxygen forms a hydrogen bond to the side chain of the conserved Lys334. Two of the hydroxyl oxygen atoms of CABP are additional ligands to Mg(II). The remaining hydroxyl group forms a hydrogen bond to the side chain of the invariant residue Ser379. Other polar interactions of the analog with the groups on the enzyme are contacts to Asn123, Thr173, the main-chain nitrogen of residue 380, and the carbamate at 201. A comparison of the crystal structures of the complexes of activated and nonactivated Rubisco with CABP shows that the metal ion has a profound influence on the mode of inhibitor binding. In the complex with nonactivated enzyme, the inhibitor binds the other way around at the active site, with the phosphate groups interchanged at their respective binding sites, as compared with the quaternary complex of activated spinach Rubisco with CABP (90). The Mg(II) ion apparently plays an important role in orienting the analog and, by inference, the substrate into the proper, e.g. catalytically competent, binding mode at the active site.

In both structures of activated L_8S_8 Rubisco with CABP, loop 6 is observed in the closed conformation, i.e. it has folded across the active site and shields the substrate from the solution. This movement of loop 6 brings the side chain of Lys334 close enough to the reaction intermediate analog to form a hydrogen bond to the 2-carboxy group of CABP.

The binding of the substrate, RuBP, to activated crystals of Rubisco from *R. rubrum* has been studied to 2.6-Å resolution (92). The substrate binds in a rather bent conformation at the active site, with one of the phosphate groups at the phosphate binding site close to loops 5 and 6. The second phosphate interacts with residue 403 from the short helix in loop 8 and with the side chain of Lys175. Because of the different position of loops 7 and 8 and α-helix 8 in the L_2 Rubisco (124), the second phosphate-binding site is shifted in relation to its position in the L_8S_8 Rubisco. As a consequence of this species-dependent conformational difference, the substrate is bound in a more bent fashion to L_2 Rubisco than in the active site of L_8S_8 Rubisco.

The C-2 oxygen atom and the C-3 hydroxyl group are ligands to the Mg(II) ion. This interaction leads, after abstraction of the C-3 proton, to the formation of the *cis*-enediol. The limited resolution of the electron-density maps does not allow the conformation at the C-3 and C-4 atom of RuBP to be established with confidence. The C-4 hydroxyl group instead of the C-3 hydroxyl group may be ligand to the metal ion. In that case, the *trans*-enediol would be formed. With the present resolution of the electron-density maps, this issue cannot be settled. The refinement of the structure of the quaternary complex of spinach Rubisco with CABP to 1.7-Å resolution should settle this issue.

The crystals of Rubisco from *R. rubrum* are inactive; this fact allowed the structure determination of the RuBP complex. The reason for the catalytic deficiency is that loop 6 is still in an open conformation. This conformation is stabilized by crystal contacts. Lys334 forms a salt link to the side chains of Glu255 and Glu259 of a neighboring molecule in the crystal lattice, thereby preventing the loop movement necessary for catalysis.

Conformational Changes During Catalysis

Comparisons of the nonactivated forms of Rubisco from *R. rubrum* (125, 126) and tobacco (22, 23) with the quaternary CABP complexes of activated Rubisco from spinach (2, 74) and tobacco (32) reveal important conformational differences around the active site. In the activated quaternary complexes of both spinach and tobacco, loop 6 is folded over the CABP molecule so that the invariant residue Lys334 interacts with one of the oxygen atoms of the carboxyl group of CABP. In addition, this residue participates in salt bridges to both the phosphate group P1 and Glu60 in the N-terminal domain of the other subunit of the dimer. This loop has a different conformation and position in the nonactivated tobacco enzyme reflected by a difference in the α-carbon positions of residue 335 of 12.3 Å. In the nonactivated *R. rubrum* enzyme, this loop is disordered (residues 330 to 341) and not visible in the electron density maps at 1.7-Å resolution.

The C terminus from residue 460 and onwards extends towards the active site and folds over loop 6 in the activated ternary complexes. In the nonactivated tobacco enzyme, some of these residues are folded differently, and the remaining ones, after residue 468, are disordered. The conformational changes of these C-terminal residues are in all probability correlated to the movement of loop 6.

Thr65, which is involved in binding the phosphate group P1, is part of a loop region in the N-terminal domain that is close to the active site in the quaternary complexes. This loop is disordered in nonactivated Rubisco from both *R. rubrum* (residues 66–76) and tobacco (residues 64–68). The N-terminal residues 9 to 21 fold over this loop in the quaternary complexes but are disordered in the nonactivated tobacco enzyme. Presumably, the ordering of both loop 64–68 and the N terminus are correlated. Conformational changes of the N and C terminus are likely to be different in L_2 Rubisco, because both the N and C terminii are quite different in sequence as well as in structure in *R. rubrum* Rubisco. The crystallographic studies on the spinach and tobacco enzymes made clear that the suggested large conformational changes upon binding of CABP, based on the low resolution structure of Rubisco from *Alcaligenes eutrophus* (59), does not occur. For the tobacco enzyme, the structures of both the nonactivated and the activated quaternary complex with CABP are known (22, 23, 32). A comparison of these two structures shows that there is no sliding mechanism, which would translate the two L_4S_4 halves of the molecule across the dimer interface of the L_2 units.

In conclusion, the following structural changes are observed when going from the nonactivated enzyme to quaternary complexes that simulate the active site after CO_2 addition. Two loop regions, one from each domain, fold over the reaction intermediate analog and provide side chains that are directly involved in binding the analog. The N and C terminii are coupled to these changes so that they in turn fold over the loop regions, locking them in position. One effect of these structural changes is to shield the reaction intermediate analog almost completely from solution; a second effect is to bring binding residues into the active site.

These conformational changes might be the reason for the observed slow turnover of the six-carbon intermediate when given to the enzyme. The intermediate must bind to the active site, and the enzyme must then adopt the catalytically competent conformation, which might be the rate-limiting step. The binding of the reaction intermediate analog, CABP, is a two step process (114). The second step has a rate constant similar to that of the measured hydrolysis of the reaction intermediate (110).

STRUCTURE AND FUNCTION

Activation

Activation involves the condensation of CO_2 with an unprotonated Lys201 (80) to form a carbamate. Examination of the electrostatic field at the active site of the nonactivated enzyme can explain the high reactivity of Lys201 as compared with other lysine side chains (88). Lys201 is in an area of high positive potential, making it prone to release a proton and react with CO_2.

Considerable effort has been directed at analyzing the metal coordination in the activated enzyme species using EPR and NMR techniques. These analyses have shown that the carbamate is stabilized by binding of Me(II) (17, 81, 84). However, prior to the X-ray structure determination, all attempts to prove direct coordination of the carbamate oxygens failed. EPR measurements on Mn(II) or Cu(II) with ^{17}O-labeled carbamate in quaternary complexes of *R. rubrum* enzyme (97, 133, 134) could not demonstrate direct coordination, and ^{13}C-NMR experiments on E-CO_2-Me(II)-2CABP (113) only suggest that the metal is within 5–6 Å of the carbamate.

The only previous evidence on the coordination of the metal ion in the activated ternary complex of Rubisco was that the EPR-spectrum of Co(II) (106, 134) is not perturbed upon binding, indicating octahedral coordination with oxygen ligands only, while E-CO_2-Cu(II) enzyme yielded nitrogen hyperfine structure (19), suggesting at least one nitrogen atom coordinated to Cu(II).

Mutation of any of the residues involved in metal ion binding results in a catalytically inactive enzyme (85). Replacement of Lys201 by a glutamic acid side chain to mimic the carbamate resulted in an enzyme devoid of activity, corroborating the importance of a correctly positioned metal ion.

Although no large conformational changes occur upon activation of the enzyme, the microenvironment of the active site is greatly changed, which can explain the large difference in physical and chemical properties between the nonactivated and activated forms of the enzyme.

Enolization

The initial step in the enolization of the substrate RuBP is the abstraction of the C-3 proton. Much effort has been directed at identifying the enzymic base involved in this step. Unfortunately, biochemical and crystallographic data disagree on the identity of this group, and a combined effort of biochemical, mutagenesis, and crystallographic methods is needed to clarify this issue.

Based on biochemical and mutagenesis data, Lys175 was suggested as the base that abstracts the C-3 proton in the first step of the enolization reaction (55, 86). The evidence for this conclusion seemed compelling. Both affinity labeling and crystallographic studies showed that Lys175 resides at the active site. Biochemical data led to the conclusion that Lys175 has an unusually low pKa value of 7.8 (54), which agrees well with the pKa of 7.5 determined from the pH dependency of the deuterium isotopic effect for proton abstraction from C-3 of the substrate (143). Site-directed mutagenesis of this residue, replacing the lysine residue with glycine, alanine, serine, glutamine, arginine, cysteine, or histidine, results in mutant proteins severely deficient in carboxylase activity (55). The Gly mutant can undergo activation and bind CABP but cannot catalyze the enolization reaction (86). Furthermore, the initial crystallographic models of the active site of Rubisco (2) did not exclude such a function for this residue.

However, as refinement of the quaternary complex of spinach Rubisco proceeded and the crystal structure of the activated complex of Rubisco from *R. rubrum* with RuBP became available, a discrepancy between the postulated role of Lys175 and the observed structure of the active site became more and more clear (74, 92). In these structures, the Nε-nitrogen atom of the side chain is about 6 Å away from the C-3 atom of the substrate. Model-building experiments cannot bring this side chain close enough for proton abstraction without destroying the conformation of loop 1. A different conformation of loop 1 would in turn influence the interactions at the subunit-subunit interface, and such a conformational change seems unlikely. In fact, crystallographic studies have revealed conformational differences between L_2 and L_8S_8 Rubisco and between the nonactivated and quaternary complex of the enzyme. However, no differences in the conformation of loop 1 in any of the crystal structures determined so far have been observed. Furthermore, this loop contains a *cis*-Pro at position 176. Conformational changes in this loop would invoke a *cis-trans* isomerization of that peptide bond. *Cis-trans* isomerizations during folding of a protein are considered to be the rate-limiting step (71) and are often catalyzed by special enzymes, *cis-trans* isomerases (37, 141). It seems very unlikely that the catalytic mechanism of Rubisco would involve a slow *cis-trans* isomerization as a necessary step along the reaction route. Based on the crystal structure of the complex of Rubisco from *R. rubrum* with RuBP is the suggestion that the Lys175 side chain acts not as a base but as an acid and that it polarizes the C-2 oxygen bond, thus facilitating the abstraction of the C-3 proton (92). Depending on whether the resulting enediol(ate) would be in the *cis* or *trans* conformation, the P1 phosphate group, His294, a water molecule, or the carbamate could be possible proton abstractors. Clearly, this issue remains to be settled and more experiments are required.

A puzzling feature of Rubisco catalysis has been linked to the enolization reaction. Higher-plant Rubisco shows a decline in activity with time, giving rise to a nonlinear rate of conversion of RuBP to phosphoglycerate (8, 76, 99, 128). The inhibition of the spinach enzyme results from the tight binding of two phosphorylated compounds at the active site. One of these inhibitors was identified as D-xylulose 1,5 bisphosphate (33). This inhibitor is formed at the active site during turn-over, most probably by a stereochemically incorrect reprotonation of the 2,3 enediol(ate).

Carboxylation

The active site Mg(II) ion plays a crucial role in the mechanism of carboxylation by Rubisco (74, 85, 92). The 2,3 enediolate, which is necessary for CO_2 addition, is stabilized by coordination of its hydroxyl groups to Mg(II). Similar 2,3 enediolates are unstable in free solution and undergo β-elimination of the C-1 phosphate group (64, 108). The transition state for CO_2 addition is in all probability stabilized by coordination of one of the carboxyl oxygen atoms to Mg(II) because such a bond is present in the complex with the reaction intermediate analog, CABP. No kinetic evidence supports the formation of a Michaelis complex with CO_2 prior to the chemical reaction (112). However, the structure of the active site of Rubisco is compatible with such a complex. The Mg(II) ion in the quaternary complex with RuBP is accessible from solution and could form a transient $Mg-CO_2$ complex with the CO_2 group in a suitable position for the subsequent chemical reaction with the C-2 atom of RuBP.

The carboxyl group of the transition state adduct is also stabilized by interactions with the positive side chain of Lys334, as deduced from the structure of the quaternary CABP complex. This residue resides at the tip of loop 6, which undergoes a major conformational change from an open to a closed form during the reaction. Mutant Rubisco molecules in which Lys334 has been changed to other residues are severely deficient in carboxylase activity and bind the competitive inhibitor 6-phosphogluconate but do not form strong complexes with CABP (132).

Chen & Spreitzer (24) isolated from *Chlamydomonas reinhardtii* a Rubisco mutant in vivo in which a residue at the base of loop 6, Val331, was replaced by Ala. These mutant Rubisco molecules show a reduction of the CO_2/O_2 specificity of 37% in favor of oxygenation. The equivalent residue in the spinach enzyme, Val331, is at the rim of the hydrophobic pocket between β-strand 6 and α-helix 6 of the α/β barrel. The side chain of Val331 interacts directly with the side chain of Thr342 in this pocket. The mutation Val331 to Ala would be expected to create a hole in this hydrophobic pocket that could alter either the position or the conformation of loop 6 and hence change details of the interaction between Lys334 and the transition state. Interestingly, an intragenic suppressor mutation has been identified in *C. reinhardtii* (24) that increases the CO_2/O_2 specificity of the mutant enzyme by 33%. In this suppressor mutant, Thr 342 has been changed to Ile. The changes in this double mutant, Val331 to Ala and Thr342 to Ile, thus at least partially restored the hydrophobic pocket and hence the role of Lys334 in differentially stabilizing the transition states for carboxylation and oxygenation. The combination Ala331 and Ile342 is present in wild-type Rubisco molecules from *Anacystis nidulans* (127).

Lys334 interacts not only with the carboxyl group of CABP in the quaternary complex but also with the side chain of Glu60. Replacement of Glu60 by the shorter side chain of Asp drastically reduces the catalytic rate (100). The effects of a longer side chain have been explored through a combination of mutation and chemical modification (129). Glu60 was first mutated to Cys, which produced a catalytically inert mutant. Catalytic activity was restored by treating the mutant with iodacetate. The Cys side chain becomes carboxymethylated and an acidic side chain is produced that contains an extra sulfur atom compared to the Glu side chain. The catalytic rate of this Rubisco molecule has decreased 10-fold compared to wild-type Rubisco, and the CO_2/O_2 specificity has changed by a factor of five in favor of oxygenation. This is the first engineered mutant with a change in specificity, and as such demonstrates the possibility of altering the carboxylation/oxygenation ratio by rational design.

SUMMARY AND PROSPECTS

In this review, we have attempted to summarize current knowledge on the relationship between the three-dimensional structure and mechanism of Rubisco. Mapping the functional relationships between specific active-site residues and the catalytic mechanism for both oxygenation and carboxylation is a necessary requirement for attempts to modify the enzyme's substrate specificity towards a higher carboxylase activity. One of the greatest obstacles in this respect is the lack of knowledge of the oxygenase reaction both in chemical and structural terms. Whereas our understanding of the carboxylation reaction is proceeding by the combined efforts of biochemical, genetic, and protein crystallographic techniques, such progress for the oxygenase activity of Rubisco is not occurring. A different approach to deduce the features responsible for the partition between the carboxylase and oxygenase activity will be the comparison of the sequences and three-dimensional structures of Rubisco with different specificity factors.

Literature Cited

1. Andersson, I., Brändén, C.-I. 1984. *J. Mol. Biol.* 172: 363–66
2. Andersson, I., Knight, S., Schneider, G., Lindqvist, Y., Lundqvist, T., et al. 1989. *Nature* 337: 229–34
3. Andersson, I., Tjäder, A.-C., Cedergren-Zeppezauer, E., Brändén, C.-I. 1983. *J. Biol. Chem.* 258: 14088–90
4. Andrews, T. J. 1988. *J. Biol. Chem.* 263: 12213–19
5. Andrews, T. J., Abel, K. M. 1981. *J. Biol. Chem.* 256: 8445–51
6. Andrews, T. J., Ballment, B. 1983. *J. Biol. Chem.* 258: 7514–18
7. Andrews, T. J., Greenwood, D. M., Yellowlees, D. 1984. *Arch. Biochem. Biophys.* 234: 313–17
8. Andrews, T. J., Hatch, M. D. 1971. *Phytochemistry* 10: 9–15
9. Andrews, T. J., Lorimer, G. H. 1985. *J. Biol. Chem.* 260: 4632–36
10. Andrews, T. J., Lorimer, G. H. 1987. In *The Biochemistry of Plants*, ed. M. D. Hatch, 10: 131–218. Orlando, FL: Academic
11. Asami, S., Takabe, T., Akazawa, T., Codd, G. A. 1983. *Arch. Biochem. Biophys.* 225: 713–21
12. Baker, T. S., Eisenberg, D., Eiserling, F. A. 1977. *Science* 196: 293–95
13. Baker, T. S., Eisenberg, D., Eiserling, F. A., Weissman, L. 1975. *J. Mol. Biol.* 91: 391–99
14. Baker, T. S., Suh, S. W., Eisenberg, D. 1977. *Proc. Natl. Acad. Sci. USA* 74: 1037–41
15. Barcena, J. A., Pickersgill, R. W., Adams, M. J., Phillips, D. C., Whatley, F. R. 1983. *EMBO J.* 2: 2363–67
16. Barraclough, R., Ellis, R. J. 1980. *Biochim. Biophys. Acta* 608: 19–31
17. Belknap, W. R., Portis, A. R. 1986. *Biochemistry* 25: 1864–69
18. Bowien, B., Meyer, F., Spiess, E., Pähler, A., Englisch, U., et al. 1980. *Eur. J. Biochem.* 106: 405–10
19. Brändén, R., Nilson, T., Styring, S. 1984. *Biochemistry* 23: 4373–77
20. Brändén, R., Nilson, T., Styring, S. 1984. *Biochemistry* 23: 4378–82
21. Calvin, M. 1956. *J. Chem. Soc.* pp. 1876–1915
22. Chapman, M., Suh, S. W., Cascio, D., Smith, W. W., Eisenberg, D. 1987. *Nature* 329: 354–56
23. Chapman, M. S., Suh, S. W., Curmi,

P. M. G., Cascio, D., Smith W. W., et al. 1988. *Science* 24: 71–74
24. Chen, X., Spreitzer, R. J. 1989. *J. Biol. Chem.* 264: 3051–53
25. Choe, H.-W., Jakob, R., Hahn, U., Pal, G. P. 1985. *J. Mol. Biol.* 185: 781–83
26. Christeller, J. T. 1981. *Biochem. J.* 193: 839–44
27. Christeller, J. T., Laing, W. A. 1978. *Biochem. J.* 173: 467–73
28. Christeller, J. T., Terzaghi, B. E., Hill, D. F., Laing, W. A. 1985. *Plant Mol. Biol.* 5: 257–63
29. Chua, N.-H., Schmidt, G. W. 1979. *J. Cell Biol.* 81: 461–83
30. Cleland, W. W. 1990. *Biochemistry* 29: 3194–97
31. Coruzzi, G., Broglie, R., Cashmore, A., Chua, N.-H. 1983. *J. Biol. Chem.* 258: 1399–1402
32. Curmi, P. M. G., Schreuder, H., Cascio, D., Sweet, R., Eisenberg, D. 1991. *J. Biol. Chem.* In press
33. Edmondson, D. L., Kane, H. J., Andrews, T. J. 1990. *FEBS Lett.* 260: 62–66
34. Ellis, R. J. 1990. *Science* 250: 954–59
35. Deleted in proof
35. Estelle, M., Hanks, J., McIntosh, L., Somerville, C. 1985. *J. Biol. Chem.* 260: 9523–26
36. Farber, G. K., Petsko, G. A. 1990. *Trends Biochem. Sci.* 15: 228–34
37. Fischer, G., Wittmann-Liebold, B., Lang, K., Kiefhaber, T., Schmid, F. X. 1989. *Nature* 337: 476–78
38. Fitchen, J. H., Knight, S., Andersson, I., Brändén, C.-I., McIntosh, L. 1990. *Proc. Natl. Acad. Sci. USA* 87: 5768–72
39. Fraij, B., Hartman, F. C. 1982. *J. Biol. Chem.* 257: 3501–5
40. Gatenby, A. A. 1984. *Eur. J. Biochem.* 144: 361–66
41. Gatenby, A. A., Van Der Vies, S. M., Bradley, D. 1985. *Nature* 314: 617–20
42. Gatenby, A. A., Van Der Vies, S. M., Rothstein, S. J. 1987. *Eur. J. Biochem.* 168: 227–31
43. Georgopoulos, C. P., Hendrix, R. W., Casjens, S. R., Kaiser, A. D. 1973. *J. Mol. Biol.* 76: 45–60
44. Gibson, J. L., Tabita, F. R. 1985. *J. Bacteriol.* 164: 1188–93
45. Goloubinoff, P., Gatenby, A. A., Lorimer, G. H. 1989. *Nature* 337: 44–47
46. Gurewitz, M., Somerville, C. R., McIntosh, L. 1985. *Proc. Natl. Acad. Sci. USA* 82: 6546–50
47. Gutteridge, S. 1990. *Biochem. Biophys. Acta* 1015: 1–14
48. Gutteridge, S., Gatenby, A. A. 1987.

Oxford Surv. Plant Mol. Cell Biol. 4: 95–135
49. Gutteridge, S., Millard, B. N. Parry, M. A. J. 1986. *FEBS Lett.* 196: 263–68
50. Gutteridge, S., Sigal, I., Thomas, B., Arentzen, R., Cordova, A., et al. 1984. *EMBO J.* 3: 2737–42
51. Haining, R. L., McFadden, B. A. 1990. *J. Biol. Chem.* 265: 5434–39
52. Hardy, R. W. F., Havelka, U. D., Quebedeaux, B. 1978. In *Photosynthetic Carbon Assimilation*, ed. H. W. Siegelman, G. Hind, pp. 165–78. New York: Plenum
53. Hartman, F. C., Larimer, W. F., Mural, R. J., Machanoff, R., Soper, T. S. 1987. *Biochem. Biophys. Res. Commun.* 145: 1158–63
54. Hartman, F. C., Milanez, S., Lee, E. H. 1985. *J. Biol. Chem.* 260: 13968–75
55. Hartman, F. C., Soper, T. S., Niyogi, S. K., Mural, R. J., Foote, R. S., et al. 1987. *J. Biol. Chem.* 262: 3496–3501
56. Hemmingsen, S., Woolford, C., Van Der Vies, S., Tilly, K., Dennis, D. T., et al. 1988. *Nature* 333: 330–34
57. Herndon, C. S., Hartman, F. C. 1084. *J. Biol. Chem.* 259: 3102–10
58. Herndon, C. S., Norton, I. L., Hartman, F. C. 1982. *Biochemistry* 21: 1380–85
59. Holzenburg, A., Mayer, F., Harauz, G., van Heel, M., Tokuoga, R., et al. 1987. *Nature* 325: 730–32
60. Houtz, R. L., Stults, J. T., Mulligan, R. M., Tolbert, N. E. 1989. *Proc. Natl. Acad. Sci. USA* 86: 1855–59
61. Incharoensakdi, A., Takabe, T., Akazawa, T. 1985. *Arch. Biochem. Biophys.* 237: 445–53
62. Incharoensakdi, A., Takabe, T., Akazawa, T. 1985. *Biochem. Biophys. Res. Commun.* 126: 698–704
63. Janson, C. A., Smith, W. W., Eisenberg, D., Hartman, F. C. 1984. *J. Biol. Chem.* 259: 11594–96
64. Jaworoski, A., Hartman, F. C., Rose, I. A. 1984. *J. Biol. Chem.* 259: 6783–89
65. Johal, S., Bourque, D. P. Smith, W. W., Suh, S. W., Eisenberg, D. 1980. *J. Biol. Chem.* 255: 8873–80
66. Jordan, D. B., Chollet, R. 1983. *J. Biol. Chem.* 258: 13752–58
67. Jordan, D. B., Chollet, R. 1985. *Arch. Biochem. Biophys.* 236: 487–96
68. Jordan, D. B., Chollet, R., Ogren, W. L. 1983. *Biochemistry* 22: 3410–18
69. Kawashima, N., Wildman, S. G. 1971. *Biochim. Biophys. Acta* 229: 749–60
70. Kettleborough, C. A., Perry, M. A., Burton, S., Gutteridge, S., Keys, A. J., et al. 1987. *Eur. J. Biochem.* 170: 335–42

71. Kiefhaber, T., Grunert, H.-P., Hahn, U., Schmid, F. X. 1990. *Biochemistry* 29: 6475–80
72. Kimball, B. A. 1982. *WCL Report* II. Washington, DC: Agric. Res. Serv., US Dept. Agric.
73. Knight, S., Andersson, I., Brändén, C.-I. 1989. *Science* 244: 702–05
74. Knight, S., Andersson, I., Brändén, C.-I. 1990. *J. Mol. Biol.* 215: 113–60
75. Krebbers, E., Seurinck, J., Herdies, L., Cashmore, A. R., Timko, M. P. 1983. *Plant Mol. Biol.* 11: 745–59
76. Laing, W. A., Christeller, J. T. 1976. *Biochem. J.* 159: 563–70
77. Larimer, F. W., Lee, E. H., Mural, R. J., Soper, T. S., Hartman, F. C. 1987. *J. Biol. Chem.* 262: 15327–29
78. Lee, E. H., Soper, T. S., Mural, R. J., Stringer, C. D., Hartman, F. C. 1987. *Biochemistry* 26: 4599–4604
79. Lorimer, G. H. 1981. *Annu. Rev. Plant Physiol.* 32: 349–83
80. Lorimer, G. H. 1981. *Biochemistry* 20: 1236–40
81. Lorimer, G. H. 1979. *J. Biol. Chem.* 254: 5599–5601
82. Lorimer, G. H. 1978. *Eur. J. Biochem.* 89: 43–50
83. Lorimer, G. H., Andrews, T. J., Pierce, J., Schloss, J. V. 1986. *Philos. Trans. R. Soc. London Ser. B* 313: 397–407
84. Lorimer, G. H., Badger, M. R., Andrews, T. J. 1976. *Biochemistry* 15: 529–36
85. Lorimer, G. H., Gutteridge, S., Madden, M. W. 1987. In *Plant Molecular Biology*, ed. D. von Wettstein, N.-H. Chua, pp. 21–31. New York: Plenum
86. Lorimer, G. H., Hartman, F. C. 1988. *J. Biol. Chem.* 263: 6468–71
87. Lorimer, G. H., Miziorko, H. M. 1980. *Biochemistry* 19: 5321–28
88. Lu, G., Lindqvist, Y., Schneider, G. 1991. *Proteins.* In press
89. Lundqvist, T., Schneider, G. 1989. *J. Biol. Chem.* 264: 3643–46
90. Lundqvist, T., Schneider, G. 1989. *J. Biol. Chem.* 264: 7078–83
91. Lundqvist, T., Schneider, G. 1991. *Biochemistry* 30: 904–8
92. Lundqvist, T., Schneider, G. 1991. *J. Biol. Chem.* 266: 12604–11
93. Martin, P. G. 1979. *Aust. J. Plant Physiol.* 6: 401–8
94. McCurry, S. D., Pierce, J., Tolbert, N. E., Orme-Johnson, W. H. 1981. *J. Biol. Chem.* 256: 6623–28
95. Miziorko, H. M. 1979. *J. Biol. Chem.* 254: 270–72
96. Miziorko, H. M., Lorimer, G. H. 1983. *Annu. Rev. Biochem.* 52: 507–35
97. Miziorko, H. M., Sealy, R. C. 1984. *Biochemistry* 23: 479–85
98. Morell, M. K., Kane, H. J., Andrews, T. J. 1990. *FEBS Lett.* 265: 41–45
99. Mott, K. A., Berry, J. A. 1986. *Plant Physiol.* 82: 77–82
100. Mural, R. J., Soper, T. S., Larimer, F. W., Hartman, F. C. 1990. *J. Biol. Chem.* 265: 6501–5
101. Musgrove, J. E., Ellis, R. J. 1986. *Philos. Trans. R. Soc. London Ser. B* 213: 419–28
102. Nagy, F., Morelli, G., Fraley, R. T., Rogers, S. G., Chua, N.-H. 1985. *EMBO J.* 4: 3063–68
103. Nakagawa, H., Sugimoto, M., Kai, Y., Harada, S., Miki, K., et al. 1986. *J. Mol. Biol.* 191: 577–78
104. Nargang, F., McIntosh, L., Somerville, C., 1984. *Mol. Gen. Genet.* 193: 220–24
105. Newman, J., Gutterridge, S. 1990. *J. Biol. Chem.* 265: 15154–59
106. Nilsson, T., Brändén, R., Styring, S. 1984. *Biochim. Biophys. Acta* 788: 274–80
107. Niogy, S. K., Foote, R. S., Mural, R. J., Larimer, F. W., Mitra, S., et al. 1986. *J. Biol. Chem.* 261: 10087–92
108. Paech, C., Pierce, J., McCurry, S. D., Tolbert, N. E. 1978. *Biochem. Biophys. Res. Commun.* 83: 1084–92
109. Pal, G. P., Jakob, R., Hahn, U., Bowien, B., Sänger, W. 1985. *J. Biol. Chem.* 260: 10768–70
110. Pierce, J., Andrews, T. J., Lorimer, G. H. 1986. *J. Biol. Chem.* 261: 10248–56
111. Pierce, J., Gutteridge, S. 1985. *Appl. Environ. Microbiol.* 49: 1094–1100
112. Pierce, J., Lorimer, G. H., Reddy, G. S. 1986. *Biochemistry* 25: 1636–44
113. Pierce, J., Reddy, G. S. 1986. *Arch. Biochem. Biophys.* 245: 483–93
114. Pierce, J., Tolbert, N. E., Barker, R. 1980. *Biochemistry* 23: 5321–28
115. Ranty, B., Lundqvist, T., Schneider, G., Madden, M., Howard, R., et al. 1990. *EMBO J.* 9: 1365–73
116. Robison, P. D., Martin, M. N., Tabita, F. R. 1979. *Biochemistry* 18: 4453–58
117. Roy, H., Bloom, M., Milos, P., Monroe, M. 1982. *J. Cell Biol.* 94: 20–27
118. Rutner, A. C., Lane, M. D. 1967. *Biochem. Biophys. Res. Commun.* 28: 531–37
119. Saver, B. G., Knowles, J. R. 1982. *Biochemistry* 21: 5398–5403
120. Schloss, J. V., Lorimer, G. H. 1982. *J. Biol. Chem.* 257: 4691–94
121. Schloss, J. V., Phares, E. F., Long, M. V., Norton, I. L., Stringer, C. D., et al. 1979. *J. Bacteriol.* 137: 490–501

122. Schneider, G., Brändén, C.-I., Lorimer, G. 1984. *J. Mol. Biol.* 175: 99–102
123. Schneider, G., Brändén, C.-I., Lorimer, G. 1986. *J. Mol. Biol.* 187: 141–43
124. Schneider, G., Knight, S., Andersson, I., Brändén, C.-I., Lindqvist, Y., et al. 1990. *EMBO J.* 9: 2045–50
125. Schneider, G., Lindqvist, Y., Brändén, C.-I., Lorimer, G. 1986. *EMBO J.* 5: 3409–15
126. Schneider, G., Lindqvist, Y., Lundqvist, T. 1990. *J. Mol. Biol.* 211: 989–1008
127. Shinozaki, K., Sigiura, M. 1983. *Nucleic Acids Res.* 11: 6957–64
128. Sicher, R. C., Hatch, A. L., Stumpf, D. K., Jensen, R. G. 1981. *Plant Physiol.* 68: 252–55
129. Smith, H. B., Larimer, F. W., Hartman, F. C. 1990. *J. Biol. Chem.* 265: 1243–45
130. Sommerville, R. C., Sommerville, S. C. 1984. *Mol. Gen. Genet.* 193: 214–19
131. Soper, T. S., Larimer, F. W., Mural, R. J., Lee, E. H., Hartman, F. C. 1989. *J. Protein Chem.* 8: 239–49
132. Soper, T. S., Mural, R. J., Larimer, F. W., Lee, E. H., Machanoff, R., et al. 1988. *Protein Eng.* 2: 39–44
133. Styring, S., Brändén, R. 1985. *Biochemistry* 24: 6011–19
134. Styring, S., Brändén, R. 1985. *Biochim. Biophys. Acta* 832: 113–18
135. Sue, J. R., Knowles, J. R. 1978. *Biochemistry* 17: 4041–44
136. Sue, J. R., Knowles, J. R. 1982. *Biochemistry* 21: 5404–10
137. Suh, S. W., Cascio, D., Chapman, M. S., Eisenberg, D. 1987. *J. Mol. Biol.* 197: 363–65
138. Tabita, F. R., McFadden, B. A. 1974. *J. Biol. Chem.* 249: 3459–64
139. Tabita, F. R., Small, C. L. 1985. *Proc. Natl. Acad. Sci. USA* 82: 6100–3
140. Takabe, T., Incharoensakdi, A., Akazawa, T. 1984. *Biochem. Biophys. Res. Commun.* 122: 763–69
141. Takahashi, N., Hayano, T., Suzuki, M. 1989. *Nature* 337: 473–75
142. Terzaghi, B. E., Laing, W. A., Christeller, J. T., Petersen, G. B., Hill, D. F. 1986. *Biochem. J.* 235: 839–46
143. Van Dyke, D., Schloss, J. V. 1986. *Biochemistry* 25: 5145–56
144. Van Der Vies, S., Bradley, D., Gatenby, A. A. 1986. *EMBO J.* 5: 2439–44
145. Voordouw, G., Van Der Vies, S. M., Bouwmeister, P. P. 1984. *Eur. J. Biochem.* 141: 313–18
146. Weissbach, A., Horecker, B. L., Hurwitz, J. 1956. *J. Am. Chem. Soc.* 76: 3611–12
147. Wildner, G. F., Henkel, J. 1979. *Planta* 169: 223–28

Annu. Rev. Biophys. Biomol. Struct. 1992. 21:145–66

MICROTUBULE DYNAMIC INSTABILITY AND GTP HYDROLYSIS

Harold P. Erickson and E. Timothy O'Brien

Department of Cell Biology, Duke University Medical Center, Durham, North Carolina 27710

KEY WORDS: tubulin, polymerization, cytoskeleton, GTP cap

CONTENTS

PERSPECTIVE AND OVERVIEW

Over the past two decades, our understanding of microtubule dynamics has progressed through three models, each postulating an increasing level of activity. First, in the early 1970s researchers demonstrated that microtubules could be reversibly assembled from soluble tubulin subunits, but at steady state the dynamics were thought to be limited to the an equilibrium exchange of subunits between the soluble pool and the microtubule ends. The length of a microtubule remained approximately constant, and only subunits very close to the end would exchange. Then in the late 1970s and

145

1056–8700/92/0610–0145$02.00

early 1980s, evidence accumulated for a more dynamic activity termed *treadmilling*. The treadmilling model postulated a constant net loss of subunits from one end and a gain at the other. The length of the microtubule would still remain constant, but all subunits would eventually exchange with the soluble pool. Finally, in 1984 a novel dynamic mechanism termed *dynamic instability* was proposed. This model states that the end of a microtubule is never in equilibrium; most of the time the microtubule is in a state of constant growth, but these episodes of elongation are interspersed with episodes of shortening. Since 1984, the phenomenon of dynamic instability has been convincingly established both in vitro and in vivo, and the model can explain the experimental data previously attributed to equilibrium exchange and treadmilling.

Figure 1*a* illustrates the phenomenon of dynamic instability using quantitative data from the study of Walker et al (75). At or near steady state, each microtubule end is in one of two phases. Most of the microtubules are in the elongation phase and continue growing at a slow, steady rate. A small fraction of the microtubules are in the rapid shortening phase, depolymerizing at a rate about 2–10 times faster than the elongation. A microtubule in either phase remains there for an extended period of time, but occasional transitions occur abruptly and stochastically. The transition from elongation to rapid shortening is termed *catastrophe*, and the reverse transition is termed *rescue*.

Mitchison & Kirschner (47, 48) first inferred dynamic instability from the measurements of fixed microtubules. The phenomenon was then vividly confirmed through direct visualization of single microtubules in vitro by Horio & Hotani (36) using dark field light microscopy and by Walker et al (75) using video-enhanced, differential interference contrast (DIC) light microscopy. This last paper and the related study of O'Brien et al (55) provide comprehensive data on the kinetics of growth rates and transition frequencies in vitro. Finally, Cassimeris et al (19) obtained similar kinetic data for interphase microtubules in living cells. Table 1 summarizes data from these studies.

What is the biological function of dynamic instability? Obviously it produces a constant redistribution of the cytoskeleton, but for what purpose? Perhaps most important is the recycling of microtubules that have missed their target. Specifically, in the mitotic apparatus, microtubules growing from the centrosome attach chromosomes and move them, but only if they spear the kinetochore (33). Those microtubules that miss the kinetochore need to be dismantled and recycled for another shot. Dynamic instability provides the mechanism. Similar redistribution of the cytoskeleton and recycling of microtubules are probably important in interphase, although the targets are not known. Schultze & Kirschner (65)

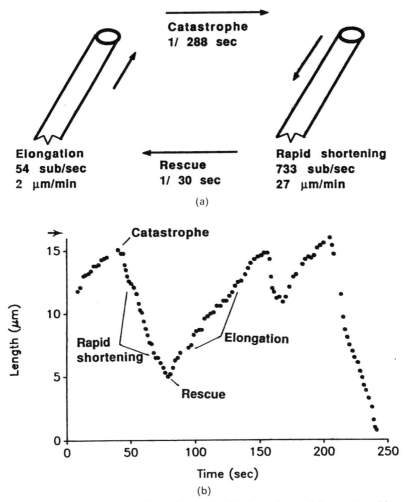

Figure 1 (*a*) The two phases, elongation and rapid shortening, and the two transitions, catastrophe and rescue, of dynamic instability. The numerical values are rates observed in vitro for the plus end (75) at 11 μM free tubulin, the estimated steady-state concentration. (*b*) Life history of a microtubule undergoing dynamic instability inside a living cell. The rates of growth and rapid shortening are constant for extended periods, and the transitions are abrupt and stochastic. From Cassimeris et al (19).

found that about 20% of the interphase microtubules are stabilized; perhaps these have hit a target in the cell cortex. The remaining dynamic microtubules are still seeking targets and being recycled.

Several excellent reviews have discussed the biological functions of

Table 1 The excursions of dynamic instability[a]

	Elongation			Rapid shortening		
	Rate (μm/min)	Time of excursion (min)	Length of excursion (μm)	Rate (μm/min)	Time of excursion (min)	Length of excursion (μm)
Plus end, 11 μM tub, 1 mM Mg	2.0	4.7	9.5	27	0.5	13.5
Minus end, 11 μM tub, 1 mM Mg	0.85	8.3	7.0	34	0.11	3.7
Plus end, 15 μM tub, 1 mM Mg	3.3	14	46	27	0.5	13.5
Minus end, 15 μM tub, 1 mM Mg	1.5	7	25	34	0.08	2.7
Plus end, 15 μM tub, 6 mM Mg	4.2	6.7	28	80	2	160
Minus end, 15 μM tub, 6 mM Mg	2.0	6.7	13.4	170	0.3	51
Plus end, in vivo	7.2	1.2	8.6	17.3	0.37	6.3

[a] Values are given for the average growth and disassembly rates, and the average time spent in each phase, as observed by DIC microscopy of single microtubules. Data are from refs. 19, 55, and 75.

dynamic instability (20, 40, 50). Carlier (14, 15) has reviewed the role of nucleotide hydrolysis in the dynamics of microtubules and actin and discusses model mechanisms. The review of Bayley (4) focuses on his "lateral cap" model, a variant of the stochastic dissociation models (75) (see Figure 3c, below). Hill (35) provides an extensive mathematical development of assembly models, including applications to dynamic instability. Salmon et al (61) reviewed the technology of video-enhanced DIC microscopy, which has been the most powerful tool for studying dynamic instability.

The present review begins by relating the modern concept of dynamic instability to the earlier concepts of equilibrium assembly and treadmilling. We then present the concept of a GTP cap as the mechanism governing the phases of dynamic instability, and briefly discuss the evolution of GTP-cap models. In spite of these many advances, a definitive and compelling model is not yet in hand. We therefore conclude by reviewing in detail three avenues of experimental work that appear most promising for unraveling the molecular mechanisms of dynamic instability: (a) kinetics of growth, shortening, and transitions as observed using video microscopy of single microtubules; (b) kinetics of GTP hydrolysis; and (c) the study of GTP analogs.

FROM EQUILIBRIUM ASSEMBLY, THROUGH TREADMILLING, TO DYNAMIC INSTABILITY

The earliest concept of microtubule dynamics was based on the classic theory of condensation polymerization of cooperative helical polymers (57) and upon experimental data such as that shown in Figure 2. When a solution of tubulin subunits is raised from 4°C to 37°C, the subunits spontaneously assemble to form microtubules. After a few minutes, the assembly reaches a stable plateau, as measured by turbidity. The microtubules appear to be in equilibrium with a pool of soluble tubulin subunits; this equilibrium concentration of free subunits has been referred to for years as the "critical concentration" (C_C) (57). We use C_C to refer to an equilibrium polymerization, and the term C_{SS} to designate the steady-state concentration of soluble subunits in the more dynamic nonequilibrium reactions.

If the microtubule were assembled through the reversible association of subunits, this equilibrium polymer would display very little dynamic activity. If a solution of polymers in equilibrium with subunits were diluted, the concentration of soluble subunits would initially fall below C_C, and polymers would then disassemble until the concentration of soluble subunits rose again to C_C. If extra soluble subunits were added, raising the

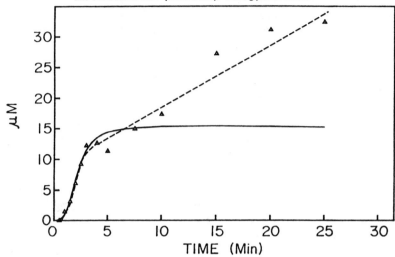

Time course: Assembly of 18.5 µM Tubulin (solid line),
and evolution of GDP (dashed line). MEM/glycerol buffer.

Figure 2   In vitro microtubule assembly followed by turbidity, and simultaneously assayed for GTP hydrolysis. At time 0, the temperature was raised to 37°C to initiate assembly. The turbidity rises to a plateau (steady state) in 4 min. GTP hydrolysis closely follows turbidity during the net assembly phase, and continues at a constant rate at steady state. From O'Brien et al (56).

concentration above C_C, they would assemble to make more polymer, until the subunit concentration fell to C_C. At equilibrium, subunits would constantly exchange on and off the ends of microtubules, but these processes would balance each other. The stochastic nature of the association-dissociation reaction would result in a slow net incorporation of new subunits at each end [proportional to the square root of elapsed time (11)] but these would never extend more than a few hundred subunits into the core of the microtubule. The concept of treadmilling provided for a much more dynamic activity. The theoretical basis of treadmilling is the polar structure of the microtubule; the opposite ends are designated plus and minus. Wegner (77) reasoned that if assembly of a polar polymer were accompanied by an irreversible chemical step like nucleotide hydrolysis, the C_C could be different at the plus and minus ends. The steady-state concentration of free subunits, C_{SS}, would lie between the C_Cs of each end. At the minus end of the microtubule, with C_C below C_{SS}, assembly would predominate, and the net gain of subunits at the minus end would be balanced by a net loss at the plus end. Thus, new subunits would be incorporated one by one at the minus end, treadmill through the micro-tubule, and eventually exit at the plus end. Experimental data for continued incorporation of subunits at steady state supported this model (42).

We now recognize that the gross effect of treadmilling can be produced by dynamic instability (26, 75). The major new feature of dynamic insta-bility is that, instead of an equilibrium exchange of one subunit at a time, dynamic instability postulates large excursions involving loss or gain of thousands of subunits in each excursion. For example, one may note from the data in Figure 1a that the average length gained during elongation, (2 μm/min $\times$ 4.8 min $= 9.6\,\mu$m), is less than that lost during rapid shortening, (27 μm/min $\times$ 0.5 min $= 13.5\,\mu$m). The plus end, over time, undergoes a net shortening, which is balanced at the minus end, where the excursions of elongation exceed those of shortening. [The specialist should also note the fundamental difference in molecular mechanism. In the Wegner tread-milling model, GTP must be hydrolyzed immediately, leaving GDP-tubu-lin at the end of the microtubule, while models for dynamic instability postulate a GTP cap at the microtubule end. With this cap, the subunit-by-subunit treadmilling mechanism cannot operate. Thus if treadmilling does occur in vivo (49), the mechanism probably involves unbalanced excursions of dynamic instability.] Mitchison & Kirschner (47, 48) dis-covered the phenomenon of dynamic instability as they tested a simple microtubule assembly system for the predictions of equilibrium assembly. They had devised a preparation of centrosomes that would nucleate micro-tubules. The centrosomes were placed in a concentrated tubulin solution and allowed to grow clusters of microtubules about 8 μm long. The micro-tubule clusters were then diluted into three different concentrations of soluble tubulin, and the lengths of the microtubules were measured after different time intervals. The classical theory predicted that the micro-tubules should grow longer when the tubulin concentration was above C_{SS} (which Mitchison & Kirschner assumed was near the C_C of the extended plus ends), and this was what they observed. The classical theory also predicted that microtubules should neither grow nor shrink when the tubulin concentration was approximately equal to C_{SS}, but they found that the microtubles continued to grow. Even more surprising was the experiment diluting the free tubulin below C_{SS}. Whereas the classical theory predicted that all microtubules should shrink at a uniform rate, Mitchison & Kirschner observed that some microtubules seemed to disappear very quickly, but those remaining continued to grow. Thus, the plus end of the microtubule extending from the centrosome can apparently exist in two states with very different C_Cs, one favoring elongation and the other favoring shortening. What is the mechanism for maintaining these very different states, and for switching between them?

THE GTP CAP

Origins and Refinements of GTP-Cap Models

The energy source that powers the constant activity of dynamic instability is almost certainly the hydrolysis of GTP. The tubulin dimer binds two molecules of guanine nucleotide. One of these is always GTP, is not exchangeable with nucleotides in solution, and is not hydrolyzed during assembly. This N-site GTP is not discussed here. The second nucleotide binding site (E site) can exchangeably bind either GTP or GDP (or other nucleotides discussed below) from solution. Microtubule assembly under most conditions requires that the E-site nucleotide be GTP, and during assembly the E-site GTP is hydrolyzed to GDP. The E-site GDP is non-exchangeable while the tubulin remains in the polymer. When the microtubule depolymerizes, the soluble tubulin can exchange the GDP for GTP and be reactivated for another cycle of assembly.

How could the energy of GTP hydrolysis be used to generate dynamic instability? The most attractive hypothesis involves some form of GTP cap. If GTP hydrolysis occurs some time after a subunit enters the microtubule lattice, the core of the microtubule will be GDP tubulin, and a small cap of GTP tubulin subunits will be maintained at the ends. The general form of this model postulates that the GTP cap is stable, favoring polymerization, while the GDP core is very labile, favoring rapid disassembly. Thus catastrophe is initiated by loss of the last GTP-tubulin subunit from the cap, and rescue is binding of a GTP subunit to recap a shortening GDP core.

The differential stability of the GTP cap and the GDP core may be related to the two conformations of the tubulin protofilament (46a). When the protofilaments are in the microtubule wall, they are necessarily straight, parallel to each other and to the axis of the microtubule. When a protofilament is freed from the lateral bonding to its neighbors, it tends to adopt a curved conformation, forming a variety of ring polymers (24a, 39a). The curved conformation is enhanced by the presence of GDP at the E site (36a), implying that the straight protofilaments in the GDP core are inherently strained. They are maintained in the straight conformation so long as they are bonded to neighbors on all sides, but when exposed at the end they peel away into the curved conformation. Thus disassembly may be driven by transition to the more favorable curved conformation. GTP tubulin, on the other hand, is relatively stable in the straight conformation (36a) and may form a stable lattice even when exposed at the end of the microtubule. Thus the E-site GTP is proposed to be an allosteric effector that favors the straight conformation, forming a stable cap (46a). A recent paper of Mandelkow et al (41a) provides striking visual evidence of curved protofilaments peeling away from disassembling microtubules, confirming the earlier negative stain observations (24a, 39a) on a time scale that is rapid and related to the phases of dynamic instability.

The size of the GTP cap is postulated, in most models, to fluctuate through stochastic processes. The actual size at any moment is important in determining the probability of catastrophe. Regardless of the specific model, the size of the GTP cap must be governed by the balance of three reactions: (*a*) the polymerization of a new GTP-tubulin subunit increases the cap size; (*b*) dissociation of a GTP-tubulin from the end of the microtubule decreases the cap size; and (*c*) hydrolysis of GTP also decreases the cap size. In most models, catastrophe occurs only when the last GTP subunit is lost. Any size cap, even a single terminal GTP-tubulin subunit, can stabilize the microtubule and keep it in the elongation phase. However, as the cap grows larger than a single subunit, the probability of achieving catastrophe decreases.

Several models for the GTP cap have been proposed, and these can be grouped into three categories (Figure 3). The ultimate test for these models is the extensive body of data from video microscopy of single microtubules. The most important data, and the most difficult for models to match, are the frequencies of catastrophe over the extended range of free tubulin concentration. Catastrophe frequency decreased only a factor of three as the free tubulin concentration was raised from 7 to 15 μM (75). In contrast, the GTP-cap models all predict a 10- to 100-fold change in catastrophe over this concentration range.

A common feature of the models generates this very steep concentration dependence: the size of the cap, and the probability of its loss, are a balance of stochastic addition and removal of GTP subunits from the cap. However, although the models fail to fit the full range of data, they can all match the frequency of catastrophe at a single concentration. This matching has led to one important conclusion, that parameters must be chosen so that the average cap is very small, no more than about eight subunits (5, 71, 75).

Probing the GTP Cap by Cutting and Diluting Microtubules

Because no specific GTP-cap model can match all the experimental data, one might question the whole idea of a cap as the regulator of dynamic instability. Perhaps catastrophe is generated, not at the end, but by some structural transformation within the microtubule. Two simple tests support the general concept that regulation is at the end, and therefore involves some kind of cap.

A first test involved cutting the microtubule in the middle. According to the model, the newly exposed ends should both be uncapped, and they

154   ERICKSON & O'BRIEN

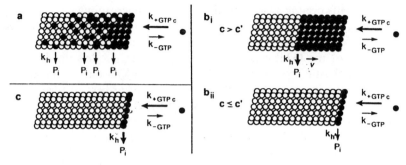

Figure 3 Models for the GTP cap (from 68). Tubulin-GTP subunits are represented by solid black circles, GDP-tubulin by open circles. The models differ in the site and mechanism of GTP hydrolysis. (*a*) Uncoupled stochastic hydrolysis. This was the original basis for the concept of a GTP cap (12, 47). GTP hydrolysis occurs randomly as a first-order reaction following incorporation of the subunit. During the initial assembly at high subunit concentration, virtually the entire polymer is GTP-tubulin. Later, the core is primarily GDP-tubulin, and the ends are primarily GTP-tubulin. (*b*) Uncoupled vectorial hydrolysis (8, 16, 46). GTP hydrolysis is enhanced by contact with a GDP-subunit, and therefore occurs almost exclusively at the interface of the GTP cap and the GDP core; moreover, this hydrolysis occurs at a constant velocity. There are two very different regimes. At high tubulin concentrations, the assembly of new subunits exceeds the rate of hydrolysis, and a substantial cap of GTP-tubulin builds up (b_i). At lower tubulin concentrations, where the assembly is slower than the hydrolysis rate, the simplest hypothesis is that the cap disappears, but then the model predicts immediate catastrophe, contrary to observation. An alternative proposal is that hydrolysis slows when only a single ring of subunits is present (b_{ii}); in this case the model reduces to that of panel *c*. (*c*) Stochastic dissociation, coupled hydrolysis (75). In this model, the cap cannot exceed a maximum size, say 13 GTP-subunits. The addition of a fourteenth GTP subunit forces the hydrolysis of the deepest one. The actual size of the cap can fluctuate from 13 to 0 subunits, depending on the stochastic balance of association and dissociation of GTP subunits. The lateral cap model (3–5) is closely related but has additional growing points and dissociation parameters.

should immediately begin rapid shortening. Walker et al (74) used a UV microbeam to cut single microtubules in vitro, observing them with DIC optics a few seconds after cutting. The observations were definitive but partly surprising. The newly exposed plus ends all began rapid shortening immediately after cutting, exactly as predicted. However, the newly exposed minus ends never shortened; they continued elongation. These investigators discussed several explanations (74), but the one we favor is that the cutting leaves the minus end in a state that is rapidly rescued. Experiments at higher Mg concentration support this speculation. At 6 mM Mg, we observed that minus-end rescue was reduced by a factor of four (55), and R. A. Walker (73a) found that a substantial fraction of cut minus ends began rapid shortening when the cutting was done in higher Mg concentrations.

Nicklas et al (52) observed essentially the same behavior, disassembly of plus ends but stable minus ends, in an in vivo cutting experiment. They used a microneedle to mechanically sever the microtubules of the mitotic spindle. The exposed plus ends showed substantial depolymerization, but the minus ends were remarkably stable. Cutting with a laser in vivo has given similar results (see 52, 69). Overall, we interpret the cutting experiments as consistent with the concept of a labile microtubule core stabilized by caps at the ends, with the severed minus end perhaps rapidly rescued.

A second test of the cap was to dilute the microtubules. If the stabilizing GTP subunits can be lost by dissociation, as predicted in most models, dilution should lead to loss of the GTP cap. Two dilution studies have now demonstrated that microtubules undergo catastrophe very quickly following dilution. Voter et al (72) concluded that all microtubules lost their caps, at both ends, in less than one second following a 15-fold dilution from steady state (to 0.5 μM free tubulin). Walker et al (76) could not achieve as rapid nor complete dilution (using a flow cell to observe single microtubules), but observed catastrophe within about 5 seconds at ~ 3.3 μM free tubulin. Extrapolation of their data to higher dilutions was consistent with the < 1-s lifetime deduced by Voter et al. Based on this lifetime, the size of the cap was estimated to be no more than 40 and 20 subunits at the plus and minus ends, respectively (72). The data are, of course, consistent with a smaller cap of 1–13 subunits.

Questions for Future Analysis and Models of the GTP Cap

We conclude this section by raising three questions not readily answered by present GTP-cap models. We hope that questions like these might lead to new insights, and eventually to a more compelling model for the mechanism of dynamic instability.

The first question is: why is the frequency of catastrophe approximately the same at the plus and minus ends? In principle, the assembly dynamics could be completely different at the two ends. The polarity problem is clearest at the molecular level: the β-tubulin subunit containing the E-site GTP (41) is exposed at one end, but at the other end it is buried in contact with an α subunit. This arrangement poses a vexing problem for model builders because different rules for coupled GTP hydrolysis generally have to be proposed for the two ends (43). We should also consider the question in terms of biology. If this type of model building is approximately correct, and different mechanisms for GTP hydrolysis indeed apply to the two ends, we must conclude that evolution has generated these separate mechanisms and finely tuned them to produce similar frequencies of catastrophe. This seems most unlikely because the minus ends are embedded in centrosomes and probably do not even exhibit dynamic instability in vivo. A mechanism that completely ignored the polarity of the lattice and necessarily produced identical frequencies of catastrophe at each end would be much more satisfying. Present models cannot provide such a mechanism.

The second question is: how can we explain the uncoupling of catastrophe from elongation rate, which is apparent in some experiments? In any model with a variable cap size, the cap should grow larger as the elongation rate increases, and one would expect a corresponding decrease in frequency of catastrophe. Indeed, in the original experiments of Walker et al (75), an increase in free tubulin was accompanied by an increase in elongation rate and a decrease in catastrophe. However, at least three observations indicate that the decrease in catastrophe is not directly coupled to elongation: (a) as mentioned above, the plus and minus ends have very different elongation rates, yet essentially the same catastrophe rates; (b) at 6.0 mM Mg, the elongation rates are twofold higher than at 0.5 mM Mg, but the catastrophe frequency did not change (55); (c) in recent experiments (54), we have found that Ca in the range of 1 mM greatly increased the frequency of catastrophe, yet did not affect the growth rate of microtubules that were still elongating. The Mg and Ca experiments argue convincingly against any model in which the cap size is proportional to elongation rate; a satisfactory model should explain how catastrophe and elongation are uncoupled and can be independently modulated.

The third question is: how does dynamic instability apply to an open microtubule sheet, comprising only a few protofilaments? Certainly these sheets, which are intermediates in the nucleation of microtubules and often persist at steady state (25, 67), must exist in a stabilized form. Parsimony would suggest that they are stabilized by the same mechanisms as the intact microtubule. Previously proposed models for a GTP cap have all been drawn for an intact helical lattice, which greatly simplifies several problems. To highlight these problems, the interested reader should try to draw a GTP cap that will stabilize a sheet of, say, four protofilaments, yet still permit elongation and lateral growth. Constructing a GTP cap for a sheet of protofilaments has yet to be considered, but may generate important new insights.

The molecular mechanism by which GTP hydrolysis produces and regulates dynamic instability is the holy grail in this field. GTP hydrolysis must certainly play the key role, and thinking has so far focused on GTP-cap models. However, none of the specific models fits all the experimental data. The basic concept of the GTP cap may be correct, but we simply have not found the correct molecular model. Alternatively, a simple cap of GTP-tubulin subunits may be fundamentally wrong. New insights are needed, and will perhaps be stimulated by new experimental approaches. The following sections review three experimental areas that may hold the key for necessary new approaches and new molecular insights.

DYNAMIC INSTABILITY IN VITRO—THE FOUR REACTIONS OBSERVED WITH VIDEO MICROSCOPY

The following descriptions and conclusions are drawn primarily from the studies of Walker et al (75), in which the behavior of single microtubules was observed over a range of concentrations of free tubulin, and O'Brien et al (55), in which both tubulin and magnesium were varied. Table 1 gives numerical values for many of the deduced growth rates. Note that to convert μm/min to subunits per second, we calculate 1625 subunits per μm.

In the elongation phase, microtubules grow at a constant rate that is directly proportional to the concentration of free subunits. A remarkable feature of the data is the negative y-intercept of the line plotting growth rate vs tubulin concentration. This observation indicates reversible association of GTP tubulin onto the growing end, where the size of the intercept gives the dissociation rate. Growth at the minus end is about one-third that at the plus end, and growth at both ends increases by about 50% as Mg is increased from 0.25 mM to 6 mM. In all cases, elongation appears to be a second-order reaction, the reversible association of GTP tubulin subunits to the growing end.

The rate of rapid shortening was found to be independent of the concentration of soluble tubulin and therefore appeared to involve a first-order dissociation of subunits from the microtubule end. The dissociating subunits must be GDP tubulin, because measurements of bulk polymer show only GDP on the E site in microtubule polymer. Walker et al (75) reported shortening at about 30 μm/min at both ends, but the study of O'Brien et al (55) revealed a much more complex situation. Although the shortening rate was constant along an extended length of most microtubules, the rate varied significantly among the microtubules in a population, and sometimes changed abruptly along a single microtubule. The wide range of shortening rates was most dramatic at higher Mg concentrations, where minus-end shortening varied from 60 to 250 μm/min. A possible explanation for the different shortening rates is that in vitro assembly produces microtubules with 13, 14, and 15 protofilaments, the number sometimes changing within a single microtubule (58, 73). Microtubules with 14 or 15 protofilaments might be significantly strained in the lattice, leading to more rapid dissociation of subunits. Alternatively, some of the shortening polymers might be open sheets or hooked microtubules (67), with very different disassembly rates.

Catastrophe occurs infrequently and apparently at random, but the transition is always abrupt at the resolution of the light microscope (i.e. an imminent transition is not preceded by a slowing growth). The frequency of catastrophe, the reciprocal of the average time of the elongation phase, decreases in an apparently linear fashion by about a factor of three over the twofold range of free tubulin concentration that could be observed experimentally. The recent dilution studies (72, 76) now extend the range to lower concentrations. Remarkably, the frequency of catastrophe at the minus end is approximately the same as at the plus end at all tubulin concentrations (75, 76) and at 6 and 1 mM Mg (55).

Rescue, like catastrophe, is infrequent, abrupt, and apparently stochastic. The experimental data are probably weakest on the rescue reaction. Although Walker et al (75) concluded that rescue was proportional to tubulin concentration, the data are very scattered, and O'Brien et al (55) could not demonstrate any significant dependence of rescue on tubulin concentration. The mechanism of rescue is therefore obscure. If it does depend on tubulin concentration it should involve a second-order association of a GTP tubulin onto the GDP core, recapping the disassembling microtubule. On the other hand, if rescue does not depend on free tubulin, it might be caused by something within the microtubule lattice, such as a defect that halted disassembly long enough for recapping, or perhaps a buried GTP-tubulin subunit. Rescue must be related in an important way to the GTP cap, but more experimental data are needed on this difficult reaction.

KINETICS OF GTP HYDROLYSIS AND A WORD ABOUT G-PROTEINS

The best kinetic data on GTP hydrolysis have been obtained by nucleotide analysis of assembly reactions at small time intervals after assembly initiation. Assembly is initiated by raising the temperature to 37°C; polymer assembly is estimated by turbidity; and samples are quenched into acid at different time points for subsequent analysis of hydrolyzed GTP. The time resolution for these pipet-determined points is 2–10 s. A typical assembly (Figure 2) shows two phases. During the net assembly phase, the first 3–4 min, GTP hydrolysis is approximately stoichiometric—one GTP is hydrolyzed per tubulin dimer incorporated into polymer—and apparently occurs simultaneously with or shortly following the incorporation of each subunit into the polymer. When steady state is reached, GTP hydrolysis continues at a constant and substantial rate. This steady-state GTP hydrolysis presumably reflects the continued assembly and disassembly of microtubules undergoing dynamic instability.

How closely is hydrolysis coupled to assembly? The early study of Carlier & Pantaloni (12) was one of the most important inspirations for the GTP-cap model because it concluded that GTP hydrolysis occurred several minutes after incorporation of the subunit. This observation was the basis for the uncoupled stochastic hydrolysis model (Figure 3a). However, the reported lag would generate a very large cap, which would be impossible to lose by stochastic processes to yield the observed frequency of catastrophe (56, 75). More recent studies by O'Brien et al (56) and Carlier et al (16) concluded that the magnitude of the lag was greatly overestimated in the earlier study. At tubulin concentrations near steady state, both studies agree that hydrolysis is closely coupled to assembly and no lag can be detected at the 2- to 10-s time resolution of the pipetting assay. Some controversy remains at higher tubulin concentrations. Carlier et al (16) reported a substantial build-up of a GTP cap at higher tubulin concentrations, and this was the basis for their second model [vectorial hydrolysis, Figure 3b; see also the paper of Caplow (46)]. In contrast, O'Brien et al (56) found that GTP hydrolysis was closely coupled to assembly at all tubulin concentrations, even up to 74 μM; i.e. there was no evidence for a buildup of a measurable GTP cap under any experimental condition.

Two recent studies used rapid and sensitive filter binding assays to look for transient incorporation of GTP into microtubules (46, 68). Melki et al (46) reported that, following incorporation of the subunit and hydrolysis of GTP, the Pi was released only very slowly from the microtubule, with a half-time of 50 s. They presented this result as consistent with their model of a GDP-Pi cap (however, one again encounters the problem that a 50-s lag would lead to very large caps, which are very difficult to lose through stochastic processes). The independent study of Stewart et al (68), using a similar filter binding assay, arrived at the opposite conclusion. They found no evidence for any transiently bound Pi, either in GTP or as a bound GDP-Pi intermediate. Technical differences in the procedures used by the two groups might explain the contradictory conclusions, and additional experimental work is needed to resolve this important controversy.

David-Pfeuty et al (23) found that if the microtubules were centrifuged out of a steady-state assembly mixture, the supernatant, comprising soluble tubulin at C_{SS}, had no remaining GTPase activity. Caplow & Shanks (10) used chemically stabilized microtubule seeds to study GTP hydrolysis at concentrations of free subunits below C_{SS}. They found that the GTPase rate depended linearly on the concentration of both microtubule seeds and of free subunits. Thus, the major hydrolysis pathway appears to require interaction of soluble GTP-tubulin with a microtubule end. An important related study is of the very prominent GTPase of tubulin-colchicine (1, 2, 62, 63). Although the tubulin-colchicine assembles into large aggregates of ring polymers, the GTP hydrolysis is apparently not coupled to this assembly. However, a separate study (34) showed that hydrolysis depends on the concentration of tubulin-colchicine. The data suggested that association with another subunit (perhaps a precursor to the larger aggregates) is required for hydrolysis. The prevailing idea from many studies is that soluble tubulin subunits do not hydrolyze GTP; hydrolysis occurs only after the subunit is incorporated into a polymer (or perhaps a dimer for tubulin-colchicine).

Analysis of steady-state GTP hydrolysis is a potentially important, but so far under-utilized, tool in dynamic instability research. Hydrolysis of GTP should equal the total rate of addition of new subunits to microtubules in the elongation phase. Buffer conditions such as 3 M glycerol or 1 M sodium glutamate, which stabilize microtubules, are generally thought to inhibit dynamic instability. However, the steady-state GTPase rate is at least as high in these buffers (29, 56) as in those in which vigorous dynamic instability is demonstrated. Even more remarkable are the effects of the drug taxol, which greatly stabilizes microtubules while only slightly reducing the steady-state GTP hydrolysis (13, 28). This result suggests that dynamic instability continues in these stabilizing buffers, and that the rate of elongation (which is coupled to GTP hydrolysis in the favored GTP-cap models) is not diminished. Because elongation must be balanced by shortening at steady state, these buffers should primarily affect catastrophe and rescue, perhaps greatly reducing the size of the excursions. Direct video microscopy of single microtubules in stabilization buffers and taxol, coupled with measurements of bulk steady-state GTP hydrolysis, may settle this speculation or may reveal new features of dynamic instability.

Many proteins besides tubulin bind and hydrolyze GTP. A large family of GTPase proteins has been identified, all of which share a consensus sequence related to GTP binding. These include G-proteins, elongation factor-Tu, and proteins involved in protein secretion and trafficking (7, 24). In all of these systems, GTP hydrolysis appears to provide a clock mechanism, activating and deactivating the protein after an extended but limited time interval. GTP hydrolysis might also be thought of as a clock in tubulin, determining the time spent in the elongation phase. Surprisingly, tubulin does not share the GTP binding consensus sequence of these other proteins (24). Therefore, tubulin is apparently not related to these other proteins and has devised its own mechanisms for GTP binding and hydrolysis. It is not surprising that the effects of GTP analogs (discussed below) may be quite different in tubulin and G-proteins. Nevertheless, the body of research on the large family of GTPases is very large (7). Many of the techniques employed in these studies could be applied to tubulin, and some of the mechanisms may be related.

One mechanistic feature seems to be shared by almost all members of the GTPase family, as well as by tubulin. The isolated, soluble GTPases hydrolyze GTP at very slow rates, but hydrolysis is greatly accelerated when the protein interacts with a separate GTPase activating protein (GAP) (7). As discussed above, soluble tubulin also has a minimal GTPase activity; GTP is hydrolyzed only after the tubulin is incorporated into polymer. Thus, tubulin may be considered to act as its own GAP, accelerating GTP hydrolysis when specific protein-protein interactions are established in the microtubule.

MICROTUBULE ASSEMBLY WITH GTP ANALOGS

Because microtubule assembly requires GTP-tubulin and the GTP is hydrolyzed in the assembly reaction, there has been considerable interest in nonhydrolyzable GTP analogs. Would these analogs support assembly, and if so would the analog microtubules be more or less stable than the GTP/GDP microtubules? If a microtubule could be assembled from a nonhydrolyzable analog, we might expect it to behave as a giant GTP cap, opening the way to otherwise impossible analyses. We first discuss weakly binding analogs, then analogs that bind more strongly, and finally aluminum and beryllium fluoride.

The most studied analogs are GMPPNP and GMPPCP, in which the oxygen bridging the β and γ phosphates is replaced with nitrogen or carbon. Since the bond lengths and angles of the terminal phosphates are very similar in the analogs and in GTP, the analogs should bind to the E site and be defective only in the hydrolysis step. Several earlier studies (reviewed in 53) gave conflicting results as to whether these analogs would support assembly. We reinvestigated the question using purified tubulin freed of all unbound nucleotide by gel filtration. This tubulin still contained one molecule of GTP bound tightly to each E site, which was sufficient for one round of assembly in the presence or absence of a large excess of analog. However, neither of the analogs would support a second cycle of assembly, and we could obtain no evidence that the analogs bound to the tubulin. The simplest interpretation, that these analogs cannot support microtubule assembly, is, however, not correct. The problem is that the affinity of these analogs for the tubulin E site is orders of magnitude weaker than that of GTP and GDP. Following our first cycle of assembly, the tubulin was left with a stoichoimetric amount of E-site GDP, which could not be competed off even by a large excess of analog. Three recent studies now provide methods for stripping the E-site GTP or GDP and replacing it with the weakly binding analogs (30, 45, 66).

Mejillano et al (45) and Seckler et al (66) developed the alkaline phosphatase technique [first used by Terry & Purich (70)] to digest the E-site GTP or GDP, and demonstrated that GMPPCP and GMPPNP could bind to the vacant E site, could support assembly of microtubules, and was incorporated into the polymer. The latter study carefully documented the rate of digestion by alkaline phosphatase and demonstrated multiple cycles of reversible assembly. Analog microtubules have not been examined yet using video microscopy, but in one study, GMPPCP eliminated the length redistribution characteristic of dynamic instability (44). Alternate procedures for stripping the E-site nucleotide are gel filtration (44) or chromatography on phenyl Sepharose (32), although the latter procedure has not yet been exploited for analog studies. The third recent analog study was that of Hamel & Lin (30), who obtained incorporation and multiple cycles of assembly by shifting to a lower pH [pH 6.1 vs the pH 6.6 used by O'Brien et al (53)]. Finally, note that ATP would also support assembly when incorporated into a vacant E site (30, 45). The ATP was hydrolyzed during the assembly reaction.

GTPγS and GTPβS, in which one of the nonbridging atoms of the γ or β phosphate are replaced by sulfur, have been important tools in G-protein work (78). Because the bridging oxygen atoms are still in place, hydrolysis can occur, but it is generally much slower than with GTP. Roychowdhury & Gaskin (59; see this paper for references to earlier studies) demonstrated formation of microtubules and sheets in the presence of GTPγS, provided the Mg concentration was 0.5–1.0 mM. At higher Mg concentrations, the analog induced rings and crystal-like aggregates of rings. Although this study did not demonstrate repeated cycles of assembly, these authors did report that the analog was incorporated into protein polymer, 0.4–0.8 mols of analog per tubulin dimer, and that the GTPγS was mostly not hydrolyzed. Other modifications of the γ phosphate, such as GTPγF (51) or bulkier substituents (39), gave analogs that bound strongly to tubulin but inhibited assembly. The GTPβS(A) and -(B) stereoisomers both supported assembly. The A isomer was hydrolyzed, but the B isomer was not (60) and is therefore a good candidate for further study.

Hamel and colleagues (27, 31) have investigated several deoxyguanosine analogs. Deoxy- and dideoxyguanosine (ddGTP) supported microtubule assembly more vigorously than GTP and were hydrolyzed. More remarkable, ddGDP also supported assembly and was incorporated into the microtubule polymer. Apparently, ddGDP displaced the GDP bound to the E site at concentrations above 0.5 mM and is therefore one of the most strongly binding of the nonhydrolyzable analogs. This analog clearly deserves additional attention.

Another analog that apparently binds strongly enough to displace the E-site GDP, and that supports multiple cycles of assembly, is GMPCPP (53, 64). Although earlier work indicated that this analog was hydrolyzed (64), recent work in our lab (H. P. Erickson & E. T. O'Brien, unpublished data) and by A. Hyman & T. J. Mitchison (personal communication) show that GMPCPP is incorporated stoichiometrically into microtubules and is not hydrolyzed. Hyman et al (38) describe a protocol for synthesizing this analog and reported that microtubules grown in an excess of this analog were extremely stable following dilution at 37°C. Although one might expect the analog microtubules to be more stable than ones grown in GTP, the apparent magnitude of this stability is surprising. First, microtubules with GMPCPP appear to be much more stable than the GTP cap itself, which was estimated to have a C_C of about 3–5 μM and a dissociation rate constant of 44 subunits/s (75). A relatively rapid dissociation rate for the GTP subunits was also deduced in dilution studies (72, 76). Second, the C_C for GMPCPP microtubules was also in the range of 3–5 μM (66); i.e. similar to that proposed for the GTP cap and much higher than that reported for GMPCPP microtubules. Further study of the possible contradictions in C_C and dissociation rates for the analog microtubules may lead to important new insights.

Aluminum and beryllium fluoride activate G-proteins, apparently by creating a kind of GTP analog from bound GDP. When the bound nucleotide is GDP, the G-protein is normally inactivated. However AlF_4^- will bind next to the β phosphate of GDP, mimicking the γ phosphate of GTP and activating the G-protein (6, 21). Three laboratories have now studied the effects of Al, Be, or Pi on microtubule assembly. Humphreys & McDonald (37) reported that AlF_x, in the presence of excess GDP, did not affect assembly. They concluded that the GDP-AlF_x complex did not function as a GTP analog in tubulin. In contrast, Carlier et al (17, 18, 22) reported that both BeF_x and AlF_x could stabilize microtubules against dilution-induced depolymerization. Beryllium bound to microtubules (but not to soluble tubulin) in a 1:1 stoichiometric ratio, and BeF_x stimulated assembly in excess GDP. This assembly was, however, quite slow and probably quite different from the assembly via GTP-tubulin; the BeF_x bound to tubulin may mimic a protein-coordinated free Pi, rather than be a GTP analog. Following this argument, Carlier and colleagues suggested that release of Pi following hydrolysis may be slow, and that a GDP-Pi cap, rather than a GTP cap, may provide the major stabilization of the microtubule end. Caplow et al (9) pursued this hypothesis using DIC light microscopy to study the effect of Pi on the dynamics of single microtubules.

In contrast to the prediction of Carlier et al, they found that 0.167 M Pi had virtually no effect on any of the parameters of dynamic instability; in particular, Pi did not slow rapid shortening, nor did it reduce the frequency of catastrophe. Thus, the direct analysis of single microtubules does not support the idea of a GDP-Pi cap. Nevertheless, the Be and Al fluorides apparently profoundly affect microtubules, and may be important tools in sorting out the complex relations of GTP hydrolysis, Pi release, and microtubule stabilization.

PROSPECTS—THE IMPORTANT QUESTIONS REMAINING

That dynamic instability describes the assembly dynamics of most micro-tubules is now well established. Many details of the reactions have been determined experimentally, providing important clues to the molecular mechanism. The energy source that powers dynamic instability must be derived from hydrolysis of GTP, and models involving a GTP cap are the most attractive. However the definitive molecular model—which should be based on simple and testable assumptions and should fit all the exper-imental data—is not yet in hand. The simple idea of a GTP cap may need just a clever modification, or it may need a complete rethinking.

New concepts are likely to come from new experimental approaches. Nonhydrolyzable analogs would seem to offer great potential. A micro-tubule polymerized completely from analog tubulin should be dynamically inactive and should behave as a pure GTP cap. Even more interesting would be a microtubule doped with a small fraction of analog subunits: would these behave as embedded GTP caps and rescue the microtubule as soon as they are exposed at the end? Or would they reveal a continued dynamics that would force us to reevaluate our ideas of the GTP cap? Also, the kinetics of GTP hydrolysis need to be studied with much higher time resolution, for example, with a quench-flow technology that could provide data on a millisecond time scale. Designing a molecular model is still the ultimate challenge, and in these efforts we should keep in mind the numerous studies of microtubule assembly accumulated over the past two decades. Although the contradictions in present data sometimes seem overwhelming, a simple molecular mechanism certainly exists. The search for this model should provide exciting biochemistry and hopefully a defini-tive mechanism within the near future.

ACKNOWLEDGMENT

We thank the UNC-Duke microtubule journal club for continued sti-mulating discussion. Supported by NIH grant GM 28553.

Literature Cited

1. Andreu, J. M., Timasheff, S. N. 1982. *Proc. Natl. Acad. Sci. USA* 79: 6753–56
2. Andreu, J. M., Wagenknecht, T., Timasheff, S. N. 1983. *Biochemistry* 22: 1556–66
3. Bayley, P., Schilstra, M., Martin, S. 1989. *FEBS Lett.* 259: 181–84
4. Bayley, P. M. 1990. *J. Cell Sci.* 95: 329–34
5. Bayley, P. M., Schilstra, M. J., Martin, S. R. 1990. *J. Cell Sci.* 95: 33–48
6. Bigay, J., Deterre, P., Pfister, C., Chabre, M. 1987. *EMBO J.* 6: 2907–13
7. Bourne, H. R., Sanders, D. A., McCormick, F. 1991. *Nature* 349: 117–27
8. Caplow, M., Reid, R. 1985. *Proc. Natl. Acad. Sci. USA* 82: 3267–71
9. Caplow, M., Ruhlen, R., Shanks, J., Walker, R. A., Salmon, E. D. 1989. *Biochemistry* 28: 8136–41
10. Caplow, M., Shanks, J. 1990. *J. Biol. Chem.* 265: 8935–41
11. Caplow, M., Zeeberg, B. 1982. *Eur. J. Biochem.* 127: 319–24
12. Carlier, M.-F., Pantaloni, D. 1981. *Biochemistry* 20: 1918–24
13. Carlier, M.-F., Pantaloni, D. 1983. *Biochemistry* 22: 4814–22
14. Carlier, M.-F. 1989. *Int. Rev. Cytol.* 115: 139–70
15. Carlier, M.-F. 1991. *Curr. Opin. Cell Biol.* 3: 12–17
16. Carlier, M.-F., Didry, D., Pantaloni, D. 1987. *Biochemistry* 26: 4428–37
17. Carlier, M.-F., Didry, D., Melki, R., Chabre, M., Pantaloni, D. 1988. *Biochemistry* 27: 3555–59
18. Carlier, M.-F., Didry, D., Simon, C., Pantaloni, D. 1989. *Biochemistry* 28: 1783–91
19. Cassimeris, L., Pryer, N. K., Salmon, E. D. 1988. *J. Cell Biol.* 107: 2223–31
20. Cassimeris, L. U., Walker, R. A., Pryer, N. K., Salmon, E. D. 1987. *BioEssays* 4: 149–54
21. Chabre, M. 1990. *TIBS* Jan. 15: 6–10
22. Combeau, C., Carlier, M.-F. 1989. *J. Biol. Chem.* 264: 19017–21
23. David-Pfeuty, T., Erickson, H. P., Pantaloni, D. 1977. *Proc. Natl. Acad. Sci. USA* 74: 5372–76
24. Dever, T. E., Glynias, M. J., Merrick, W. C. 1987. *Proc. Natl. Acad. Sci. USA* 84: 1814–18
24a. Erickson, H. P. 1974. *J. Supramol. Struct.* 2: 393–411
25. Erickson, H. P., Voter, W. A. 1986. *Ann. N. Y. Acad. Sci.* 466: 552–65
26. Farrell, K. W., Jordan, M. A., Miller, H. P., Wilson, L. 1987. *J. Cell Biol.* 104: 1035–46

27. Hamel, E., del Campo, A. A., Lin, C. M. 1983. *Biochemistry* 22: 3664–71
28. Hamel, E., del Campo, A. A., Lowe, M. C., Lin, C. M. 1981. *J. Biol. Chem.* 256: 11887–94
29. Hamel, E., del Campo, A. A., Lowe, M. C., Waxman, P. G., Lin, C. M. 1982. *Biochemistry* 21: 503–9
30. Hamel, E., Lin, C. M. 1990. *Biochemistry* 29: 2720–29
31. Hamel, E., Lustbader, J., Lin, C. M. 1984. *Biochemistry* 23: 5314–25
32. Hanssens, I., Baert, J., Van Cauwelaert, F. 1990. *Biochemistry* 29: 5160–65
33. Hayden, J. H., Bowser, S. S., Rieder, C. L. 1990. *J. Cell Biol.* 111: 1039–45
34. Heusele, C., Carlier, M.-F. 1981. *Biochem. Biophys. Res. Commun.* 103: 332–38
35. Hill, T. L. 1987. *Linear Aggregation Theory in Cell Biology.* New York: Springer
36. Horio, T., Hotani, H. 1986. *Nature* 321: 605–7
36a. Howard, W. D., Timasheff, S. N. 1986. *Biochemistry* 25: 8292–8300
37. Humphreys, W. G., MacDonald, T. L. 1988. *Biochem. Biophys. Res. Commun.* 151: 1025–32
38. Hyman, A., Drechsel, D., Kellogg, D., Salser, S., Sawin, K., et al. 1991. *Methods Enzymol.* 196: 478–85
39. Kirsch, M., Yarbrough, L. R. 1981. *J. Biol. Chem.* 256: 106–11
39a. Kirschner, M. W., Williams, R. C., Weingarten, M., Gerhart, J. C. 1974. *Proc. Natl. Acad. Sci. USA* 71: 1159–63
40. Kirschner, M., Mitchison, T. 1986. *Cell* 45: 329–42
41. Linse, K., Mandelkow, E.-M. 1988. *J. Biol. Chem.* 263: 15205–10
41a. Mandelkow, E.-M., Mandelkow, E., Milligan, R. A. 1991. *J. Cell Biol.* 114: 977–91
42. Margolis, R. L., Wilson, L. 1981. *Nature* 293: 705–11
43. Martin, S. R., Schilstra, M. J., Bayley, P. M. 1991. *Biochim. Biophys. Acta Gen. Subj.* 1073: 555–61
44. Mejillano, M. R., Barton, J. S., Himes, R. H. 1990. *Biochem. Biophys. Res. Commun.* 166: 653–60
45. Mejillano, M. R., Barton, J. S., Nath, J. P., Himes, R. H. 1990. *Biochemistry* 29: 1208–16
46. Melki, R., Carlier, M.-F., Pantaloni, D. 1990. *Biochemistry* 29: 8921–32
46a. Melki, R., Carlier, M.-F., Pantaloni, D., Timasheff, S. N. 1989. *Biochemistry* 28: 9143–52

47. Mitchison, T., Kirschner, M. 1984. *Nature* 312: 237–42
48. Mitchison, T., Kirschner, M. 1984. *Nature* 312: 232–37
49. Mitchison, T. J. 1989. *J. Cell Biol.* 109: 637–52
50. Mitchison, T. J., Sawin, K. E. 1990. *Cell Motil. Cytoskelet.* 16: 93–98
51. Monasterio, O., Timasheff, S. N. 1987. *Biochemistry* 26: 6091–99
52. Nicklas, R. B., Lee, G. M., Rieder, C. L., Rupp, G. 1989. *J. Cell Sci.* 94: 415–23
53. O'Brien, E. T., Erickson, H. P. 1989. *Biochemistry* 28: 1413–22
54. O'Brien, E. T., Erickson, H. P., Salmon, E. D. 1990. J. *Cell Biol.* 111: 388a–3880 (Abstr.)
55. O'Brien, E. T., Salmon, E. D., Walker, R. A., Erickson, H. P. 1990. *Biochemistry* 29: 6648–56
56. O'Brien, E. T., Voter, W. A., Erickson, H. P. 1987. *Biochemistry* 26: 4148–56
57. Oosawa, F., Kasai, M. 1962. *J. Mol. Biol.* 4: 10–21
58. Pierson, G. B., Burton, P. R., Himes, R. H. 1978. *J. Cell Biol.* 76: 223–28
59. Roychowdhury, S., Gaskin, F. 1986. *Biochemistry* 25: 7847–53
60. Roychowdhury, S., Gaskin, F. 1988. *Biochemistry* 27: 7799–7805
61. Salmon, T., Walker, R. A., Pryer, N. K. 1989. *BioTechniques* 7: 624–33
62. Saltarelli, D., Pantaloni, D. 1982. *Biochemistry* 21: 2996–3006
63. Saltarelli, D., Pantaloni, D. 1983. *Bio-*

64. Sandoval, I. V., Weber, K. 1980. *J. Biol. Chem* 255: 6966–74
65. Schulze, E., Kirschner, M. 1986. *J. Cell Biol.* 102: 1020–31
66. Seckler, R., Wu, G.-M., Timasheff, S. N. 1990. *J. Biol. Chem.* 265: 7655–61
67. Simon, J. R., Salmon, E. D. 1990. *J. Cell Sci.* 96: 571–82
68. Stewart, R. J., Farrell, K. W., Wilson, L. 1990. *Biochemistry* 29: 6489–98
69. Tao, W., Walter, R. J., Berns, M. W. 1988. *J. Cell Biol.* 107: 1025–35
70. Terry, B. J., Purich, D. L. 1980. *J. Biol. Chem.* 255: 10532–36
71. Voter, W. A., O'Brien, E. T., Erickson, H. P. 1987. *Biophys. J.* 51: 214a
72. Voter, W. A., O'Brien, E. T., Erickson, H. P. 1991. *Cell Motil. Cytoskelet.* 18: 55–62
73. Wade, R. H., Chrétien, D., Job, D. 1990. *J. Mol. Biol.* 212: 775–86
73a. Walker, R. A. 1989. *Microtubule dynamic instability in vitro.* PhD thesis. Univ. N.C., Chapel Hill
74. Walker, R. A., Inoué, S., Salmon, E. D. 1989. *J. Cell Biol.* 108: 931–37
75. Walker, R. A., O'Brien, E. T., Pryer, N. K., Soboeiro, M. F., Voter, W. A., et al. 1988. *J. Cell Biol.* 107: 1437–48
76. Walker, R. A., Pryer, N. K., Salmon, E. D. 1991. *J. Cell Biol.* 114: 73–81
77. Wegner, A. 1976. *J. Mol. Biol.* 108: 139–50
78. Yamanaka, G., Eckstein, F., Stryer, L. 1985. *Biochemistry* 24: 8094–8101

Annu. Rev. Biophys. Biomol. Struct. 1992. 21:167–98

NMR STRUCTURE DETERMINATION IN SOLUTION: A Critique and Comparison with X-Ray Crystallography

Gerhard Wagner, Sven G. Hyberts, and Timothy F. Havel

Department of Biological Chemistry and Molecular Pharmacology, Harvard Medical School, 240 Longwood Avenue, Boston, Massachusetts 02115

KEY WORDS: NMR distance geometry, protein conformation, protein flexibility

CONTENTS

PERSPECTIVES AND OVERVIEW

The natural environment of most proteins is an aqueous solution. Despite this fact, researchers have only been able to observe proteins in their native habitat in the past decade. This advance was made possible by the development of new strategies and techniques in nuclear magnetic resonance (NMR) (cf. 127). To date, the structures of about 100 proteins

167

1056–8700/92/0610–0167$02.00

of up to 157 amino acid residues have been determined using these techniques, with a precision that in at least some cases rivals that of the established crystallographic methods (see e.g. 11, 25). Although the debate about where the limits of NMR spectroscopy may lie is considerable, few would say that these limits have been reached.

While the most important distinction between NMR and crystallography lies in the nature of their samples, there are several other basic differences. Consequently, the meaning and significance of the structures themselves is quite different. Unfortunately, the existence of several superficial similarities in the two structure-determination procedures, e.g. the use of Fourier techniques and of simulated annealing structure refinement, tends to obscure these differences. This leads to the danger that, by using or adapting techniques originally designed for crystallography in NMR structure analysis, the unique information that NMR can provide will not be fully utilized.

One distinctive feature of NMR is that each cross peak in a NMR spectrum contains direct information on a single torsion angle or distance within the protein. In contrast, each individual peak in a diffraction pattern contains information on the entire structure and cannot be interpreted without taking the rest of the peaks into account at the same time. This interpretation requires taking the spatial Fourier transform of the diffraction pattern. The Fourier transforms used in NMR, however, convert time-dependent signals and perturbations into frequency-dependent peaks; subsequently, the geometric information contained in these peaks must be extracted from them by other means.

Similarly, while the result of a crystallographic refinement is usually presented as a single spatial structure that minimizes the R-factor (and deviations from ideal covalent geometry), the result of a distance geometry calculation is usually presented as an ensemble of structures compatible with the NMR data. This different presentation of structures emerges from the very different theoretical frameworks in which the data available from these two techniques must be interpreted. In crystallography, differences in structures are leveled out by destructive interference in the diffractogram and show up only in the B-factors. Thus, fitting a molecular model to the electron density naturally yields a single most likely structure; the attempts to represent electron density plots by ensembles of structures have been relatively few (55, 132). In contrast, the effects of mobility upon NMR data are much more complicated and diverse, and proteins are probably more mobile in solution than they are in crystals. Fortunately, we can establish reasonable bounds on the effects of mobility on the NMR data, which leads to a representation of the structure by an ensemble of conformations lying within those bounds.

Despite these differences, NMR provides several valuable independent checks on the accuracy of crystallographic results and has already detected errors in several X-ray structures. Even when no actual errors have occurred, however, NMR structures have the advantage of being definitively free of artifacts resulting from crystallization. Although both NMR and X-ray structures generally exhibit the same overall chain fold, often some of the surface residues have been perturbed by intermolecular contacts in the crystal. Because the surfaces of proteins are where they interact with other proteins, with their ligands, or with DNA, these differences, although small, are likely to be biologically relevant. Other advantages of NMR include its ability to estimate the time scales of intramolecular motions (27, 97, 100) and its ability to characterize the conformations of bound ligands (cf. 2, 28, 29, 48, 49, 96).

Several recent reviews of protein structure determination by NMR spectroscopy, emphasizing the collection and interpretation of the data, have appeared (6, 30, 39, 79, 118, 128). The book by Wüthrich (127) provides an excellent introduction to this subject. Other reviews have been published that emphasize computational procedures that are used (16, 22, 62, 76, 107). Numerous books on the fundamentals of NMR spectroscopy are also available (e.g. 1, 15, 47, 91, 110). The purpose of the present review is to compare the methodology and structures available from NMR with those of crystallography. We begin with an account of the data and procedures by which protein structures are determined from NMR spectra, with emphasis on the features that distinguish them from those used in crystallography. This discussion is followed by a survey of previous NMR structure determinations in which the investigators made a detailed comparison with the corresponding crystal structures. Finally, we present a new comparison of the NMR data and structures for the elastase inhibitor eglin c with the X-ray structures of the complex of this protein with the proteases subtilisin and thermistase.

THE STRUCTURAL INTERPRETATION OF NMR DATA

The overall strategy commonly used for protein-structure determination by NMR proceeds as follows. First, each ^{1}H resonance must be assigned to specific protons within the molecule. Then, the cross peaks observed in the two-dimensional (2D) spectra must be assigned and interpreted geometrically as contraints[1] on the interatomic distances and on the torsion

---

[1] The term "restraints" is also used almost interchangably with "constraints"; properly speaking, restraints are the potential functions used to maintain consistency with the constraints during optimization and simulated annealing.

angles about single bonds. This purely geometric information is combined with that available from the primary structure, other experiments and/or database searches, and then used as input for distance geometry calculations, which produce molecular models consistent with the constraints. Finally, the resultant structures may then be energy minimized or otherwise refined to eliminate structural irregularities while maintaining consistency with the experimental constraints.

The Resonance Assignment Problem

ASSIGNMENTS AND PHASES   In the analysis of molecular structure using NMR, the first step on which everything else depends is the assignment of resonances. In certain respects, this problem is analogous to the phase problem in X-ray crystallography, in which the individual reflections in the diffraction pattern must be assigned a phase. In the resonance assignment problem, however, the individual nuclei (predominantly protons) must be assigned resonance frequencies. In neither case is any meaningful structural interpretation possible until one overcomes the assignment hurdle, but the methods actually used to solve the phase and resonance assignment problems necessarily have little in common.

THE SEQUENTIAL ASSIGNMENT STRATEGY   The original, and most direct, approach to solving the assignment problem is to isotopically label the protein at specific sites (80). Because of the great labor and expense involved, this method is currently used only as a last resort. The first really practical method of solving the problem, known as the sequential assignment method (45), had to await the development of two-dimensional NMR methods (9, 120, 123, 124, 130). Figure 1 illustrates this method.

There are essentially two important classes of ^{1}H-^{1}H 2D NMR experiments, each of which provides quite different information. In the two-dimensional correlated spectroscopy (COSY) -type experiments, the cross peaks occur only between protons that are neighbors in the covalent structure. As a rule, in these experiments only protons that are separated by not more than three chemical bonds are connected by cross peaks. By tracing these connectivities through the spectrum, the resonances can be grouped into the spin systems characteristic of the individual amino acids, as indicated by the solid boundaries drawn in Figure 1. Many techniques that complement COSY and provide additional information have since been developed, such as relayed coherence transfer spectroscopy (RELAY) (102, 116) and total correlation spectroscopy (TOCSY) (19).

The other class of experiments is exemplified by 2D nuclear Overhauser enhancement spectroscopy (NOESY). These spectra provide information about protons that are close together (usually $\leqslant 4.5$ Å) in space. In the

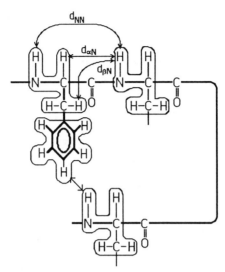

Figure 1 The strategy for structure determination via homonuclear 2D NMR experiments. The protons enclosed by solid boundaries form spin systems that can be identified via COSY-type experiments (COSY, RELAY, TOCSY, HOHAHA). The connectivities between the spin systems obtained by NOESY experiments are indicated by arrows between protons. These are used not only for the sequential assignments, but also to obtain the numerous long-range distance constraints that are the basis for constructing 3D models of the protein via distance geometry programs.

classical sequential assignment strategy, this experiment is used to establish sequential connectivities between the spin systems of the individual residues ($d_{\alpha N}$, d_{NN}, and $d_{\beta N}$ in Figure 1) (9, 124, 131). In addition, the NOESY experiment provides the numerous distance constraints, particularly between protons that are far apart in the sequence, needed for the actual structure calculations (see below).

MULTIDIMENSIONAL, MULTIPLE RESONANCE EXPERIMENTS   In proteins with more than 100 amino acid residues, the above sequential assignment method becomes difficult to use because of the extensive overlap of the many peaks in the 2D spectra. Fortunately, if the protein can be uniformly labeled with ^{13}C and/or ^{15}N (e.g. if the protein has been cloned and can be overexpressed), the investigator can overcome this crowding of the 2D ^{1}H-^{1}H spectra by dispersing the spectra in a third or even a fourth dimension (7, 34, 50, 77, 78, 94, 133). The principles behind these techniques are more fully described as follows (see also 33):

The protons connected in the 2D spectra are attached to either carbon or nitrogen, and these multiple resonance techniques require that the protein be uniformly labeled with ^{13}C or ^{15}N. In the latter case, the crowded 2D spectrum can be decomposed into different layers, where each layer contains only those cross peaks that connect pairs of protons bonded to a nitrogen atom (for example along the horizontal axis) with a particular ^{15}N resonance frequency. If the protein can also be uniformly labeled with ^{13}C, this three-dimensional (3D) layer can be further simplified by dispersing the resonances along the vertical axis in a fourth dimension, in which the different layers are characterized by the frequencies of the attached carbons. By these means, researchers have assigned the resonances to the protons in the covalent structure of proteins of up to 186 residues (38, 71, 112).

Above about 20 kilodaltons (kDa), however, dipole-dipole relaxation increasingly broadens the resonances (cf. 91). This broadening makes experiments involving homonuclear coherence transfer steps ineffective, since these require line widths not much larger than the ^1H-^1H coupling constants (COSY, TOCSY). Recently developed experiments that promise to substantially alleviate this problem are triple resonance experiments, which make use of the larger one-bond coupling constants (^1H-^{13}C, ^1H-^{15}N, ^{13}C-^{13}C, and ^{13}C-^{15}N) (51, 70–73, 83, 84). These allow intraresidue and sequential assignments via one-bond connectivities independent of the nuclear Overhauser effects (NOEs), and thus independent of the polypeptide conformation (83). The combination of these multidimensional and multiple resonance techniques has tremendously increased the power of NMR, so that the determination of the structures of 30-kDa proteins now appears feasible.

ASSIGNMENT OF NOESY CROSS PEAKS   Once as many resonances as possible have been assigned, one must assign as many cross peaks in the NOESY spectra as possible to pairs of resonances along the main diagonal. Because more than one resonance can occur with almost exactly the same frequency, this problem can also be very difficult, and in the past the information available from many NOESY cross peaks had to be omitted from the initial calculations because these ambiguities could not be resolved on the basis of the experimental data alone. Fortunately, the above-mentioned 3D and 4D heteronuclear experiments also provide nearly complete assignments of NOESY cross peaks (77, 78). The assignment of about five interresidue NOEs per residue, on the average, yields reliable but low-precision structures; the best structures to date have ~15–18 interresidue NOEs per residue assigned.

MISSING AND ERRONEOUS ASSIGNMENTS   In all but the best possible circumstances, some resonances and cross peaks will generally remain unassigned even after most of the above methods have been tried. These generally involve protons in highly mobile parts of the molecule, or else those far out on long side chains where a long sequence of connectivities through the crowded aliphatic region of the spectrum would have to be followed to assign them. Although one should certainly try to assign all the resonances and cross peaks, in practice a few missing assignments do not greatly reduce the overall precision of the structure determination. As seen later on, erroneous assignments are the greater danger.

Geometric Interpretation

QUALITATIVE NOE CONSTRAINTS   Once all the cross peaks have been assigned, the geometric information they contain must be extracted. This step plays a somewhat similar role to the calculation of electron density plots in crystallography: In both cases, the basic theory on which the experiments are based must be called upon in order to derive the raw geometric information needed for the subsequent calculations. The most important structural information available from NMR is the distance information inherent in the NOESY cross peaks [nuclear Overhauser effects (NOEs)]. In principle, the volumes of the cross peaks in 2D or higher dimensional NOE spectra connecting two protons i and j are proportional to the inverse sixth power of their internuclear distance r_{ij}^{-6}. In practice, the constants of proportionality are influenced in several ways by the local dynamics of the protein, while the actual peak volumes correspond to averages over the ensemble of different conformations undergoing rapid exchange in solution.

Thus, the quantitative interpretation of cross-peak volumes (even disregarding the many difficulties associated with measuring them precisely) is often not practical. Instead, a highly conservative approach has been widely adopted, in which the volumes of the cross peaks are interpreted in terms of lower and upper bounds on the interatomic distances. Although such a conservative interpretation of the data sacrifices some precision for the sake of certitude, the fact that many more such distance constraints are generally available than internal degrees of freedom leads to a surprising overall degree of conformational restriction (64).

Because it decays so rapidly with increasing interproton distance, the mere presence of a NOE between two protons can be taken to mean that the distance between them is quite small, usually less than 4.5 Å. Because of the possibilities of peak overlap and local mobility, the absence of a NOE does not necessarily mean that the distance between a pair of protons exceeds these limits. In addition, the investigator should make sure that the transfer of magnetization that gives rise to the NOE does not result from spin diffusion. This occurs when the magnetization is transferred from the first proton i to an intermediate proton k, and then from k to the other proton j. Under these conditions, the actual distance between i and j could be significantly larger than it would be if the transfer were direct. This phenomenon can be controlled by keeping the mixing time small, but only at the expense of reducing the overall sensitivity of the NOESY experiment.

QUANTITATIVE NOE CONSTRAINTS   Because the volumes of NOESY cross peaks at short mixing times are, assuming the molecule is perfectly rigid, proportional to the inverse sixth power of the interproton distances, in principle one can derive more precise distance constraints from the volumes. The constant of proportionality can be determined by measuring the volumes of the NOESY cross peaks for pairs of protons whose distances are strongly restricted by the covalent structure (e.g. geminal pairs). In large proteins, the attainable precision is limited to the signal-to-noise ratio that can be obtained at mixing times sufficient to eliminate spin diffusion, the severe peak overlap, and the unknown effects of molecular mobility.

In the past, therefore, NOEs have usually been quantified at only three levels: strong, medium, and weak. Another approach to realistically quantitating the precision that has recently been used is to add and subtract the estimated uncertainty in the volume measurements from each such measurement (S. Hyberts, M. Goldberg, T. Havel & G. Wagner, in preparation). When these uncertainties in the volumes are converted into uncertainties in the distances as the inverse sixth root, one obtains a pair of curves giving the minimum and maximum distance compatible with the uncertainties as a function of intensity. These two curves are trumpet shaped, meaning they diverge rapidly as the cross-peak intensity falls off. Other, more sophisticated approaches are under evaluation (114).

STEREOSPECIFIC ASSIGNMENTS   Another important step to improving the precision of the structure is to obtain stereospecific assignments of methylene protons and geminal methyl groups. These cannot be obtained from COSY/TOCSY-type experiments alone. If it is not possible to identify which proton is which, the distance constraints used must be loose enough to account for both possibilities. These constraints are usually generated by placing a "pseudoatom" halfway between the pair that can serve as a reference point for the distance constraints. One can then correct the constraints by adding to them the distance between the pseudoatom and the protons (129). If, however, the various cross peaks can be definitively assigned to one or the other of the pair of protons, this correction can be avoided and some information on the orientation of the pair relative to the rest of the molecule is obtained. Empirically, it has been found that such stereospecific assignments lead to a significant improvement in the precision of protein structures determined from NMR data (44, 58, 62).

In the past, stereospecific assignments of β-methylene protons and γ-methyl groups have been obtained by analyzing H^{α}-H^{β} vicinal coupling constants, by the quantitative interpretation of intraresidue and sequential NOEs (68, 104), or by searching structural data bases (from X-ray structures) for conformations that give NOE patterns similar to the experimental ones (58, 93). Recently, new methods for measuring heteronuclear vicinal ^{15}N-H^{β} coupling constants (84, 118) have significantly facilitated stereospecific assignments of the β-methylene protons, while at the same time characterizing the rotomeric state of the torsion angle χ^1 (23, 118) (see also below). Stereospecific assignments of geminal methyl groups have also been obtained through selective carbon labeling, taking advantage of the biosynthesis pathways of amino acids (90). At present, methylene protons farther out in the side chains and the α-protons of glycine residues are stereospecifically assigned only by examination of the ensembles computed without this information to see which of the two possibilities seems to be a consequence of the remaining data. In our opinion, this procedure is highly prone to error, and should only be used with extreme caution.

HYDROGEN-BOND CONSTRAINTS   Another, less direct source of distance constraints comes from the fact that protons involved in hydrogen bonds can often be identified from NMR studies. In this case, two types of studies are particularly useful. In the first, the protein is dissolved in D_2O, and the rate at which the exchangable proton resonances decay is monitored. Those involved in hydrogen bonds will exchange more slowly (117). The other approach monitors the chemical shifts of protons during titration of the sample. Unfortunately, neither approach tells us the identity of the other atom involved in the hydrogen bond, although this can in some cases be inferred from nearby NOEs or from the known patterns of hydrogen bonds in regular secondary structures [which can be identified by direct inspection of the NMR data (cf. 9)]. For this reason, NMR is inferior to crystallography with respect to its ability to characterize hydrogen bonds. Recent achievements in using NMR to identify amide protons bound to internal waters (26, 95) only partially alleviate the problem, because we still have no way to find out which amide protons are hydrogen bonded to the same water molecule.

TORSION-ANGLE CONSTRAINTS   The multiplet structure of NMR resonances resulting from scalar coupling often contains information concerning the torsional angles. The couplings of interest here are three-bond couplings; in particular $^3J(H^{\alpha}, H^N)$ is related to the angle ϕ, and $^3J(H^{\alpha}, H^{\beta})$

and $^3J(N, H^\beta)$ are related to χ^1. These relations have been calibrated on known structures (42, 98) and are given below (in Hertz).

$$^3J(H^\alpha, H^N)\phi = 6.4\cos^2(\phi - 60°) - 1.4\cos(\phi - 60°) + 1.9$$

$$^3J(H^\alpha, H^{\beta 2})\chi^1 = 9.5\cos^2(\chi^1 - 120°) - 1.6\cos(\chi^1 - 120°) + 1.8$$

$$^3J(H^\alpha, H^{\beta 3})\chi^1 = 9.5\cos^2\chi^1 - 1.6\cos\chi^1 + 1.8$$

$$^3J(N, H^{\beta 2})\chi^1 = -4.5\cos^2(\chi^1 + 120°) + 1.2\cos(\chi^1 + 120°) + 0.1$$

$$^3J(N, H^{\beta 3})\chi^1 = -4.5\cos^2(\chi^1 - 120°) + 1.2\cos(\chi^1 - 120°) + 0.1$$

The measurement of these coupling constants in the 2D proton spectra of large proteins is not trivial, since the resonances can be much broader than the coupling constants. Moreover, as can be seen from the equations, the determination of the torsion angles from coupling constants is ambiguous, in that one value of the coupling constant could result from as many as four different values of the angle. However, ϕ angles are usually negative, so that large couplings (9 Hz) are indicative of extended structures, and small couplings (4 Hz) are typical of helical structures.

The χ^1 angles of residues with β-methylene groups can be characterized from the four coupling constants listed above: First, one assumes (as is usually the case) that the side chain is either in one of the three staggered conformers ($\chi^1 = +60°$, $-60°$ or $180°$) or that it is jumping rapidly between these three rotomers with roughly equal populations. Together with the two possible stereospecific assignments of the β-methylene protons, these four states give rise to eight distinct patterns of coupling constants, which makes it possible to identify the rotomeric state while making the stereospecific assignments (as described previously). In particular, this analysis enables us to decide whether the side chain has a well-defined χ^1 angle, or is mobile around the C^α-C^β bond (see Figure 2). This analysis can also be extended to side chains with a β-methine group.

Recently, significant progress was made in measuring the above coupling constants even in large proteins, provided they can be ^{13}C and ^{15}N enriched (83, 85, 108, 118, 122). As shown by a comparison of the results obtained for eglin c (see below), one can determine the χ^1 rotomer states of this protein more reliably using the above method than using crystallography. Nonetheless, one should remember that these methods cannot determine the exact range of values accessible to the angle. The practice of imposing narrow ranges on the torsion angles designed to keep them in the nearly staggered states usually observed in refined crystal structures may make the structure look better, but it involves assumptions that are not a direct consequence of the NMR data.

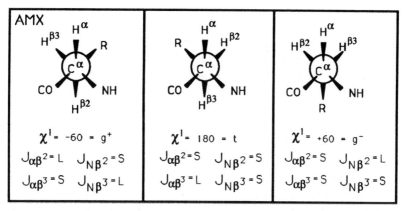

Figure 2 Diagrams showing how the patterns of $^3J(N, H^\beta)$ and $^3J(H^\alpha, H^\beta)$ coupling constants can be used to identify the rotational state of the χ^1 angle while simultaneously stereo-specifically assigning the β-methylene protons. In a nonrotating side chain, the H^α and the H^βs, or the N and the H^βs, are either *gauche* or *trans*, leading to small or large coupling constants, respectively. Small and large means ~ 3.4 and 12.9 Hz for the homonuclear couplings and -0.4 and -5.7 Hz for the heteronuclear couplings, respectively. If the side chain is jumping between the three rotamer states with equal populations, the averaged homonuclear and heteronuclear coupling constants are expected to be ~ 6.6 and -2.2 Hz, respectively.

PRECISION VERSUS ACCURACY   In deriving both distance and torsion-angle constraints, one must tread a fine line between two possible errors. On one hand, if one is too cautious, the ranges of distances and angles used will be too wide, resulting in an ensemble of structures that does not realistically reflect the actual solution ensemble. On the other hand, if one is not critical enough, the accepted constraints will exclude some of the structures present in significant concentration, including quite possibly the most populated conformer. The former error gives rise to excessive imprecision while the latter results in inaccuracy. Because inaccuracy is clearly much less desirable than imprecision, one should generally err on the side of being too cautious (if possible). The overall quality of a NMR structure determination is not simply proportional to the precision, but also depends upon the accuracy of the constraints, the quality of the convergence obtained in the distance geometry calculations, the number of structures computed, and the method of structural refinement.

Distance Geometry Algorithms

DISTANCE GEOMETRY VERSUS ELECTRON-DENSITY FITTING   The computation of ensembles consistent with the geometric constraints is in some ways analogous to fitting the polypeptide chain to the electron-density plot in crystallography. Once again, however, the methods used in NMR are quite different from those used in crystallography. Because a large portion of the NMR data available for proteins can be interpreted in terms of bounds on distances, the computer programs used to compute conformational ensembles are widely known as distance geometry programs.[2] A wide variety of such programs are available, and a detailed description of them would be outside the scope of this review (for accounts, see 18, 54, 59, 62, 63, 76, 88, 92, 107). Here, we only describe how these programs are used in protein structure determination from NMR data.

SAMPLING CONFORMATION SPACE   Once the individual cross peaks have been interpreted geometrically, the problem of describing the set of conformations consistent with this interpretation needs to be solved. Because this interpretation consists of ranges of allowed values for a subset of the distances and angles in the protein, the set of conformations generally contains a continuum of possibilities. Thus, it is not possible to find the coordinates of all these conformations but only a representative sample or ensemble. At this stage of the analysis, no attempt is made to identify any single structure as being, in some sense, the best. Instead, the entire ensemble is studied in order to find out what structural features are present in all its members, and hence are uniquely determined by the NMR data. Note that when the NMR data is combined with the fixed bond lengths, angles, chiralities, and so on, in the protein, many geometric properties may be determined that are not direct consequences of the NMR data itself.

In computing conformational ensembles from NMR data, one should sample as widely as possible. If one does not, the precision of the ensemble may seem to be higher than it actually is, which might lead to the conclusion that certain geometric features of the protein are consequences of the data when in fact they are artifacts of poor sampling. [Havel (61, 62) discusses this problem in detail and how it can be solved.] Even an unbiased ensemble, however, should be large enough to ensure that essentially all significantly different conformations consistent with the constraints have been found. This requirement can be checked by verifying that the average of the root mean square deviation (rmsd) and other measures of the differences in the ensemble (see below) have stabilized and do not change significantly as more structures are added to the ensemble. In our experience, this stabilization generally requires 40 to 50 structures.

---

[2] We use the term *distance geometry program* not for any particular algorithm, but rather for any program designed to solve the purely geometric problem of finding molecular conformations compatible with distance and chirality constraints, including torsion-angle constraints.

VIOLATIONS OF THE CONSTRAINTS   Unlike crystallographic calculations, in which the goal is to attain the lowest R-factor compatible with the signal-to-noise ratio, the goal of distance geometry is to obtain a random sample from the set of all conformations consistent with the constraints. Thus in principle, the structures in this ensemble should contain no violations of the constraints whatsoever. Molecules as large as proteins, however, seldom meet this criterion. First, perfect convergence is very difficult to obtain in such large numerical problems. Second, the constraints themselves may be geometrically inconsistent, meaning that no conformation simultaneously satisfies them all. With our current methods of generating conformational ensembles, the former problem is not usually serious (62). When the latter problem occurs, it usually results from a mistake in the assignment procedure (or a typographical error). Thus, knowing what sort of convergence to expect from the distance geometry program in use when the data is consistent can be a very useful means of catching such errors.

Inconsistencies in the constraints, however, can also be caused by motional averaging, in which two or more distinct conformations give rise to a set of NOEs and/or coupling constants that cannot simultaneously occur in any one of them. Even if this effect does not result in noticeable convergence problems, the near-fit to the inconsistent constraints will often be nearly unique. This in turn gives rise to the danger that one will conclude that the conformation is more precisely defined than it actually is (115). Fortunately, this problem is not usually serious in practice; if it were, inconsistent constraints would be encountered much more often than they actually are. Including a meaningful convergence analysis of the results of any distance geometry calculation, which demonstrates that none of the above problems are serious, remains very important. The usual practice of reporting only the rms average NOE constraint violation, or the sum of squares of the violations, is woefully inadequate because an average of 0.05 Å is not serious if it arises from a dozen or so 0.1-Å violations, but is if it results from even a single 1.0-Å violation.

QUANTITATING THE PRECISION   The most widely used and, we feel, most useful measure of precision is the average of the rmsd (for definitions, see 64, 105) between all pairs of structures in the ensemble. This property of the ensemble has received considerable study and is relatively well understood (61). When computed for the α-carbon atoms or the heavy backbone atoms alone, it provides a very good idea of how precisely the overall chain fold is determined by the NMR data. The relation of this number to the precision of an X-ray structure is at present a matter of conjecture, but it is generally assumed that a mean α-carbon rmsd of 1.0 Å corresponds to a precision of about 2.0 Å; the general relation will certainly be nonlinear.

Graphs of the local average rmsd among all sets of four contiguous atoms along the chain as a function of sequence number have also been used to measure local variability (64). Sometimes, however, it is preferable to maintain the global alignment of the structures and plot the rms distances between corresponding pairs of atoms in the different structures. Other investigators prefer to compare the structures with a "mean" structure calculated by averaging their coordinates in an optimum alignment [or by averaging their distances, as described by Hyberts et al (S. Hyberts, M. Goldberg, T. Havel & G. Wagner, in preparation)]. In this case, one should expect values about 30% lower than the values between structures. Some investigators have attempted to correlate these local values with crystallographic B-factors (17, 27).

Another measure of local variability is the rms difference in various classes of torsion angles, most notably ϕ and ψ. This measurement can be averaged over all residues or plotted as a function of residue number (64). Recently, we have been using an angular order parameter, S, defined as the norm of the average of a set of unit vectors in the plane whose angles with the x-axis equal the values of a particular torsion angle in each member of the ensemble. Two-dimensional plots, e.g. scatter plots of the residues in the ϕ, ψ plane or matrix plots of the ranges of distances in the ensemble, have also proven useful.

When viewing such projections of the results, one should keep in mind that they are but a means of throwing out hopefully irrelevant information so that what is relevant can be clearly seen. Unfortunately, what is actually relevant may be difficult to predict in advance, and hence there is no substitute for computer graphics as a means of visualizing the entire ensemble of structures. Usually, the structures are superimposed on one another so as to minimize the rmsd among them, thus obtaining a common orientation and origin. This procedure generally produces a tube of backbone conformations surrounded by a cloud of side chains, and gives one an excellent overview of the results of one's computations.

Refinement of NMR Structures

Because the variations in the relative positions of the atoms in the ensembles of structures obtained from distance geometry calculations are typically of order 1 Å, a variety of techniques have been applied to further reduce the uncertainty. These techniques fall into two basic categories. In the first, the conformation-dependent energy of the molecule is taken as an inverse measure of the quality of the structure, and those structures that minimize this energy (and remain consistent with the NMR data) are sought after. In the second, one back-calculates the NMR observables directly from the structure together with a simple model of its dynamics, and attempts to optimize the fit of the structure to the data directly. Although these back-calculations are necessarily quite different from those used in crystallography, the basic idea and philosophy behind such best-fit procedures is identical to (indeed, derived from) the extensive structure refinements now performed in X-ray crystallography (e.g. 22).

Experience with energy refinement (e.g. 106) has shown that most if not all of the structures obtained from distance geometry calculations can readily be minimized to a reasonably low energy, even without the use of restrained dynamics. Although any structure with an energy more than a few $k_B T$ above the lowest energy could in principle be eliminated, the total negative energy is only a measure of average quality. Hence, even a good structure could be very bad in some parts, and vice versa. In addition, unless restraints are used to enforce the geometric constraints derived from the NMR data, the constraint violations will generally increase markedly on energy minimization. Restrained energy minimization does lead to a marked improvement in the distribution of torsion angles, however, and in some cases, restrained dynamics has improved the sampling of conformation space over what was available from some early distance geometry algorithms (43).

One can approach the problem of modifying the conformation of a protein so that the experimental and back-calculated NOESY spectra agree in several ways (13, 14, 89, 131), and describing them all is outside the scope of this review. Suffice to say that these methods all assume that the protein has but a single, rigid conformation in solution so that its motion can be adequately described as a randomly reorienting sphere or cylinder. Then the coefficients in the linear system of ordinary differential equations that describes the NOE cross-peak volumes as a function of mixing time can be calculated analytically, and the equations solved by a variety of integration schemes (53). The various back-calculation methods available differ primarily in how they modify the structure so that the experimental and back-calculated peak volumes agree. In principle, one can also include other experimental data in these refinements, such as the coupling constants obtained from the torsion angles via the Karplus relation, though to our knowledge this has yet to be done.

In closing this section, we emphasize again that it may not always be desirable to summarize all our knowledge of a protein with a single conformation. Although the single-structure approximation is simpler and hence easier to understand than is the full continuum of possible conformations for a protein, the single-structure approximation may often be more misleading than it is illuminating. This is particularly true if, as is widely believed, the flexibility of proteins is necessary to their biological functions. In such cases, an ensemble of structures, like that obtained from distance geometry, may be a more meaningful way of representing the structural implications of the NMR data.

COMPARISONS OF X-RAY STRUCTURES WITH NMR STRUCTURES

We begin this section with a brief summary of all the methods that could be used to compare the results of NMR and X-ray studies of protein structure, and then provide a survey of those cases in which these methods have been used for such comparisons. First, we survey those comparisons in which no significant differences were found, either because they did not exist or because the NMR data were not complete enough to identify them. Next, we survey some cases in which the differences observed are believed to result from errors in the interpretation of either the NMR or the X-ray data. Next is an account of the few cases in which the differences have been shown to be both significant and real. Finally, we present a detailed comparison of several different crystal structures of the proteinase inhibitor eglin c with the NMR data and structures we have obtained.

Comparing NMR Data with Crystallographic Results

One can compare NMR data with the results of crystallographic investigations in three ways. In the first approach, one computes an ensemble of structures consistent with the geometric constraints derived from the NMR data, and then compares the NMR structures with the corresponding crystal structure to see if the crystal structure is a representative member of the ensemble or, if not, in what ways the crystal structure is distinct. In the second approach, one compares the crystal structure with the geometric constraints derived from the NMR data to see if it satisfies them. In the third approach, one back-calculates the NMR observables directly from the crystal structure and compares them with the actual experimental data. We refer to these as comparisons based on structures, constraints, and data, respectively.

Comparisons based on structures rely on the same statistical methods used to analyze the ensembles obtained from distance geometry calculations (see above). If the deviations between the crystal structure and the ensemble of NMR structures all exceed the deviations among the ensemble itself, clearly the crystal structure is not a typical member of the ensemble. Most comparisons of crystal structures and NMR ensembles to date, however, have been simple visual examinations, in which one superimposes each member of the NMR ensemble onto the crystal structure so as to minimize the coordinate deviation, and then uses computer graphics to find those regions in which the crystal structure appears to lie outside the cloud of structures in the ensemble. Though certainly effective, this method is labor intensive and subject to operator bias. A more analytic approach examines the crystal structure to see if its torsion angles lie within the range of values observed in the ensemble (10).

The advantage of the comparison of structures is that it may enable the researcher to detect differences in conformational features for which no constraints were available. Comparisons based on constraints, on the other hand, have the advantage that they can be performed prior to doing any structure calculations. For example, the absence of an interproton contact in the crystal structure, i.e. an interproton distance exceeding ~ 5 Å, where a direct NOE is clearly observed in the solution structure, is a good indication of a significant difference between the two. Unfortunately, because long-range NOEs are sensitive primarily to the overall chain fold, large differences are rarely observed in them. Fortunately, the three-bond J-coupling constants available from COSY and other NMR experiments are related to the structure in a relatively simple way and are highly sensitive to the local conformational state of the backbone and side chains.

Comparisons based on data are done by back-calculating the NMR observables from the crystal structure, which may then be directly compared with the experimental data. In principle, these comparisons can be done even before the experimental data have been interpreted as geometric constraints. The disadvantage is that one must make several simplifying assumptions to make the back-calculation computationally tractable, and thus one must check carefully that any differences observed in the data indeed result from differences in the structure rather than the shortcomings of these assumptions.

The simplest and hence most reliable example of a comparison based on data uses the homonuclear J-couplings (see e.g. 111) that can be readily predicted from the Karplus relation. Recent improvements in methods of predicting chemical shifts can also be used to check the consistency of the results of crystallographic studies, e.g. ring current shifts (3, 56, 125) and the downfield shifts that accompany hydrogen bonding or salt-bridge formation (99, 121). Perhaps the most promising comparison based on data is the comparison of back-calculated and observed NOESY cross-peak intensities. This comparison could be combined with a comparison of the coupling constants using a recently developed method (N. Beeson & G. Wagner, in preparation) to reproduce the entire NOESY spectrum from the back-calculated cross-peak volumes and coupling constants. To our knowledge, however, these sorts of comparisons have not yet been attempted.

No Significant Differences

EARLY NMR STRUCTURES   The first NMR structures of proteins were of relatively low precision, and no detailed comparisons were possible or attempted except as a check on the NMR structures. This group of proteins includes BUSI IIA, the first NMR structure determined for a protein with no known crystal structure (126). The structure was compared with two close homologues of BUSI IIA, however, and the interior backbone and side-chain atoms were found to be remarkably similar considering the low precision of this early NMR structure. This group of proteins also includes the bovine pancreatic trypsin inhibitor (BPTI) (119), carboxypeptidase inhibitor (CPI) (36), and barley serine proteinase inhibitor-2 (BSPI-2) (35). In all three cases, the average rmsds of the NMR structures to the X-ray structures were on the order of 2.0 Å, which were comparable to the differences among the NMR structures themselves.

The presently available NMR structure of BPTI (119) is of low precision, so a detailed comparison between it and the X-ray structure cannot be made. However, early comparisons of the X-ray structure with the pH titration shifts observed in the NMR spectra indicated subtle differences between the solution and crystal structures. Specifically, the pH titration of lysine side chains at low ionic strength indicated that the side chain of Lys41 forms a hydrogen bond with the hydroxyl group of Tyr10 (21). In the crystal, this interaction is absent because an arginine side chain from a neighboring molecule in the crystal intercalates between these two side chains. However, quantitative distance information cannot be obtained from titration experiments. Also, the pH titration curves in solution of the C-terminal carboxyl group of Ala58 indicate that a salt bridge exists with the N terminus, while in the crystal structure the distance between the two titrable groups is ~ 8 Å (20). This difference is plausible because of the very different ionic strengths used in solution and for crystallization.

TENDAMISTAT   The structure of the α-amylase inhibitor tendamistat was determined independently and in parallel using NMR (75) and X-ray crystallization (101), and a detailed comparison of both structures was subsequently published (10). The average rmsd between the mean NMR structure and the X-ray structure for the well-defined residues 5 to 73 is 1.05 Å, while the rmsd between these residues in the NMR structures is 0.85 Å. The displacements are larger at external loops than in the interior, but displacements between the NMR and the X-ray structure larger than the displacements between the NMR structures were found only at a few positions on the protein surface. The torsion angles of the X-ray structure were compared with the ranges of torsion angles observed in the NMR structures, and generally found to be within the NMR ranges. Finally, the

X-ray phases were solved with the NMR structures and refined (17), which lowered the backbone rmsd between the two structures from 1.03 Å to 0.26 Å. No significant local conformational differences between these two structures were found except for the side chain of Gln52.

PLASTOCYANIN AND THIOREDOXIN   A high-precision structure of reduced thioredoxin has been determined (46) and compared with the X-ray structure of the oxidized protein. No significant differences were found except for the active site, which differs by the oxidation state of the disulfide. A more detailed comparison, however, has not appeared. Similarly, high-precision structures of plastocyanins from several different sources have been determined, again without the publication of detailed comparisons with the X-ray structures (86, 87).

INTERLEUKIN 1β Interleukin 1β is the largest protein for which a NMR structure has been determined to date (33, 37). X-ray structures of this protein have also been independently determined in two laboratories (52, 103). The structures are very similar, but no detailed comparisons between crystal and solution structures are yet available. Nonetheless, displacements in the backbone position of a loop around residues 32–36 of up to 1 Å were observed. This loop is on the protein surface, and the differences may result from crystal-packing effects.

HEN EGG WHITE LYSOZYME   A detailed comparison has been made for hen egg white lysozyme (111), comparing primarily the measured coupling constants with the values expected from the torsion angles in a 1.2-Å resolution neutron diffraction crystal structure of triclinic lysozyme (81), together with a 2.0-Å X-ray structure of tetragonal type 2 lysozyme (60). The differences between the experimental coupling constants $^3J(H^N\text{-}H^\alpha)$ and values estimated from the two crystal structures, as calculated using the calibration of the Karplus equations obtained by Pardi et al (98), in no case imply a ϕ-angle difference larger than 30°, and the average rms difference between the experimental and simulated coupling constants is only 0.88 Hz. The side-chain χ^1 angles of 57 residues were also compared with the homonuclear coupling constants and intraresidue NOEs. For 41 of these, complete agreement with the crystal structures was found, while for the other 16 residues, the NMR data indicated rotational averaging about the χ^1 angle. All these residues are on the protein surface, and differences between the χ^1 values between the two crystal structures indicate that the particular orientation of many of these side chains in the individual crystal structures may actually be artifacts of crystallization. No other comparisons of the solution and crystal structures of lysozyme have been made so far.

Spurious Differences and Unresolved Cases

In a few cases, major differences were originally reported between X-ray structures and NMR structures, and later turned out to be result from erroneous interpretations of the data. These include histidine-containing protein (HPr) (74) and metallothionein-2 (MT-2) (109). For the latter, subsequent reinvestigation of the X-ray structure resulted in better agreement with the NMR structures (113). A significant difference has also been found between the X-ray and NMR structure of α-bungarotoxin (5), which is manifested in the observation that several distances in the X-ray structure are inconsistent with observed NOEs. The reason for these differences is not yet known, but the X-ray structure appears to be inconsistent with the established regularities of protein structure (5). Together, these examples show that NMR plays an important control function by providing a completely independent check on the accuracy of crystallographic studies.

Verifiable Significant Differences

THE INFLAMMATORY PROTEINS C5a AND C3a   The most outstanding case in which differences between crystal and solution structures have been demonstrated involves the C5a and C3a proteins (134). C5a and C3a are homologous proteins. To our knowledge, only C3a can be crystallized, and a crystal structure is available (66). The solution structures of both C3a and C5a have been determined using NMR and exhibit a bundle of four helices containing residues 4–12, 18–26, 34–39, and 46–63 (in the C5a numbering). The crystal structure, however, clearly lacks the N-terminal helix, and the crystal lattice lacks the space for it. This helix is very well defined in the NMR structure of C5a and folds back onto the core of the protein, as shown directly by the many strong NOEs between this helix and the rest of the protein. In C3a, this helix appears to be much less stable, and the NOEs between the N-terminal helix and the rest of the molecule are much weaker. The NOEs are nevertheless sufficient to determine the orientation of this helix relative to the rest of the protein, which is similar to that found in C5a (24). Interestingly, the mutation of residue 26 in C5a from an alanine to the methionine found in C3a destabilizes the N-terminal helix. These studies imply that crystallization destroys the labile N-terminal helix in C3a, whereas this helix is more stable in C5a, and this stability prevents the protein from crystalizing in this space group.

Another significant difference between the crystal and solution structures of these proteins is found in the C-terminal helix. The C terminus is the active site of the protein. In solution, this helix appears frayed after residue 63, while in the crystal it extends farther out and ends in a β-turn. The loss of structure in solution is observed in both C5a and C3a. In the crystal, however, the C-terminal helix seems to be stabilized by favorable contacts with neighboring molecules in the unit cell. Thus we see that crystallization can either destabilize or stabilize parts of a protein structure. The latter has particularly important implications for characterization of active sites. In the NMR structures of proteinase inhibitors, hormones, and growth factors, the active sites often appear disordered even though they are ordered in the X-ray structures. This makes sense because mobility should facilitate recognition via induced fit. The ordered structure frozen out of the solution ensemble by crystallization, however, may not correspond to a biologically active conformation. In such cases, the NMR ensemble may actually be more relevant because it should include not only the bound conformation, but also the conformations involved in recognition and binding.

INTERLEUKIN 8   Probably the most detailed comparison between a NMR structure and an X-ray structure made to date is for the protein interleukin 8 (IL-8) (31, 32). IL-8 is a small homodimer of 2×8 kDa. Clore et al (25) determined the NMR structure, and Baldwin et al (4) solved the X-ray structure using the NMR structure to determine the phases. The rmsd between the X-ray structure and the NMR structure for the well-defined part of the molecule (residues 7–72) was 1.1 Å for the backbone atoms and 1.6 Å for all atoms. Even in this well-defined region, the rms distance between the aligned X-ray and NMR structures is sometimes as large as 3 to 4 Å. Residues 4–6 are disordered in the NMR structure but well ordered in the X-ray structure. The reason for this difference appears to be the salt bridge observed in the crystal structure between Glu4 in one subunit and Lys23′ in the other; in the solution structure, this salt bridge has been replaced by one between Glu29 and Lys23′. Another difference was found in the loop comprising residues 31 to 36. His33 accepts a hydrogen bond from the backbone amide bond of Gln8 in the NMR structure but donates a hydrogen bond to the backbone carbonyl group of Glu29 in the X-ray structure. This difference could plausibly be explained by contacts with another molecule in the crystal that prevent the formation of the hydrogen bond seen in solution.

The quaternary structures are also signifcantly different: Two helices sitting on top of an extended β-sheet structure are separated by 14.8 Å in solution but only 11.1 Å in the crystal. This difference could be seen by comparing the observed NOEs with those expected from the crystal structure. The crystal structure of the homologous platelet factor 4 (PF4), on the other hand, has the same interhelix distances as seen the NMR structure of IL-8, suggesting that these differences are mainly a consequence of crystal packing. This is a good example of the susceptibility of proteins to large-scale deformations by intermolecular interactions in the crystal.

The side-chain χ^1 angles in the interior of IL-8 were generally very similar to the crystal structure, while the χ^1 angles of 10 residues on the surface differed significantly. For another eight surface residues, the NMR data (homonuclear coupling constants $^3J_{\alpha\beta}$) indicated motional averaging about the χ^1 angle, even though the side chains in the X-ray structure were placed in a single rotamer state. They may have adopted a single rotomer in the crystal state, but the difference may also have resulted from the intrinsic difficulty of identifying multiple conformations of side chains using X-ray crystallography.

In an attempt to make the NMR results directly comparable to the X-ray results, an analog of the crystallographic B-factor was constructed from the rmsd values of the NMR structure using the relation $B = 8\pi^2\bar{u}^2$, where $\bar{u}$ was replaced with the average rms distance to the corresponding average position (4). The comparison with the X-ray B-factor showed similar trends, while the NMR B-factors were approximately twice as high. This is not unreasonable because the crystal packing may reduce mobility. However, more experience with these comparisons will be needed to establish their validity.

A Detailed Comparison of Eglin C with Four Crystal Structures

The elastase inhibitor eglin c provides another interesting comparison of a NMR structure in solution with several different X-ray structures of the same protein, although the NMR studies were done on the free inhibitor while the X-ray studies were performed on complexes with proteases (subtilisin Carlsberg, subtilisin Novo, and thermistase). There are five independent X-ray structure determinations of eglin c (12, 41, 57, 65, 82), and in two of these the structure was actually solved twice, each time in a different space group (57, 65), resulting in seven different crystal structures of eglin c in all. We had access to four of the coordinate sets (12, 57, 65, 82), which are described below.

PRECISION OF THE NMR STRUCTURE OF EGLIN C   The NMR structure of the free inhibitor was determined on the basis of 947 NOE distance constraints, 417 of which were quantified in NOESY spectra with a mixing time of 50 ms. In addition, 38 ϕ-angle constraints were obtained from measurements of the coupling constants $^3J(H^N\text{-}H^\beta)$, and 41 χ^1 angle constraints were obtained from measurements of the coupling constants $^3J(H^\alpha\text{-}H^\beta)$ together with the heteronuclear coupling constants $^3J(N\text{-}H^\beta)$ (69). The structures were calculated using the distance geometry program DG-II (62), and the energy was refined with the program DISCOVER from BIOSYM®

Technologies using the AMBER potentials. The NOE constraints were maintained by suitable restraints, but for technical reasons no torsion-angle constraints were included. What follows is a preliminary account of the results we have obtained thus far; a more complete account is forth-coming (S. Hyberts, M. Goldberg, T. Havel & G. Wagner, in preparation).

A total of 75 structure calculations were carried out, of which 64 achieved sufficiently low error function values to be considered acceptable. None of these 64 structures violated any distance constraints by more than 0.3 Å. Figure 3 shows a superposition of the 64 structures accepted. These structures were aligned along a canonical average structure to avoid bias towards any single structure in the ensemble. This canonical structure was obtained by averaging the squared distances, which were then used as input for the EMBED program (40). Only the well-defined residues 8–38 and 51–68 were used for the alignment. The mean α-carbon rmsd between these residues and the average structure was 0.43 Å, while the mean α-carbon rmsd between the computed structures themselves was 0. 61 Å. Figure 4 shows a plot of the rms distance to the average structure vs sequence, while the solid lines in Figure 5 show the order parameters for the torsion angles ϕ, ψ, and χ^1.

THE PRECISION OF THE X-RAY STRUCTURES   The structure of Bode et al (12) of the complex with subtilisin Carlsberg was refined with a reciprocal space refinement procedure with energy restraints using 44,500 reflections in the resolution range 10.0–1.2 Å to an R-factor of 0.18. The structure of McPhalen & James (82) of the complex with subtilisin Carlsberg used 27,094 reflections in the resolution range 8.0–1.8 Å and was refined to an

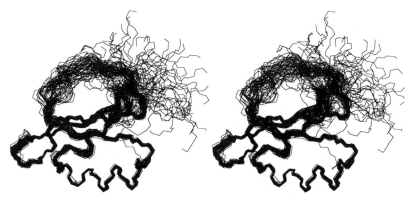

Figure 3   Superposition of the 64 backbone NMR structures of eglin c that were accepted after DC-II calculations (in stereo).

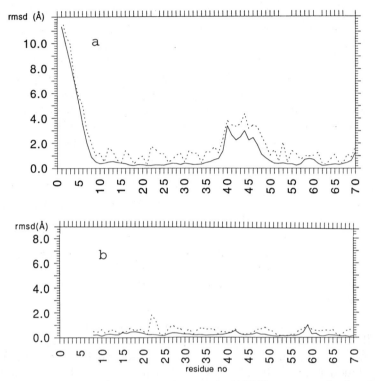

Figure 4 (*a*) Average rmsds vs sequence between the 64 NMR structures of eglin c. The rmsds were calculated relative to the canonical structure. (*b*) Average rmsds of the four X-ray structures to their mean coordinates. In both *a* and *b*, the solid line represents the heavy atoms of the backbone, and the broken line represents all heavy atoms of backbone and side chains.

R-factor of 0.136. The structure of Gros et al (57) of the complex with thermistase was refined with restrained molecular dynamics methods using reflections to 1.98-Å resolution to an R-factor of 0.165. Heinz et al (65) determined the structure from crystals in two space groups as a complex with subtilisin Novo and using reflections to 2.4-Å resolution. The structure of Dauter et al (41) of the complex with thermistase was at 1.8-Å resolution, again using crystals from two different space groups. We had access to coordinates from the first four of these structure determinations, which collectively covered three different space groups. The average α-carbon rmsd between these X-ray structures is 0.455 Å. Thus, the precision of the X-ray structures is apparently better than that of the NMR structures, but not by much. The structures of Bode et al (12) and McPhalen

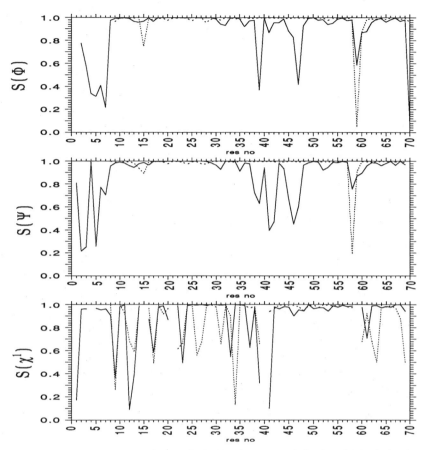

Figure 5 Order parameters S for the dihedral angles ϕ, ψ, and χ^1. The solid line is for the 64 NMR structures; the dotted lines represent the four X-ray structures.

& James (82) are the most similar and were determined in the same space groups. Figure 6 shows a superposition of the four X-ray structures with one of the NMR structures, using the same residues for alignment as in Figure 3. Obviously, the X-ray structures are more similar to each other than to the NMR structures. Table 1 lists the average rmsds between the X-ray structures and the NMR structures; Figure 4*b* shows the rms distances of the ensemble of the four X-ray structures to their mean coordinates; and the dotted lines in Figure 5 show the order parameters for the torsion angles ϕ, ψ, and χ^1 in the X-ray ensemble.

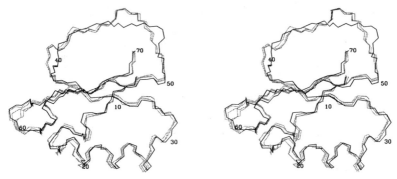

Figure 6   Superposition of the backbones of the four X-ray structures of eglin c (*thin line*) with the NMR structure with lowest energy after restrained energy minimization (*thick line*).

COMPARISON OF THE BACKBONE CONFORMATIONS   Figure 6 shows that the backbones of the NMR structures and the X-ray structures are indeed very similar; the only exception is the proteinase binding loop. This is not surprising because the crystal structures were solved for proteinase complexes while the NMR structures were determined for the free inhibitor. The hairpin loop at the apex of the antiparallel β-sheet around residue 60 (left) is, however, remarkable. The average torsion angles ϕ and ψ in the NMR structures indicate the presence of a type I turn for the residues 58–61. This observation agrees with two of the X-ray structures (57, 82), while the other two structures have a type II turn at residues 57–60. We also observe that the side chain of Thr60 has a χ^1 angle of around 180° in all the NMR structures, while the X-ray structures have values of $+60°$ or $-60°$. Obviously, the rmsd in the loop region is larger in the X-ray structures than in the NMR structures.

Table 1   Average rmsds between the backbone atoms (N, C^α, C') among the NMR structures and between the NMR structures and each of the X-ray structures for alignment of the residues 8–38 and 51–68[a]

	DG-II	B	H	G	M
DG-II	0.61	0.85	0.87	0.85	0.85
B			0.48	0.56	0.23
H				0.51	0.50
G					0.45

[a] The X-ray structures are abbreviated B [Bode et al (12)], H [Heinz et al (65)], G [Gros et al (57)], and M (McPhalen & James (82)]. DG-II stands for the 64 structures of the DG-II runs.

COMPARISON OF THE TORSION ANGLES   A comparison of the angular order parameters S of the crystal structures and the NMR structures (Figure 5) shows that the torsion angles are in most but not all cases better defined in the X-ray structures. Figure 7 shows a plot of the ranges of χ^1 angles in the NMR structures vs the sequence (dotted lines), along with the values in the crystal structures (solid lines). In most cases, the side chains are in the same rotamer state in X-ray and NMR structures. In Ser9, Val13, and Glu39, both the NMR and X-ray structures have disordered (different) χ^1 angles. Surprisingly, the side chain of Val13 is buried in the protein interior. Nevertheless, the coupling constants exhibit averaged values and clearly indicate that this side chain is jumping between different rotamer states. The fact that the crystal structures exhibit χ^1 values in different rotamer states (Figure 7) indicates that this side chain may be rotating in the crystal as well. Figure 8 shows the strand from Ser8 to Tyr24, which contains two of these disordered side chains, for both the X-ray and NMR structures.

In Thr26, Leu27, Val34, Thr60, Val62, Val63, and Val69, all of the NMR structures have the same rotamer state while the crystal structures exhibit various rotamer states, indicating that crystal contacts may change these side-chain orientations. A reverse situation occurs when the crystal structures agree on a single rotamer state but the NMR structures have an undefined χ^1 angle, i.e. Leu37, Ser41, Asn61. Also, in Val43 and Leu47, all the NMR structures have χ^1 in the same rotamer state, but all the X-ray structures agree on a different rotamer state. Both of these

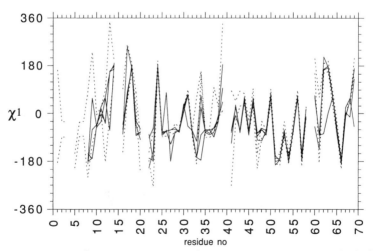

Figure 7   Ranges of χ^1 angles in the NMR structures (*dotted lines*) and values in the four crystal structures (*solid lines*).

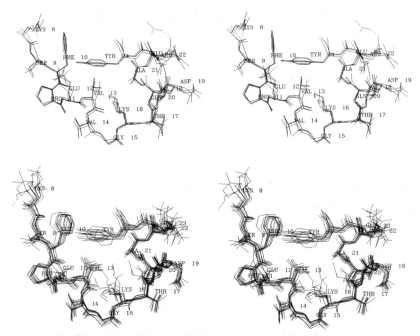

Figure 8   (*Top*) Stereo view of the strand Ser8 to Tyr24 of the four X-ray structures; (*bottom*) same strand for the 10 best NMR structures. In both cases, only those parts of the structures shown were aligned.

residues are in the proteinase-binding loop, implying that these side chains reorient upon proteinase binding.

CONCLUSION

The precision with which the NMR structures of small proteins can now be determined approaches that of moderately good X-ray crystal structures. In the protein interior, the structures obtained from the highest quality NMR data can be as precise as all but the very best X-ray structures, whereas the surface residues often appear disordered in solution and hence in the NMR structures derived from solution data. Unlike crystallography, however, the conformation does not have to be virtually unique before NMR can tell us anything about it; if only certain qualitative features, such as the rotomeric state of some of the χ^1 angles, are well defined in the solution ensemble, NMR data can still be used to characterize them.

The main differences between the NMR and X-ray structures of proteins are in fact usually found on protein surfaces. In the case of eglin c, the validity of these differences is supported by the fact that X-ray structures determined in different crystal forms exhibit differences in their surface residues (both main chain as well as side chain) that are sometimes as large or larger than the differences seen within the NMR structures. This observation is most likely the result of intermolecular contacts in the crystals. Thus, the apparent high precision of a single crystal structure on the protein surface has little relevance if not compared with other crystal forms because it does not represent the mobility of the protein surface.

Because the mobility of active sites probably plays an important role in biomolecular recognition, we feel that the ability of NMR to detect and even (to some extent) characterize mobility is one of its great strengths. Thus, even though very few large differences have been found between the NMR and X-ray structures of proteins, the smaller differences are probably biologically relevant. The more interesting active sites on protein surfaces are usually much less well defined and more mobile than the less interesting scaffold of the protein core.

ACKNOWLEDGMENTS

This review was written with the financial support of NIH grant GM-38608 and NSF grant DMB-9007878 to G. Wagner and NIH grant GM-38221 to T. Havel.

Literature Cited

1. Abragam, A. 1961. *Principles of Nuclear Magnetism.* Oxford: Oxford Univ. Press. 599 pp.
2. Albrand, J. P., Birdsall, B., Feeney, J., Roberts, G. C. K., Burgen, A. S. V. 1979. *Int. J. Biol. Macromol.* 1: 37–41
3. Asakura, T., Nakamura, E., Asakawa, H., Demura, M. 1991. *J. Magn. Reson.* 93: 355–60
4. Baldwin, E. T., Weber, T. T., St. Charles, R., Xuan, J.-C., Appella, E., et al. 1991. *Proc. Nat. Acad. Sci. USA* 88: 502–6
5. Basus, V. J., Billeter, M., Love, R. A., Stroud, R. M., Kuntz, I. D. 1988. *Biochemistry* 27: 2763–71
6. Bax, A. 1989. *Annu. Rev. Biochem.* 58: 223–56
7. Bax, A., Clore, G. M., Driscoll, P. C., Gronenborn, A. M., Ikura, M., Kay, L. E. 1990. *J. Magn. Reson.* 87: 620–28
8. Deleted in proof
9. Billeter, M., Braun, W., Wüthrich, X. 1982. *J. Mol. Biol.* 155: 321–46
10. Billeter, M., Kline, A. D., Braun, W., Huber, R., Wüthrich, K. 1989. *J. Mol. Biol.* 206: 677–87
11. Billeter, M., Qian, Y., Otting, G., Muller, M., Gehring, W. J., Wüthrich, K. 1990. *J. Mol. Biol.* 214: 183–97
12. Bode, W., Papamokos, E., Musil, D. 1987. *Eur. J. Biochem.* 166: 673–92
13. Boelens, R., Koning, T. M. G., van der Mael, G. A., van Boom, J. H., Kaptein, R. 1990. *J. Magn. Reson.* 82: 290–308
14. Borgias, B. A., James, T. L. 1988. *J. Magn. Reson.* 79: 493–512
15. Bovey, F. A. 1988. *Nuclear Magnetic Resonance Spectroscopy.* New York: Academic. 653 pp. 2nd ed.
16. Braun, W. 1987. *Q. Rev. Biophys.* 19: 115–57
17. Braun, W., Epp, O., Wüthrich, K., Huber, R. 1989. *J. Mol. Biol.* 206: 669–76
18. Braun, W., Go, N. 1985. *J. Mol. Biol.* 186: 611–26

19. Braunschweiler, L., Ernst, R. R. 1983. *J. Magn. Reson.* 53: 521–28
20. Brown, L. R., DeMarco, A., Richarz, R., Wagner, G., Wüthrich, K. 1978. *Eur. J. Biochem.* 88: 87–95
21. Brown, L. R., DeMarco, A., Wagner, G., Wüthrich, K. 1976. *Eur. J. Biochem.* 62: 103–7
22. Brünger, A. T., Karplus, M. 1991. *Acc. Chem. Res.* 24: 54–61
23. Bystrov, V. 1976. *Prog. Nucl. Magn. Reson. Spectrosc.* 10: 41–81
24. Chazin, W. J., Hugli, T. E., Wright, P. E. 1988. *Biochemistry* 27: 9139–48
25. Clore, G. M., Appella, E., Yamada, E., Matsushima, K., Gronenborn, A. M. 1990. *Biochemistry* 29: 1689–96
26. Clore, M. G., Bax, A., Wingfield, P. T., Gronenborn, A. M. 1990. *Biochemistry* 29: 5671–76
27. Clore, M. G., Driscoll, P. C., Wingfield, P. T., Gronenborn, A. M. 1990. *Biochemistry* 29: 7387–7401
28. Clore, M. G., Gronenborn, A. M. 1983. *J. Magn. Reson.* 53: 423–42
29. Clore, M. G., Gronenborn, A. M. 1990. *Biochem. Pharm.* 40: 115–19
30. Clore, M. G., Gronenborn, A. M. 1991. *Annu. Rev. Biophys. Biophys. Chem.* 20: 29–63
31. Clore, M. G., Gronenborn, A. M. 1991. *J. Mol. Biol.* 217: 611–20
32. Clore, M. G., Gronenborn, A. M. 1991. *J. Mol. Biol.* 217: 611–20
33. Clore, M. G., Gronenborn, A. M. 1991. *Science* 252: 1390–99
34. Clore, G. M., Gronenborn, A. M. 1991. *Prog. Nucl. Magn. Reson. Spectrosc.* In press
35. Clore, M. G., Gronenborn, A. M., Kjaer, M., Poulsen, F. M. 1987. *Protein Eng.* 1: 313–18
36. Clore, M. G., Gronenborn, A. M., Nilges, M., Ryan, C. A. 1987. *Biochemistry* 26: 8012–23
37. Clore, M. G., Wingfield, P. T., Gronenborn, A. M. 1991. *Biochemistry* 30: 2315–23
38. Clubb, R., Thanabal, V., Osborne, C., Wagner, G. 1991. *Biochemistry* 30: 7718–30
39. Cooke, R. M., Campbell, I. D. 1988. *BioEssays* 8: 52–56
40. Crippen, G. M., Havel, T. F. 1978. *Acta Crystallogr.* A34: 282–84
41. Dauter, Z., Betzel, C., Hohne, W. E., Ingelman, M., Wilson, K. S. 1988. *FEBS Lett.* 236: 171–78
42. De Marco, A., Llina, M., Wüthrich, K. 1978. *Biopolymers* 17: 2727–42
43. De Vlieg, J., Scheek, R. M., van Gunsteren, W. F., Berendsen, H. J. C., Kaptein, R., Thomason, J. 1988. *Proteins*

Struct. Funct. Genet. 3: 209–18
44. Driscoll, P. C., Gronenborn, A. M., Clore, G. M. 1989. *FEBS Lett.* 243: 223–33
45. Dubs, A., Wagner, G., Wüthrich, K. 1978. *Biochem. Biophys. Acta* 577: 177–94
46. Dyson, H. J., Gippert, G. P., Case, D. A., Holmgren, A., Wright, P. E. 1990. *Biochemistry* 29: 4129–36
47. Ernst, R. R., Bodenhausen, G., Wokaun, A. 1986. *Principles of Nuclear Magnetic Resonance in One and Two Dimensions.* Oxford: Oxford Univ. Press. 610 pp.
48. Feeney, J. 1990. *Biochem. Pharmacol.* 40: 141–52
49. Fesik, S. W. 1989. In *Computer Aided Drug Design,* ed. T. J. Perun, C. L. Probst, pp.133–84. New York: Marcel Decker
50. Fesik, S. W., Zuiderweg, E. R. P. 1988. *J. Magn. Reson.* 78: 588–93
51. Fesik, S. W., Zuiderweg, E. R. P. 1990. *Q. Rev. Biophys.* 23: 39–96
52. Finzel, B. C., Clancy, L. L., Holland, D. R., Muchmore, S. W., Watenpaugh, K. D., Einspahr, H. M. 1989. *J. Mol. Biol.* 209: 779–91
53. Forster, M. J. 1991. *J. Comput. Chem.* 12: 292–300
54. Gippert, G. P., Yip, P. F., Wright, P. E., Case, D. A. 1990. *Biochem. Pharmacol.* 40: 15–22
55. Glover, I., Haneef, I., Pitts, J., Wood, S., Moss, D., et al. 1983. *Biopolymers* 22: 293–304
56. Glushka, J., Lee, M., Coffin, S., Cowburn, D. 1989. *J. Am. Chem. Soc.* 111: 7716–22
57. Gros, P., Betzel, C., Dauter, Z., Wilson, K. S., Hol, W. G. J. 1989. *J. Mol. Biol.* 210: 347–67
58. Güntert, P., Braun, W., Billeter, M., Wüthrich, K. 1989. *J. Am. Chem. Soc.* 111: 3997–4004
59. Güntert, P., Braun, W., Wüthrich, K. 1991. *J. Mol. Biol.* 217: 517–30
60. Handoll, H. H. G. 1985. *Crystallographic studies of proteins.* PhD Thesis. Oxford Univ.
61. Havel, T. F. 1990. *Biopolymers* 29: 1565–86
62. Havel, T. F. 1991. *Prog. Biophys. Mol. Biol.* 56: 43–78
63. Havel, T. F., Wüthrich, K. 1984. *Bull. Math. Biol.* 46: 673–98
64. Havel, T. F., Wüthrich, K. 1985. *J. Mol. Biol.* 182: 281–94
65. Heinz, D. W., Priestle, J. P., Rahuel, J., Wilson, K. S., Grüter, M. G. 1991. *J. Mol. Biol.* 217: 353–71
66. Huber, R., Scholze, H., Paques, E. P.,

Deisenhofer, J. 1980. *Hoppe Seyler's Z. Phys. Chem.* 361: 1389–99
67. Deleted in proof
68. Hyberts, S. G., Marki, W., Wagner, G. 1987. *Eur. J. Biochem.* 164: 625–35
69. Hyberts, S. G., Wagner, G. 1990. *Biochemistry* 29: 1465–74
70. Ikura, M., Kay, L. E., Bax, A. 1990. *Biochemistry* 29: 4659–67
71. Kay, L. E., Clore, G. M., Bax, A., Gronenborn, A. M. 1990. *Science* 249: 411–14
72. Kay, L. E., Ikura, M., Bax, A. 1990. *J. Am. Chem. Soc.* 112: 888–89
73. Kay, L. E., Ikura, M., Tschudin, R., Bax, A. 1990. *J. Magn. Reson.* 89: 496–514
74. Klevit, R. E., Waygood, B. E. 1986. *Biochemistry* 25: 7774–81
75. Kline, A. D., Braun, W., Wüthrich, K. 1986. *J. Mol. Biol.* 189: 337–42
76. Kuntz, I. D., Thomason, J. F., Oshiro, C. M. 1989. *Methods Enzymol.* 177: 159–204
77. Marion, D., Driscoll, P. C., Kay, L. E., Wingfield, P. T., Bax, A., et al. 1989. *Biochemistry* 28: 6150–56
78. Marion, D., Kay, L. E., Sparks, S. W., Torchia, D. A., Bax, A. 1989. *J. Am. Chem. Soc.* 111: 1515–17
79. Markley, J. 1989. *Methods Enzymol.* 176: 12–64
80. Markley, J. L., Putter, I., Jardetzky, O. 1968. *Science* 161: 1249–51
81. Mason, S. A., Bentley, G. A., McIntyre, G. J. 1984. In *Neutrons in Biology*, ed. B. P. Schoenborn, pp. 323. New York: Plenum
82. McPhalen, C. A., James, M. N. C. 1988. *Biochemistry* 27: 6582–98
83. Montelione, G. T., Wagner, G. 1989. *J. Am. Chem. Soc.* 111: 5474–75
84. Montelione, G. T., Wagner, G. 1990. *J. Magn. Reson.* 87: 183–88
85. Montenlione, G. T., Winkler, M. E., Rauenbuehler, P., Wagner, G. 1989. *J. Magn. Reson.* 82: 198–204
86. Moore, J. M., Case, D. A., Chazin, W. J., Gippert, G. P., Havel, T. F., et al. 1988. *Science* 240: 314–17
87. Moore, J. M., Chazin, W. J., Powls, R., Wright, P. E. 1988. *Biochemistry* 28: 7806–16
88. Nerdal, W., Hare, D. R., Reid, B. R. 1988. *J. Mol. Biol.* 201: 717–39
89. Nerdal, W., Hare, D. R., Reid, B. R. 1989. *Biochemistry* 28: 10008–21
90. Neri, D., Szyperski, T., Otting, G., Senn, H., Wüthrich, K. 1989. *Biochemistry* 28: 7510–16
91. Neuhaus, D., Williamson, M. P. 1989. *The Nuclear Overhauser Effect in Structural and Conformational Analysis.*

New York: VCH
92. Nilges, M., Clore, G. M., Gronenborn, A. M. 1988. *FEBS Lett.* 229: 317–24
93. Nilges, M., Clore, G. M., Gronenborn, A. M. 1990. *Biopolymers* 29: 813–22
94. Oschkinat, H., Griesinger, C., Kraulis, P. J., Sorensen, O. W., Ernst, R. R., et al. 1988. *Nature* 322: 374–76
95. Otting, G., Wüthrich, K. 1989. *J. Am. Chem. Soc.* 111: 1871–75
96. Otting, G., Wüthrich, K. 1990. *Q. Rev. Biophys.* 23: 39–96
97. Palmer, A. G., Rance, M., Wright, P. E. 1991. *J. Am. Chem. Soc.* 113: 4371–80
98. Pardi, A., Billeter, M., Wüthrich, K. 1984. *J. Mol. Biol.* 180: 741–51
99. Pardi, A., Wagner, G., Wüthrich, K. 1923. *Eur. J. Biochem.* 137: 445–54
100. Peng, J. W., Thanabal, V., Wagner, G. 1991. *J. Magn. Reson.* 94: 82–100
101. Pflugrath, J. W., Wiegand, G., Huber, R. 1986. *J. Mol. Biol.* 189: 383–86
102. Piantini, U., Sorensen, O. W., Ernst, R. R. 1982. *J. Am. Chem. Soc.* 104: 6800–1
103. Priestle, J. P., Schär, H.-P., Grütter, M. 1989. *Proc. Natl. Acad. Sci. USA* 86: 9667–71
104. Rance, M., Bodenhausen, G., Wagner, G., Wüthrich, K., Ernst, R. R. 1985. *J. Magn. Reson.* 62: 497–510
105. Rao, S. T., Rossmann, M. G. 1973. *J. Mol. Biol.* 76: 241–56
106. Schaumann, T., Braun, W., Wüthrich, K. 1990. *Biopolymers* 29: 679–94
107. Scheek, R. M., van Gunsteren, W. F., Kaptein, R. 1989. *Methods. Enzymol.* 177: 204–18
108. Schmieder, P., Thanabal, V., McIntosh, L. P., Dahlquist, F. W., Wagner, G. 1991. *J. Am. Chem. Soc.* 113: 6323–24
109. Schultz, P., Worgotter, E., Braun, W., Wagner, C., Vasak, M., et al. 1988. *J. Mol. Biol.* 203: 251–68
110. Slichter, C. P. 1990. *Principles of Magnetic Resonance.* Berlin: Springer-Verlag. 655 pp. 3rd ed.
111. Smith, L. J., Sutcliffe, M. J., Redfield, C., Dobson, C. M. 1991. *Biochemistry* 30: 986–96
112. Stockman, B., Nirmala, N. R., Wagner, G., Delcamp, T. J., DeYarman, M. T., Freisheim, J. H. 1991. *Biochemistry.* In press
113. Stout, C. D., McRee, D. E., Robbins, A. H., Collett, S. A., Williamson, M., Xuong, X. H. 1989. *Abstr. Int. Chem. Congr. Pacific Basin Soc.* Honolulu, HI, Dec. 18–22
114. Thomas, P. D., Basus, V. J., James, T. L. 1991. *Proc. Natl. Acad. Sci.* 88: 1237–41

115. Torda, A. E., Scheek, R. M., van Gunstren, W. F. 1990. *J. Mol. Biol.* 214: 223–35
116. Wagner, G. 1983. *J. Magn. Reson.* 55: 151–56
117. Wagner, G. 1983. *Q. Rev. Biophys.* 16: 1–57
118. Wagner, G. 1990. *Prog. Nucl. Magn. Reson. Spectrosc.* 22: 101–39
119. Wagner, G., Braun, W., Havel, T. F., Schaumann, T., Go, N., Wüthrich, K. 1987. *J. Mol. Biol.* 196: 611–39
120. Wagner, G., Kumar, A., Wüthrich, K. 1981. *Eur. J. Biochem.* 114: 375–84
121. Wagner, G., Pardi, A., Wüthrich, K. 1983. *J. Am. Chem. Soc.* 105: 5948–49
122. Wagner, G., Schmieder, P., Thanabal, V. 1991. *J. Magn. Reson.* 93: 436–40
123. Wagner, G., Wüthrich, K. 1982. *J. Mol. Biol.* 155: 347–66
124. Wider, G., Lee, K. H., Wüthrich, K. 1982. *J. Mol. Biol.* 155: 367–88
125. Williamson, M. P. 1990. *Biopolymers* 29: 1423–31
126. Williamson, M. P., Havel, T. F.,

Wüthrich, K. 1985. *J. Mol. Biol.* 182: 295–315
127. Wüthrich, K. 1986. *NMR of Proteins and Nucleic Acids.* New York: Wiley. 292 pp.
128. Wüthrich, K. 1990. *J. Biol. Chem.* 265: 22059–62
129. Wüthrich, K., Billeter, M., Braun, W. 1983. *J. Mol. Biol.* 169: 949–61
130. Wüthrich, K., Wider, G., Wagner, G., Braun, W. 1982. *J. Mol. Biol.* 155: 311–19
131. Yip, P., Case, D. A. 1989. *J. Magn. Reson.* 83: 643–48
132. Yu, H. A., Karplus, M., Hendrikson, W. A. 1985. *Acta Crystallogr.* B41: 191–201
133. Zuiderweg, E. R. P., Fesik, S. W. 1989. *Biochemistry* 28: 2387–91
134. Zuiderweg, E. R. P., Nettesheim, D. G., Fesik, S. W., Olejniczak, E. T., Mandecki, W., et al. 1990. In *Frontiers of NMR in Molecular Biology*, ed. D. Live, I. M. Armitage, D. Patel, pp. 75–87. New York: Wiley-Lyss

Annu. Rev. Biophys. Biomol. Struct. 1992. 21:199–222

FEMTOSECOND BIOLOGY

Jean-Louis Martin and Marten H. Vos

Laboratoire d'Optique Appliquée, INSERM U275, Ecole Polytechnique
ENSTA, 91120 Palaiseau, France

KEY WORDS: femtosecond spectroscopy, heme proteins, reaction center

CONTENTS

PERSPECTIVES AND OVERVIEW

The primary steps of biochemical processes take place within proteins and
protein complexes. Redox changes, conformational changes, and local
structural changes induced by ligand binding may occur on a femtosecond
time scale, after external triggering. These changes may be very complex
and result from long-distance interactions, which are characteristic for
protein functions. Examples of such processes are oxygen dissociation
and association in hemeproteins, transmembrane electron transport in

199

1056–8700/92/0610–0199$02.00

photosynthetic bacterial reaction centers, and isomerization of the retinal chromophore in bacteriorhodopsin.

The development of femtosecond laser spectroscopy (97, 98) and its direct application by biophysicists in the past 10 years has been crucial for our knowledge of ultrafast processes. In fact, optical spectroscopic techniques are the only dynamical experimental tools presently available for visualizing such processes in real time. Other spectroscopic techniques suffer from fundamental [electron paramagnetic resonance (EPR)] or technical (X-ray diffraction) restrictions that prevent a femtosecond time resolution. Temporal resolution in the visual frequency range now reaches the Heisenberg limit, where it is determined by the required spectral resolution.

Apart from just the higher time resolution, a more fundamental difference separates the spectroscopy of protein complexes in the femtosecond time range and longer time ranges. Within a protein, mechanical perturbations are essentially localized on a time scale of 100 fs; acoustic dispersion takes place in the picosecond time range. Therefore, the initial vibrational perturbation of a protein system is much better characterized when using a femtosecond light pulse than when using longer pulses. More explicitly, when the coupling to the probed reaction is efficient, a femtosecond excitation may in principle synchronize a molecular ensemble at the level of the vibrational phase of the coupled mode(s). This action may lead to a significant population of transition states along the reaction coordinates. Hence, femtosecond techniques allow one to study directly the transport of energy by vibrational coupling between different parts of the protein. On the other hand, if on a femtosecond time scale, delocalized perturbations are observed, the coupling mechanism must be electronic in nature.

Both triggering and probing of the systems can be achieved only by using light; this limits the processes that can be studied. Of course, systems in which light is physiologically used, such as photosynthetic and retinal pigment-protein complexes, are ideally suited for optical techniques. But processes in proteins with optically active cofactors (often porphyrins), such as hemeproteins, can also be followed optically. Furthermore, the (ultraviolet) absorption of amino acid residues allows the study of the protein dynamics itself.

Although concepts from solid-state physics may sometimes be useful in understanding biological systems, the collective character of most of the reactions in proteins requires more specific treatment. The combination of extreme speed, long-distance range, and high efficiency of the ultrafast processes in biological material is not found in other condensed-phase material, presenting a challenge for many workers in the field. Apparently, the occurrence of ultrafast processes is strongly related to the specific structure of the protein and protein-cofactor complexes. So, experimental dynamical results are discussed in view of structural information, obtained with steady-state spectroscopic techniques, and in view of theoretical predictions, such as molecular dynamics simulations. Also, the development of genetic engineering techniques (18), now enabling the manipulation of biological structures on the level of single amino acid residues, has yielded a tool for externally varying structural parameters. In this field, collaborations between genetic engineers and theoretical physicists are not uncommon.

Fleming reviewed the pioneering applications of femtosecond spectroscopy in a broad spectrum of fields in chemical and biochemical physics in 1986 (31). Reviews by Hochstrasser & Johnson in 1988 (46) and by Holzwarth in 1989 (50) cover processes in the femtosecond-to-nanosecond time scale in the same fields as we address here. We restrict ourselves to the truly femtosecond processes, i.e. those occurring in a time scale up to a few picoseconds, and focus on a few biophysical questions that have received considerable recent attention. First we briefly describe the main experimental techniques used in this field to acquaint the nonspecialized reader with the possibilities and restrictions of these techniques. Then we address results on various biological systems, emphasizing hemeproteins and photosynthetic reaction centers [retinal photochemistry was recently reviewed by Mathies et al in this series (77)], and discuss general mechanisms of femtosecond biology.

EXPERIMENTAL TECHNIQUES

As stated in the previous section, optical pulses are required for triggering and also for subsequent monitoring of processes taking place in the femtosecond time scale; no optical or electronic detection devices are available with response times less than several picoseconds. Several reviews (31, 98) are available on the techniques of femtosecond pulse generation and manipulation. Here, we restrict ourselves to a short description of the techniques most used in ultrafast biophysical research. We show that the complementarity of the time and frequency domains is a central point in understanding these techniques. As an example for a complete system, Figure 1 shows the experimental setup currently employed in our laboratory for transient absorption measurements.

Generation and Amplification of Femtosecond Pulses

Generation of pulses with a pulse length of 30–100 fs is achieved by mode-locking techniques, generally using ring cavities. In the most commonly used, the colliding pulse mode-lock technique (34) (Figure 1), a (con-

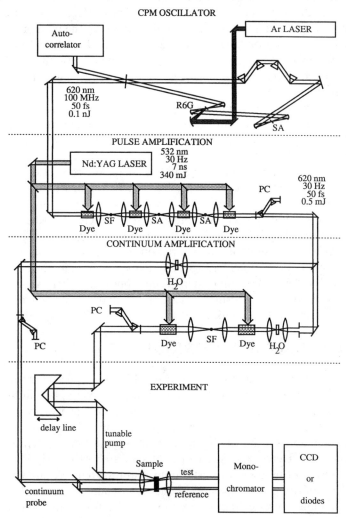

Figure 1 Scheme of an experimental setup used for femtosecond transient absorption spectroscopy. The spectrum of the pump pulse is tunable by the choice of the dyes in the amplification of the continuum. The temporal length of the pulses depends on the spectrum and generally is shorter than the fundamental pulse. Abbreviations are: SA, saturable absorber; SF, spatial filtering; PC, pulse compression.

ventionally liquid) gain medium is continuously pumped. Passive mode-locking and pulse shortening is achieved by a saturable absorber, which is reached simultaneously by two counter propagating pulses in each round. Alternatively, active mode-locking can be achieved by synchronously pumping the gain medium (or media) with (picosecond) pulses. In the latter case, the cavity length must be equal to that of the pump laser. Here the saturable absorber acts only to shorten the pulse. When generating such short pulses, the limiting factor is pulse broadening by group velocity dispersion. Such effects are minimized by using mirror optics rather than lenses, by using very thin dye jets, and by compensating the unavoidable dispersion within the cavity to first order through the use of dispersive prisms (35). The oscillator output consists of pulses in the pico- to nano-joule regime, spaced at about 12 ns, depending on the cavity length. Amplification to the micro- or millijoule regime can be achieved in multiple stages by synchronous pumping with a nanosecond or picosecond pulse laser at a lower repetition rate.

As a whole, the techniques for generating femtosecond pulses are now becoming rather standard and commercially available, a development that will be enhanced by the arrival of femtosecond oscillators with a solid-state amplification medium, Titanium Sapphire (39). The attention of experimentalists now focuses on the optimal manipulation of the pulses for their specific applications.

All techniques discussed here are of the pump-probe type, in which the pulse is split after amplification. The pump pulse may be used directly if its spectrum is convenient, but if this is not the case, the investigator can amplify part of a generated continuum. In this technique, the pulse is focused on a cell containing water or a water-alcohol mixture to produce a continuous spectral range (white light) by nonlinear processes such as self-phase modulation that are not yet fully understood. The desired part of the spectrum is then selected and amplified in one or more additional stages using appropriate dyes (72). The temporal width of the pump pulse is usually limited by the bandwidth of the amplification medium and/or by spectral restrictions of the sample and is in the order of 40 fs after compensation for chirp induced by optical components between continuum generation and sample.

Transient Absorption Spectroscopy

When performing transient absorption spectroscopy, one aims at following the spectral evolution either by monitoring the kinetics at certain wavelengths or by taking entire spectra at certain pump-probe delay times. In both cases, a spectrally broad probe pulse is required. This pulse is conventionally obtained by continuum generation in a water cell, as explained above, sometimes in combination with re- (and pre-)compression of the pulse. In a recently introduced technique, the investigator induces in an optical fiber a chirp that can be subsequently compressed to a pulse as short as 6 fs (33). Mathies and coworkers used such an arrangement to study the femtosecond spectral evolution of bacteriorhodopsin (76). Note that for the probe pulse, in contrast to the pump pulse, the pulse length has no lower limits that relate to the spectral resolution, because wavelength selection or dispersion can be achieved after passing the sample.

In transient spectroscopy, the delay time between pump and probe is varied with an optical delay line. The two beams are focused on the sample nearly colinearly, so that the probe beam can still be detected separately.

Transient Raman Spectroscopy

Two traditional protein vibrational spectroscopy techniques, Raman and infrared absorption spectroscopy, have been extended to the sub-picosecond time domain. Here, the complementarity of time and frequency is clear and imposes more severe restrictions on the time resolution than transient absorption spectroscopy in the submicrometer wavelength domain. In Raman spectroscopy, the spectrum of the probe pulse is necessarily very narrow, as its width directly determines the resolution of the transient Raman spectrum. For instance, a spectral resolution of 30 cm^{-1} (~ 0.5 nm at 450 nm) correspond to pulses of 500 fs. Further, the intensity of the probe pulses should be sufficient (but not actinic) to accumulate the generally weak transient Raman spectra within a reasonable time. For this reason, techniques of amplification of the continuum similar to those for the pump pulse are used, in combination with frequency-doubling techniques, to obtain the desired spectral selection. Petrich et al described the first subpicosecond Raman apparatus and used it to identify the nature of primary processes in hemoglobin (92).

Transient Infrared Absorption Spectroscopy

In the past three years, time-resolved infrared (IR) spectroscopy has been extended to the subpicosecond regime (2–5, 38, 45, 53). The basic setup is the following: A visible femtosecond pulse initiates the reaction as in a standard femtosecond absorption experiment. The probe is a continuous-wave (CW) IR light either from a tunable diode or a CO laser. Gated detection of the CW IR probe enables the femtosecond time resolution. The transmitted IR light is mixed with a femtosecond visible pulse in a nonlinear crystal; the resulting up-converted visible light is proportional to the transmitted IR intensity over the temporal window defined by the gating pulse. Transient infrared spectroscopy in the femtosecond time scale was first applied in biology to follow the free CO molecule in hemoglobin after its photodissociation from the heme (3).

Fluorescence Up Conversion

Fleming and colleagues (40, 96) and Hochstrasser et al (88, 89) extended fluorescence depolarization techniques, which are particularly suited to studying dynamics of rotational motion, to the femtosecond time domain. The time resolution is achieved by gating the fluorescent light emitted by the sample. The interaction in a nonlinear crystal between the fluorescence and a gating pulse derived from the pump pulse produces a pulse at the sum frequency. The time evolution of the up-converted signal is determined by the temporal overlap of the gating pulse and the fluorescence. This technique is called fluorescence up conversion. A time resolution of 200–250 fs has been achieved (40, 89).

Some related techniques need to be mentioned here, although they are not be discussed in any detail. First, the subpicosecond techniques, photon echo spectroscopy (43) and coherent anti-Stokes Raman spectroscopy (CARS) (65), are applied to specific biological systems. These techniques make explicit use of the coherence of laser light (108) and can monitor electronic dephasing processes. Here, the monitored process may even occur on a time scale shorter than the pulse width. Second, the complementarity of time and frequency domains implies that results from high resolution frequency techniques [such as hole-burning spectroscopy (54)] can be Fourier transformed and interpreted in the time domain.

HEMEPROTEIN DYNAMICS

Excited-State Photophysics

Obviously, light is not a natural ingredient of hemoglobin biochemistry. When using light-pulse activation in such a system, one must first characterize the induced nonphysiological processes. Using femtosecond pulses, we have shown (73–75, 92, 93) that photodissociation of the ligand occurs in less than 50 fs with a quantum yield of approximately unity, irrespective of whether the ligand is CO, O_2, or NO. The ground-state unligated heme species appears in 300 fs. Two short-lived species are formed upon ligand photodissociation. We have assigned these species to excite states of the unligated heme and labeled them Hb_I^* and Hb_{II}^* (Figure 2). Hb_I^* may represent a species in which the heme is already partially domed and that decays in 300 fs to the ground-state, unligated species (93). Hb_{II}^* is populated via a competitive channel with a yield strongly dependent on the nature of the ligand. This channel is very efficient when the ligand is

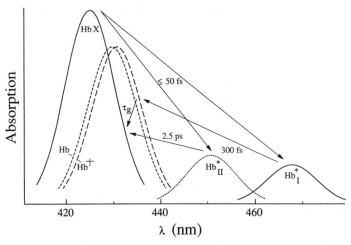

Figure 2 Generalized absorption spectra of heme proteins and their photoproducts. The diagram is labeled for hemoglobin, but is equally applicable to myoglobin and protoheme, provided that the associated shapes and positions of the deoxy-like species (+) are taken into account. X denotes the ligand (O_2, CO, or NO). The excited-state unligated species Hb_I^* and Hb_{II}^* are formed in less than 50 fs from the photoexcited HbX; their relative amounts depend on X. The deoxy-like species is formed from Hb_I^* in 300 fs; Hb_{II}^* decays to the ground state in 2.5 ps. The term τ_g reflects the time constant(s) for geminate recombination.

NO or O_2. The lifetime of the Hb_{II}^* species is 2.5 ps and corresponds to recombination of O_2 and NO. This ultrafast recombination of a significant fraction of the dissociated ligand with this highly reactive species is in part at the origin of the low yield of photodissociated O_2- and NO-heme compounds as measured on a microsecond time scale. Petrich et al (93) first suggested that the fast recombination results from a planar heme geometry in Hb_{II}^*; this proposition is in agreement with recent sub-picosecond resonance Raman spectroscopy of oxyhemoglobin (102).

After a few picoseconds, the deoxy-like species, $Hb^\dagger$, is the only remaining (transient) species. This species represents the first identified intermediate state on the physiological pathway between the ligated conformation and the deoxy structure. In hemoglobin, and not in myoglobin, the spectrum of the $Hb^\dagger$ species is distorted with respect to equilibrium unligated Hb. The slow relaxation of this distortion (nanosecond to microsecond) is attributed to the constraint in the hemoglobin tetramer that results from an ultrafast increased interaction between the (at least partially) domed heme and its proximal environment. The time scale of the relaxation corresponds to the time required for the change in quaternary structure of the hemoglobin molecule (47).

Excess Energy and Vibrational Cooling

The absorption of a photon by a heme should in principle result in a significant increase in temperature. In femtosecond experiments, the typical wavelength of the photon used for dissociation is 585 nm. The energy of a 585-nm photon is 49 kcal/mol. Because the Fe-C bond dissociation energy is about 22 kcal/mol (56), an excess photon energy of 27 kcal/mol is available. According to molecular dynamics simulations (42), a 27-kcal/mol excess energy results in a temperature increase of about 200 K. In an early experiment using femtosecond resonance Raman spectroscopy, we observed that the initial downshift of the v_4 transition relaxes within a few picoseconds, suggesting a cooling of the heme on this time scale (92). This finding is in the range predicted by the simulations and in agreement with recent experiments on heme cooling that monitored the transient anti-Stokes spectrum (66). Assuming thermal distribution of vibrational energy, these authors estimate a temperature of 20 K above room temperature within their 10-ps resolution. Combining these different results, we can conclude that cooling of the heme must be faster than 10 ps.

Structural Dynamics of Hemoglobin and Myoglobin

Detailed information about structural dynamics of the protein environment of the heme is obtained with spectroscopy of vibrational rather than electronic transitions. Petrich et al (92) used the v_4 transition of the heme as a probe in a subpicosecond Raman study of hemoglobin. They observed that, upon CO photodissociation after relaxation (i.e. re-upshift) of the initial downshift of the v_4 transition resulting from vibrational cooling (see above), a downshift occurs with a time constant of approximately 30 ps. This latter downshift is thought to reflect the response of the protein to doming of the heme (92); in particular, the proximal histidine tilts with respect to the heme plane (37). This interpretation is in agreement with findings from earlier picosecond transient Raman studies by Findsen et al (28, 29), who showed that the v_{Fe-His} stretching mode appears after 25 ps in hemoglobin, but not in myoglobin (see also 44, 91), and indicates that strain energy that is initially stored in the Fe-His bond generates a deoxy-like change at the $\alpha_1\beta_2$ contacts in about 30 ps. Thus, these techniques enable one to follow the directed flow of strain energy.

Ligand Dynamics in Hemoglobin and Myoglobin

After the ultrafast photodissociation, ligands may rebind to the heme. The time scale of this geminate recombination depends on the ligand. Recombination of CO takes place on the time scale of nanoseconds and slower, whereas recombination of NO and O_2 occurs mainly on the picosecond time scale. The latter time scale is also accessible for molecular dynamics simulations. Thus, the NO geminate recombination process is well suited for direct comparison between simulated and experimental observables.

NO geminate recombination is nonexponential at room temperature (90). This behavior may in principle result from (a) a distribution of substates, as originally proposed by Frauenfelder and coworkers (6) for the nonexponential kinetics of CO rebinding at low temperature, or (b) a time-dependent recombination barrier associated with structural rearrangement of the heme protein, or both. Petrich et al (90) recently reported a combined study of NO recombination in hemes using femtosecond absorption spectroscopy and of rearrangements of the heme and its environment after ligand photodissociation using molecular dynamics simulations. This study showed that several structural rearrangements occur in the time range of 50 fs to 100 ps, i.e. on the same time scale as NO recombination, suggesting that a time-dependent activation barrier plays an important role in the nonexponential kinetics. The presence of several intermediates in the escape pathway of CO after photodissociation is well illustrated in the molecular dynamics trajectory shown in Figure 3 (J.-C. Lambry & J.-L. Martin, unpublished results).

Dynamics of Photodissociated CO in Cytochrome Oxidase

Recently, the studies of ligand dynamics on the femto- and picosecond time scale in hemeproteins were extended to eukaryotic cytochrome oxidase. Cytochrome oxidase contains two heme centers, cytochrome a and cytochrome a_3, to which exogenous ligands may bind, and two copper centers Cu_A and Cu_B. The presence of two heme centers and the fact that the structure of this important protein is not known in detail somewhat complicate the interpretation of transient absorption data. The spectroscopic features reflecting the heme photophysics can be studied separately in the unligated enzyme (100); they can be ascribed mainly to cytochrome a and are similar to those in hemoglobin and myoglobin (see above).

As could be expected from the ligand dissociation studies in hemoglobin

———————————————————————————→

Figure 3   Molecular dynamics simulation of the pathway of CO in myoglobin after photodissociation with negligible excess energy. Each drawn step is 50 fs; the total trajectory is 100 ps. The CO ligand clearly resides in three distinct intermediate states during this trajectory. In this specific simulation, the transitions from the first to the second state and from the second to the third state take place after, respectively, 36 ps and 65 ps. Each figure shows the entire trajectory; the position of the nearest amino acid residues is averaged over the residence time in the first (*A*), second (*B*), and third (*C*) state.

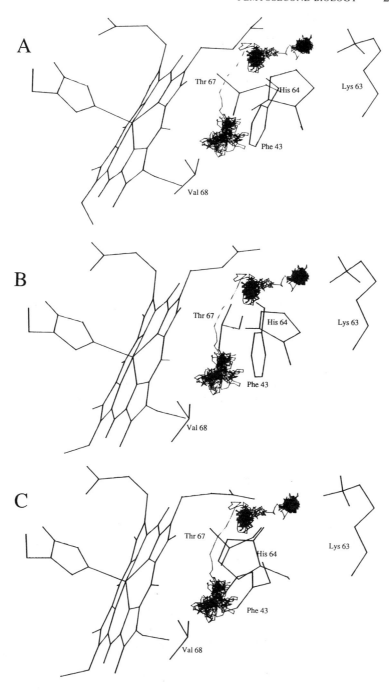

and myoglobin, dissociation of CO from cytochrome a_3 in the CO-ligated enzyme takes place in less than 100 fs (100). Picosecond infrared spectroscopy revealed that CO then very rapidly binds to the Cu_B center: this process takes less than 1 ps (25). Apparently, the Cu_B center acts as a ligand shuttle (107); CO is released to solution in 1.5 μs (24). The transient absorption spectrum shows significant changes in the cytochrome a_3 center upon photodissociation of CO and a subsequent relaxation with a time constant of 6 ps (100). The nature of this relaxation remains to be determined. More studies on eukaryotic and bacterial cytochrome oxidase, including subpicosecond Raman spectroscopy, are needed to gain further understanding of these ultrafast processes.

PRIMARY CHARGE SEPARATION IN PHOTOSYNTHETIC BACTERIAL REACTION CENTERS

Properties of the Reaction Center

The key processes of photosynthetic energy conversion occur in the so-called reaction center. The very fast (~ 17 Å in ~ 3 ps) and highly efficient (quantum yield near unity) primary electron transport step has been studied with a variety of direct and indirect techniques and has, in addition, gained considerable theoretical attention. Several reviews on the structure and the electron transport properties of reaction centers are available (11, 27, 59, 85, 86). We briefly describe the structure of the reaction center and introduce the current main research topics, which are discussed in light of the most recent dynamical data.

The reaction center is a membrane-bound pigment-protein complex. In purple bacteria, four bacteriochlorophylls (P_L, P_M, B_L, and B_M), two bacteriopheophytins (H_L and H_M), and one or two quinones (Q) are bound to two reaction center subunits, L and M. Reaction centers from two species, *Rhodopseudomonas viridis* and *Rhodobacter sphaeroides*, have been crystallized, and their structure has been resolved using X-ray diffraction (1, 19). The arrangement of the cofactors is very similar in both species; Figure 4 shows this arrangement for *R. viridis*. The center displays approximate C_2 symmetry; the C_2 axis runs through the center of two neighboring bacteriochlorophylls at the periplasmic side of the complex and through a nonheme iron atom at the cytoplasmic side of the complex. The Q_Y absorption bands of the six bacteriochlorin pigments are in the near-infrared. It is generally agreed that in the ground state P_L and P_M have a strong excitonic interaction; they are usually referred to as P. The lowest absorption band of the reaction-center pigment complex is assigned to the

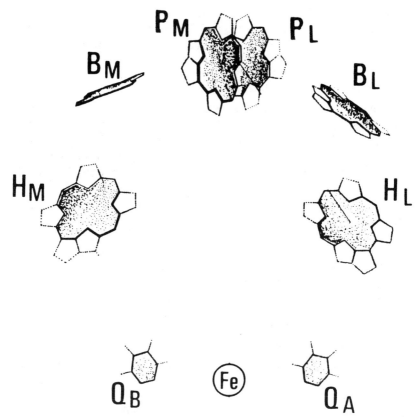

Figure 4 Arrangement of cofactors in reaction centers of purple bacteria. P_L, P_M, B_L, and B_Ms are bacteriochlorophylls; H_L and H_M are bacteriopheophytins; Q_A and Q_B are quinone secondary acceptors. The arrangement shows near C_2 symmetry with the C_2 axis running through P and the nonheme iron. The distance between P and H_L is ~ 17 Å.

lower exciton band of P, when regarded as a strict dimer, and is located, at room temperature, at 960 nm and 870 nm for *R. viridis* and *R. sphaeroides*, respectively. The other pigments presumably also interact with each other and with the surrounding protein matrix. The extent of these interactions and, not unimportantly, the mixing of charge-transfer states with the ground state and excited state(s) of the complex are still subject to debate (for reviews see 36, 41, 87).

The symmetry of the reaction centers is not complete. The L and M subunits are not completely homologous and the chromophore orientation is also slightly dissymmetrical (20, 21). The asymmetry is directly reflected in the function as there is much evidence that electron transport results in the reduction of H_L, but not of H_M (59, 83, 86). This observation indicates that structural details play an important role in the primary electron transfer processes.

The Identity of the Primary Electron Acceptor

Since the mid 1970s, researchers have known that a photoproduct P^+I^- formed within a few picoseconds (55, 95) in which I was ascribed to a bacteriopheophytin and P to bacteriochlorophyll (26). The first data with subpicosecond pulses with which the formation kinetics of this state could be adequately determined date from the mid 1980s. Woodbury et al (106), using pulses of 0.8 ps at 610 nm that excited the ensemble of bacteriochlorophyll Q_X bands, found a charge separation time of 4 ps in *R. sphaeroides*, whereas Martin and coworkers, using pulses of 150 fs and exciting directly in the near-infrared Q_Y band of P, reported a charge separation time of 2.8 ps for both *R. sphaeroides* (70) and *R. viridis* (14) (all at room temperature). Both groups concluded from their data that the electron transfer step $P^* \rightarrow P^+H_L^-$ is a one-step process. This conclusion was based on the fact that the same kinetic constant could describe within the experimental error the kinetics at several wavelengths, reflecting P^* decay (in its stimulated emission); the rise of the electrochromic bandshift around 800 nm due to charge separation; and the reduction of H_L (bleaching of its ground state and formation of the bacteriopheophytin anion band). These studies seemed to make clear that no intermediate state $P^+B_L^-$, with a lifetime longer than that of P^*, forms prior to $P^+H_L^-$, as had been previously suggested on the basis of picosecond spectroscopy (99).

The scheme of primary electron transport that emerges from these data, one step from P to H_L, is surprisingly simple in view of the complex hexachromophore structure of the reaction center. Conventional electron transport theory (36, 41, 87) cannot explain such a fast, long distance, one-step reaction. The identity of the primary electron acceptor (B_L or H_L) and the very nature of the primary electron transfer events are highly controversial. Several different mechanisms have been proposed on the basis of additional experiments and theoretical arguments.

A superexchange mechanism has gained considerable attention (10, 83, 105). In this model, the state $P^+B_L^-$ acts as virtual state (with a free energy above that of P^*) that facilitates electron transfer from P to H_L. Alternatively, a sequential two-step mechanism, in which the state $P^+B_L^-$ acts as a real intermediate but is depleted much faster than it is formed, could also explain the data (68). Such a mechanism does not fit in the general picture of stepwise stabilization of sequentially longer-lived photoproducts, as is found throughout the slower range of processes of photosynthetic energy stabilization. However, the basis for such a picture, i.e. quasi equilibrium between the different states, may not apply at very short time scales. Experiments on reaction centers of *R. sphaeroides* at room temperature by Zinth and coworkers revealed the presence of small kinetic phases with a time constant of ~ 0.9 ps, i.e. faster than P* decay (48, 49). These results clearly show that the kinetic picture is more complicated than outlined above. The experiments were interpreted in terms of the above-mentioned sequential model, with B_L as the primary electron acceptor, reduced in 3.5 ps and reoxidized in 0.9 ps [0.65 ps in *R. viridis* (22, 23)]. However, this mechanism is not generally accepted. An experimental result crucial for the identification of the proposed intermediate state as $P^+B_L^-$, the polarization of the kinetics in the bacteriochlorin anion band at 665 nm (48), could not be reproduced in other laboratories (17, 62; J.-L. Martin, J.-C. Lambry, M. H. Vos & J. Breton, unpublished results). Also, when $P^+B_L^-$ forms as a separate intermediate state, its accumulation should be possible under conditions where reduction of H_L is prevented. No evidence for a population of $P^+B_L^-$ was found in the D_{LL} mutant of *Rhodobacter capsulatus*, which lacks H_L (13).

Very recently, femtosecond spectroscopy of reaction centers at cryogenic temperatures, with pulses of 45 fs, revealed that the optical transients are modulated by damped oscillations, with periods of ~ 0.5–2.0 ps (103). These oscillations presumably reflect low frequency, and hence collective, vibrational motion of the protein matrix. The expression of these modes in the absorption and stimulated emission of the pigment complex shows that (*a*) the vibrational modes are not relaxed on the time scale of electron transport (vibrational dephasing, but not necessarily relaxation, takes place in ~ 1–2 ps) and (*b*) the electronic configuration of the complex is very sensitive to the protein conformation. Despite the fact that extreme care must be taken on a phenomenological level when analyzing femtosecond data of reaction centers with a linear reaction scheme, these data indicate that electron transport may be coherently coupled to low frequency protein modes, because an oscillation with a period of about 2 ps is seen in the decay kinetics of stimulated emission. Figure 5 shows a model of coherent (or better, phase persistent) electron transport in terms of motion of wave packets on an anharmonic potential energy surface in the excited state P*, which is consistent with the observed stimulated emission data.

The proposition of coupling of electron transport to low frequency, nonrelaxed, vibrational modes offers some interesting consequences. Using the collective character of such protein vibrations, the charge transfer process may be visualized as a charge distribution, oscillating over the pigment-protein complex, including the accessory bacteriochlorophylls B_L

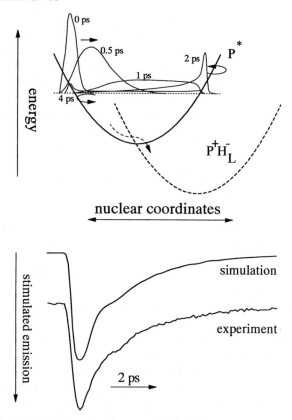

Figure 5 Wave packet motion on the potential energy surface of the P* state of a bacterial reaction center following excitation with an 80-fs pump pulse. The wave packet (average vibrational energy 9 cm^{-1}) broadens because of anharmonicity. To model the excitation at 870 nm in *R. sphaeroides* (i.e. in the high energy side of the ground-state absorption band), an excess energy of 500 cm^{-1} was taken. Electron transport may be coupled to such modes. To model this coupling, a one-way transition zone to the charge-separated state was introduced at the bottom of the well (activationless electron transfer). The experimental stimulated emission could be well simulated with these parameters. Good simulations could also be obtained when a small activation barrier was introduced.

and B_M. In contrast to the conventional electron transfer picture (8, 69), the probability of charge separation upon single passage of the transition zone is near unity, i.e. such a reaction would be near-adiabatic. Such a reaction is not stochastic in nature and the classical concept of a rate constant becomes meaningless.

Coupling of electron transport to coherent low frequency modes remains to be proved or falsified. Regardless of this, another major point arises from the sheer observation of low frequency vibrational modes: the importance of long-distance interactions in the pigment-protein complex in femtosecond processes. The transient spectrum in functional reaction centers, observed within 100 fs after excitation in the lower exciton band at low temperature, also shows such interactions: one observes marked changes in the entire Q_Y spectral range, including the bacteriopheophytins (104). Furthermore, spectral evolution is observed on a time scale less than a few hundred femtoseconds, notably in the B band region (104). This evolution cannot result from two-step sequential electron transfer (the spectral characteristics of the intermediate state would be unphysical). They may reflect relaxation of intramolecular vibrational modes, changes in the charge transfer character, and/or rearrangements of protein side groups within the excited state. An electronic relaxation occurring in less than 100 fs, which has been observed in a photon echo experiment (81, 82), may well reflect the same process. Also, molecular dynamics simulations have shown that, upon charge displacement, the protein relaxes within 300 fs by rearrangement of small protein side groups (101).

Mutant reaction centers that lack H_L show much less marked changes in the $t = 0$ fs transient spectrum and almost no ultrafast spectral relaxation (104). This may indicate that these features are functional in the primary electron transfer process.

Altogether, a rather more complicated picture appears of early events in photosynthetic reaction centers than sketched in the early femtosecond papers (12, 14, 15, 60, 70, 106). Other observations may be related. For instance, in analyzing kinetics of *R. sphaeroides* reaction centers, Kirmaier & Holten (61) found a wavelength dependence in the 750- to 830-nm region. They postulated a distribution of reaction-center conformers to explain their results. However, in this wavelength region, kinetics faster than those of the primary charge separation prominently occur both at low temperature (104) and at room temperature (48, 49); these kinetics presumably biased the fits (in the first few hundred femtoseconds, no datapoints were shown). Chan et al (17) observed that the kinetics of bleaching of the Q_X band of H_L are slower than the decay of the stimulated emission. These data were analyzed in terms of a previously proposed (13) reaction scheme of parallel two-step sequential and one-step direct electron transport. On the other hand, nonsingle exponential decay has been resolved for the kinetics of stimulated emission, which more directly reflects P*, in *Chloroflexus aurantiacus* (7, 71) (the nonexponentiality is more apparent at low temperature) and *R. sphaeroides* (103, 104). Becker et al (7) proposed a dynamic heterogeneity, which interconverts more slowly at lower temperatures, to explain their data on *C. aurantiacus*. Other explanations of nonexponential kinetic behavior are discussed below.

An observation of a somewhat different nature may be related to the strong electronic coupling of pigments: the transfer of excitation energy within the reaction center takes place within 100 fs (12, 14, 15). This time is much faster than would be expected on the basis of Förster weak coupling theory (51). Apparently, to understand the femtosecond dynamics of the reaction center complex, treatment as a hexamer (in interaction with the protein matrix) is more appropriate than the classical treatment in terms of a dimer and four monomers.

Temperature Dependence of the Charge Separation Reaction

Fleming et al (32) systematically studied the temperature dependence of the primary charge separation reaction. The overall rate constant speeds up from 2.8 ps at room temperature to 1.2 ps for *R. sphaeroides* and 0.7 ps for *R. viridis* upon cooling to 8 K. The same trend was observed in reaction centers of the green sulfur bacterium *C. aurantiacus* (7) (7 ps at room temperature and a fast phase of about 3 ps at 80 K). The weak temperature dependence is generally ascribed to the activationless character of the reaction (9, 11, 32).

For *R. sphaeroides* and *R. viridis*, the temperature dependence has been modeled (32) in terms of the thermally averaged Franck-Condon factor (8), thus assuming coupling to vibrationally relaxed modes and nonadiabatic electron transfer (weak coupling), using a single mode representation. This approach yielded a very good description for *R. sphaeroides* (80 cm^{-1} mode, electronic coupling constant 24 cm^{-1}), but showed deviations for *R. viridis*. This discrepancy might arise from an increase in the electronic coupling constant by thermal contraction of the protein (9, 11, 32) or from the use of a single-mode representation (11). However, the use of a weak coupling model itself may not be justified. To reconcile a 80–100 cm^{-1} coupling mode with a rate constant of 0.7 ps, one must assume that the reaction is nearly adiabatic (32), which is internally inconsistent with the a priori assumption of weak coupling. Furthermore, the experimental finding of modes of ~ 80 cm^{-1} that are not completely dephased (and thus certainly not relaxed) on the time scale of electron transport (103) indicates that the assumption of thermal equilibrium may not be valid. Therefore, the validity of the above approach may be questioned.

Alternatively, one could consider the model in which electron transport is near-adiabatically coupled to low frequency vibrational modes (Figure 5). Stronger dephasing (and possibly relaxation) at higher temperature is consistent with the experimental findings (103). Stronger dephasing would lead to (*a*) a longer average delay time before the transition zone is reached and (*b*) a faster loss of coherence between the electronic matrix element and vibrational motion (cf. 52) at higher temperature. Both effects would slow down the overall reaction (again, care should be taken with the notion of a reaction rate in this case). Of course, in this picture, changes in the electronic coupling constant due to thermal contraction may also play a role.

If the precursor of electron transport is a vibrationally hot excited state (at least at low temperature), a small activation barrier (i.e. $\lambda > -\Delta G$, where λ is the reorganizational energy, ΔG the free energy difference) initially may not hinder efficient electron transport. This possibility may underlie the finding that the effect of an external electric field [which raises the activation energy in a classical picture (69)] on the primary charge separation reaction is much smaller than expected on the basis of a classical treatment (67). Also, a small activation barrier may be the origin of the observed multiphasic decay of P* (7, 71, 103, 104). Vibrational relaxation that competes with electron transfer would then lead to an increasing effect of this barrier, resulting in a decrease of the net efficiency of P* depletion with time. This explanation is consistent with the finding that the effect is more prominent in reaction centers performing slower electron transport (7) (see below) [electron transport of *C. aurantiacus* is two to three times slower than in *R. sphaeroides*, both at room temperature and at cryogenic temperatures (7, 71)]. An alternative explanation within this model is that dephasing of the oscillations originates in an anharmonic potential energy surface (cf. Figure 5); in this case, the time-averaged transition probability would be different for different vibrational levels.

The slower secondary electron transport reaction (reoxidation of bacteriopheophytin by quinone), which takes 100–200 ps and has a rather similar temperature dependence (64), cannot be treated with this mechanism, because thermalization presumably has taken place for all modes on this time scale.

Mutant Reaction Centers

A useful approach to study structure-function relationships is to vary the protein structure by site-directed mutagenesis (18). Mutants with local alterations may be divided into those in which the pigment composition (*a*) is not or (*b*) is modified. To the former group belongs a set of mutants in which a tyrosine (M210 in *R. sphaeroides*, M208 in *R. capsulatus*) in close contact with P, B_L, and H_L is replaced. Replacement by isoleucine, leucine, phenylalanine, or threonine slows down the primary electron transfer step at room temperature three- to sixfold (16, 30, 84). Wild-type *C. aurantiacus*, which has a leucine at this position (and one bacteriochlorophyll replaced by a bacteriopheophytin), also exhibits somewhat slower primary electron transport than wild-type purple bacteria (7, 71). Hence, this residue appears to be important in the fine tuning of the primary charge separation, but not crucial for the charge separation to take place. The effect of the different mutations, as well as the lack of effect that replacement by histidine has (16), indicate that both the aromaticity and the capability of hydrogen bonding determine the influence of this tyrosine (16, 84).

Surprisingly, in *R. capsulatus*, replacement of the phenylalanine at the homologous location in the inactive branch (L181) by tyrosine speeds up the initial reaction (3.5 to 2.1 ps), and interchanging the tyrosine at M208 and the phenylalanine at L181 has no great overall effect (16). No wrong-way electron transfer was detected in these cases (16). These results indicate that (*a*) both residues have a similar influence (16) and (*b*) the speed of primary electron transfer is not completely optimized in wild-type reaction centers.

The temperature dependence of the primary charge separation reaction in the mutants is also of interest. The general trend is that slowing down of the reaction is correlated with an increase in dk/dT (16, 84) (dk/dT is negative for wild-type, see above), i.e. that slowing down results from the breakdown of activationlessness. Also, at low temperature, the reaction becomes more nonexponential (16, 84). These findings support the model of electron transport coupled to low frequency vibrational modes, discussed above.

Mutants with altered pigment composition have also been studied. Replacement of the histidine ligand to P_M (M200 in *R. capsulatus*, M202 in *R. sphaeroides*) with leucine results in the replacement of the P_M bacteriochlorophyll with a bacteriopheophytin, i.e. in a heterodimer primary donor P (18). Upon excitation of reaction centers of this mutant, within 350 fs a state forms with a significant charge-transfer character. This state is very unstable: 50% of this state falls back to the ground state with about the same time constant as charge separation (~ 30 ps) (57, 63, 78–80). Qualitatively similar effects were observed in an opposite heterodimer mutant (replacement of the P_L bacteriochlorophyll by bacteriopheophytin) (80). Conversely, when the leucine ligand to H_L (L214 in *R. capsulatus*) is replaced by histidine, the H_L bacteriopheophytin converts to bacteriochlorophyll (58). This bacteriochlorophyll acts as a primary acceptor with a high quantum yield (the lifetime of P* is only two times longer as in wild-type), but the recombination from this state is high ($\sim 40\%$). So, in these mutants electron transport is seriously perturbed, indicating that the pigment composition, at least of the active branch [although no mutants with modifications in B_L are available yet (18)], is important for optimal efficiency of primary charge separation processes. The pigment composition of the inactive branch may be less critical. Electron transport in wild-type reaction centers of *C. aurantiacus*, which incorporate a bacteriopheophytin at the location of B_M in purple bacteria (7 and references therein), is fully efficient, although somewhat slower than purple bacteria (7, 71).

Recently, mutants with more global modifications were also constructed. Partially symmetrizing the reaction-center protein by duplicating the D helix of the L chain to the M chain in *R. capsulatus* leads to a complete loss of H_L (94). Some relevant properties of this D_{LL} mutant are discussed in the above sections. The long-lived character of the excited state of this mutant (71) facilitates the study of protein vibrational modes reflected in the kinetics. The frequencies of these modes in the D_{LL} mutants are somewhat different from those in *R. sphaeroides* R-26 reaction centers (103), which may reflect differences in global structure.

In summary, the single local mutations lift the activation barrier somewhat but, if the pigment composition is not altered, do not drastically alter the efficiency of primary electron transport ($P^+H_L^-$ still forms at a rate much faster than classical electron transport theory predicts). This may indicate that the global structure of the protein matrix is vital for the charge separation to occur, whereas the local structure, on the level of single residues, optimizes the reaction and allows for binding of the right pigments. This hypothesis might for instance be tested with mutants with an altered global rigidity but intact pigment composition.

CONCLUDING REMARKS

We have discussed recent advances in the understanding of ultrafast processes in biological systems. The overview is not exhaustive and is biased by the authors' present main research interests. However, a more general picture of the mechanisms of femtosecond biology may be extracted. After femtosecond excitation, the mechanical interaction of the perturbed chromophore with the local environment is probed. The directed and possibly collective motion that is of physiological importance to the biological system can then be followed. Additionally, in multiple-chromophore systems, evolution of electronic interactions can be observed. Combined efforts with rapidly developing computational and experimental methods will be needed for a very detailed understanding of the structural evolution of protein systems on a short time scale.

Most results in femtosecond spectroscopy discussed in this review have been obtained using light in or near the visible region. Those techniques will certainly be further exploited in the near future. Additionally, extensions of the spectrum of ultrafast spectroscopy to both the infrared (vibrational spectroscopy) and the ultraviolet (motion of amino acid residues) are currently introduced in biophysical research. Both techniques are especially useful for studying structural motion. An exciting further development will be, of course, the generation of femtosecond X-ray pulses to take snap shots of the entire protein structure.

ACKNOWLEDGMENTS

We gratefully acknowledge our collaborators J.-C. Lambry (molecular dynamics simulations and femtosecond spectroscopy), J. Breton (bacterial reaction centers), D. C. Youvan and S. G. Robles (site-directed mutagenesis of bacterial reaction centers), C. Poyart (hemoglobin and myoglobin), P. O. Stoutland and W. H. Woodruff (cytochrome oxidase), and N. Yamada and B. Bohn (technical assistance). M. H. V. is recipient of a grant from the EEC SCIENCE Program and is also affiliated with the Service de Biophysique, Centre d'Etudes Nucleuires de Saclay, Gif-sur-Yvette.

Literature Cited

1. Allen, J. P., Feher, G. 1984. *Proc. Natl. Acad. Sci. USA* 81: 4795–99
1a. Amesz, J., ed. 1987. *Photosynthesis.* Amsterdam: Elsevier
2. Anfinrud, P., Han, C.-H., Hansen, P. A., Moore, J. N., Hochstrasser, R. M. 1988. *Ultrafast Phenom.* 6: 442–46
3. Anfinrud, P., Han, C.-H., Hochstrasser, R. M. 1989. *Proc. Natl. Acad. Sci. USA* 86: 8397
4. Anfinrud, P., Han, C.-H., Lian, T., Hochstrasser, R. M. 1990. *J. Phys. Chem.* 95: 1180–84
5. Anfinrud, P., Han, C.-H., Lian, T., Hochstrasser, R. M. 1991. *J. Phys. Chem.* 95: 574–78
6. Austin, R. H., Beeson, K. W., Eisenstein, L., Frauenfelder, H., Gunsalus, C. 1975. *Biochemistry* 14: 5355–77
7. Becker, M., Middendorf, V., Nagarajan, V., Parson, W. W., Martin, J. E., Blankenship, R. E. 1991. *Biochim. Biophys. Acta* 1057: 299–312
8. Bixon, M., Jortner, J. 1986. *J. Phys. Chem.* 90: 3795–3800
9. Bixon, M., Jortner, J. 1988. *Chem. Phys. Lett.* 159: 17–20
10. Bixon, M., Jortner, J., Michel-Beyerle, M. E. 1991. *Biochim. Biophys. Acta* 1056: 301–15
11. Boxer, S. G. 1990. *Annu. Rev. Biophys. Biophys. Chem.* 19: 267–99
12. Breton, J., Martin, J.-L., Fleming, G. R., Lambry, J.-C. 1988. *Biochemistry* 27: 8267–84

13. Breton, J., Martin, J.-L., Lambry, J.-C., Robles, S. J., Youvan, D. C. 1991. See Ref. 82a, pp. 293–302
14. Breton, J., Martin, J.-L., Migus, A., Antonetti, A., Orszag, A. 1986. *Proc. Natl. Acad. Sci. USA* 83: 5121–25
15. Breton, J., Martin, J.-L., Petrich, J., Migus, A., Antonetti, A. 1986. *FEBS Lett.* 209: 37–43
16. Chan, C. K., Chen, L. X. Q., DiMagno, T. J., Hanson, D. K., Nance, S. L., et al. 1991. *Chem. Phys. Lett.* 176: 366–72
17. Chan, C. K., DiMagno, T. J., Chen, L. X. Q., Norris, J. R., Fleming, G. R. 1991. *Proc. Natl. Acad. Sci. USA.* In press
18. Coleman, W. J., Youvan, D. C. 1990. *Annu. Rev. Biophys. Biophys. Chem.* 19: 333–67
19. Deisenhofer, J. P., Epp, O., Miki, K., Huber, R., Michel, H. 1984. *J. Mol. Biol.* 180: 385–98
20. Deisenhofer, J. P., Michel, H. 1989. *Science* 245: 1463–73
21. Deisenhofer, J. P., Michel, H. 1991. *Annu. Rev. Biophys. Biophys. Chem.* 20: 247–66
22. Dressler, K., Finkele, U., Lauterwasser, C., Hamm, P., Holzapfel, W., et al. 1991. See Ref 82a, pp. 135–140
23. Dressler, K., Umlaut, E., Schmidt, S., Hamm, P., Zinth, W., Buchanan, S., Michel, H. 1991. *Chem. Phys. Lett.* 183: 270–76
24. Dyer, R. B., Einarsdottir, O., Killough,

P. M., Lopez-Garriga, J. J., Woodruff, W. H. 1989. *J. Am. Chem. Soc.* 111: 7659–61
25. Dyer, R. B., Peterson, K. A., Stoutland, P. O., Woodruff, W. H. 1991. *J. Am. Chem. Soc.* 113: 6276–77
26. Fajer, J., Brune, D. C., Davis, M. S., Forman, A., Spaulding, L. D. 1975. *Proc. Natl. Acad. Sci. USA* 72: 4956–60
27. Feher, G., Allen, J. P., Okamura, M. Y., Rees, D. C. 1989. *Nature* 339: 111–16
28. Findsen, E. W., Friedman, J. M., Ondrias, M. R., Simon, S. R. 1985. *Science* 229: 661–65
29. Findsen, E. W., Scott, T. W., Chance, M. R., Friedman, J. M., Ondrias, M. R. 1985. *J. Am. Chem. Soc.* 107: 3355–57
30. Finkele, U., Lauterwasser, C., Zinth, W., Gray, K., Oesterhelt, D. 1990. *Biochemistry* 29: 8517–21
31. Fleming, G. R. 1986. *Annu. Rev. Phys. Chem.* 37: 81–104
32. Fleming, G. R., Martin, J.-L., Breton, J. 1988. *Nature* 333: 190–92
33. Fork, R. L., Brito Cruz, C. H., Becker, P. C., Shank, C. V. 1986. *Opt. Lett.* 12: 483–85
34. Fork, R. L., Greene, B. I., Shank, C. V. 1981. *Appl. Phys. Lett.* 38: 671–72
35. Fork, R. L., Martinez, O. E., Gordon, J. P. 1984. *Opt. Lett.* 9: 150–52
36. Friesner, R. A., Won, Y. 1989. *Biochim. Biophys. Acta* 977: 99–122
37. Gelin, B. K., Karplus, M. 1977. *Proc. Natl. Acad. Sci. USA* 74: 801–5
38. Glownia, J. H., Misewich, J., Sorokin, P. P. 1987. *Chem. Phys. Lett.* 137: 491–95
39. Goodberlet, J., Wang, J., Fujimoto, J. G., Schulz, P. A. 1989. *Opt. Lett.* 14: 1125–27
40. Hansen, J. E., Rosenthal, S. J., Fleming, G. R. 1990. *Ultrafast Phenom.* 7: 548–50
41. Hanson, L. K. 1988. *Photochem. Photobiol.* 47: 903–21
42. Henry, E. H., Eaton, W. A., Hochstrasser, R. M. 1986. *Proc. Natl. Acad. Sci. USA* 83: 8982–86
43. Hesselink, W. H., Wiersma, D. A. 1981. *J. Chem. Phys.* 75: 4192–97
44. Hochstrasser, R. M. 1989. *Ber. Bunsenges. Phys. Chem.* 93: 239–45
45. Hochstrasser, R. M., Anfinrud, P. A., Diller, R., Han, C., Iannone, M., et al. 1990. *Ultrafast Phenom.* 7: 429–33
46. Hochstrasser, R. M., Johnson, C. K. 1988. See Ref. 54a, pp. 357–417
47. Hofrichter, J., Sommer, J. H., Henry, E. R., Eaton, W. A. 1983. *Proc. Natl.*

Acad. Sci. USA 80: 2235–39
48. Holzapfel, W., Finkele, U., Kaiser, W., Oesterhelt, D., Scheer, H., et al. 1989. *Chem. Phys. Lett.* 160: 1–7
49. Holzapfel, W., Finkele, U., Kaiser, W., Oesterhelt, D., Scheer, H., et al. 1990. *Proc. Natl. Acad. Sci. USA* 87: 5168–72
50. Holzwarth, A. R. 1989. *Q. Rev. Biophys.* 22: 239–326
51. Jean, J., Chan, C. K., Fleming, G. R. 1988. *Isr. J. Chem.* 28: 169–75
52. Jean, J., Friesner, R. A., Fleming, G. R. 1991. *Ber. Busenges. Phys. Chem.* 95: 253–58
53. Jedju, T. M., Rothberg, L., Labrie, A. 1988. *Opt. Lett.* 13: 961–63
54. Johnson, S. G., Tang, D., Jankowiak, R., Hayes, J. M., Small, G. J., Tiede, D. M. 1989. *J. Phys. Chem.* 93: 5953–57
54a. Kaiser, W., ed. 1988. *Ultrashort Laser Pulses and Applications.* Berlin: Springer
55. Kaufmann, K. J., Dutton, P. L., Netzel, T. L., Leigh, J. S., Rentzepis, P. M. 1975. *Science* 188: 1301–4
56. Keyes, M. H., Falley, M., Lumry, R. J. 1971. *J. Am. Chem. Soc.* 93: 2035
57. Kirmaier, C., Bylina, E. J., Youvan, D. C., Holten, D. 1989. *Chem. Phys. Lett.* 159: 251–57
58. Kirmaier, C., Gaul, D., DeBey, R., Holten, D., Schenck, C. C. 1991. *Science* 251: 922–27
59. Kirmaier, C., Holten, D. 1987. *Photosynth. Res.* 13: 225–60
60. Kirmaier, C., Holten, D. 1988. *FEBS Lett.* 239: 211–18
61. Kirmaier, C., Holten, D. 1990. *Proc. Natl. Acad. Sci. USA* 87: 3552–56
62. Kirmaier, C., Holten, D. 1991. *Biochemistry* 30: 609–13
63. Kirmaier, C., Holten, D., Bylina, E. J., Youvan, D. C. 1988. *Proc. Natl. Acad. Sci. USA* 85: 7562–66
64. Kirmaier, C., Holten, D., Parson, W. W. 1985. *Biochim. Biophys. Acta* 810: 33–48
65. Leonhardt, R., Holzapfel, W., Zinth, W., Kaiser, W. 1987. *Chem. Phys. Lett.* 133: 373–77
66. Lingle, R., Xu, X., Zhu, H., Yu, S.-C., Hopkins, J. B. 1991. *J. Am. Chem. Soc.* 113: 3992–94
67. Lockhart, D. J., Kirmaier, C., Holten, D., Boxer, S. G. 1990. *J. Phys. Chem.* 1990: 6987–95
68. Marcus, R. A. 1987. *Chem. Phys. Lett.* 133: 471–77
69. Marcus, R. A., Sutin, N. 1985. *Biochim. Biophys. Acta* 811: 265–322
70. Martin, J.-L., Breton, J., Hoff, A. J.,

Migus, A., Antonetti, A. 1986. *Proc. Natl. Acad. Sci. USA* 83: 957–61
71. Martin, J.-L., Lambry, J.-C., Ashokkumar, M., Michel-Beyerle, M. E., Feick, R., Breton, J. 1990. *Ultrafast Phenom.* 7: 514–28
72. Martin, J.-L., Migus, A., Poyart, C., Lecarpentier, Y., Antonetti, A., Orszag, A. 1982. In *Picosecond Phenomena*, ed. K. B. Eisenthal, R. M. Hochstrasser, W. Kaiser, A. Lauberau, 3: 294–97. Berlin: Springer
73. Martin, J.-L., Migus, A., Poyart, C., Lecarpentier, Y., Astier, R., Antonetti, A. 1983. *Proc. Natl. Acad. Sci. USA* 80: 173–77
74. Martin, J.-L., Migus, A., Poyart, C., Lecarpentier, Y., Astier, R., Antonetti, A. 1983. *EMBO J.* 2: 1815–19
75. Martin, J.-L., Migus, A., Poyart, C., Lecarpentier, Y., Astier, R., Antonetti, A. 1984. *Ultrafast Phenom.* 4: 1447–51
76. Mathies, R. A., Brito Cruz, C. H., Pollard, W. T., Shank, C. V. 1988. *Science* 240: 777–79
77. Mathies, R. A., Lin, S. W., Ames, J. B., Pollard, W. T. 1991. *Annu. Rev. Biophys. Biophys. Chem.* 20: 491–518
78. McDowell, L. M., Gaul, D., Kirmaier, C., Holten, D., Schenck, C. C. 1991. *Biochemistry* 30: 8315–22
79. McDowell, L. M., Kirmaier, C., Holten, D. 1990. *Biochim. Biophys. Acta* 1020: 239–46
80. McDowell, L. M., Kirmaier, C., Holten, D. 1991. *J. Phys. Chem.* 95: 3379–83
81. Meech, S. R., Hoff, A. J., Wiersma, D. A. 1986. *Chem. Phys. Lett.* 121: 287–92
82. Meech, S. R., Hoff, A. J., Wiersma, D. A. 1986. *Proc. Natl. Acad. Sci. USA* 83: 9464–68
82a. Michel-Beyerle, M. E., ed. 1991. *Reaction Centers of Photosynthetic Bacteria.* Berlin: Springer
83. Michel-Beyerle, M. E., Plato, M., Deisenhofer, J., Michel, H., Bixon, M., Jortner, J. 1988. *Biochim. Biophys. Acta* 932: 52–70
84. Nagarajan, V., Parson, W. W., Gaul, D., Schenck, C. 1990. *Proc. Natl. Acad. Sci. USA* 87: 7888–92
85. Parson, W. W. 1982. *Annu. Rev. Biophys. Bioeng.* 11: 57–80
86. Parson, W. W. 1987. See Ref. 1a, pp. 43–61
87. Pearlstein, R. M. 1987. See Ref. 1a, pp. 299–317
88. Pereira, M. A., Share, P. E., Sarisky, M. J., Hochstrasser, R. M. 1990. *Ultrafast Phenom.* 7: 438–40
89. Pereira, M. A., Share, P. E., Sarisky, M. J., Hochstrasser, R. M. 1991. *J. Chem. Phys.* 94: 2513–22
90. Petrich, J. W., Lambry, J.-C., Kuczera, K., Karplus, M., Poyart, C., Martin, J.-L. 1991. *Biochemistry* 30: 3975–87
91. Petrich, J. W., Martin, J.-L. 1989. *Chem. Phys.* 131: 31–47
92. Petrich, J. W., Martin, J.-L., Houde, D., Poyart, C., Orszag, A. 1987. *Biochemistry* 26: 7914–23
93. Petrich, J. W., Poyart, C., Martin, J.-L. 1988. *Biochemistry* 27: 4049–60
94. Robles, S. J., Breton, J., Youvan, D. C. 1990. *Science* 248: 1402–5
95. Rockley, M. G., Windsor, M. W., Cogdell, R. J., Parson, W. W. 1975. *Proc. Natl. Acad. Sci. USA* 72: 2251–55
96. Ruggiero, A. F., Todd, D. C., Fleming, G. R. 1990. *J. Am. Chem. Soc.* 112: 1003–14
97. Shank, C. V. 1986. *Science* 233: 1276–80
98. Shank, C. V. 1988. See Ref. 54a, pp. 5–34
99. Shuvalov, V. A., Klevanik, A. V. 1983. *FEBS Lett.* 160: 51–55
100. Stoutland, P. O., Lambry, J.-C., Martin, J.-L., Woodruff, W. H. 1991. *J. Phys. Chem.* 95: 6406–8
101. Treutlein, H., Schulten, K., Niedermeier, C., Deisenhofer, J., Michel, H., DeVault, D. 1988. In *The Photosynthetic Bacterial Reaction Center, Structure and Function*, ed. J. Breton, A. Verméglio, pp. 369–77. New York: Plenum
102. Van den Berg, R., El-Sayed, M. A. 1990. *Biophys. J.* 58: 931–37
103. Vos, M. H., Lambry, J.-C., Robles, S. J., Youvan, D. G., Breton, J., Martin, J.-L. 1991. *Proc. Natl. Acad. Sci. USA* 88: 8885–89
104. Vos, M. H., Lambry, J.-C., Robles, S. J., Youvan, D. G., Breton, J., Martin, J.-L. 1992. *Proc. Natl. Acad. Sci. USA.* In press
105. Warshel, A., Creighton, S., Parson, W. W. 1988. *J. Phys. Chem.* 92: 2697–2701
106. Woodbury, N. W., Becker, M., Middendorf, D., Parson, W. W. 1985. *Biochemistry* 24: 7516–21
107. Woodruff, W. H., Einarsdottir, O., Dyer, R. B., Bagley, K. A., Palmer, G., et al. 1991. *Proc. Natl. Acad. Sci. USA* 88: 2588–92
108. Zinth, W., Kaiser, W. 1988. See Ref. 54a, pp. 235–77

Annu. Rev. Biophys. Biomol. Struct. 1992. 21:223–42

INTRAMEMBRANE HELIX-HELIX ASSOCIATION IN OLIGOMERIZATION AND TRANSMEMBRANE SIGNALING

B. J. Bormann

Department of Immunology, Boehringer Ingelheim Pharmaceuticals, Inc., Ridgefield, Connecticut 06877

D. M. Engelman

Department of Molecular Biophysics and Biochemistry, Yale University, New Haven, Connecticut 06511

KEY WORDS: dimerization, protein interaction, receptor conformation, signal transduction, receptor structure

CONTENTS

1056–8700/92/0610–0223$02.00

INTRODUCTION

Many functions of cell surface membranes are carried out by proteins that are integrated across the lipid bilayer. These transbilayer proteins serve a large and diverse array of important biological functions critical for cell survival. Although investigators using cDNA cloning have deduced the sequences of numerous transmembrane proteins in the past several years, precise information regarding these proteins' secondary, tertiary, and quaternary structure is very limited (1). Moreover, the mechanisms by which these transmembrane proteins function, transmitting solutes or information across the lipid bilayer, are even less well defined (79).

In this review, we describe how a two-stage model of protein folding and helix-helix association (73) can be applied to models of signal transduction for proteins that contain a single transmembrane domain. We provide some general discussion of transmembrane structures and theoretical models as to their role in signaling. The focus is not on the primary formation or membrane insertion of the helices but on their assembly with other helices to form tertiary and quaternary structures. We present the emerging evidence that many single helix proteins oligomerize to transduce information to the cytoplasmic domain and the functional attributes of oligomerization and relate this evidence to recent structure discussions (72).

FOLDING OF MULTIHELIX TRANSMEMBRANE PROTEINS

Multiple-helix proteins as a group include molecules such as bacteriorhodopsin, rhodopsin, the anion transporter channels, sugar transporters, ATPases, and receptors including those that bind substance K, lutropin, follicle stimulating hormone, and the muscarinic receptor family (31, 42, 76, 105). The amino acid sequences of multiple helix proteins predicted from cDNA sequences allow provisional models for their arrangement in the membrane (105). Hydropathy profiles and related algorithms can predict the location of the putative transmembrane segments reasonably well. The secondary structure of the aqueous domains of the extracellular and intracellular loops connecting the transmembrane helices can also be predicted somewhat less successfully (26, 42, 104). However, we have no useful algorithm to predict the tertiary arrangement of helices. Although all possible arrangements may be considered as formal possibilities, certain specific arrangements appear to be likely, as described below for bacteriorhodopsin.

To be useful, a view of folding necessarily contains a set of assumptions, several of which are made in this review. The first assumption is that transmembrane proteins are folded in a stable state regardless of the specific mechanism of insertion into the bilayer. Second, the transmembrane orientation of proteins is stable, and such proteins do not flip from one side of the bilayer to the other (70). And last, the intramembranous domains of the transmembrane proteins are assumed to be α-helices where they contain hydrophobic regions sufficient to span a bilayer. The energy considerations of the hydrogen-bonding properties of a hydrophobic α-helix in an apolar environment indicate such helices (26). Obvious exceptions to this assumption are the transmembrane domains of the porins (111), which are β-barrels defining aqueous channels across bacterial outer membranes, but porins do not have the hydrophobic sequences characteristic of transmembrane helices.

Energetics of Folding in Two Stages

The transmembrane domains of multiple-helix proteins are characterized by hydrophobic stretches of about 20 amino acids. The primary structures indicate that each of the transmembrane domains might be independently stable as a separate transbilayer structure interacting with only the nonpolar region of the lipid bilayer. In folded proteins, such as bacteriorhodopsin or reaction centers, the conformation of these segments is altered little from that which would be predicted as the conformation and transbilayer locus of the separate entities. Therefore, the interaction energies producing the tertiary structure of the folded molecule may not be as strong as those stabilizing the helices. The separation of the folding of independent helices from their association in higher order structures divides the energy constraints into two stages. Based on this view, a two-stage model of helix formation followed by helix-helix association was recently proposed by Popot & Engelman (73). Although the present review does not repeat the rationale of this model in detail, the general principles and arguments must be reiterated as they are the basis for the proposal that oligomerization and transmembrane signaling of single-helix membrane proteins may involve helix-helix interactions inside the bilayer.

In simple terms, the two-stage model predicts that a protein such as bacteriorhodopsin, which has seven transmembrane domains (41), could first fold each α-helix to an independent, stable conformation across a bilayer and then assemble these transmembrane helices into a tertiary structure in which the helices are not much altered. The first stage can be accounted for by the hydrophobic effect and hydrogen bonding that lead to the stability and conformation of the helices. Association of the helices, the second stage, requires the participation of other factors including polar interactions, links between helices, links to extra-membrane domains or other proteins such as cytoskeletal proteins, interactions with prosthetic groups, and packing effects. Much experimentation has focused upon bacteriorhodopsin in order to test the propositions of the helix-association model.

Bacteriorhodopsin Folding

Strong evidence in favor of the two-stage folding model has come from studies of the refolding and functional activity of proteolytically cleaved bacteriorhodopsin. Bacteriorhodopsin can be functionally reconstituted from proteolytic fragments in a variety of environments (41, 46, 48, 58, 74). When two proteolytic fragments are separately incorporated into two populations of lipid vesicles, each fragment forms a set of transbilayer helices. When the two populations of vesicles are fused, bacteriorhodopsin reforms from the association of the fragments and is functionally active (74). The crystal structure of such renatured molecules is indistinguishable from that of the native molecule at low resolution (75).

The significance of these kinds of experiments is that although the separate domains of bacteriorhodopsin are refolded under conditions that greatly differ from those occurring in vivo, the structures of the separate pieces are close to those expected if each helix forms independently. Furthermore, side-to-side interaction of the helices can occur as demonstrated by the fact that subunits recognize each other and form a folded molecule. The two-stage hypothesis predicts these data. Each individual helix must appropriately form and span the membrane prior to the association with neighboring helices to yield the complex, biologically active structure. These data also call attention to the role of polar forces and packing effects in helix-helix interactions. In this regard, helices are known to engage in detailed close packing (1, 22, 77, 115), and this packing interaction must overcome the entropy that favors helix separation (73).

Two-Stage Folding and Single-Helix Proteins

At the level of the lipid bilayer, the energetics required for packing helical transmembrane regions of a multiple-helix protein into a subunit are not different from packing transmembrane domains of separate single-helix proteins into an oligomer because stable helices can be regarded as folding domains (72). This is illustrated by the bacteriorhodopsin experiments in which refolded bacteriorhodopsin fragments behave as the two subunits of a heterodimer (73). The initial formation of independently stable helices is therefore critical for both multiple- and single-helix proteins. As a rule, genomic intron segments never occur in the coding sequence for transmembrane regions (47), supporting the idea that the helices are important domains. Furthermore, proteins such as the major intrinsic channel protein (MIP) contain tandem sequence repeats indicative of the evolution of multiple-helix proteins from ancestral single-helix homodimers (111). The oligomerization of single-helix proteins is also probably of significance in signaling, as we discuss below.

TOPOLOGY OF SINGLE-HELIX PROTEINS

A wide variety of transmembrane proteins have a single apparent helix, including the influenza virus hemagglutinins, the histocompatability antigens, the tyrosine kinase growth factor receptor family, immunoglobulin, the T-cell receptor, and the integrin receptor families (19, 72). Receptor proteins can be segregated into three chemically distinct domains: extracellular, transmembrane, and cytoplasmic. Notable diversity is found in the primary and secondary structures of the extra- and intracellular domains of these transbilayer proteins. However, the transmembrane segments generally are similar in length and hydrophobicity.

The transmembrane segments of single-helix proteins are composed of approximately 20 hydrophobic and uncharged amino acids, and are probably helical. The simplest argument for helicity comes from consideration of the geometry necessary to cross the lipid bilayer with about 20–22 amino acids. Twenty amino acids packed into an α-helical secondary structure would fold into six helical loops and extend about 30 Å, the length of the nonpolar region of an average lipid bilayer. Studies designed to test the minimum number of apolar residues needed for a protein to be stably maintained in the membrane showed that a lower limit of 12–14 amino acids maintains membrane insertion. This finding leaves open issues as to whether the thickness of the membrane can be locally dictated by the length of the transmembrane segment, whether potentially charged residues can be stably integrated into the bilayer, or whether alternative secondary structures might maintain the integrity of the transmembrane segments (21, 37). The energy cost of burying a potentially charged residue in its uncharged form can be offset by the net energy of burying the nonpolar residues of a 20-amino acid helix (26). When single-helix proteins are studied using circular dichroism in the presence of detergents, the transmembrane segments give spectra characteristic of α-helices (19).

SIGNALING THROUGH THE BILAYER

Given that the transmembrane regions of single-helix proteins are similar in overall composition, secondary structure, and length, it remains a conceptual problem to explain how signals are transmitted through the transmembrane helices and cellular functions are activated. When a simple

receptor such as that for the epidermal growth factor (EGFR) is bound
to its ligand, EGF, the calculated stoichiometry of ligand binding to
receptor is 1 : 1 (81, 98, 106). However, a Scatchard analysis of this binding
event reveals nonlinear plots indicative of two receptor populations of
different affinities. About 5% of the total receptor population is considered
high affinity, and the remainder are low affinity (52). Given these observations for numerous single-helix membrane receptors, what is the physical
difference, if any, between a high affinity receptor and a low affinity
receptor if the primary and secondary structure of these receptors are
identical?

Monomolecular Models

Several models have been advanced to explain signal transduction and
high versus low affinity receptors based on monomeric receptors. We argue
that such mechanisms are unlikely given the fluidity and deformability of
the lipid bilayer. Bilayer fluidity has been explored by several means, and
was well established at an early date (85). The viscosity of a lipid bilayer
is approximately 1 centipoise, the approximate viscosity of olive oil. Molecular diffusion both of proteins and of lipids when they are unconstrained
by linkage to other macromolecules is rapid. Further, the bilayer is known
to be deformable; a thickness change of 30% corresponds to only about
1 kT in energy (62). Measurements of bacteriorhodopsin aggregation
suggest that this local deformability is used to accommodate rather large
mismatches between the hydrophobic thickness of a transmembrane protein and the thickness of the lipid bilayer (61). Thus, any proposed mechanism must be framed in terms of the deformable, fluid environment in
which membrane proteins reside.

One mechanism assumes that a single helix can independently transmit
information via an allosteric change in the α-helix. This model of single-
helix transmission would include models that suggest that the α-helix
unfolds, breaking one or more of its hydrogen bonds. The chain of energetic causality is not closely reasoned in such models, since the energy for
local bilayer deformation is small compared to the energy required to
break a hydrogen bond (5–6 kcal per mole) (73). A related mechanism
posits that prolines within the α-helix may undergo *cis-trans* isomerization
upon ligand binding (10), redirecting the protein chain. This model also
suggests that proline carbonyl groups can act as intramembranous cation
binding sites, the binding of which might also activate second messenger
systems. Again, the energetic details of such mechanisms are not spelled
out. To be credible, such proposals must invoke either known mechanisms
derived from studies of related structures in other proteins or have a
complete rationale in terms of the resistive as well as active elements in

the causal chain. Such arguments have not yet been put forward, and it is unclear how the events would be carried out in a fluid environment.

A third mechanism is based on the idea that a rotation of the helix in the membrane would change the relative geometry of the cytoplasmic domain. This model seems particularly unlikely given the fluidity of the lipid bilayer, because the helix is already in a low viscosity environment that permits rapid rotational diffusion (85).

A fourth mechanism, which might be referred to as the push-pull model, suggests that ligand binding causes in the extracytoplasmic domain a conformational change that either pulls or pushes on the transmembrane helix, thereby altering the cytoplasmic domain and triggering signaling. Given the deformability of the lipid bilayer (62), the proposed mechanism is far more likely to result in a change in the local bilayer thickness than a conformational change in the protein. The low energy of such deformation events would not provide sufficient specificity for information transfer to occur without a very high noise background.

The single-molecule models are diagrammed schematically in Figure 1.

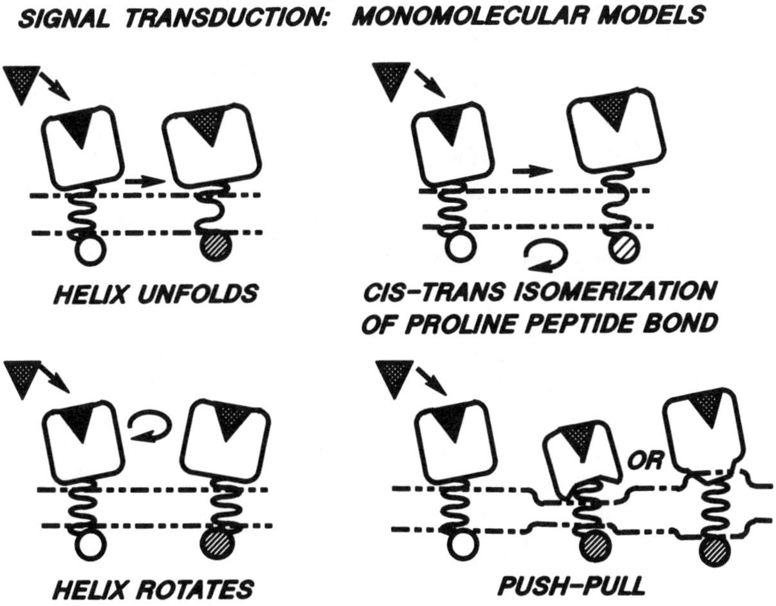

Figure 1 Signal transduction: single helix models. The schematic diagram shown suggests four mechanisms of transmitting information through the bilayer via a single-helical domain. Each diagram depicts the conformation of the receptor before and after interaction with ligand. The models, described in the text, suggest that the helix unfolds, proline peptide bonds isomerize, the helix rotates, and that the helix is pushed or pulled.

Given the known properties of lipid bilayers and the failure at this point to reason a causal chain in such an environment, none of these models seems a strong hypothesis for a mechanism of low noise information transfer across a membrane.

Oligomerization Models

The second general concept of signaling through the transmembrane region requires more than a single-molecule receptor. One such model proposes that receptors are in an equilibrium between monomeric and oligomeric states. In the presence of a signal, the ligand molecule either physically bridges two receptor molecules or binds to a single receptor ectodomain, possibly changing the conformation of the ectodomain, to stabilize dimerization or oligomerization. In an oligomerization event, the sum of three energies is involved: the interaction of the ectodomains, the interaction of the transmembrane domains, and the interaction of the cytoplasmic domains. Thus, the alteration induced by receptor binding need only displace the sum of these energies to give a favorable free energy for interaction, which might be accomplished either by an additional favorable interaction of ectodomains or by a relaxation of an unfavorable interaction. Either mechanism of ligand action would result in the creation of a new oligomeric structure in the cytoplasm, which could trigger signaling. This hypothesis also predicts that, upon release of ligand, the oligomers would dissociate and return to their basal state of equilibrium. A difficulty with this model concerns the rapid diffusion kinetics of proteins in lipid, which would suggest that monomeric receptors might frequently collide and produce a signal background from transient oligomers. This would, in effect, compromise the controls or constraints on receptor activation that are overcome by ligand binding. However, the difficulty is avoided in the mechanism involving the removal of unfavorable interactions between the ectodomains as a consequence of ligation.

A corollary of the oligomerization model incorporates an oligomerization step with a subsequent allosteric global conformational change of the receptor complex upon interaction with ligand. This allosteric or conformational change could be a ligand-induced rotation of one subunit of the dimer in opposition to the other, creating a new relationship of cytoplasmic domains, and might require a close association or contact with all or some of the receptor domains. This model would also include receptors that exist as oligomeric, heterodimeric, or covalently linked dimers in their basal state, which would bind ligand and signal by an allosteric change. Figure 2 shows schematic diagrams of the multiple-helix models.

OLIGOMERIZATION MODELS

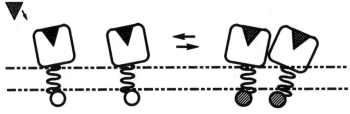

PROXIMITY/ ASSOCIATION DISSOCIATION

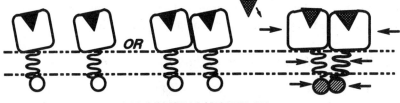

ALLOSTERIC/CONTACT

Figure 2   Oligomerization models. The upper schematic diagram suggests an association-dissociation equilibrium that favors oligomerization of proximal receptors in the presence of ligand (*top, right*). The lower diagram suggests that receptors may exist as monomers or oligomers and may oligomerize and/or alter their conformation by an allosteric mechanism in the presence of ligand. The conformational activation of the receptors would involve close association of all of the domains of the receptor protein as signified by the small arrows in the diagram.

EXAMPLES OF OLIGOMERIZATION AND SIGNAL TRANSDUCTION

Oligomerization and conformational change have been studied using a variety of methods in many biological systems. These methods include covalent cross-linking by insertion of unpaired cysteine residues, chemical cross-linking, separations by sucrose gradients, column chromatography or electrophoresis under nondenaturing conditions, and the construction and expression of truncated, mutated, and chimeric receptors. Studies of the statistical probability of protein-protein interaction in membranes involving the limited volume of the membrane and the true concentration of bilayer proteins present predict that the likelihood that membrane proteins would form oligomers is a million-fold greater than the probability that these proteins would exist in isolated states (35).

Examples of oligomeric signaling also include covalently linked dimers, like the insulin receptor, and heterodimeric proteins such as the integrin family of molecules. The glycophorin A protein is a stable dimer under a variety of conditions in vitro (10), and rotary shadowing techniques have also shown it to be a dimer (25). Complex receptors such as the T-cell receptor, lutropin receptor, and follicle stimulating hormone receptor are also thought to exist as dimers (76, 86).

In a study designed to assess the mechanism of signal transduction in the bacterial aspartate receptor, unpaired cysteines were used to replace charged residues in various locations in the ecto-, transmembrane, and cytoplasmic domains (28). Upon stimulation with ligand, significant changes were observed in the rate of disulfide-bond formation at most of the locations that the cysteines were placed. This is direct evidence for a ligand-induced global conformational change affecting large structural portions of the receptor during transmembrane signaling.

The Tyrosine Kinase Receptor Family

The family of tyrosine kinase receptors is proposed to transduce signals by oligomerization and allosteric conformational changes after binding to ligand (99). This family includes the epidermal growth factor (EGFR), platelet-derived growth factor (PDGFR), colony stimulating factor (CSFR), and insulin receptors, and the HER2/neu and trk protooncogene-coded proteins (2, 40, 49, 97, 98, 100).

The EGFR and PDGFR have been postulated to exist at an equilibrium between monomers and dimers and to rapidly and reversibly form dimers upon stimulation with ligand (40, 113). The EGF and PDGF receptors have been chemically cross-linked in the presence of ligand on living cells, membrane preparations, and highly purified receptor preparations (6, 13, 16). The amount of covalently cross-linked EGF-induced dimer correlates with the concentration of ligand (29). The EGF-receptor has been studied using nondenaturing gel electrophoresis and sucrose gradient centrifugation and found to exist as monomers and noncovalent dimers with a significant increase in the amount of dimer in the presence of EGF (113). The dimeric fraction is of higher affinity for ligand and demonstrates higher levels of phosphorylation (8). Sedimentation analysis of the PDGFR has indicated that it exists exclusively as a dimer in the presence of ligand. The dimerizing effects of EGF and PDGF are both reversible and saturable (6, 113). These data support the hypothesis that oligomerization is necessary for signal transduction. The observation that several of the ligands for members of this family are bivalent, such as PDGF and CSF-1, suggests that these ligands are designed to mediate dimerization of neighboring receptors (38, 40, 83). Furthermore, if the bivalent ligand is a heterodimer, as found for PDGF, it may serve as a selective control by the cell that mediates which second messenger pathway is activated depending on the composition of the ligand (99). The EGF ligand, however, is monomeric, which suggests that the ligand may not be simply bridging the receptor but instead may induce a conformational change (36).

A signaling mechanism using dimerization would also imply the possible existence of hybrid complexes between structurally similar receptors such as the α- and β-type PDGFR, EGFR, and HER2/*neu* or insulin and insulin-like growth factor receptor (IGF-1-R). Researchers have demonstrated hybrid complexes in several cases. PDGFR α forms heterodimers with PDGFR β, and insulin receptor forms a heterodimer with the IGF-1 receptor (87, 95). The EGFR-HER2/*neu* hybrid complex has also been detected by chemical cross-linking and immunoblotting (34, 103). It is not yet known if these hybrid receptors are functionally active (99).

Phosphorylation of the cytoplasmic domain on tyrosine appears to release an internal constraint by establishing a conformation of the receptor that is competent to interact with and phosphorylate many cellular substrates (99). The PDGFR, EGFR, and insulin receptor all reportedly phosphorylate between receptors (43, 99). For example, PDGF can stimulate a kinase-inactive β subunit when expressed with a normal α subunit (51, 95). The HER2/*neu* is also known to be a substrate of the EGFR (53, 90). Evidence indicates that synergistic interactions between HER2/*neu* and EGFR occur. When EGFR is coexpressed with nontransforming *neu* protein, the cells transform, while neither protein individually expressed has this effect (56). The EGFR when cotransfected with a kinase-negative point mutation becomes phosphorylated. These data are evidence for intermolecular phosphorylation, but cannot differentiate between intra- and interoligomeric mechanisms (44).

Some data suggest that the EGFR can signal via a single-helix mechanism. Purified EGFR preparations reportedly exist as inactive dimers that dissociate to active monomers upon binding ligand and ATP (7, 13). This report is supported by the observation that the EGFR isolated from human placenta, which is totally monomeric, is fully active (57, 71). Preparations of monomeric EGFR can also be activated under artificial conditions, for example in the presence of 0.25 M ammonium sulfate (57, 71). Furthermore, recent studies using resonance energy transfer in living cells, in contrast to membrane preparations, show no evidence of microaggregation (14). The lack of microaggregation in living cells suggests that the receptor may be constrained by neighboring proteins or cytoskeletal elements; such interactions could overcome the difficulties with monomolecular mechanisms mentioned above. Furthermore, a signal mechanism based on an inactive dimer and active monomer is plausible.

TOPOLOGY OF INTERACTIONS IN OLIGOMERS FOR SIGNALING

If oligomerization and allosteric conformational change of receptors is required upon ligand binding to trigger signaling, what portions of the receptor molecule are required to participate? Is the interaction of a part of a receptor with an intact receptor sufficient to form an oligomer and/or trigger signaling? These questions have been studied by constructing truncated and chimeric receptors that delete or replace specific domains.

Ectodomains

We have several examples of an association site residing in the ectodomain of transmembrane proteins. Hemagglutinin lacking a transmembrane and cytoplasmic domain can form a trimer (23, 25). However, this oligomer derives significant stability from transmembrane-domain interactions, suggesting that the domain also has a complementary site (23). Histocompatibility-locus antigen heavy chains lacking transmembrane and cytoplasmic domains can form heterodimeric complexes with β2-microglobulin (59). Soluble ectodomains derived from the cell adhesion molecule CD11b/CD18, a heterodimer, can form a soluble heterodimer when the ectodomains of each subunit are secreted from cotransfected cells (20). Peptides derived from the ectodomain of histocompatibility complex class I antigens are able to associate with the ectodomain of the insulin receptor and inhibit the activation of the receptor without inhibiting the binding of insulin (39).

Chemical cross-linking has shown that soluble ectodomains of the insulin, epidermal growth factor, and platelet-derived growth factor receptors associated with their respective native ectodomains when the soluble forms were coexpressed or incubated with the intact receptors in the presence of ligand (4, 96, 110). The soluble ectodomains inhibited the stimulation of the intact receptors by a mechanism other than competition for ligand. These observed associations of the ectodomains were specific. For example, the EGFR ectodomain did not inhibit the function of the PDGF, insulin, or HER2/*neu* receptors (4).

Constructs of the PDGF-receptor that contain the transmembrane and ectodomains have been made to look at the effect of a membrane-bound ectodomain. In the presence of ligand, this construct could form a heterodimer with full-length PDGFR as well as a truncated homodimer (96, 110). Neither the truncated homodimer nor the heterodimer with the wild-type receptor was functionally activated by ligand, as assayed by tyrosine phosphorylation and calcium mobilization. The data presented clearly show that the ligand-dependent association of the ectodomain segments of the tyrosine kinase receptor family is insufficient to induce the appropriate conformational change in the cytoplasmic segment and trigger the tyrosine kinase activity. Thus, an activating conformational change in the receptor may require the association of the transmembrane and cytoplasmic domains in coordination with the ectodomains.

Transmembrane and Cytoplasmic Domains

Other examples show that the transmembrane domain has a significant role in mediating oligomerization. The best example is the demonstration that a synthetic peptide corresponding to the transmembrane domain of glycophorin A can compete for the full-length molecule in order to form a heterodimer comprised of a subunit of full length and a subunit of peptide (9). This reaction was also determined to be sequence specific because peptides corresponding to homologous but nonidentical transmembrane domains did not inhibit the dimerization (9). The deletion of the transmembrane domain of gp160, the envelope glycoprotein of HIV-1, causes the protein to lose its propensity to dimerize (94). Manolios et al (65) recently demonstrated that the transmembrane sequence of the α-chain of the T-cell receptor is critical for the α-chain to associate with the CD3 δ-chain subunit of the T-cell receptor. A subdomain in this transmembrane segment, which contained two charged residues, was requisite for the T-cell receptor assembly, and the charge motif could be placed in an unrelated receptor transmembrane domain and restore assembly of the T-cell receptor subunits (18).

Replacement of the transmembrane domain of the PDGF receptor with that of the EGF receptor abolished ligand-mediated signaling of the PDGF receptor, indicating that the transmembrane domain plays a significant role in signaling (57). Replacement of the transmembrane domain of the neural growth factor receptor with the transmembrane domain of the EGFR inhibited the neural outgrowth of transfected cells, indicating that critical information was contained in the transmembrane domain sequence of the nerve growth factor (NGF) receptor (112). Proteolytic removal of the ectodomains of chicken asialoglycoprotein receptors have shown that the transmembrane domain mediates homodimerization of this receptor (63). Truncation of the ectodomain of the *c-ros* protooncogene product in viruses, the EGFR, and the nontransforming *neu* protein, constructs similar to the *v-erb-B* avian oncoprotein (24), activates tyrosine kinase activities. This observation suggests that the ectodomains may act to sterically hinder the transmembrane and cytoplasmic domains from close contact, which would be overcome by binding to ligand (3, 5, 32, 69). The transmembrane domains are required for this amplified activity because the cytoplasmic domains expressed alone in baculovirus systems have extremely low activity (45, 107).

A recent study that specifically addressed the signaling mechanism by the EGFR transmembrane domain found that truncation of the trans-membrane segment by six amino acids, the insertion of a charged residue similar to the *neu* protein mutation, and the placement of three proline residues in the transmembrane region had no effect on signaling (12). These mutations suggest that the monomolecular push-pull and rotational models are not relevant for the EGFR.

In the case of the *neu* protein, a single point mutation in the trans-membrane domain of the 185-kilodalton (kDa) protooncogene protein, valine to glutamic acid, induces transforming activity (2). Modeling and chemical cross-linking data suggest that this point mutation induces dimer-ization and subsequent transformation (91, 108, 109). The glutamic acid can be replaced by a glutamine and weakly by an aspartic acid but no other residues. Also, the glutamic acid residue cannot be moved from the location where it occurs without complete loss of transforming activity (3). The entire ectodomain and large portions of the cytoplasmic domain can be removed using molecular techniques with no diminution of trans-forming activity (3). The recent report of a valine-to-isoleucine point mutation in the transmembrane domain of amyloid precursor protein in patients with familial Alzheimer's disease has led to the speculation that a dimerizing event similar to that seen with the *neu* protein may be involved (33, 93).

Finally, a close association of the cytoplasmic domain, perhaps mediated by cytoskeletal proteins, may also play a part in signal transduction (78). Studies on the low density lipoprotein (LDL) receptor showed that the 30 terminal residues in the cytoplasmic domain were essential for the for-mation and stability of LDL receptor dimers (101). In the tyrosine kinase family, a chimeric molecule that contained the ectodomain of the EGFR with the PDGFR transmembrane and cytoplasmic domain lost activity from deletions in the cytoplasmic domain that were not the tyrosine kinase domain (27). This result was interpreted as indicating that regions of the cytoplasmic domain had important conformational effects on the tyrosine kinase domain.

Cotransfection of wild-type PDGF receptor with a truncated mutant that lacks a cytoplasmic domain led to dimerization and hetero-dimerization with full length PDGF receptor, but the heterodimer was not active. These data indicate that a close association of the ectodomain and transmembrane domain was not sufficient to activate the tyrosine kinase, suggesting a role for the close association of the cytoplasmic domain.

Constructs that placed the ectodomain of the EGFR onto the *v-erb-B* oncoprotein were not transforming except for deletions in the cytoplasmic domain that constitutively activated the receptor (66). And finally, a recent report indicated that tyrphostin molecules, which inhibit the tyrosine kinase activity of the EGFR, did not affect dimerization of the receptors (88). The data presented show that the propensity of specific receptors for oligomerizing and transducing signals may reside in a necessary allosteric change or in a close association in each of the three domains of the receptor.

MODELS OF TRANSMEMBRANE DOMAIN INTERACTION   In surveys of proteins known to oligomerize, such as the trimeric structure of influenza virus hemagglutinin or the heterodimeric structure of the class II MHC antigens, the transmembrane regions are fairly well conserved across species. This indicates an evolutionary constraint on the sequence of the transmembrane segments. For example, in a survey of 20 hemagglutinins from several species, only one or two possible amino acids are allowed in some positions in the transmembrane domain, and these positions are spaced every 4 amino acids. The same motif is also found in Rous sarcoma virus gp37 and the poly-Ig receptor (60). As another example, there is remarkable identity between the different heavy-chain transmembrane regions of the MHC class II antigens as well as between the light chain hydrophobic regions (50). The juxtamembrane segments are not conserved, which suggests that a transmembrane association of the heavy and light chains produces a distinct selective pressure on the allowable composition of the transmembrane segments. The same observations have also been made for membrane IgG1, IgG2a, IgM, and the glycophorins (50).

Researchers have generally concluded that the tyrosine kinase receptor family has unremarkable transmembrane sequences (114). However, the transmembrane domain of the PDGF-receptor, for example, is highly conserved across species (110). Various models have been proposed to explain the propensity of the transforming *neu* protein to dimerize. Studies using conformational energy analyses based on empirical conformational energies for polypeptides programs (80) predicted that the non-transforming *neu* protein had a sharp bend at the valine position 664. In the transforming protein, this position is mutated to a glutamic acid and this study predicted that the glutamic acid allowed the transmembrane domain to form an α-helix (11). Gullick & Sternberg (57) have proposed that the side chain of the glutamic acid is protonated because of the hydrophobic environment and could form hydrogen bonds in the bilayer. This model also predicts a close packing of the α-helices to allow the formation of an interreceptor hydrogen bond (15).

In a survey of the transmembrane domain of members of the tyrosine

Table 1   Survey of transmembrane domains with small aliphatic side-chain cluster motif[a]

0	1	2	3	4															
A	L	I	**V**	G	T	L	S	G	T	I	F	F	I	L	L	I	I	F	L	C3B/C4B RECEPTOR
G	I	I	**L**	G	L	L	L	V	V	V	A	I	A	G	G	V	L	L	W	Fc RECEPTOR, p51
G	L	V	**L**	A	A	G	A	M	A	V	A	I	A	R						POLY Ig RECEPTOR
G	S	S	**I**	G	G	L	L	L	L	A	L	I	T	A	V	L	Y	K		ALPHA p150/95
P	I	V	**A**	G	V	V	A	G	I	V	L	I	G	L	A	L	L	I		BETA-3 INTEGRINS
G	V	M	**A**	G	V	I	G	T	I	L	L	I	S	Y	G	I	R			GLYCOPHORIN A
G	L	T	**V**	G	L	V	G	I	I	I	G	T	I	F	I	L	K			HLA-DR ALPHA
G	F	V	**L**	G	L	L	F	L	G	A	G	L	F	I	Y	F	R			HLA-DR BETA
S	A	V	**V**	G	M	S	L	L	A	L	I	S	I	F	A	S	C	Y	M	SEMLIKI FOREST VIRUS E2
G	G	V	**A**	G	L	L	L	F	I	G	L	G	I	F	F	C	V	R		T4 T-CELL SURFACE PROTEIN
A	A	I	**V**	G	G	T	V	A	G	I	V	L	I	G	I	L	L	L	V	BETA SUBUNIT LFA-1, MAC-1

[a] A random survey of the transmembrane helices using the small aliphatic side-chain motif suggested by Sternberg & Gullick (92) was performed. The sequences shown are representative of large families of receptors that contain this motif. The residues that include the sequence in the motif are shown in bold type. C3B/C4B receptor (55); the Fc receptor, p51 (84); Poly Ig receptor (67); Alpha subunit of p150/95 (17); β-3 integrin subunit (30); glycophorin A (68); HLA-DR antigens α and β subunits (50); Semliki Forest virus protein E2 (102); T-cell T4 (CD4) protein (64); β subunits of LFA-1 and MAC-1 (54); and human cellular adhesion molecule-1 (89).

kinase receptor family, Sternberg et al (92) observed that clusters of small aliphatic side-chain residues were conserved in a motif. As glycines are infrequent in transmembrane regions, this motif appears to be significant (82). A survey of random transmembrane proteins, shown in Table 1, demonstrates that this motif is not particular to the tyrosine kinase receptor family but can also be found in the integrin and immunoglobulin families. The motif is found, for the most part, in receptor proteins known to form homo- or heterodimers. The exceptions to this rule are the observation of this motif in the CD4 and ICAM-1 molecules, neither of which is, at present, known to dimerize.

SUMMARY AND CONCLUSIONS

In spite of our greatly expanded knowledge of the primary structures of transbilayer receptor proteins, our knowledge of the tertiary and quaternary structures that define the biological activity of these receptors is scant. If we assume that the transmembrane regions of receptor proteins form stable α-helices regardless of the mechanism of insertion, a two-stage model of protein folding can be applied. For a multiple-helix protein, the two-stage model would predict that stable helical formation would be followed by an association of the helices to form the appropriate tertiary/quaternary structure. The two-stage model of protein folding is supported by various experiments with bacteriorhodopsin demonstrating that separate proteolytic fragments of bacteriorhodopsin can be refolded separately and can specifically recognize each other in order to associate and form a biologically active molecule.

At the level of the bilayer, we propose that the energetics required for the association and packing of the helical transmembrane regions of a multiple-helix protein should not be significantly different from the association of separate single-helix proteins into an oligomer. Given the homogeneity in primary and secondary structure of the transmembrane regions of single-helix proteins, the association of multiple monomers may physically define high vs low affinity states and be a plausible mechanism of signal transduction.

Increasing data suggest that oligomerization of receptor proteins may be involved in signal transduction. The transmembrane domains of receptor proteins appear to contain information critical to signaling and may be involved in a close contact site between receptors. This observation allows the two-stage model of protein folding for multiple-helix proteins to be directly applied to the oligomerization of single-helix receptor proteins. In addition, significant data suggest that the ectodomains and cytoplasmic domains are also involved in signaling and oligomerization of receptor molecules. In effect, the present data suggest that the most plausible model, both mechanistically and energetically, is one that includes both oligomerization and a global allosteric conformational change involving all of the defined domains of the receptor molecule.

An oligomerization/conformational change model would predict that new sites of close contact would occur between the domains of the receptor molecule, some of which may be between the transmembrane helices. Therefore, experimenters should be able to generate peptides or small molecules that can specifically interfere with either the oligomerization or generation of new close-contact sites involved in the conformational change of the receptor that leads to signaling. In this way, specific receptors might be targeted for inhibition or possibly activation using binding events inside the bilayer.

ACKNOWLEDGMENTS

B. J. Bormann wishes to gratefully acknowledge the efforts of Drs. P. Jayaraj, J. Woska, P. Reilly, T. Kishimoto, and S. Marlin in the preparation of various portions of the manuscript. D. M. Engelman is grateful for support by the NIH, NSF, Boehringer Ingelheim, the National Foundation for Cancer Research, and to J.-L. Popot for discussions.

Literature Cited

1. Altenbach, C., Marti, T., Khorana, H. G., Hubbell, W. L. 1990. *Science* 248: 1088–92
2. Bargmann, C. I., Hung, M. C., Weinberg, R. A. 1986. *Cell* 45: 649–57
3. Bargmann, C. I., Weinberg, R. A. 1988. *EMBO J.* 7: 2043–52
4. Basu, A., Raghunath, M., Bishayee, S., Das, M. 1989. *Mol. Cell. Biol.* 9: 671–77
5. Birchmeier, C., Birnbaum, D., Waitches, G., Fasano, O., Wigler, M. 1986. *Mol. Cell. Biol.* 6: 3109–16
6. Bishayee, S., Majumdar, S., Khire, J., Das, M. 1989. *J. Biol. Chem.* 264: 11699–11705
7. Biswas, R., Basu, M., Sen-majumdar, A., Das, M. 1985. *Biochemistry* 24: 3795–3802
8. Boni-Schnetzler, M., Pilch, P. F. 1987. *Proc. Natl. Acad. Sci. USA* 84: 7832–36
9. Bormann, B. J., Knowles, W. J., Marchesi, V. T. 1989. *J. Biol. Chem.* 264: 4033–37
10. Brandl, C. J., Deber, C. M. 1986. *Proc. Natl. Acad. Sci. USA* 83: 917–21
11. Brandt-Rauf, P. W., Rackovsky, S., Pincus, M. R. 1990. *Proc. Natl. Acad. Sci. USA* 87: 8660–64
12. Carpenter, C. D., Ingraham, H. A., Cochet, C., Walton, G. M., Lazar, C. S., et al. 1991. *J. Biol. Chem.* 266: 5750–55
13. Carraway, K. I., Koland, J. G., Cerione, R. A. 1989. *J. Biol. Chem.* 264: 8699–8707
14. Carraway, K. L., Cerione, R. A. 1991. *J. Biol. Chem.* 266: 8899–8906
15. Chothia, C., Levitt, M., Richardson, D. 1981. *J. Mol. Biol.* 145: 215–50
16. Cochet, C., Kashles, O., Chambaz, E. M., Borrello, I., King, C. R., et al. 1988. *J. Biol. Chem.* 263: 3290–95
17. Corbi, A. L., Miller, L. J., O'Connor, K., Larson, R. S., Springer, T. A. 1987. *EMBO J.* 6: 4023–28
18. Cossen, P., Lankford, S. P., Bonifacino, J. S., Klausner, R. D. 1991. *Nature* 351: 414–16
19. Crise, B., Ruusala, A., Zagouras, P., Shaw, A., Rose, J. K. 1989. *J. Virol.* 63: 5328–33
20. Dana, N., Fathallah, D. M., Arnaout, M. A. 1991. *Proc. Natl. Acad. Sci. USA* 88: 3106–10
21. Davis, N. G., Boeke, J. D., Model, P. 1985. *J. Mol. Biol.* 181: 111–21
22. Deisenhofer, J., Epp, O., Miki, K., Huber, R., Michel, H. 1985. *Nature* 318: 618–24

23. Doms, R. W., Helenius, A. 1986. *J. Virol.* 60: 833–39
24. Downward, J., Yarden, Y., Mayes, E., Scrace, G., Totty, N., et al. 1984. *Nature* 307: 521–27
25. Doyle, C., Sambrook, J., Gething, M.-J. 1986. *J. Cell Biol.* 103: 1193–1204
26. Engelman, D. M., Steitz, T. A., Goldman, A. 1986. *Annu. Rev. Biophys. Biophys. Chem.* 15: 321–53
27. Esser, V., Russell, D. W. 1988. *J. Biol. Chem.* 263: 13276–81
28. Falke, J. J., Koshland, D. E. 1987. *Science* 237: 1596–1600
29. Fanger, B. O., Stephens, J. E., Staros, J. V. 1989. *Fed. Proc. Fed. Am. Soc. Exp. Biol.* 3: 71–75
30. Fitzgerald, L. A., Steiner, B., Rall, S. C. Jr., Lo, S., Phillips, D. R. 1987. *J. Biol. Chem.* 262: 3936–39
31. Froshauer, S., Green, G. N., Boyd, D., McGovern, K., Beckwith, J. 1988. *J. Mol. Biol.* 200: 501–11
32. Gamett, D. C., Tracey, S. E., Robinson, H. L. 1986. *Proc. Natl. Acad. Sci. USA* 83: 6053–57
33. Goate, A., Chartier-Harlin, M.-C., Mullan, M., Brown, J., Crawford, F., et al. 1991. *Nature* 349: 704–6
34. Goldman, R., Levy, R. B., Peles, E., Yarden, Y. 1990. *Biochemistry* 29: 11024–28
35. Grasberger, B., Minton, A. P., DeLisi, C., Metzger, H. 1986. *Proc. Natl. Acad. Sci. USA* 83: 6258–62
36. Greenfield, C., Hils, I., Waterfield, M. D., Federwisch, W., Wollimer, A., et al. 1989. *EMBO J.* 8: 4115–24
37. Guan, J. L., Ruusala, A., Cao, H., Rose, J. K. 1988. *Mol. Cell Biol.* 8: 2869–74
38. Hammacher, A., Mellstrom, K., Heldin, C.-H. 1989. *EMBO J.* 8: 2489–95
39. Hansen, T., Stagsted, J., Pedersen, L., Roth, R. A., Goldstein, A., et al. 1989. *Proc. Natl. Acad. Sci. USA* 86: 3123–26
40. Heldin, C.-H., Ernlund, A., Rorsman, C., Ronnstrand, L. 1989. *J. Biol. Chem.* 264: 8905–12
41. Henderson, R., Unwin, P. N. T. 1975. *Nature* 257: 28–32
42. Hollenberg, M. D. 1991. *Fed. Proc. Fed. Am. Soc. Exp. Biol.* 5: 178–86
43. Honegger, A. M., Kris, R. M., Ullrich, A., Schlessinger, J. 1989. *Proc. Natl. Acad. Sci. USA* 86: 925–29
44. Honegger, A. M., Schmidt, A., Ullrich, A., Schlessinger, J. 1990. *Mol. Cell. Biol.* 10: 4035–44

45. Hsu, C.-Y. J., Mohammadi, M., Nathan, M., Honegger, A., Ullrich, A., et al. 1991. *Cell Growth Differ.* 12: 191–200

46. Huang, K. S., Bayley, H., Liao, M.-J., London, E., Khorana, H. G. 1981. *J. Biol. Chem.* 256: 3802–9

47. Jennings, M. L. 1989. *Annu. Rev. Biochem.* 58: 999–1027

48. Jubb, J. S., Worcester, D. L., Crespi, H. L., Zaccai, G. 1984. *EMBO J.* 3: 1455–61

49. Kaplan, D. R., Hempstead, B. L., Martin-Zanca, D., Chao, M. V., Parada, L. F. 1991. *Science* 252: 554–58

50. Kaufman, J. F., Auffray, C., Korman, A. J., Shackelford, D. A., Strominger, J. 1984. *Cell* 36: 1–13

51. Kelly, J. D., Haldeman, B. A., Grant, F. J., Murray, M. J., Siefert, R. A., et al. 1991. *J. Biol. Chem.* 266: 8987–92

52. King, A. C., Cuatrecasas, P. 1982. *J. Biol. Chem.* 257: 3053–60

53. King, C. R., Borrello, I., Bellot, F., Comoglio, P., Schlessinger, J. 1988. *EMBO J.* 7: 1647–51

54. Kishimoto, T. K., O'Connor, K., Lee, A., Roberts, T. M., Springer, T. A. 1987. *Cell* 48: 681–90

55. Klickstein, L. B., Wong, W. W., Smith, J. A., Weis, J. H., Wilson, J. G., et al. 1987. *J. Exp. Med.* 165: 1095–1112

56. Kokai, Y., Myers, J. N., Wada, T., Brown, V. I., LeVea, C. M., et al. 1989. *Cell* 58: 287–92

57. Koland, J. G., Cerione, R. A. 1988. *J. Biol. Chem.* 263: 2230–37

58. Kouyama, T., Kimura, Y., Kinosita, K. Jr., Ikegami, A. 1981. *J. Mol. Biol.* 153: 337–59

59. Krangel, M. S., Pious, D., Strominger, J. L. 1984. *J. Immunol.* 132: 2984–91

60. Lazarovits, J., Shia, S.-P., Ktistakis, N., Lee, M.-S., Bird, C., et al. 1990. *J. Biol.Chem.* 265: 4760–67

61. Lewis, B. A., Engelman, D. M. 1983. *J. Mol. Biol.* 166: 203–10

62. Lipowsky, R. 1991. *Nature* 349: 475–81

63. Loeb, J. A., Drickamer, K. 1987. *J. Biol. Chem.* 262: 3022–29

64. Maddon, P. J., Littman, D. R., Godfrey, M., Maddon, D. E., Chess, L., et al. 1985. *Cell* 42: 93–104

65. Manolios, N., Bonifacino, J. S., Klausner, R. D. 1990. *Science* 249: 274–77

66. Massoglia, S., Gray, A., Dull, T. J., Munemitsu, S., Kung, H.-J., et al. 1990. *Mol. Cell. Biol.* 10: 3048–55

67. Mostov, K. E., Friedlander, M., Blobel, G. 1984. *Nature* 308: 37–43

68. Murayama, J., Tomita, M., Hamada, A. 1982. *J. Membr. Biol.* 64: 205–15

69. Neckameyer, W. S., Shibuya, M., Hsu, M.-T., Wang, L.-H. 1986. *Mol. Cell. Biol.* 6: 1478–86

70. Nicolson, G. 1976. *Biochim. Biophys. Acta* 457: 57–108

71. Norwood, I. C., Davis, R. J. 1988. *J. Biol. Chem.* 263: 7450–53

72. Popot, J.-L., de Vitry, C. 1990. *Annu. Rev. Biophys. Biophys. Chem.* 19: 369–403

73. Popot, J.-L., Engelman, D. M. 1990. *Biochemistry* 29: 4031–37

74. Popot, J.-L., Gerchman, S.-E., Engelman, D. M. 1987. *J. Mol. Biol.* 198: 655–76

75. Popot, J.-L., Trewhella, J., Engelman, D. M. 1986. *EMBO J.* 5: 3039–44

76. Reichert, L. E. Jr., Dattatreyamurty, B., Grasso, P., Santa-Coloma, T. A. 1991. *Trends Pharmacol. Sci.* 12: 199–203

77. Richards, F. 1977. *Annu. Rev. Biophys. Bioeng.* 6: 151–76

78. Roy, L. M., Gittinger, C. K., Landreth, G. E. 1989. *J. Cell. Phys.* 140: 295–304

79. Ruestow, P. C., Levinson, D. J., Catchatourian, R., Sreekanth, S., Cohen, H., et al. 1980. *Arch. Intern. Med.* 140: 1115–16

80. Scheraga, H. A. 1984. *Carlsberg Res. Commun.* 49: 1–55

81. Schlessinger, J. 1988. *Biochemistry* 27: 3119–23

82. Schulz, G. E., Schirmer, R. H. 1978. In *Principles of Protein Structure*, ed. G. E. Schulz, R. H. Schrimer, pp. 10–16. New York: Springer-Verlag. 378 pp.

83. Seifert, R. A., Hart, C. E., Phillips, P. E., Forstrom, J. W., Ross, R., et al. 1989. *J. Biol. Chem.* 264: 8771–78

84. Simister, N. E., Mostov, K. E. 1989. *Nature* 337: 184–87

85. Singer, S. J., Nicolson, G. L. 1972. *Science* 175: 720–31

86. Sojar, H. T., Bahl, O. P. 1989. *J. Biol. Chem.* 264: 2552–59

87. Soos, M. A., Siddle, K. 1989. *Biochem. J.* 263: 553–63

88. Spaargaren, M., Defize, L. H. K., Boonstra, J., deLaat, S. W. 1991. *J. Biol. Chem.* 266: 1733–39

89. Staunton, D. E., Marlin, S. D., Stratowa, C., Dustin, M. L., Springer, T. A. 1988. *Cell* 52: 925–33

90. Stern, D. F., Kamps, M. P. 1991. *EMBO J.* 7: 995–1001

91. Sternberg, M. J. E., Gullick, W. J. 1989. *Nature* 339: 587–87

92. Sternberg, M. J. E., Gullick, W. J. 1990. *Protein Eng.* 3: 245–48

93. Tanzi, R. E., Hyman, B. T. 1991. *Nature* 350: 564–64

242 BORMANN & ENGELMAN

94. Thomas, D. J., Wall, J. S., Hainfeld, J. F., Kaczorek, M., Booy, F. P., et al. 1991. *J. Virol.* 65: 3797–3803
95. Treadway, J. L., Morrison, B. D., Soos, M. A., Siddle, K., Olefsky, J., et al. 1991. *Proc. Natl. Acad. Sci. USA* 88: 214–18
96. Ueno, H., Colbert, H., Escobedo, J. A., Williams, L. T. 1991. *Science* 252: 844–47
97. Ullrich, A., Bell, J. R., Chen, E. Y., Herrera, R., Petruzzelli, L. M., et al. 1985. *Nature* 313: 756–61
98. Ullrich, A., Coussens, L., Hayflick, J. S., Dull, T. J., Gray, A., et al. 1984. *Nature* 309: 418–25
99. Ullrich, A., Schlessinger, J. 1990. *Cell* 61: 203–12
100. Ushiro, H., Cohen, S. 1980. *J. Biol. Chem.* 255: 8363–65
101. van Driel, I. R., Davis, C. G., Goldstein, J. L., Brown, M. S. 1987. *J. Biol. Chem.* 262: 16127–34
102. Vaux, D. J. T., Helenius, A., Mellman, I. 1988. *Nature* 336: 36–42
103. Wada, T., Qian, X., Greene, M. I. 1990. *Cell* 61: 1339–47
104. Wallace, B. A., Cascio, M., Mielke, D. L. 1986 *Proc. Natl. Acad. Sci. USA* 83: 9423–27
105. Ward, W. H. J., Timms, D., Fersht, A. R. 1990. *Trends Pharmacol. Sci.* 11: 280–84
106. Webwe, W., Betrics, P. J., Gill, G. N. 1984. *J. Biol. Chem.* 259: 14631–36
107. Wedegaertner, P. B., Gill, G. N. 1989. *J. Biol. Chem.* 264: 11346–53
108. Weiner, D. B., Kokaj, Y., Wada, T., Cohen, J. A., Williams, W. V., et al. 1989. *Oncogene* 4: 1175–83
109. Weiner, D. B., Liu, J., Cohen, J. A., Williams, W. V., Greene, M. I. 1989. *Nature* 339: 230–31
110. Williams, L. T. 1989. *Science* 243: 1564–70
111. Wistow, G. J., Pisano, M. M., Chepelinsky, A. B. 1991. *Trends Biol. Sci.* 16: 170–71
112. Yan, H., Schlessinger, J., Chao, M. V. 1991. *Science* 252: 561–63
113. Yarden, Y., Schlessinger, J. 1987. *Biochemistry* 26: 1443–51
114. Yarden, Y., Ullrich, A. 1988. *Biochemistry* 27: 3113–18
115. Yeates, T. O., Komiya, H., Rees, D. C., Allen, J. P., Feher, G. 1987. *Proc. Natl. Acad. Sci. USA* 84: 6438–42

Annu. Rev. Biophys. Biomol. Struct. 1992. 21:243–65

PROTEIN FOLDING STUDIED USING HYDROGEN-EXCHANGE LABELING AND TWO-DIMENSIONAL NMR

S. Walter Englander and Leland Mayne

The Johnson Research Foundation, Department of Biochemistry and Biophysics, University of Pennsylvania, Philadelphia, Pennsylvania 19104-6059

KEY WORDS: molten globule, folding intermediate

CONTENTS

243

1056–8700/92/0610–0243$02.00

OVERVIEW AND PERSPECTIVES

Soon after the demonstration that protein molecules could fold spontaneously without external guidance (29), C. Levinthal (51) pointed out a
fundamental problem. Even a small protein has access to an enormous
number of possible conformational states, which could not be searched
through in a random way in any reasonable length of time. Dill (14) has
reduced this number to 10^{15} conformations for a 100-residue protein, but
the problem remains. Apparently, the nascent random chain polypeptide
must be guided through some predetermined folding pathway to find its
native structure.

Much effort has been expended in the attempt to characterize protein-
folding pathways. Yet some of the most basic issues concerning folding
processes are still before us. Does protein folding follow a linear sequence
of defined intermediate structures, or is the pathway heterogeneous so that
folding can proceed through a few or even many alternative pathways?
What kinds of structural intermediates and kinetic barriers determine
folding pathways? How does the one-dimensional amino acid sequence
code for not only the final three-dimensional native structure, but also for
the pathway, perhaps involving many nonnative intermediate structures,
that leads to the final structure? Discovery of the principles that determine
protein-folding pathways and equilibrium structure has become a central
preoccupation of protein chemists (1, 10, 12, 13, 15, 16, 32, 36, 37, 43, 44,
46, 58, 59, 63, 66, 71–73, 77, 78, 85, 86, 89, 90).

As with any biochemical pathway, one can hope to understand protein
folding by isolating intermediates in some folding pathways and examining
their structures. Protein-folding intermediates, however, present a special
problem. They have only transient existence and usually cannot be isolated
for study. Nevertheless, experiments that can secure direct structural information on kinetic intermediates have been devised. Also, kinetic intermediates have been sought in an indirect sense by attempting to find
and characterize equilibrium intermediate forms that may mimic possible
kinetic intermediates.

Two approaches aiming for direct structural information on kinetic
intermediates have so far been exploited. Creighton and his colleagues
have been able to isolate intermediates on the folding pathway of pancreatic trypsin inhibitor, a small 58-residue protein with 3 disulfide bridges,
by the covalent trapping of 1- and 2-disulfide intermediate forms. From
this pioneering work, several insights have emerged (10, 11). However, for
the majority of proteins, which do not use multiple disulfide bonds, this
particular option does not exist.

Here we are concerned with a second mode of covalent trapping, a labeling method that can use the exchangeable hydrogens of a protein as probes of structure and structure change. Many hydrogens, distributed throughout every protein structure, continually exchange with solvent hydrogens. The wide dynamic range of exchange rates contains detailed information on structure and structural energy, resolved to the level of individual amino acid residues. Hydrogen exchange[1] (HX) labeling experiments exploit this behavior to label selectively the sites one wishes to identify and study. Two-dimensional nuclear magnetic resonance spectroscopy (2D NMR) can then be used to determine the HX labeling pattern at high resolution (30, 99).

Hydrogen-exchange labeling methods were initially developed for studies of structure and dynamics in stable protein systems (22). Kinetic labeling selects sites on the basis of their HX rates (9, 28). Functional labeling selects sites that change in HX rate, for example in an allosteric transition (24, 53). Recently, specially designed HX experiments have been used to label kinetic folding intermediates in a structure-sensitive way and even to resolve the time-dependent formation of structure. Hydrogen isotope label can be emplaced with millisecond time resolution and then can be trapped by adjusting solution and structural conditions. Lengthy sample preparation and 2D NMR analyses can then be done to identify the labeled sites and their isotopic occupancy, and thus obtain fairly detailed information on structure and dynamics.

The encouraging results so far achieved recommend the use of HX labeling for more widespread studies. The design and successful execution of HX labeling experiments depend upon the expert manipulation of the hydrogen-exchange reaction, and the proper interpretation of these kinds of data may be less than obvious. This article illustrates the broad repertoire and experimental power available for these approaches and considers some of the problems of experimental design and interpretation that such studies must face.

THE DETERMINANTS OF PROTEIN-HYDROGEN EXCHANGE

The continual exchange with solvent of peptide-group NHs[1] and polar side-chain hydrogens does not simply occur spontaneously. These reac-

---

[1] Hydrogen exchange is often referred to as proton exchange. We prefer the more general term because exchange experiments often involve deuterons and tritions as well as protons. Similarly, the peptide group is often referred to, especially in the NMR literature, as the NH. Proteins contain three kinds of amides: the primary amide side chains of asparagine and glutamine, the peptide group secondary amide, and the tertiary amide of prolyl residues. It therefore seems best to refer to the peptide group by its specific name.

tions must be catalyzed by solvent acids and bases. Especially important for exchange of the peptide NHs are specific acid and base, i.e. H_3O^+ and OH^- ions. Polar side chains, owing to their less extreme pKs, may also be catalyzed by general acids and bases, such as the pH buffers used in protein experiments. The much slower exchange of carbon-bound hydrogens can, in the context of folding experiments, be ignored. In structured proteins, the exchange of many hydrogens is greatly slowed. Here, we briefly review the major determinants of these rates at the chemical and structural levels.

Hydrogen-Exchange Chemistry

Figure 1 shows the H-D exchange behavior of freely exposed peptide NH in D_2O as a function of pD, recently recalibrated (39) in the random chain model, poly-D,L-alanine. Exchange rates vary linearly with H^+ and OH^- ion concentrations, and a pH-independent mechanism becomes apparent only near the pH of minimum rate, around pH 3. Equation 1 describes this behavior. Rate constants are in Figure 1.

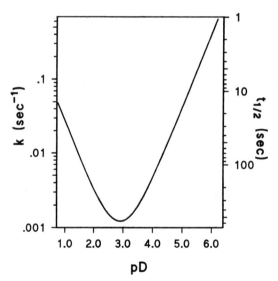

Figure 1   Exchange behavior for random chain poly-D,L-alanine (NH in D_2O at 20°C) (39). The second-order specific acid and specific base rate constants (k_A and k_B in Equation 1) are, respectively, 0.27 $M^{-1}s^{-1}$ and $5.7 \times 10^8 \, M^{-1}s^{-1}$. The first-order pH-independent reaction rate constant (k_W) is $5.6 \times 10^{-4} \, s^{-1}$. The term $[D^+]$ is taken as the apparent value ($[D^+] = 10^{-pD}$), uncorrected for the glass electrode deuterium isotope artifact, and $[OD^-]$ is computed using $K_D = [D^+][OD^-] = 10^{-15.14}$.

$$k_{ch}[cat] = k_A[D^+] + k_B[OD^-] + k_W \qquad\qquad 1.$$

Hydrogen-exchange rates are sensitive to temperature. The present best estimates of activation energies for peptide NH exchange near room temperature are 14 kcal for specific acid catalysis and 17.5 kcal for specific base catalysis (20, 27). The HX rates of individual peptide NHs are sensitive to the electron-withdrawing character of their nearest neighbor side chains; these effects have been calibrated (62, 79). HX rates can also be affected by local charged groups (42), by organic cosolvents (21), and by denaturants (52).

This information is necessary for interpreting protein HX experiments in terms of structure and stability and also shows how HX rates can be shifted at will over a large dynamic range. Under conditions in which most proteins are stable, from pH 5 to 9 and from 0°C to 40°C, the exchange of unstructured peptide NH with solvent proceeds with halftimes between 0.1 ms and 100 s. Structurally involved peptide NH can be far slower, by many orders of magnitude. Therefore, the manipulation of HX rate via pH and temperature in a folding experiment can selectively label, with a time resolution of milliseconds, sites that are not slowed by structure. Yet the hydrogen isotope label deposited in this way can be stably maintained for days in the refolded protein, allowing time-consuming sample processing and 2D NMR analysis of the labeling to be performed.

The exchange of polar side-chain hydrogens may provide additional probe points within a protein. This resource is limited. Side-chain hydrogens are often not assigned in the ^{1}H-NMR spectrum. Also, most are not involved in blocking hydrogen bonds and tend to exchange rapidly, especially as caused by catalysis by buffer acids and bases. A special case, the indole NH of tryptophan, is often resolved even in one-dimensional (1D) NMR spectra, and may well be buried, hydrogen bonded, and slowly exchanging (67, 96). HX rates for the unprotected indole hydrogen have been calibrated (64, 94).

The reader can find further discussion of protein-related HX chemistry elsewhere (3, 25, 70, 98), and the chemical principles of proton transfer reactions have been reviewed (18, 19).

Protein Structural Physics

Hydrogen bonding can greatly slow hydrogen exchange, even when the bond is at the protein surface. This conclusion is implied by the chemistry of proton-transfer reactions, which requires hydrogen-bond formation between the exchanging group and the HX catalyst (18). The vast majority of identified slowly exchanging peptide-group NHs participate in hydrogen bonding, although in crystallographic models, a few slowly exchanging

NHs appear to be sequestered from solvent interaction without apparent hydrogen bonding (perhaps bound water molecules play a role). The detection of structure and structure formation in protein-folding experiments can be taken as largely synonymous with the formation of hydrogen bonding.

What are the mechanisms by which structurally blocked hydrogens in proteins manage to exchange with solvent? Minimally, hydrogen-bond breakage (or hydrogen-bond distortion sufficient to allow fruitful hydrogen bonding to HX catalysts) appears necessary for exchange to occur. Transient hydrogen-bond breakage as a determinant of hydrogen exchange was considered in the early work of Linderstrøm-Lang and his coworkers (35). Subsequent protein studies have provided evidence for the concerted breakage of neighboring hydrogen bonds in some cases, implying a role for small-scale, cooperative structural distortions, referred to as local unfolding (22).

In this view, the HX rate of a structure-blocked hydrogen relates to the parameters of the governing structural opening as in Equation 2a.

$$k_{ex} = k_{op}k_{ch}[cat]/(k_{op} + k_{cl} + k_{ch}[cat]) \qquad 2a.$$

$$k_{ex} \approx K_{op}k_{ch}[cat] \qquad 2b.$$

Here k_{op} and k_{cl} are structural opening and reclosing rate constants, and $k_{ch}[cat]$ may be assumed to be the same as the rate calibrated for freely exposed groups (Figure 1). Equation 2b gives the usual limiting case encountered in proteins, where structure is stable ($k_{op} < k_{cl}$) and the chemical exchange reaction is slow relative to structural reclosing ($k_{ch}[cat] < k_{cl}$). Here, k_{op}/k_{cl} equals K_{op}, the equilibrium constant for local structural unfolding. This second-order behavior, in which the rate depends on catalyst concentration ([cat]), has been called the EX2 case (35). Since $k_{ch}[cat]$ is known from the chemical calibrations noted before, the measurement of k_{ex} yields K_{op}. When chemical exchange is faster than reclosing, HX appears to be unimolecular (EX1) (35) and exhibits the rate of the structural opening reaction. EX1 reactions are rarely seen in stable proteins (82, 88), but may (or may not) occur under the conditions of some protein refolding experiments.

For an EX1 reaction, the HX rate relates to the activation energy for opening. For EX2 reactions, Equation 3a connects measurable HX rates with structural stability (K_{op}) and therefore with structural stabilization free energy ($\Delta G°$).

$$\Delta G° = -RT \ln K_{op} = -RT \ln(k_{ex}/k_{ch}[cat]) \qquad 3a.$$

$$\delta \Delta G^{\circ} = -RT\delta \ln K_{op} = -RT\ln (k_{ex}, 1/k_{ex}, 2) \qquad\qquad 3b.$$

In protein folding experiments, the experimentally derived HX slowing or protection factor, $P = k_{ch}[cat]/k_{ex} \approx 1/K_{op}$, relates to local structural stability in this sense. When a structure change occurs, e.g. when a segment is strained or loses a stabilizing crosslink, transient unfolding of the segment is promoted, and its hydrogen-bonded NHs will exchange more rapidly. The increase in HX rate measures the change in stabilization free energy, according to Equation 3b, which is valid so long as the free energy of the unfolded state has not been changed. These relationships appear to provide a general probe for measuring the free energy of local structural stability (Equation 3a) and the change in free energy (Equation 3b), and can be applied not only to native proteins but even to fractions of structure in transiently present folding intermediates.

A variety of models for the mechanism of slow protein hydrogen exchange focus generally on the fact of burial within the protein as a determinant of slow hydrogen exchange and on the need for penetration by solvent catalysts to the site of the NH (7, 55, 65, 76, 97). These accessibility-penetration models are qualitative in nature and generally suggest no quantitative or even measurable correlations between HX rate and definable structural parameters. Thus, framing experimental tests for their validity has been difficult.

Available results obtained by methodologies that can measure the HX behavior at identified peptide NH sites often exhibit HX behavior consistent with local unfolding reactions. These results include the apparently concerted exchange of neighboring peptide-group NHs in some, but not all, α-helical segments (47, 53, 54, 95), the concerted change in such sets in response to local structural modifications (53, 54, 60), and the semiquantitative correlation between free energy values found by HX and other methods. The present situation appears to be that local unfolding reactions account for slow protein hydrogen exchange in some cases. The more complete picture remains to be determined.

Summary

The exchange rate of freely exposed peptide-group NHs depends on pH, temperature, and nearest-neighbor side chains. These effects are well-understood, have been calibrated, and allow for the manipulation of HX rates over a wide range. Hydrogen bonding slows HX rates for reasons that are clear in light of the chemical mechanisms of exchange. The exchange process appears to require hydrogen-bond breakage, which may often occur in small concerted unfolding reactions. In this case, HX rates are related to the free energy of local structural stability.

HX-LABELING STUDIES OF STRUCTURE AND STRUCTURE CHANGE

Kinetic Labeling in Myoglobin

Selective hydrogen-exchange labeling dates back to early experiments that used kinetic labeling with low resolution H-T exchange to study especially the non-hydrogen-bonded NH at the surface of myoglobin (28). To selectively label and thus resolve the fast NH, myoglobin was subjected to exchange-in in tritiated water for only a short period (~ 10 HX halftimes for free peptides). Exchange-out of the partially labeled protein produced an HX curve in which the normally occurring large background of slower NHs do not appear. This made it possible to clearly distinguish and measure the fast NHs. Their number was equal to that expected from the X-ray model, and their rate was close to that expected for free peptide NH (28, 62). These results tended to alleviate prior concerns that NH exchange in proteins is subject to uncontrolled effects that could render HX rates meaningless, i.e. unpredictable slowing due to water structure at the protein surface and/or unpredictable speeding due to catalysis by nearby polar side chains (45, 50).

Kinetic-labeling experiments were later extended (9) to selectively study different subpopulations among the hydrogen-bonded peptide NHs in myoglobin—the relatively fast, intermediate, and quite slow NHs—and to specifically portray the response of each to solvent conditions. The results provided evidence that progressively slower NHs tend to exchange by way of transient protein distortions that expose progressively more surface to the solvent, as might be expected for local unfolding reactions (Equation 2).

Functional Labeling in Hemoglobin

In more sophisticated functional labeling experiments, selective labeling and trapping methods were developed to study allosteric structure change in hemoglobin. These experiments continue to use tritium labeling, gel filtration, and scintillation counting because hemoglobin is too large for NMR analysis. Functional labeling uses a sequence of steps involving exchange-in, change in functional state, and an exchange-out chase (24, 53). These operations cause allosterically involved sites, those that change their HX rate in the allosteric transition, to become self-selectively labeled. One can then define the position in the protein of the tritium-labeled allosterically sensitive segments using medium-resolution proteolytic fragmentation and fragment-separation methods (2, 21, 23, 84) under conditions that make HX chemistry slow (low pH and temperature). The HX rate of each defined set can be measured in either allosteric form, with or without specific allosteric effectors, and as a function of specific chemical or mutational modifications, placed locally or remotely.

These techniques have been used to identify allosterically sensitive segments, to study several detailed allosterically involved interactions, and to measure their allosteric free energy contributions and interrelationships (21, 24, 53, 54, 56, 60). Also, these experiments have produced results that appear to require a local unfolding model for the HX process.

Summary

HX-labeling experiments have been done with myoglobin and hemoglobin in different modes. In addition to the information obtained on protein function and HX behavior, this work showed that hydrogen exchange can be performed under any chosen conditions, functionally interesting sites can be induced to self-selectively label, the label can be trapped in a slowly exchanging form, and subsequent time-consuming processing and analysis can be done under any other chosen conditions. These unusual characteristics make the hydrogen-exchange labeling method useful for a variety of protein studies.

HX-LABELING STUDIES OF EQUILIBRIUM FOLDING INTERMEDIATES

One now appreciates that the two-state paradigm of protein structure is in a sense an artifact of the extreme conditions one normally uses to observe the native $\rightleftharpoons$ denatured transition. Under strongly native or strongly denaturing conditions, partially folded intermediates are unlikely to be seen. It has now proven possible to populate alternative states under mild conditions that selectively destabilize the globally integrated native state relative to partially folded forms. A number of proteins when mildly destabilized assume a kind of liquid-like state that has been discussed in terms of a form named the molten globule (17, 31, 46, 69, 74, 75), thought to be intermediate in structure between the native and unfolded states. The molten globule is unavoidably somewhat imprecisely defined (75), and a variety of nonnative forms that may or may not meet all the criteria have been placed in this category.

The structure of these forms can provide insights concerning the equilibrium and kinetic determinants of protein folding. However, detailed structural information has been lacking. The dynamic flexibility and marginal stability of structural intermediates makes them unlikely candidates for crystallographic study. It also degrades NMR chemical shift dispersion and nuclear Overhauser effect (NOE) interactions, making NMR structural studies difficult. As a result, no such structures have been solved.

These forms can be studied using nonperturbing HX labeling, at whatever condition the protein system requires. Recent studies of folding intermediates have used a kinetic-labeling approach to distinguish hydrogen-bonded and non-hydrogen-bonded sites. The common plan has been to place the protein in mildly destabilizing acid conditions and expose it to hydrogen exchange in D_2O. The H-D exchange pattern is then trapped by shifting the protein to the native state under solution conditions that make HX slow. Analysis using 2D NMR, done in the native state for a series of samples labeled for various time periods, can then recognize the presence or absence of hydrogen bonding in many peptide NHs in the intermediate. The same approach has been used to determine the HX rate of sites that are hydrogen bonded in the intermediate in order to measure structural stability.

Results Available

HX labeling experiments (4) with α-lactalbumin showed that a number of NHs maintained slow exchange in the molten globule state. At pD 2, these sites remain [1]H-labeled after 10 h in D_2O, indicating an HX slowing factor of 100 or more. On return to the native state, these sites show NH-NH NOESY cross peaks characteristic of a helical segment with eight sequential residues. This segment therefore appears to maintain its hydrogen-bonded helical conformation in the low pH molten globule. Also, magnetization transfer experiments were performed in the unfolding transition region (pH 7.4, 65°C), where conformational exchange between native and molten globule states is fairly fast. Here several aromatic side chains, apparently some of those in the same "hydrophobic box" region of the native protein that involves the stable helix, maintained a strongly perturbed chemical shift in the nonnative form. Baum et al (4) conclude that the hydrophobic core of the protein is at least in part maintained in the intermediate states obtained both at low pH and at high temperature.

HX labeling experiments have been done with an equilibrium folding intermediate of apomyoglobin (34). Myoglobin (Mb) forms a box of eight helical segments, named A to H, built to contain the central heme group. When the heme is removed to form apomyoglobin (apoMb), the helical content diminishes [according to circular dichroism (CD) spectra]. The apoprotein exhibits a partial unfolding transition in mild acid; the helix content falls from 55 to 35%. Hughson et al (34) subjected apoMb to H-D exchange labeling, both at pD 6.0 above the acid transition (native apoMb) and at pD 4.2 in the partially folded intermediate. Protein concentration was kept low to avoid irreversible aggregation. The label was trapped through renaturation (heme added, pH raised); the protein was concentrated; and 2D NMR was applied to serial samples to determine the HX rates of about 40 available probe NHs in the native and the intermediate apoMb forms. Whereas all the probe NHs are slowly exchanging in native apoMb (P ranges from ~ 10 to $> 10^5$), only helices A, G, and H have protected NHs in the intermediate, with $P \approx 10$. For helix E, P approximately equals 1. No information was available for C, D, and F. Hughson et al (34) propose that the apoMb intermediate forms a partially folded structure with helices A and G docked against helix H, as in the native protein.

HX-labeling experiments were performed with acid cytochrome c, which behaves like a typical molten globule (31, 32). Initial experiments (38) were done under high salt (1.5 M NaCl, pD 2.2, 20°C) conditions, where cytochrome c is compact and relatively stable (33). The protein was exposed to HX labeling in D_2O for various time periods (2 min to 500 h) and then submitted to 2D NMR analysis, which could measure the ^1H label trapped at 44 hydrogen-bonded peptide NH sites. All the NHs that are normally slowly exchanging in the 3 major helices of the native protein ($P = 10^5$–10^9) are also slow in the molten globule, with HX protection factors between 30 and 3000. About half of the 15 measurable NHs involved in irregular hydrogen bonding in the native protein show protection factors close to unity, i.e. these hydrogen bonds are either broken in the compact molten globule or have very little stability.

Surprising results were obtained (39) with cytochrome c at lower salt concentration, which deshields and further destabilizes the heavily charged protein (pD 2.2; charge $= +24$ in 104 residues). In 0.02 M NaCl, the protein is greatly expanded (as evidenced by viscosity, fluorescence quenching), perhaps to twice its native extent. The amino acid side chains and much of the main chain are dynamically disordered (as shown by NMR); the single centrally buried tryptophan is exposed to solvent (fluorescence); and most of the tertiary structural hydrogen bonds and some hydrogen bonds at helix termini are broken (HX labeling). Yet the protein retains 85% of its native helical content (CD spectra). The helix present involves the same residues that are helical in the native state, with protection factors between 10 and 30 (HX labeling). Jeng & Englander (39) suggest that the helical segments in the expanded form of acid cytochrome c exist as part of native-like midsized folding units that are larger than a single helix (because the helical segments alone are known to be structureless when isolated) but much smaller than the whole protein.

Interpretational and Experimental Problems

Do non-hydrogen-bonded peptide NHs in these poorly understood protein forms in fact exchange at the expected free peptide rate? If exchange is generally slower than expected, for any unforeseeen reason, then only the

NHs trapped in the refolded native state will spuriously suggest native-like structure in the destabilized form. Here, available results are encouraging. Earlier experiments (28) that used kinetic labeling to study the non-hydrogen-bonded peptide NHs in native myoglobin measured normal free peptide HX rate behavior (see above). In the expanded acid form of cytochrome *c*, 1D NMR was used (39) to directly record an overall HX curve for all the peptide NHs in acid cytochrome *c*. The results showed a large number of fast NHs exchanging at about the rate expected for free peptides; the number of slow NHs was close to the number measured to be trapped in the reformed native state. Kinetic refolding experiments with ribonuclease A (93) similarly suggest that the HX rate of free peptide NH in folding intermediates is normal (see below).

How does one obtain a picture of structure from individual slowly exchanging NHs? Some pattern must be observed among many NHs. For example, if multiple sequential NHs that normally occur in a helix are found to be slowed in some nonnative form, the slow NHs actually measured are probably helical in the experimental structure. One's view is limited, however; only NHs that are slowly exchanging in the native protein can be trapped, and only those with assigned NMR resonances can be identified. It seems dangerous to extrapolate from a few slow NHs to the integrity of a whole helix. For example, native-like helices present in acid cytochrome *c* appear to have lost some of their end residues (39). Helices that might be inferred to be fully formed in apomyoglobin on the basis of a limited number of probes would exceed the helical content indicated by CD (6).

Severe experimental problems arise in working with highly charged proteins at low pH and low salt concentration where molten globule structures have most often been studied. The Helmholtz double layer of the protein can effectively bind a large fraction of the anions added and exclude cations, and thus disturb both salt and pH. Jeng & Englander (39) describe the special handling necessary to control these parameters, and also to avoid perturbing the HX labeling pattern when switching to the acid condition and back to the native state. These problems and also the protein aggregation problem can be minimized by performing the HX experiment at low protein concentration, then trapping the hydrogens and reconcentrating the protein for the NMR analysis.

Comments

Available results show that HX labeling and trapping methods can define elements of structure even in tenuously structured protein forms. The native-like elements found in several partially structured proteins indicate that these forms are indeed intermediates between the native and unfolded states. HX results for the expanded form of cytochrome c and the apo-myoglobin intermediate, and other results with fragments of basic pancreatic trypsin inhibitor (68), show that the formation of considerable native-like structure does not require the compact molten globule form, which apparently represents but one possible format for the intermediate, liquid-like state of proteins. These results suggest that proteins more generally may be composed of mid-sized folding units, fairly small, submolecular, native-like structures that have independent stability. If true, this concept has rather broad implications (39). Kinetic folding intermediates may involve the same kind of mid-sized folding units (see below).

HX-LABELING STUDIES OF KINETIC FOLDING INTERMEDIATES

R. L. Baldwin and his coworkers conceived and demonstrated the use of hydrogen-exchange labeling to study protein refolding. Building on the selective tritium labeling methods described above, the early work used low resolution H-T exchange. A pH-competition labeling mode (87) and a pH-pulse labeling mode (5, 41) were developed in experiments with ribonuclease A. Kuwajima et al (48) demonstrated the potential of H-D exchange for high resolution study of individual hydrogen sites by utilizing NMR analysis. A study of refolding in pancreatic trypsin inhibitor (83) used the pH competition method and rapid mixing techniques with detection by one-dimensional (1D) NMR. These approaches have matured with the further development of the pH pulse-labeling experiment together with high resolution 2D NMR analysis (8, 81, 92, 93).

pH Competition Mode

In the pH competition experiment, protein refolding and HX labeling are initiated simultaneously. When refolding is performed at low pH where exchange is slow, the refolded native structure simply traps the initial isotope. At higher pH, HX proceeds more rapidly, and some exchange occurs before hydrogen bonds can be reformed. Half of a given site will be labeled when its HX rate and hydrogen bond-formation rate are equal. Knowledge of the free peptide rate at this solution condition (Equation 1) can then reveal the folding rate.

A central problem for competition experiments is that change in the independent variable, pH, may also perturb the folding pathway and the stability of intermediates. An experimental advantage is that only one mixing step is necessary. The experiment has been described in some detail (40, 80).

pH Pulse Mode

The pH-pulse labeling mode can effectively use the many HX probes in a protein to dissect the details of protein-folding behavior. Unlike the pH competition experiment, the entire time-dependent folding process is monitored at a constant solution condition. As for HX experiments in general, the refolding experiment can be done under any solution condition, which can be chosen to help stabilize possible intermediates (e.g. low temperature, neutral pH), and even to include additives such as helper enzymes. One can subsequently reisolate the experimental protein in a suitably HX-trapped condition in order to prepare samples for NMR analysis.

The protein can be initially unfolded in denaturant in D_2O, so that the peptide sites are all NDs. In a first mixing step, the solution is diluted to initiate folding. To avoid further large dilutions, the first dilution can be into H_2O at a pH and temperature sufficiently low that folding is initiated but exchange labeling does not yet occur. After some folding time, t_f, a labeling pulse in the form of a sharp pH increase is applied (small volume addition), so that D-to-H exchange becomes fast. Peptide sites still available for exchange at t_f become labeled with H (if the pulse intensity is great enough). Sites already hydrogen bonded at t_f are protected and remain as NDs (unless pulse intensity is too great). The labeling pulse is terminated by quenching to low pH (small volume addition). The protein then folds to completion. At each site trapped by hydrogen bonding in the reformed native state, the H/D ratio established by the labeling pulse at t_f can then be read out using 2D NMR spectroscopy. Results at a series of t_f values then can trace out the history of hydrogen-bond formation at each peptide NH trapped in the native state.

The use of a three-stage rapid mixing device lends special advantages, although two stages can be used (8, 61). With a third mixer, the length of the labeling pulse can be controlled so that the intensity of the pulse can be set at will. Pulse intensity can be defined as $I_p = \Delta t_p / \tau_{ex,p} = k_{ex,p} \times \Delta t_p$, the ratio of pulse time (Δt_p) and HX lifetime ($\tau_{ex,p}$) at the pulse condition. Here, $k_{ex,p}$ equals $1/\tau_{ex,p}$ equals $k_{ch}[cat]$ from Equation 1. At pH 9 and 10°C, the free peptide lifetime is ~ 3 ms (Equation 1 with temperature and average Molday effects), so a 30-ms pulse corresponds to an intensity of 10. Pulse intensity in this range is great enough to ensure the labeling of free peptide sites but small enough to minimize the labeling of slower, hydrogen-bonded sites. Such a short interrogation pulse is unlikely to perturb the structure labeled during its course. A short labeling pulse can also reveal the presence of eccentric behavior. For example, the formation, loss, and reformation of hydrogen bonding could be observed. The initial formation of intermediates with nonnative hydrogen-bonding patterns might be detected. However, the analysis for detailed folding behavior and for folding intermediates depends upon the presence of fortuitously placed kinetic barriers, or barriers that can be purposely engineered (57).

One can vary the pulse intensity (I_p) to test the stability of particular intermediates and their change in stability as folding progresses. When the pulse intensity is decreased at constant t_f, labeling should fall off when $I_p \approx 2$, about pH 8.3 for a 30-ms pulse at 10°C, since the fraction of free NHs not labeled is $\exp(-I_p)$. Udgaonkar & Baldwin (93) observed this behavior in ribonuclease, which suggests that free peptide NH exchange is normal in folding intermediates. If pulse intensity is increased, sites already hydrogen bonded will begin to be labeled when $K_{op}I_p \approx 0.15$. This relationship can be used to estimate K_{op} (Equation 2b) and thus can estimate the stability of local folded structure in a folding intermediate (ΔG°_{op} in Equation 3). The energy analysis (Equation 3) assumes that HX in the intermediate is determined in an EX2 manner. This assumption deserves some consideration. Does exchange occur by an EX1 or EX2 mechanism?

Interpretation of Pulse-Labeling Curves

One can present pulse-labeling results as in Figure 2, which plots the course of ^{1}H labeling as a function of the folding time, t_f. As t_f increases, protection against labeling increases, and proton occupancies measured in 2D NMR spectra decrease. For simplicity, these graphs show possible results for a four-proton protein, with time on a logarithmic scale to illustrate folding events over a realistically broad time range. Folding may proceed from the unfolded state (U) through a simple linear sequence of intermediates (I_i) to the native state (N), as follows: $U \rightarrow I_1 \rightarrow I_2 \rightarrow N$. Again, folding may be heterogeneous; different fractions of U may follow alternative, parallel paths: $U_1 \rightarrow N; U_2 \rightarrow I \rightarrow N$. These steps are in principle reversible, but for most kinetic events seen here, the back reaction will be slower than the short labeling pulse used.

Certain principles are helpful in guiding the interpretation of protection curves. Folding may appear to be a concerted, two-state, $U \rightarrow N$ reaction (Figure 2a). Here, all the probe sites achieve 100% protection at the same rate, in a single first-order kinetic step. The protection rate observed represents the rate at which molecules cross the rate-limiting barrier preceding N. Other energy barriers and intermediate structures undoubtedly occur, but they are transparent to these measurements.

Figure 2b reflects a simple sequential pathway ($U \rightarrow I \rightarrow N$) in which an intermediate that has formed hydrogen bonds A and B is populated before hydrogen bonds C and D are formed. A and B attain 100% protection with the same time constant. The presence of a partially folded intermediate is

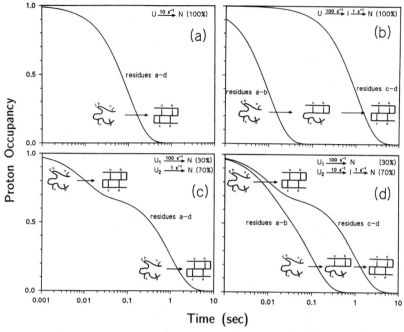

Figure 2 Idealized HX pulse-labeling results for a four-hydrogen bond protein that folds as in the pathways indicated: (*a*) concerted; (*b*) sequential with one intermediate state; (*c*) two heterogeneous, parallel paths with concerted folding; (*d*) two parallel paths with one intermediate in the slower path.

revealed when different probes show different degrees of protection at a given folding time, i.e. they follow a different time course, as in Figure 2*b*. This condition is analogous to the ratio test for equilibrium folding intermediates (49, 91). The labeling results further reveal the identity of residues hydrogen bonded in the formation of a populated intermediate.

For an intermediate to be well populated, it must occupy an energy well in the reaction surface that is lower than all prior wells, and the barrier blocking its further progress must be larger than all prior barriers (trough to peak) (26). Because this condition is a difficult one, most folding intermediates are not seen, and elements that appear to form simultaneously, such as hydrogen bonds A and B in Figure 2*b*, may well reflect independent folding steps that are merely kinetically indistinguishable. In testing for the stability of an intermediate (variation of pulse intensity), one appreciates that the population being tested may be spread over more than one structural well.

The search for molecular intermediates is complicated by the ubiquitous presence of population heterogeneity, with independent parallel pathways. Heterogeneity is indicated when less than 100% of a given probe is protected in a given first-order step ($U_1 \rightarrow I_1$ at k_1; $U_2 \rightarrow I_1$ or I_x at k_2; where $k_1 \neq k_2$). In different fractions of the protein population, a given amino acid residue forms hydrogen bonds at different rates. Any subpopulation may then still exhibit two-state folding (as in Figure 2a) or more interesting behavior (as in Figure 2b). In Figure 2c, the system is heterogeneous, but each folding step involves all the NHs ($U_i \rightarrow N$). Intermediates are not visible. In Figure 2d, the earliest step involves all the NHs in 30% of the molecular population and appears concerted. In a kinetically distinct subpopulation (70% of the molecules), the presence of a partially folded intermediate is revealed by the fact that different probes follow a different time course. A sequential pathway can artifactually mimic heterogeneity when protection against labeling is incomplete, either because the labeling pulse is too strong or because a protected state is in rapid equilibrium with an incompletely protected state ("rapid" being relative to the pulse time).

Results Available

RIBONUCLEASE A   Udgaonkar & Baldwin (92, 93) used pH pulse labeling to study refolding of RNase A. This protein has a large β-sheet structure and three short helices (named helix 1, 2, and 3), and is stabilized by four disulfide bonds. In initial experiments (92), these investigators initiated refolding of the denatured, disulfide-intact protein by using a 10-fold dilution from guanidine (D_2O) into D_2O (pD 9, 5°C), and used a long (10-s) labeling pulse (sixfold dilution into H_2O at pH 9). In subsequent experiments (93), the initial dilution was into H_2O (pH 4, 10°C), and a short pulse was used (37 ms, pH 9 and 10, 1.5-fold dilution). The final 2D NMR COSY analysis could follow 27 probe NHs and drew on the completed ^1H NMR assignments of RNase A. This work enhances prior H-T exchange labeling and optical studies that revealed a three-part population heterogeneity, including a fast component ($U_F \rightarrow N$; $\tau = 40$ ms; 20% of the population) and a slow component ($U_SI \rightarrow N$; $\tau = 50$ s; 15% of the population). Both these components appeared to fold to the native state in kinetically two-state reactions. A major component (65%) displayed more kinetic structure, with an early hydrogen-bonded intermediate and a late native-like intermediate ($U_SII \rightarrow I_1 \rightarrow I_N \rightarrow N$).

The pH pulse-labeling studies make the population heterogeneity obvious. The very fast and very slow components are cleanly displayed. The more recent study (93) focuses on the major, multistep path (65% of the population). Two probe residues in helix 1, the N-terminal helix of native RNase, achieve protection against HX labeling in one kinetic step ($\tau = 1$ s). At this same rate, tyrosine absorbance changes signal tertiary structure formation and the development of I_N. The presence of a partially folded molecular intermediate is shown by the fact that other residues, in the extended β-sheet, are protected in a different manner. These NHs fold in two heterogeneous components; 40% of the total population in a faster group ($\tau \approx 20$ ms) and 25% in a slower group with a time constant of ~ 1 s, close to that seen for helix 1 and tertiary structure formation. The behavior of the major 65% phase is similar to that in Figure 2d, except that in RNase A the phase with the common rate is the slower one. These results document a partially folded intermediate (I_1) with the extensive β-sheet structure and perhaps also helices 2 and 3 largely intact, but helix 1, which forms later, is missing at this point.

The stability of the I_1 structure evolves during the 0- to 400-ms time interval. In experiments that varied the intensity of the labeling pulse, a 37-ms pulse was used at pH 9 and pH 10. The β-sheet structure in I_1 is resistant to labeling at pH 9. At pH 10, incomplete protection is seen initially (protection factor $P = 1/K_{op} \approx 250$), but stability increases to full protection ($P > 1000$) over a 400-ms period.

Finally, Udgaonkar & Baldwin (93) systematically tested the stability of structure present at $t_f = 400$ ms by varying the pulse pH from 7.6 to 11. The labeling achieved falls off for all peptide NHs below pH ~ 8.5; the 37-ms pulse becomes too weak to label fully all the free NHs, as expected. At pH above 10, some already structured sites start to label (probably because of local unfolding); others do not, indicating the considerable overall stability ($P > 10^4$) of the intermediate structure present ($I_1 + I_N$).

CYTOCHROME c Roder et al (81) used pH pulse labeling to study refolding of cytochrome c. Folding was initiated by dilution from guanidine (D_2O) into H_2O at pH 6 and 10°C. A 50-ms labeling pulse was used at pH 9 (small dilution). The 2D NMR COSY analysis followed 35 peptide NHs.

An early phase in cytochrome c refolding, within the ~ 3-ms dead time of the mixing apparatus, involves ~ 20% of every NH, indicating rapid folding of this component to a near-native state. At longer times, one sees several heterogeneous subfractions. Sites in the N-terminal and C-terminal helices simultaneously gain protection in three parallel steps with time scales of about 20 ms (40%), 400 ms (20%), and 4 s (20%). Similar time constants are seen for the decrease in fluorescence of the single tryptophan (Trp59), which is quenched in the native protein by proximity to the heme. Population heterogeneity is also seen for sites in the 60s helix, the short 70s helix, and the centrally buried indole NH. These sites become protected, perhaps in a concerted manner, in at least two different phases (~ 80 ms and 4 s). The behavior is like that in Figure 2d, but with more steps.

These results show that an early molecular intermediate occurs in which the N- and C-terminal helices are largely formed before much of the rest of the structure (40% of the population, ~ 20 ms). In the native protein, these helices interact. Thus, the early intermediate may well be native-like and rate-limited by the effective docking of the two nascent helices. This situation, in which concerted formation of the terminal helices is followed in time by the 60s and 70s helices and the Trp59 tertiary probe, seems to repeat at longer times, but these events are difficult to disentangle. The pulse intensity used in these experiments indicates that the early folding intermediate has an equilibrium stability constant greater than 50.

BARNASE   Bycroft et al (8) used two-stage rapid mixing with a long (~ 10 s) pH labeling pulse to study the refolding of barnase (pD 8.5, 25°C) after dilution from guanidine. Of the 29 peptide NHs slow enough to be measured at the trapping and NMR conditions used, 25 are in secondary structural elements (helix, sheet, turn) and 4 represent tertiary interactions. The formation of tertiary packing was also monitored using the change in fluorescence of three tryptophan residues. The results exhibit both population heterogeneity and a molecular intermediate, but the simplicity of the patterns found allow these to be rather fully described.

A very slow phase ($t_{1/2} = 8.5$ s) that includes 20% of every peptide site was not followed in this work. All the secondary structure probes are protected in two faster phases (as in Figure 2c). The first phase (~ 20–40% of each secondary structural NH) proceeds essentially within the mixing dead time. The second phase (~ 30–60% of each secondary structural NH) shows a rate constant of ~ 10–30 s^{-1}. Impressively, all four tertiary NH probes and also one residue in a reverse turn achieve protection at a common, somewhat slower rate, ~ 5 s^{-1}. This rate is closely equal to that for regaining the tryptophan fluorescence amplitude. (This description omits some interesting details.)

The first, very fast phase has two possible interpretations. Bycroft et al suggest that the fast phase involves the whole population (excluding the very slow fraction) in a relatively unstable folded intermediate, in (rapid) equilibrium with the unfolded state, so that peptide NH sites become partially labeled. In the second phase, stable helices and sheets are formed from this complex. Alternatively, according to the diagnostic criteria described before, the first and the second phases may represent independent fractions of a twofold heterogeneous molecular population (as in Figure 2c). These alternatives might be distinguished by varying the pulse intensity via pH, and observing the effect on the apparent size of the fast phase. Whether or not some tertiary bonds also form in the very fast phase seems ambiguous.

In any case, clearly the more or less complete secondary structure of barnase forms in a concerted way, while tertiary interactions follow in a slower phase. (In the view favored by Bycroft et al, the unstable fast form represents an additional intermediate.) The overall secondary structure-tertiary structure comparison resembles Figure 2*b*. A transient molecular intermediate is indicated in which almost all the secondary structural hydrogen bonds are intact, but tertiary hydrogen bonds are largely absent. The large-scale intermediate seen in RNase A seems similar though less complete. These intermediates seem to be kinetic analogs of the equilibrium form (39) seen in acid cytochrome *c* at low salt concentration (secondary structure intact, tertiary bonds broken), and perhaps, more generally, are analogs of molten globules.

Summary

HX-labeling experiments in the pH-pulse mode show that protein folding can be remarkably fast. A near-native form can be reached within milliseconds. Experimental analysis of the folding process on the millisecond-to-second time scale depends upon the presence of kinetic barriers that avoid apparent two-step folding. A common barrier produces molecular intermediates; disparate barriers produce population heterogeneity that makes analysis more difficult. Results available exhibit an early, native-like two-helix intermediate in cytochrome *c*, an extensive, native-like, *β*-sheet-plus-helix intermediate in RNase A, and a late native-like molten globular intermediate in barnase. These differences appear to reflect chance differences in the placement of the determining kinetic barriers. Requirements for observing kinetic folding intermediates are difficult to satisfy, so most intermediates are not seen, and intermediates that are seen often represent the sum of multiple preceding steps.

POSTSCRIPT

This review discusses the current status of hydrogen-exchange labeling approaches and their utility for studying protein forms that are less than fully native. The chemical and physical bases of these approaches are rather well understood. The HX techniques and the high resolution 2D NMR analysis required for this work are now routine. We have considered how these methods are being used to characterize structure in equilibrium folding intermediates and in kinetic intermediates that must be caught in-flight in refolding experiments.

Perhaps the most suggestive general result of all this work, obtained in both equilibrium and kinetic experiments, is that submolecular, native-like folding intermediates exist and have independent, intrinsic stability. Although the integrated structure of native proteins has been considered to be the irreducible unit of stability, emerging results now suggest that proteins may be composed of simpler, more primitive units. These structural units, perhaps conserved through evolution from primeval protein forms, may provide the essential intermediates in protein folding pathways and the fundamental building blocks of protein structure.

ACKNOWLEDGMENTS

This work was supported in part by NIH research grants DK11295 and GM31847.

Literature Cited

1. Alber, T. 1989. *Annu. Rev. Biochem.* 58: 765–98
2. Allewell, N. M. 1983. *J. Biochem. Biophys. Methods* 7: 345–57
3. Barksdale, A. D., Rosenberg, A. 1982. *Methods Biochem. Anal.* 28: 1–113
4. Baum, J., Dobson, C. M., Evans, P. A., Hanley, C. 1989. *Biochemistry* 28: 7–13
5. Brems, D. N., Baldwin, R. L. 1984. *J. Mol. Biol.* 180: 1141–56
6. Breslow, E. 1991. *Chemtracts Biochem. Mol. Biol.* 2: 34–38
7. Bryan, W. D. 1970. *Recent Prog. Surf. Sci.* 3: 101–20
8. Bycroft, M., Matouschek, A., Kellis, J. T., Serrano, L., Fersht, A. R. 1990. *Nature* 346: 488–90
9. Calhoun, D. B., Englander, S. W. 1985. *Biochemistry* 24: 2095–2100
10. Creighton, T. 1990. *Biochem. J.* 270: 1–16
11. Creighton, T. E. 1978. *Prog. Biophys. Mol. Biol.* 33: 231–97
12. Creighton, T. E. 1991. *Current Opinion Struc. Biol.* 1: 5–16
13. DeGrado, W. F. 1988. *Adv. Protein Chem.* 39: 51–124
14. Dill, K. A. 1985. *Biochemistry* 24: 1501–9
15. Dill, K. A., Shortle, D. 1991. *Annu. Rev. Biochem.* 60: 795–825
16. Dobson, C. M. 1991. *Curr. Opin. Struct. Biol.* 1: 22–27
17. Dolgikh, D. A., Gilmanshin, R. I., Brazhnikov, E. V., Bychkova, V. E., Semisotnov, G. V., et al. 1981. *FEBS Lett.* 136: 311–15
18. Eigen, M. 1964. *Angew. Chem. Int. Ed. Eng.* 3: 1–19
19. Eigen, M., Kruse, W., Maas, G., DeMaeyer, L. 1964. In *Progress in Reaction Kinetics*, ed. G. Porter, 2: 286. Oxford: Pergamon
20. Englander, J. J., Calhoun, D. B., Englander, S. W. 1979. *Anal. Biochem.* 92: 517–24
21. Englander, J. J., Rogero, J. R., Englander, S. W. 1985. *Anal. Biochem.* 147: 234–44
22. Englander, S. W. 1975. *Ann. N. Y. Acad. Sci.* 244: 10–27
23. Englander, S. W., Calhoun, D. B., Englander, J. J., Kallenbach, N. R., Liem, R. K. H., et al. 1980. *Biophys. J.* 32: 577–90
24. Englander, S. W., Englander, J. J. 1983. In *Structure and Dynamics: Nucleic Acids and Proteins*, ed. E. Clementi, R. H. Sarma, pp. 421–34. Guilderland, NY: Adenine
25. Englander, S. W., Kallenbach, N. R. 1984. *Q. Rev. Biophys.* 16: 521–655
26. Englander, S. W., Milne, J. 1992. In *Protein Structure and Function*, ed. Z. H. Zaidi. Karachi/New York: Twel. In press
27. Englander, S. W., Poulsen, A. 1969. *Biopolymers* 7: 329–39
28. Englander, S. W., Staley, R. 1969. *J. Mol. Biol.* 45: 277–95
29. Epstein, C. J., Goldberger, R. F., Anfinsen, C. B. 1963. *Cold Spring Harbor Symp. Quant. Biol.* 27: 439–49
30. Ernst, R. R., Bodenhausen, G., Wokaun, A. 1986. *Principles of Nuclear Magnetic Resonance in One and Two Dimensions.* Oxford: Clarendon
31. Fink, A. L., Calciano, L. G., Goto, Y., Palleros, D. R. 1990. In *Current Research in Protein Chemistry: Techniques, Structure, and Function*, ed. J. J. Villafranca, pp. 417–24. New York: Academic
32. Goldenberg, D. P. 1988. *Annu. Rev. Biophys. Biophys. Chem.* 17: 481–507
33. Goto, Y., Calciano, L. J., Fink, A. L. 1990. *Proc. Natl. Acad. Sci. USA* 87: 573–77

34. Hughson, F. M., Wright, P. E., Baldwin, R. L. 1990. *Science* 249: 1544–48
35. Hvidt, A., Nielsen, S. O. 1966. *Adv. Protein Chem.* 21: 287–386
36. Jaenicke, R. 1991. *Biochemistry* 30: 3147–61
37. Janin, J. 1991. *Curr. Opin. Struct. Biol.* 1: 42–44
38. Jeng, M.-F., Englander, S. W., Elove, G. A., Wand, A. J., Roder, H. 1990. *Biochemistry* 29: 10433–37
39. Jeng, M.-F., Englander, S. W. 1991. *J. Mol. Biol.* 221: 1045–61
40. Kim, P. S. 1986. *Methods Enzymol.* 131: 136–56
41. Kim, P. S., Baldwin, R. L. 1980. *Biochemistry* 19: 6124–29
42. Kim, P. S., Baldwin, R. L. 1982. *Biochemistry* 21: 1–5
43. Kim, P. S., Baldwin, R. L. 1990. *Annu. Rev. Biochem.* 59: 631–66
44. King, J. 1989. *Chem. Eng. News* 67: 32–54
45. Klotz, I. M., Frank, B. H. 1965. *J. Am. Chem. Soc.* 87: 2721–28
46. Kuwajima, K. 1989. *Proteins* 6: 87–103
47. Kuwajima, K., Baldwin, R. L. 1983. *J. Mol. Biol.* 169: 299–324
48. Kuwajima, K., Kim, P. S., Baldwin, R. L. 1983. *Biopolymers* 22: 59–67
49. Labhardt, A. M., Baldwin, R. L. 1979. *J. Mol. Biol.* 135: 231–44
50. Leichtling, B. H., Klotz, I. M. 1966. *Biochemistry* 12: 4026–37
51. Levinthal, C. 1968. *J. Chem. Phys.* 65: 44–45
52. Loftus, D., Gbenle, G. O., Kim, P. S., Baldwin, R. L. 1986. *Biochemistry* 25: 1428–36
53. Louie, G., Thao, T., Englander, J. J., Englander, S. W. 1988. *J. Mol. Biol.* 201: 755–64
54. Louie, G., Englander, J. J., Englander, S. W. 1988. *J. Mol. Biol.* 201: 765–72
55. Lumry, R., Rosenberg, A. 1975. *Colloq. Int. C. N. R. S. Eau Syst. Biol.* 246: 55–63
56. Mallikarachchi, D., Burz, D. S., Allewell, N. M. 1989. *Biochemistry* 28: 5386–91
57. Matoushek, A., Kellis, J. T., Serrano, L., Bycroft, M., Fersht, A. R. 1990. *Nature* 346: 440–45
58. Matthews, B. W. 1991. *Curr. Opin. Struct. Biol.* 1: 17–21
59. Matthews, C. R. 1991. *Curr. Opin. Struct. Biol.* 1: 28–35
60. McKinnie, R. E., Englander, J. J., Englander, S. W. 1991. *J. Chem. Phys.* In press
61. McPhie, P. 1982. *Biochemistry* 21: 5509–15
62. Molday, R. S., Englander, S. W., Kallen,

63. Montelione, G. T., Scheraga, H. A. 1989. *Acc. Chem. Res.* 22: 70–76
64. Nakanishi, M., Nakamura, H., Hirakawa, A. Y., Tsuboi, M., Nagamura, T., Saijo, Y. 1978. *J. Am. Chem. Soc.* 100: 272–76
65. Nakanishi, M., Tsuboi, M., Ikegami, A. 1973. *J. Mol. Biol.* 75: 673–82
66. Nall, B. T. 1990. In *Protein Folding: Deciphering the Second Half of the Genetic Code*, ed. L. M. Gierasch, J. King, pp. 188–207. Washington: Am. Assoc. Adv. Sci.
67. O'Neil, J. D. J., Sykes, B. D. 1989. *Biochemistry* 28: 6736–45
68. Oas, T. G., Kim, P. S. 1988. *Nature* 336: 42–48
69. Ohgushi, M., Wada, A. 1983. *FEBS Lett.* 164: 21–24
70. Perrin, C. L., Lollo, C. P. 1984. *J. Am. Chem. Soc.* 106: 2754–57
71. Privalov, P. L. 1989. *Annu. Rev. Biophys. Biophys. Chem.* 18: 47–69
72. Privalov, P. L. 1990. *Crit. Rev. Biochem.* 25: 281–305
73. Privalov, P. L., Gill, S. J. 1988. *Adv. Protein Chem.* 39: 191–234
74. Ptitsyn, O. B. 1987. *J. Protein Chem.* 6: 272–93
75. Ptitsyn, O. B., Pain, R. H., Semisotnov, G. V., Zerovnik, E., Razgulyaev, O. I. 1990. *FEBS Lett.* 262: 20–24
76. Richards, F. M. 1979. *Carlsberg Res. Commun.* 44: 47–63
77. Richards, F. M. 1991. *Sci. Am.* 264: 54–63
78. Richardson, J. S., Richardson, D. C. 1989. *Trends Biochem. Sci.* 14: 304–9
79. Robertson, A. D., Baldwin, R. L. 1991. *Biochemistry* 30: 9907–14
80. Roder, H. 1989. *Methods Enzymol.* 176: 446–73
81. Roder, H., Elöve, G. A., Englander, S. W. 1988. *Nature* 335: 700–4
82. Roder, H., Wagner, G., Wüthrich, K. 1985. *Biochemistry* 24: 7396–7407
83. Roder, H., Wüthrich, K. 1986. *Proteins* 1: 34–42
84. Rosa, J. J., Richards, F. M. 1979. *J. Mol. Biol.* 133: 399–416
85. Schellman, J. A. 1987. *Annu. Rev. Biophys. Biophys. Chem.* 16: 115–37
86. Schmid, F. X. 1991. *Curr. Opin. Struct. Biol.* 1: 36–41
87. Schmid, F. X., Baldwin, R. L. 1979. *J. Mol. Biol.* 135: 199–215
88. Segal, D. M., Harrington, W. F. 1967. *Biochemistry* 6: 768–87
89. Sharp, K. A., Honig, B. 1990. *Annu. Rev. Biophys. Biophys. Chem.* 19: 301–32
90. Shortle, D. 1989. *J. Biol. Chem.* 264: 5315–18

91. Tanford, C. 1968. *Adv. Protein Chem.* 23: 122–282
92. Udgaonkar, J. B., Baldwin, R. L. 1988. *Nature* 335: 694–99
93. Udgaonkar, J. B., Baldwin, R. L. 1990. *Proc. Natl. Acad. Sci. USA* 87: 8197–8201
94. Waelder, S. F., Redfield, A. G. 1977. *Biopolymers* 16: 623–29
95. Wagner, G., Wüthrich, K. 1982. *J. Mol.* *Biol.* 160: 343–61
96. Wand, A. J., Roder, H., Englander, S. W. 1986. *Biochemistry* 25: 1107–14
97. Woodward, C. K., Hilton, B. D. 1979. *Annu. Rev. Biophys. Bioeng.* 8: 99–127
98. Woodward, C. K., Simon, I., Tuchsen, E. 1982. *Mol. Cell. Biochem.* 48: 135–60
99. Wüthrich, K. 1986. *NMR of Proteins and Nucleic Acids.* New York: Wiley

Annu. Rev. Biophys. Biomol. Struct. 1992. 21:267–92

THE PERMEATION PATHWAY OF NEUROTRANSMITTER-GATED ION CHANNELS

Henry A. Lester

Division of Biology, California Institute of Technology, Pasadena, California 91125

KEY WORDS: synapse, nicotinic acetylcholine receptor, neurotransmitter receptor, open-channel blockers, site-directed mutagenesis

CONTENTS

PERSPECTIVES AND OVERVIEW

The group of neurotransmitter-gated ion channels includes (*a*) cation channels gated by acetylcholine (ACh), glutamate, ATP, and serotonin and (*b*) anion channels gated by GABA, glycine, ACh (invertebrates), and histamine (invertebrates). I doubt that more than one or two additional neurotransmitters will be found that directly gate ion channels, although

267

1056–8700/92/0610–0267$02.00

additional receptor subtypes gated by the above known transmitters are often discovered. The same neurotransmitters also activate, with quite different kinetics and pharmacology, a distinct class of receptors that have seven transmembrane helices and in turn activate G proteins; this chapter does not treat the seven-helix receptor family. Ligand-dependent ion channels are presently thought to perform several distinct functions: (a) ligand binding; (b) gating, the conformational transitions that open and close the channel; (c) desensitization; and (d) permeation. This chapter focuses on permeation and is motivated by much recent data from site-directed mutagenesis and peptide chemistry showing that permeation occurs in regions of the protein that are at least partially distinct from those subserving the other three functions. My attempt at a unified treatment is of course based on the structural similarity suggested by recent cDNA sequencing and protein chemical data for neurotransmitter-gated channels; these similarities suggest that this group represents a superfamily (see e.g. 22, 145). Many incisive previous reviews have treated channels gated by neurotransmitters and by intracellular ligands (18, 22, 55, 60, 97, 125, 145, 154).

Most ligand-dependent cation channels are less selective than voltage-dependent cation channels. Ligand-gated anion channels are rather nonselective as well—indeed, GABA and glycine channels show a measurable permeability for cations (122). As is also true for the voltage-gated channels, no studies report pharmacological or genetic manipulations that grossly affect the selectivity of ligand-gated channels, e.g. that change cation to anion channels. Such manipulations, when successfully performed and interpreted, will represent a triumph of the site-directed mutagenesis approach. Mutations that produce subtle changes in acetylcholine receptor selectivity have, however, recently been studied (29, 30, 81, 152).

Transmembrane Topology and Primacy of the M2 Region

The adult muscle ACh receptor is a pseudosymmetric pentamer with subunit composition $\alpha_2\beta\gamma\delta$. Other members of the neurotransmitter-gated receptor superfamily are probably pentamers as well (10a). Each subunit has at least four putative membrane-spanning regions (M1 through M4). This chapter reviews the evidence that the M2 region (Figure 1) lines at least part of the conduction pathway. Certain contrary facts are also cited below and must be explained. An elegant recent review provides hypothetical diagrams of the M2 region at atomic resolution for the ACh channel and homologous regions for GABA and glycine channels (145). In the view Figure 1C presents of the ACh receptor in its open conformation, the five M2 α-helices line the conducting pore like sheaves of wheat, slightly askew to create a point of closest approach. At the extracellular vestibule, some fixed charges affect ion flux. The open-channel blocker,

QX-222, penetrates from the external solution partially into the tapering channel, so that its nonpolar aromatic moiety and its polar charged moiety interact most strongly with residues at position 10' and 6', respectively. Permeant ions also interact with residues at position 6'. The taper of the channel prevents QX-222 from reaching the next turn, at position 2'. Here and at the next turn—position −1'—the channel is narrowest, and amino-acid side chains interact most strongly with permeant ions. As ions continue to flow inward, they experience a broadening channel, but conductance can still be affected by residues at position −4'.

Classes of Molecular Manipulation

The rapid progress of recent years derives directly from four new classes of molecular manipulation: (a) DNA sequencing and site-directed mutagenesis, (b) protein sequencing, (c) patch-clamp measurements of channel conductance, and (d) patch-clamp measurements of single channels during local anesthetic molecule block. This chapter shows how these experiments are used to test the postulated structures and mechanisms, particularly for the ACh receptor. It also provides a comparative view of the complementary information from other neurotransmitter-gated ion channels.

Practical Relevance

Biophysical and structural analysis of the permeation pathway may lead to knowledge that is useful in neurobiological or clinical contexts. Rectification in the current-voltage relation of neurotransmitter receptors might influence encoding properties of neurons (92). The flux of Ca^{2+} through neuronal ACh channels might influence many processes ranging from transmitter release to gene activation (reviewed in 38). At N-methyl-D-aspartate (NMDA) receptors, Ca^{2+} influx might underlie some forms of memory and learning (79) as well as ischemic damage (28).

CLASSES OF MEASUREMENT

This section describes the conclusions that can be drawn from several classes of experiments on neurotransmitter-gated channels. The organization follows a recent chapter describing permeation through voltage-gated channels (90). The reader should consult that chapter and the book by Hille (62) for the theoretical basis of the electrophysiological experiments.

Reversal Potentials

The measurement of reversal potentials is a null technique that gives a single value; it has wide application because it is sensitive to neither block nor saturation in the channel. For instance, macroscopic reversal potential measurements are possible under conditions in which single-channel cur-

A

		-4'				-1'			2'				6'			9'	10'								20'
ACh	α1	D	S	G		E	K	M	T	L	S	I	S	V	L	L	S	L	T	V	F	L	L	V	I	V	E
	β	D	A	G		E	K	M	G	L	S	I	F	A	L	L	T	L	T	V	F	L	L	L	L	A	D
	γ	K	A	G	G	Q	K	C	T	V	A	T	N	V	L	L	A	Q	T	V	F	L	F	L	V	A	K
	δ	D	C	G		E	K	T	S	V	A	I	S	V	L	L	A	Q	S	V	F	L	L	L	I	S	K
	α7	D	S	G		E	K	I	S	L	G	I	T	V	L	L	S	L	T	V	F	M	L	L	V	A	E
5HT3		D	S	G		E	R	V	S	F	K	I	T	L	L	L	G	Y	S	V	F	L	I	I	V	S	D
GABA	α	E	S	V	P	A	R	T	V	F	G	V	T	T	V	L	T	M	T	T	L	S	I	S	A	R	N
GLY		D	A	A	P	A	R	V	G	L	G	I	Y	T	V	L	Y	M	T	T	Q	S	S	G	S	R	A
GluR1		D	Q	S	N	E		F	G	I	F	N	S	L	W	F	S	L	G	A	F	Q	Q	G	C		D

B

COND	X	X	X	X		X
SEL		X	X			X
QX				X	X	
NCI		X		X	X	

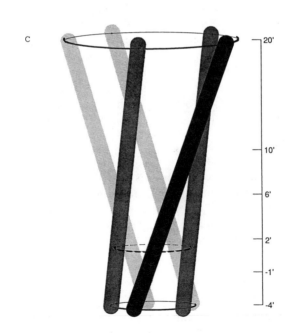

C

rents are too small to be measured (29, 30). For ligand-gated channels in particular, permeabilities measured by reversal potentials decrease monotonically with hydrated radius or other measures of molecular size (6, 42); therefore the narrowest region of the channel is usually identified with the highest energy barrier that an ion must traverse in crossing the membrane.

Because several previous studies of ACh receptors suggested that single-channel conductance was most strongly affected by mutations at the 2' or the −1' position (26, 71), these positions seemed likely candidates for the narrowest region of the channel. It also seemed most promising to examine effects of mutations on the relative permeability P_{Tris}/P_{Na}, as Tris is a slightly permeant ion. Several mutations at the 2' position, but not at the 6', 10', nor 14' positions, did in fact render Tris relatively less permeant than in the wild-type receptor, without appreciable changes in the permeability to Na^+ (29, 30). The total range of manipulations in these experiments was roughly threefold, from $P_{Tris}/P_{Na} = 0.36$ to 0.11. Thus, the 2' position is apparently near the narrowest region of the channel. A surprising result was the ratio of 0.36 for wild-type mouse ACh channels, compared with the ratio of 0.18 obtained for the frog muscle channels (6, 42). Yet Cohen et al (29) measured P_{Tris}/P_{Na} for the wild-type *Torpedo californica* ACh channel in the oocyte system and obtained 0.22, close to the value for frog; thus among wild-type ACh channels, this parameter displays differences that cannot be explained by the M2 sequence alone. The amino acids at the −1' position were not systematically mutated by Cohen et al (29); however, the single mutation reported, δE-1'Q, decreased P_{Tris}/P_{Na} nearly threefold. Interestingly, the mouse $\alpha\beta\gamma$ receptor (obtained by omitting δ-subunit mRNA from the injection mixture), but not the $\alpha\beta\delta$

Figure 1   The M2 region of neurotransmitter-gated channels. (*A*) Aligned sequences in the M2 region of the mouse muscle α, β, γ, and δ subunits, the chick neuronal $\alpha7$ subunit [which forms homooligomeric channels (33)], a $5HT_3$ receptor (105a), α subunits from the GABA and glycine receptors, and the GluR1 kainate/AMPA receptor (the latter sequence is the least similar in the group and the alignment is therefore tentative). Underlining shows a periodicity of 3.5, which would align the residues in a stripe along one face of the helix. Underlining agrees well with the location of boxed residues, or their homologs in the *T. californica* receptor, which have been localized to the conduction pathway by types of experiments shown in *B*. (*B*) Abbreviations are: COND, conductance; SEL, selectivity; QX, QX-222 blockade; NCI, noncompetitive inhibitor binding. (*C*) Schematic diagram of the region surrounding the permeation pathway. The five rods each represent an α-helix that extends from position −4' to 20'. The distance from the center of each helix to the center of the channel is arbitrarily set to 5 Å at position 1' (*dotted circle*). Each helix is tilted 20° in a plane tangent to the circumference at this point, yielding a taper in both directions away from position 1'. Assuming 3.6 residues/turn and 5.4 Å/turn, the diagram shows that position 20' is 26.8 Å away axially from the narrowest region and has a diameter of 10.9 Å; position −4' is 7.5 Å away and has a radius of 5.5 Å. The vertical scale at right shows positions discussed above (*A*) and in the text.

receptor, was characterized by a very low P_{Tris}/P_{Na} ratio (29, 30). Other work suggests that the omitted γ or δ subunit is replaced by the δ or γ subunit, respectively (P. Charnet, C. Labarca & H. A. Lester, submitted). Because the γ subunit has a Gln residue at the $-1'$ position, the $\alpha\beta\gamma$ receptor is like the δE-1'Q mutation at the $-1'$ position; the result is thus consistent with the large effect the $-1'$ position has on selectivity.

The mutations generated by Imoto et al (69) (described in detail below) were later subjected to reversal potential analyses that clearly showed the primacy of the $-1'$ position versus the $-4'$ and $20'$ positions (81). The δE-1'Q mutation changed the P_{Cs}/P_K ratio to 0.77 from the wild-type value of 1.10; smaller changes also occurred in the P_{Na}/P_K ratio. On the other hand, at the $-4'$ and the $20'$ positions, four charge changes were required to affect the P_{Na}/P_K ratio.

CALCIUM PERMEABILITY   Table 1 summarizes some studies that determine the Ca^{2+} permeability of neurotransmitter-gated channels, mostly on the basis of reversal potential measurements. A useful generalization is that there appear to be three classes of Ca^{2+} permeabilities: (a) undetectably low, (b) comparable to that for Na^+, and (c) much higher than Na^+ (the last class includes NMDA receptors only). Friel & Bean (50) have presented a lucid discussion of the possible artifacts in measuring Ca^{2+} permeability of channels gated by extracellular ATP, which would be expected to chelate Ca^{2+}. Although non-NMDA glutamate receptors are often considered impermeable to Ca^{2+}, the recent study by Hollmann et al (63) should be consulted for literature references to previous studies of non-NMDA receptors that reported Ca^{2+}-permeable non-NMDA responses in neurons.

Table 1 Measured Ca^{2+} permeabilities for some neurotransmitter-gated channels

Agonist	Tissue/source	P_{Ca}/P_{Na}	G_{Ca}/G_{Na}	Reference
ACh	Muscle/electroplaque	0.6–1.0	0.4–0.6	38, 85, 95
ACh	Muscle	0.2		6
ACh	Neuronal	0.93	∼0.5	47
ACh	*Aplysia* neurons		0.13	14
Kainate/AMPA	GluR2+GluR1 or GluR2+GluR3	N.D.[a]	N.D.[a]	63
Kainate/AMPA	GluR1+GluR3 or GluR1 or GluR3	∼1[b]	0.3–0.7	63
NMDA	Mouse neurons	7.5–10.6		12, 112
ATP	Smooth muscle	∼3		20
5-HT	NG108-15 cells	<0.076		156

[a] Not detectable.
[b] Calculated from the data in Ref. 63 by Dr. B. N. Cohen, assuming $P_K/P_{Na} = 1$.

STREAMING POTENTIALS   Dani (36) has measured changes in reversal potential of ACh channels during exposure to osmotic pressure gradients. The results are interpreted in terms of the number of water molecules associated with a single permeant cation and, in turn, reveal the length of the narrowest region of the channel (90). This length is rather small—3–6 Å—in agreement with other measurements that show a highly localized selectivity filter.

Current-Voltage Relations

Single-channel measurements are the preferred method for determining current-voltage relations for open channels; however, in some cases, the venerable technique of voltage-jump relaxations, which yield instantaneous current-voltage relations, has been useful (1, 118, 137). In general, neurotransmitter-gated cation channels are thought to involve fewer binding sites, ionic interactions within the channel, and deviations from independence than do the more highly selective voltage-gated channels. For both ACh and NMDA channels (12), conductances have a Q_{10} of 1.5 to 1.6, as though they were determined by free diffusion. However, when conductances for monovalent metal ions are studied in detail for ACh channels, their sequences are different from free-solution mobilities or hydrated radii, which correlate well with permeability relations. Instead, conductances peak for K^+ and decline for Rb^+ and Cs^+ (81, 133, 152). Therefore the channel is more complex than a simple water-filled pore.

An early paper on ACh noise analysis established that the extrajunctional receptors of embryonic and denervated muscle have roughly 2/3 the conductance of the adult, junctional form (119), in addition to a roughly threefold-greater channel duration. When Mishina et al (114) discovered that these differences were explained by the substitution of the ε for the γ subunit in bovine muscle, researchers hoped that chimeric ε/γ subunits would allow investigators to pinpoint the amino acid residues responsible for the difference. However, it proved simpler to exploit the differences between the conductances conferred by the bovine and T. californica δ subunits, which are more homologous to each other than are the ε and γ subunits. Thus, chimeric bovine/T. californica δ subunits helped to localize one determinant to a region including the M2 segment and of the adjoining putative extracellular region (70). Investigators began site-directed mutagenesis studies in this region, motivated by (a) the chimera results, (b) the region's highly conserved nature (Figure 1A), and (c) emerging data on covalent labeling by channel blockers in this region.

RINGS OF CHARGE FLANK THE M2 REGION   Imoto et al (69) undertook mutagenesis of conserved acidic residues flanking M2, partially based on the following rationale. When permeant cation concentrations are decreased at ACh channels, the conductance decreases more slowly than predicted by a model in which saturation at a given site governs conductance (37). Also, conductances are reduced by low concentrations of divalent cations. The most straightforward explanation for these effects, which also occur at voltage-gated Na^+ channels, is the presence of net negative charge that brackets the pore.

In important experiments that localized at least part of this charge, Imoto et al (69) made single-channel recordings of ACh receptors mutated at positions $-4'$, $-1'$, $0'$, $20'$, $21'$, and $23'$ and expressed in various hybrid combinations in *Xenopus laevis* oocytes. The strongest effects on conductance were obtained at position $-1'$, with weaker effects at positions $-4'$ and $20'$. At each of these positions, many residues have acidic side chains (Figure 1A). Results may be summarized as follows. 1. When negative charges were removed at positions $-4'$ and $20'$, the current-voltage relations displayed decreased conductance and increased rectification consistent with the appearance of a new energy barrier near the internal or external surface (positions $-4'$ and $20'$, respectively). Such a barrier could consist of a narrow region, a change in dipole moment, or a change in charge—anything that makes ions pause as they move through the channel (90). The rate of change was such that neutralizing one charge decreased the conductance by roughly 15% of the wild-type conductance; effects twice this size were observed for negative-to-positive mutations or for mutations in the α subunit, which is present in two copies. The αE20'K or αE20'R mutations were equivalent to four changes in charge and reduced the conductance to about half the wild-type value. 2. At position $-1'$, conductance changes were larger, with a 50% decrease in conductance upon removal of a single negative charge in the α, β, and δ subunits. The increased rectification was roughly as strong as for mutations at position $-4'$, suggesting that positions $-4'$ and $-1'$ are electrically close to each other. However, the γQ-1'K mutation produced an even greater 75% decrease in conductance and little rectification. Thus, the residue at position $-1'$ in the γ subunit occupies a special position. In a further study with these same mutations, some of these effects were much more prominent for Cs^+ and Rb^+ than for the smaller ions, particularly at the δ subunit: for the wild-type channel, the Cs^+ conductance is greater than the K^+ conductance, but this order is reversed for δE-1'Q. Thus, these mutations actually change the selectivity of the channel (81). More recent data show that the anomalous effects of γ subunit mutations are produced by the additional amino acid residue between positions $-1'$ and $-2'$ (S. Numa, personal communication). 3. Single-channel rectification caused by intracellular and extracellular Mg^{2+} was reduced by removal of negative charges at positions $-4'$ and $20'$, respectively.

The concept of charged rings that control cation current through the channel has some predictive value. 1. Anion-permeable ligand-gated channels lack the rings at the crucial position $-1'$, although they contain charged rings of the same sign as the ACh channel at positions $-4'$ and, for the $\beta2$ subunit of the GABA receptor, at position $20'$. The ring at position $24'$ is negatively charged in some ACh receptor subunits and positively charged in all known anionic channels. The positively charged ring at $0'$, which does not affect ACh channel conductance, has the same sign in anion channels. 2. Different single-channel conductances of mouse-*T. californica* ACh receptor hybrids are consistent with differences in the rings at position $-4'$ (γ subunit) and $20'$ (γ and δ subunits) (157), as is the difference between the $\alpha\beta\gamma\delta$ and $\alpha\beta\epsilon\delta$ receptors (69). 3. To establish the stoichiometry of the chick neuronal $\alpha4/n\alpha1$ hybrid receptor (the rat equivalent would be called $\alpha4\beta2$), Cooper et al (32) made mutations at residue $20'$. The mutated subunits, $\alpha4E20'K$ and $n\alpha1K20'E$, conferred the expected decreases and increases, respectively, on the single-channel conductances at high negative potentials (32). Coexpression of the normal and mutated subunits produced distinctive populations of receptors with distinct conductances between the values for the normal and mutated receptors. The number of intermediate conductances was consistent with a complex containing two $\alpha4$ and three $n\alpha1$ subunits, as might be expected on other grounds (10a, 97). 4. For the muscle receptor lacking a γ subunit, Charnet et al deduced that the pentameric complex contains an additional δ subunit, on the basis of the single-channel conductance and the charges in the rings (P. Charnet, C. Labarca & H. A. Lester, submitted). 5. An Arg residue in kainate/α-amino-3-hydroxy-5-methyl-4-isoxasole propionate (AMPA) receptors—near the putative external face of the channel—produces a rectification that decreases inward currents (150) and completely blocks Ca^{2+} permeation (67). In Figure 1A, this residue is in M2 at position $15'$; in other alignments, it is in the extracellular region between M2 and M3.

POLAR GROUPS LINE THE CHANNEL BETWEEN THE CHARGED RINGS   While the Gottingen-Kyoto collaborators investigated the charged rings at both ends of the M2 helices (69), the Caltech group independently investigated the role played by the several rings of polar but uncharged residues within the M2 helices themselves (88). Positions $2'$, $6'$, and $10'$ are especially rich in Ser (and a few Thr) residues, and mutation of these residues produces more dramatic effects as one moves inward ($10'$ to $2'$), presumably because of the taper. Although removal of just one of these residues at positions $10'$ and $6'$ dramatically affected open-channel blocker binding (see below), removal of up to three residues at position $10'$ failed to affect current-voltage relations at all (26). At position $6'$, a clear inward rectification occurred when three Ser residues (two on α, one on δ) were mutated to Ala (88).

At position 2', current-voltage relations are also sensitive to mutations, as first shown by Charnet et al (26). Significantly, many more mutations at position 2' than at 6' or 10' failed to express (26, 29), possibly because no current could flow at all (although neither antibody labeling nor α-bungarotoxin binding were done to confirm the expression of unresponsive receptors). Outward currents were, however, clearly decreased in the δS2'A and $\alpha_{T2'A}\beta_{G2'S}$ mutant hybrids, consistent with the idea that position 2' is a narrow region of the channel near the cytoplasmic surface. Villarroel et al (152) extended these observations for the rat muscle ACh channel as follows. The αThr2' residue was mutated to Val, Ala, and Gly. The channel conductance decreased with side-chain volume for the larger permeant ions, such as Rb^+ and Cs^+, but not for the smaller Na^+ nor for NH_4^+, which has special hydrogen-bonding properties. It was concluded that larger ions such as Cs^+ experience friction with the side chain at position 2' that may limit ion conduction.

CHARGE IN THE VESTIBULE AND ON THE MEMBRANE SURFACE   Although some of the excess net negative charge bracketing the ACh channel pore is at positions $-4'$ and 20', some investigators have called attention to a possible role played by charges in the presumed extracellular amino-terminus of the channel, where at least 200 amino-acid residues are localized (and many more in the case of kainate/AMPA receptors) (36). The vestibule extends some 50 Å above the membrane surface and tapers from a diameter of 70–80 Å down to <20 Å at the membrane surface (145, 147). The cation-selective ACh channels have an excess negative charge of approximately -50 on the amino acid residues in this region; the charge is roughly equal and opposite for the anion-selective channels of GABA and glycine receptors (reviewed in 145). Clearly, conductance values for receptors mutated at some or all of these residues would be interesting. Surface-charge effects play a measurable but small role in ion permeation at neurotransmitter-gated channels (16, 95).

MULTIPLE CONDUCTANCE STATES   Nearly every neurotransmitter-gated channel has multiple conductance states. What do these states tell us about the structure of the permeation pathway? One class of multiple states are presumably caused by distinct subunit compositions; where such cases have been analyzed, they reinforce present concepts about the control of channel conductance by rings of charge (32, 84, 151; P. Charnet, C. Labarca & H. A. Lester, submitted).

In recordings that reveal interconversion among subconductance states during a single opening, different subunit compositions cannot be invoked and one must instead consider conformational changes in the conduction pathway (34, 61, 71). For substates created by D-tubocurarine blockade, we can conclude that the vestibule of the channel is so large that a D-tubocurarine molecule can occupy it and partially occlude current flow (146). For the present, however, subconductance states give no specific information about the structure of the open channel.

In a recent study on the $\alpha 7$ neuronal ACh homooligomeric channel, the L9'T mutation produced an additional single-channel conductance level, possibly corresponding to a desensitized state that does not conduct at all in the wild-type receptor (129a). The new state has several interesting properties. Further study of this and similar mutations may show how the M2 region can rearrange to produce multiple conductance states.

Anomalous Mole-Fraction Effects

Anomalous mole-fraction effects are generally thought to reflect the presence of more than one binding site within a channel (reviewed recently in 90). No reports clearly indicate such effects for cationic channels gated by neurotransmitters, but the anion channels gated by GABA and by glycine clearly exhibit an anomalous mole-fraction effect for mixtures of Cl^- and SCN^- (23). A tentative explanation for this difference between cationic and anionic channels is that the known anionic channels have a longer Ser- and Thr-rich stretch within the M2 region; such residues occupy perhaps five adjacent turns of the postulated α-helix, versus roughly three for the known cation channels (Figure 1). Thus, the anion channels could have room for additional binding sites. The GABA and glycine-gated channels show remarkable similarities with regard to mole-fraction effects, selectivity, sequences, and conductance sequences. Indeed, in both cases, the conductance sequences are the inverse of the permeability sequences from reversal potential measurements, again suggesting the presence of binding sites within the channel (23).

GABA and glycine channels, like many nominal anion-selective channels, have a measurable cation permeability (122). Perhaps the cation permeability arises because the hydroxyl side chains that line the pore resemble those of cation channels.

Blockade Within the Channel by Organic Ions and Local Anesthetics

DEVELOPMENT OF THE OPEN-CHANNEL BLOCKADE CONCEPT   Local anesthetics in clinical use are tertiary amines and can permeate membranes in their uncharged form; in their charged form, they primarily block voltage-gated Na^+ channels from the cytoplasmic surface. However, procaine and its quaternary ammonium analogs constitute major tools in the mapping of neurotransmitter-gated channels as well. The first series of studies on ionophoretic application of blocking drugs noted that brief (~ 20 ms) pulses of procaine blocked ACh responses and that the blockade disappeared much more rapidly than did that of D-tubocurarine (40). The brief action can now be understood by the fact that procaine has a lower affinity for closed channels than does D-tubocurarine and would therefore not be subject to buffering of diffusion (11).

During the 1960s, Armstrong and his colleagues developed the concepts of voltage-dependent open-channel blockade by quaternary ammonium ions and their derivatives at voltage-dependent K^+ channels. Interestingly, in some of the earliest voltage-clamp experiments on endplate currents (e.p.c.s), procaine had voltage-dependent effects on endplate current waveforms (54). A hypothesis proposed that Na^+ and K^+ passed through distinct channels, both controlled by the agonist, and that procaine selectively blocked the Na^+ channels. This explanation became untenable with the demonstrations that (*a*) a wide spectrum of waveform changes were produced by various procaine and lidocaine derivatives; (*b*) some derivatives produced a small tail of endplate current that far outlasted the original current; and (*c*) the noise variance vanished at the reversal potential (19, 39, 82, 103, 143, 144). Instead, A. B. Steinbach presciently proposed that the blocking drugs were binding to the receptor after the agonist bound and activated it, to produce a state of lower conductance but longer lifetime (144). One important aspect of this scheme is that the binding of the blocker proceeds with kinetics similar to those of channel gating—a situation that has provided experimental, analytic, and computational challenges for a generation of membrane biophysicists. Steinbach also introduced the quaternary ammonium lidocaine derivatives, QX-222 and QX-314 (which we simply term QX), as suitable reagents for such studies. One advantage of these reagents is that they do not permeate membranes; they act only on the external surface of the receptor (64). Because the blockers share several structural features with ACh, Steinbach also suggested that they bound at the agonist site (143); this latter hypothesis is probably not true.

In 1975, Adams (2) brilliantly united the Armstrong and Steinbach views with the following model:

> ... part of the procaine molecule (presumably the cationic head) can transiently bind to and block open but not closed endplate channels. The early component of the procaine e. p. c. tail therefore represents channels either being blocked, or closing in the normal manner. The later component arises because as the open but blocked channels progressively unblock (procaine dissociating) they are left in the open state, and only close again at the normal rate. Also, they may again be blocked by procaine before closing has occurred.... Since the postulated binding is within the channel and is partly cou-

lombic, the binding rate constants will be voltage-dependent [155]. The model therefore agrees that the procaine e. p. c. will be affected by membrane potential, in a manner that agrees with experiment....

The proposed kinetic scheme is thus (see also Figure 2),

$$\text{closed} \underset{\alpha}{\overset{\beta}{\rightleftharpoons}} \text{open} \underset{F}{\overset{G\,[Q]}{\rightleftharpoons}} \text{open} \cdot \text{blocked}$$

Scheme 1

In Scheme 1 and subsequent schemes, α and β are composite rate constants for channel opening, incorporating both agonist binding and conformational changes; and G and F are the forward and reverse binding rates for the blocker. Adams calculated 10^7 M^{-1} s^{-1} and 300 s^{-1}, respectively, for procaine (corresponding to a dissociation constant of 30 μM for the open state), but pointed out that these parameters depend on the membrane potential (Figure 2). Essentially all aspects of Scheme 1 have been verified in subsequent studies, except that procaine itself may also act by binding to closed states of the channel (4). Therefore, many subsequent investigators have employed QX-222, which binds only to the open state of the channel under the appropriate conditions. Clearly, many organic cations can block open ACh channels; the list includes (a) most agonists themselves at sufficiently high concentration (8, 106, 141); (b) the classical competitive antagonist, D-tubocurarine (31); (c) arginine, dimethyldiethylammonium, and Tris (134); (d) guanidine derivatives (46); and (e) most known local anesthetics.

During the late 1970s, the open-channel blockade model was investigated with the appropriate electrophysiological techniques as they were developed. Neurally evoked endplate currents and spontaneous miniature endplate currents, in the presence of these drugs, decayed with at least two exponential components, including one faster and one slower than the single component in the absence of drug (9, 10, 19, 131, 132). Noise analysis in the presence of local anesthetics or QX revealed two components, with corner frequencies higher and lower than the single control value (15, 76, 131, 132). Voltage-jump relaxations with procaine and QX again showed two exponential components with time constants that flanked the normal values (4, 15, 80, 107). In double-pulse ionophoretic experiments, the use dependence was as expected if the block affected open channels and was slowly reversible (3, 7, 77). A light-activated open-channel blocker rapidly terminated postsynaptic currents and blocked steady-state currents even though it was created after the channels opened (93). The amplitudes and rates of these kinetic components depended on blocker concentration in a manner consistent, for the most part, with the open-channel blockade model (reviewed in 5); but the generation of biophysicists who received

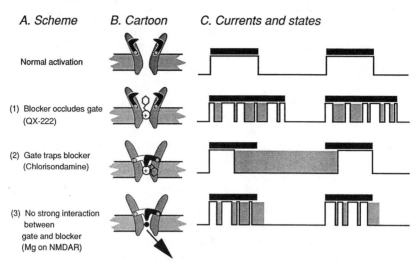

Figure 2 The varieties of open-channel block. (*A*) Short descriptions of the three schemes presented more fully in the text, with examples in parentheses. (*B*) Cartoons showing how the blocker and the gates might interact. The blockers do not accurately portray real molecules but merely show a general charged moiety and a general aromatic moiety for Schemes 1 and 2 and a simple ion (such as Mg^{2+}) for Scheme 3. (*C*) Idealized single-channel current traces are shown for normal activation and for cases where the channel is blocked roughly half the time in each scheme. The upward deflections denote current flow. The shaded areas denote periods when the blocker is bound. The channel is assumed to have two gates, which must both be open. The heavy bars above the traces denote the open state. In all cases, a bound blocker prevents current flow. In Scheme 1, the bound blocker occludes the closing of the gates. In Scheme 2, the closed gates trap the blocker in the channel; soon after the gates reopen, the blocker leaves and current then flows. Scheme 3 resembles Scheme 1 while the gates are open, but unlike in Scheme 1, the gate can close on the blocker. Unlike Scheme 2, Scheme 3 allows the blocker to leave the channel while the gates are closed.

their training with these painstaking analyses understood that the resolution of the experiments did not allow decisive answers to certain questions: (*a*) Does channel conductance fall to zero when the blocker is bound? (*b*) Can the channel close when the blocker is bound?

Scheme 1, in conjunction with single-channel measurements, allows the investigator to do physical chemistry at the level of individual ligand-receptor interactions. Therefore, open-channel blockade by QX was chosen as the topic for the first detailed study using single-channel recording (120), even before the gigaohm seal was discovered. The records showed: (*a*) that QX-222 modified a single opening to provide a burst of briefer openings that alternated with interruptions of current flow; (*b*) that during these interruptions less than 5% of the normal current flowed (and perhaps no current at all); (*c*) that the brief openings became briefer and the bursts longer at higher [QX-222]; (*d*) that these kinetic changes were greater at more negative potentials. All these findings are predicted by the open-channel blockade scheme if the channel cannot close when the blocker is bound. With QX-314, the data were consistent with previous suggestions that the blocked state lasts much longer than for QX-222. After the discovery of the gigaohm seal, Neher (117) repeated some of these measurements at higher resolution and refined the upper limit for the conductance of the blocked state to less than 1/144 that of the open state. He also found evidence for two departures from the simple sequential model for [QX-222] > 40 μM. First, the blocked state displayed a double exponential distribution of lifetimes, and second, the time integral of the openings decreased to less than the control value. Apparently, the channel can close on the bound QX-222 molecule, perhaps by the trapping effect described below.

SITE-DIRECTED MUTAGENESIS OF THE QX-222 BINDING SITE   In the mid-1980s, site-directed mutagenesis and oocyte expression became the appropriate techniques for investigating the interaction between open-channel blockers, exemplified by QX-222, and the receptor channel. Researchers hoped that the specificity of site-directed mutagenesis would complement the molecular precision of the single-channel measurements on open-channel blockade. To identify promising residues for mutagenesis, the Caltech group noted the body of literature on noncompetitive inhibitors at ACh channels. When we began the site-directed mutagenesis experiments in 1987, position 6′ was the appropriate first choice, as outlined in the next major section.

Mutant subunits of the mouse muscle ACh receptor (α, β, γ, δ) at positions 2′, 6′, and 10′ were expressed in oocytes and assessed for their ability to change the binding kinetics of QX-222 (26, 88). F and G (Scheme 1) were measured directly from single-channel measurements (120), and the equilibrium dissociation constant $K_Q = F/G$ was measured with an independent set of electrophysiological experiments on macroscopic voltage-jump relaxations (4). Although the voltage-clamp circuit could not resolve the fast macroscopic inverse relaxation (4) associated with the direct QX-222-receptor interaction, it was possible to study the slow relaxation component whose time constant τ_Q is given by $\tau_Q = \tau(1+[\text{QX-222}]/K_Q)$. The results showed that (a) substitution of Ala for Ser residues at position 6′ increased K_Q at a rate of 30–50% per substitution; (b) Ser or Thr to Ala substitutions at position 10′ had roughly equal but opposite effects; (c) the effects on QX-222 binding were minimal for mutations at position 2′, although many of the mutant hybrids failed to express; (d) the substitutions affected K_Q by changing F only—there were no major effects on the forward binding rate G; (e) none of the mutations changed the voltage sensitivity of binding, implying that the binding site for QX-222 remains at a position that senses 65–75% of the electrical distance across the membrane. It was concluded that the aromatic, hydrophobic moiety of the QX-222 molecule interacts with the side chains at position 10′, and that the charged quaternary ammonium moiety interacts preferentially with the side chains at position 6′.

The concept that an open-channel blocker interacts with adjacent α-helical turns, which are 5.4 Å apart, explains previous observations that many local anesthetics and related molecules possess aromatic and amino moieties separated by this approximate distance (26). The channel lumen at positions 10′ and 6′ seem best described as annuli whose properties are averaged from those of individual side chains. The lack of effects at position 2′ probably arises because the channel's taper prevents the blocking drug from penetrating to this point.

OTHER ASPECTS OF QX-222 ACTION   The QX-222 results paint a self-consistent picture of blocker-channel interactions, but many questions remain. How would binding be affected by groups other than Ser, Thr, or Ala? Do positions other than 2′, 6′, or 10′ play a role in binding? Recently, it was found that the L9′T mutation produces a special conductance state that is insensitive to QX-222 (129a). Another recent study shows that the forward binding rate for channel block by ACh itself depends much less on temperature than do other kinetic processes (140). This observation agrees with many previous suggestions that forward binding is diffusion-limited for open-channel blockers. Is the forward binding rate nonetheless sensitive to the groups near the mouth of the channel, such as positions 14′, 16′, or 20′? There is no systematic study on whether the blocker can be knocked off the channel by permeant ions. Such effects have been observed for many channel blockers at voltage-dependent channels and would yield an interesting picture of ion-channel-blocker interactions.

OPEN-CHANNEL BLOCKADE AT NEURONAL AChR CHANNELS   Neuronal acetylcholine receptors (AChR) with cation channels share some sequence homology with muscle receptors, particularly in the M2 region; yet the pharmacology of open-channel blockade displays some differences in detail with the muscle receptor. Recent studies show that the precise pharmacology of neuronal receptor hybrids varies with the particular α and β subunit, possibly because of differences in channel blockade (102). The best-studied open-channel blocker at neuronal ACh channels is hexamethonium (13, 21, 25, 58, 127), a compound that shows little or no open-channel blockade at muscle receptors and acts instead as a rapidly equilibrating competitive antagonist (128, 129). (On the other hand, QX-222 blocks the α4β2 neuronal receptor at least an order of magnitude more poorly than it does the muscle receptor.) The forward binding rate for hexamethonium at neuronal receptors varies among receptor subtypes but is in the range of $10^7 \text{ M}^{-1}\text{ s}^{-1}$ (25, 127) and increases with hyperpolarization at a rate of e-fold per 56 mV (127), like the equivalent parameter for open-channel blockers at muscle receptors. The exact electrical position of the binding site must be determined from the voltage dependence of the equilibrium binding affinity; this is unknown because the trapping phenomenon described next vitiates measurements of the voltage dependence of the dissociation rate.

TRAPPING IN ACh CHANNELS   Hexamethonium seems to remain bound to neuronal ACh channels for a longer time than the average channel duration. The estimate for F from Scheme 1 is about 4 s^{-1}, yielding $F/G = 0.4\ \mu\text{M}$ (25). However, there is a qualitative departure from Scheme 1 because the ACh channel can close on hexamethonium, trapping it for several seconds (Figure 2) (58). Similar phenomena occur for chlorisondamine and several other channel blockers at ACh channels in crustacean and frog muscle (98, 99, 116).

$$\text{closed} \underset{\alpha}{\overset{\beta}{\rightleftharpoons}} \text{open} \underset{F}{\overset{G\,[Q]}{\rightleftharpoons}} \text{open} \cdot \text{blocked} \underset{\beta'}{\overset{\alpha'}{\rightleftharpoons}} \begin{array}{c}\text{closed} \cdot \text{blocked} \\ \text{(trapped)}\end{array}$$

Scheme 2

If repetitive pulses of agonist are applied, trapping produces a use-dependent blockade, as also seen for blockers trapped by the inactivation gate at voltage-dependent channels (62). When agonist is reapplied and the channel reopens, the blocker can leave the channel, particularly at depolarized voltages where the blocker's affinity is reduced. Although α' and β', the rate constants for closing and opening of the blocked channels, are nonzero in contrast to Scheme 1, it is not known whether these parameters equal those for the unblocked channels α and β. Although Lingle (99) found no evidence for trapping of QX-222, Neher (117) found that the muscle receptor can close on QX-222 under some conditions. Site-directed mutagenesis experiments might aid in defining the mechanism of location of trapping at neuronal ACh channels.

NMDA CHANNEL BLOCKERS   Several classes of molecules, including phencyclidine/ketamine and analogs, benzomorphan (σ) opiates, bicyclic amines such as MK-801, and diarylguanidines (78) are noncompetitive NMDA receptor antagonists. In direct binding experiments, these drugs share a common site on the receptor, distinct from the agonist site but enhanced by agonist binding (reviewed in 154; see also section on noncompetitive inhibitors). Additionally, their binding is competitive with that of Mg^{2+}, which also binds within the channel (66). In general, these compounds exert voltage- and use-dependent block, as though they interact most strongly with the open channel and allow the receptor to trap them. The forward binding rate G for the open channel is $\sim 3 \times 10^7$ M^{-1} s^{-1}—very close to that for QX at the muscle ACh channel, and the lifetime $1/F$ is on the order of seconds—like that for QX-314 at the ACh channel (66, 78). Depolarization in the presence of the agonist drives the blockers off the channels (49, 66), recapitulating (from my cholinocentric viewpoint) trapping experiments for hexamethonium and chlorisondamine at ACh channels.

Considering the similarities with channel-blocker actions that occur at the ACh channel, one of the many MK-801 (87) or diarylguanidine (78) derivatives will probably be used to map out the conduction pathway now that NMDA receptors have been cloned and expressed and can be subjected to site-directed mutagenesis experiments (115a). Choline is another good candidate for a pure open-channel blocker, but it blocks with such low affinity that the kinetics would not be resolvable (12). One should also evaluate whether the many blockers of epithelial Cl^- channels include a suitable probe for GABA or glycine channels.

Covalent Labeling by Channel Blockers

Many investigations have shown that acetylcholine receptors can be blocked by a wide variety of drugs that do not bind directly at the ligand site; these drugs are generally termed noncompetitive inhibitors (NCIs). An open-channel blocker is one type of NCI. ACh receptors exist in several affinity states for agonists, and some noncompetitive inhibitors favor a transition to one of these high-affinity states in membrane fragments or receptors purified from *T. californica* electric organ (55, 75, 145). Undoubtedly, some of these high-affinity states are desensitized and therefore not of direct interest for ion channel permeation. However, according to Scheme 1, open-channel blockers increase the time that the agonist is bound to the receptor without changing the forward binding rates for the agonist; therefore, such blockers also increase the affinity of the agonist (83). When primary amino acid sequences were determined from cDNA cloning during the early 1980s, it became important to identify the particular residue(s) labeled by a covalently bound NCI.

Therefore, several diligent groups developed criteria for proof that a noncompetitive inhibitor is an open-channel blocker: (*a*) The binding should depend on the activation by ligand. This analysis requires time-resolved measurements, often using light-activated covalent ligands, in which the NCI binding site is revealed within a few milliseconds after agonist application and follows the approximate dose-response relation for activation. In particular, investigators wished to distinguish this concentration and time dependence from the much slower desensitization process that appears at lower agonist concentration. (*b*) The labeling should be blocked by known open-channel blockers. (*c*) For charged NCIs such as QX, binding should depend on voltage in the expected fashion. Usually this criterion cannot be tested decisively in studies on membrane fragments. Also in electrical measurements, several uncharged blockers fulfill most criteria for open-channel blockade. Molecules in this class include some barbiturates (3), benzocaine (80, 123), and at concentrations <300 nM, chlorpromazine (24). Their forward binding rates G are typically 3- to 10-fold smaller than for the QX compounds, as though the uncharged blockers are not accelerated by the membrane field.

Several groups have identified binding sites for noncompetitive inhibitors. [^{3}H]Chlorpromazine labels γThr2′, αSer6′, βSer6′, γSer6′, δSer6′, βLeu9′, and γLeu9′; criteria *b* and probably *c* are established, but some questions surround criterion *a* (56, 57, 130). [^{3}H]Triphenylmethylphosphonium labels αSer6′, βSer6′, and δSer6′; again criteria *b* and probably *c* are established, but *a* was not established.

Recently, several other amino-acid residues were identified as covalently labeled by NCIs. [^{3}H]Quinacrine azide meets all three criteria (41). Although the precise site has not been determined, the labeled residue is on the α subunit of *T. californica*, in a peptide fragment corresponding to amino acid residues 208–243. This fragment contains the M1 helix but not the M2 helix. Karlin (75) has presented arguments that the quinacrine azide molecule is too small to span the distance from the M1 region to the binding sites at position 6′ found by other investigators; instead, he suggests that there are two distinct open-channel blocker sites. In another study (126), [^{3}H]meproadifen mustard, a cationic open-channel blocker, labeled *T. californica* αGlu20′ (residue #262), which is presumably at the extracellular end of M2 and 2.1 nm from position 6′ (the probe itself is at most only 1.4 nm long). Of the three criteria, *a* is problematic, although the agonist dose dependence is more appropriate to activation than to desensitization; *b* is established, and *c* is not established (104).

Blockade Within the Channel by Inorganic Ions

Many studies show that Ca^{2+} interferes with monovalent cation flux through ACh and NMDA channels. However, Mg^{2+}, Co^{2+}, Mn^{2+}, and Ni^{2+} occupy a special position in ion channel biophysics because their water substitution rates are 10^3 to 10^4 times slower than those for other common ions (62); as a possible result, these cations block many types of ion channels. Mg^{2+} in particular has been studied in detail as an open-channel blocker and seems to play this role at NMDA and other neurotransmitter-gated channels.

RECTIFICATION AT NEURONAL AChR CHANNELS   In many [but not all (100, 142)] neurons and in *Electrophorus electricus* electroplaques, macroscopic ACh-induced currents display pronounced inward rectification (21, 25, 68, 91, 108, 135); instantaneous current-voltage relations show the same direction of rectification, suggesting that rectification arises at least partially from single-channel conductance rather than from gating (25, 68, 91, 108). The effect persists when the receptors are expressed in oocytes (21, 25). Ifune & Steinbach (68) studied PC-12 cells and found that single channels passed reduced outward current if Mg^{2+} bathed the internal surface, but without Mg^{2+}, these channels displayed linear current-voltage relations. In rat sympathetic neurons, Mathie et al (108) also found that internal Mg^{2+} blocks single channels, as though the binding site is 76% of the electrical distance toward the external surface of the membrane. Because of this voltage dependence, the internal Mg^{2+} site is probably not at position $-4'$, where mutations modify Mg^{2+} blockade of muscle receptors (69). Perhaps the site is at position $20'$. The relief of blockade at more positive potentials suggests that the blocking ion can permeate through the channel as well: the barrier on the cytoplasmic side of the binding site is not infinitely high. In retrospective support of Mg^{2+} blockade, *E. electricus* electroplaques displayed the strongest rectification under conditions that allowed influx of divalent cations (89).

Careful analysis suggests that macroscopic rectification of the ACh-induced currents is not fully explained by rectification at the single-channel level; presumably gating also contributes (68, 108, 136).

Mg^{2+} BLOCKADE OF NMDA RECEPTOR CHANNELS   Early investigations on NMDA receptors demonstrated a voltage-dependent block by extracellular Mg^{2+} and related ions (17, 109–111, 121) and showed that Scheme 1 cannot describe the blockade because bursts do not become longer at higher [Mg^{2+}]. Most available data suggest that the channel can close on the bound Mg^{2+} ion but cannot trap it; perhaps the bound Mg^{2+} ion can dissociate to the intracellular surface (see Figure 2).

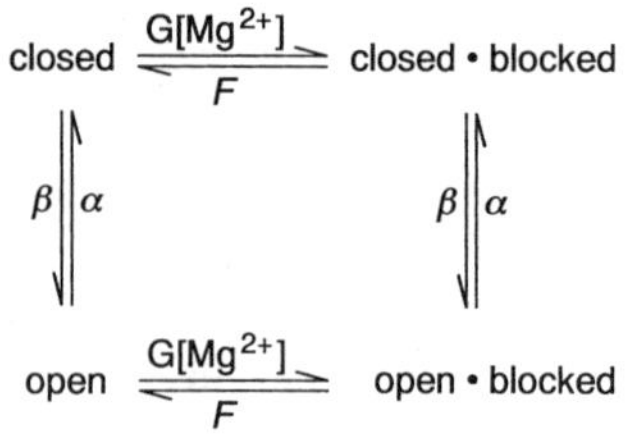

$$\text{closed} \underset{F}{\overset{G[Mg^{2+}]}{\rightleftharpoons}} \text{closed} \cdot \text{blocked}$$

$$\beta \Updownarrow \alpha \qquad\qquad\qquad \beta \Updownarrow \alpha$$

$$\text{open} \underset{F}{\overset{G[Mg^{2+}]}{\rightleftharpoons}} \text{open} \cdot \text{blocked}$$

Scheme 3

For simplicity, we have omitted a second blocked state that depends neither on Mg^{2+} nor on other ions present in the test solutions (72, 73).

Within the framework of Scheme 3, the forward binding rate G for Mg^{2+} block is $\sim 10^6 \, M^{-1} \, s^{-1}$ and increases e-fold for 17–21 mV at more negative potentials (16, 72, 73). Mg^{2+} remains bound for a fraction of a millisecond at 0 mV $(1/F)$ and longer at more negative potentials, at a rate of e-fold for 47–50 mV (16, 72, 73). The combined voltage dependences correspond to a binding site at an electrical distance about 80% of the way through the membrane. Thus, the Mg^{2+} binding site in the NMDA channel is at roughly the same electrical distance as the QX binding site in the nicotinic receptor, but binding proceeds roughly 10-fold more slowly. Agreement with this model over several orders of magnitude in $[Mg^{2+}]$ assures that Mg^{2+} blocks directly by binding within the channel, rather than indirectly by inducing a conformational change that would block the channel (73).

In another similarity with ACh channels, Mg^{2+} also blocks NMDA channels from the internal surface (74, 121). Is the site the same as that reached by external Mg^{2+}? The answer is not straightforward. Because the off rate F for the two blocked states differed substantially, Johnson & Ascher (74) argued that they were distinct. However, for the site accessed by internal Mg^{2+}, the voltage dependence of the blocking rates gave blockade at $\sim 35\%$ of the electrical distance across the membrane, which actually locates this site external to the blocking site accessed by external Mg^{2+}. This discrepancy was explained by suggesting that multiple ion occupancy within the channel distorted the measurements, tending to enhance the voltage sensitivities obtained. Thus the external and internal sites would be $< 80\%$ and $< 35\%$ of the way from the external and internal surfaces, respectively.

STRUCTURAL STUDIES OF ION BINDING   X-ray scattering using five-wavelength anomalous dispersion shows that a few Tb(III) ions bind to the *T. californica* ACh receptor in a region within the bilayer. These binding sites have been interpreted as lying within the pore itself and would therefore be useful in mapping the structure of the M2 region (45).

Peptide Channel Models

Artificial peptides that are Ser- or Thr-rich, like the M2 region, form channels in lipid bilayers (86). A 23-mer beginning at position $-5'$ of the *T. californica* M2δ sequence forms channels with conductance near that of ACh receptors (124). In later work, tethered tetramers synthesized with M2 peptides attached to a carrier template showed ACh receptor-like conductance, Ca^{2+} selectivity, and blockade by QX-222 (115). Furthermore, the S6′A substitution decreased the single-channel conductance, in a manner similar to that for mouse ACh receptor channels (88). The M1 peptides did not form detectable channels. Artificial peptide channels thus continue to serve as powerful alternative systems for studying permeation pathways.

Does the Conduction Pathway Move in Gating?

Our ignorance about the nature of gating transitions stands in sharp contrast to the evidence reviewed above about the localization of the permeation pathway. During normal synaptic transmission, most ligand-gated channels open within a few microseconds after binding agonist (94) and remain open for milliseconds. Events are probably a bit slower at NMDA channels. However, gating events in the most general sense— current fluctuations, openings, and closings of neurotransmitter-gated channels—occur over a time scale of microseconds to tens of seconds. A pertinent question is whether any of these events involve changes in the shape of the conduction pathway itself. More specifically, do the M2 regions change shape or move relative to each other (148)? We simply do not know the answers to these questions. The fastest events, termed open-channel noise, do not seem correlated with normal gating (138, 139).

There are now hints of a structural basis for the slowest events, such as desensitization. A desensitized state may involve altered interactions between the γ and δ subunits (149). Binding of ^{125}I TID is also altered for the γ subunit during desensitization (113, 153), again suggesting a structural change. Agonist-sensitive photolabeling by the same compound occurs in the β and δ M2 regions (153a). Mutations of a highly conserved Leu residue at position 9' in the homopentameric α7 neuronal ACh channel render the desensitized state conducting, suggesting that the M2 region is indeed involved in the structural transition(s) of desensitization (129a).

Perhaps tilting or sliding of the M2 region underlies agonist-triggered channel opening as well (148). This idea gains some support from site-directed mutagenesis. For instance, the βF6'S mutation changes single-channel duration by several fold (88); the same is true for mutations in a Cys residue in the M1 region that, in the standard models, might contact M2 roughly at its midpoint (101).

For a working hypothesis about agonist-triggered gating, however, we should also consider the ball-and-chain models now being worked out for voltage-gated channel inactivation in several laboratories. Such mechanisms reject concerted transitions in the channel protein as a whole and invoke motions of specific domains that physically occlude the conduction pathway at one end. For voltage-gated channels, the inactivation flap is at the cytoplasmic surface; for neurotransmitter-gated channels, I would postulate that it is part of the large extracellular amino-terminal region of the protein.

THEORETICAL APPROACHES

Structural data on neurotransmitter-gated channels are presently limited in resolution to $\sim$20 Å. However, the detailed interactions that govern permeation probably require description with a resolution of ~ 1 Å. To obtain further insights, investigators have modeled the permeation pathway (open channel) at several levels. (*a*) Many workers construct barrier and binding-site models to explain their current-voltage data. One or two binding sites, flanked by two or three barriers, are invoked for cation channels (43, 81, 95, 96, 105). Complex phenomena such as anomalous mole-fraction effects in anion channels require at least two binding sites flanked by three barriers (23). (*b*) Some models include explicit formulations for charge densities at the vestibule (35, 37, 81). (*c*) Selectivity sequences are interpreted in terms of the energies for dehydration and coulombic interaction, using Eisenman's models (62). (*d*) Structural hypotheses about the conformation of the M2 region at the atomic level attempt to provide qualitative explanations for experimental data (51, 65). Earlier hypotheses (48, 59) featured the charged amphipathic MA regions, now thought to be intracellular. (*e*) Some structural models have also served as the basis for simulations of free energy experienced by probe ions as they move through the channel (44, 52, 53).

CONCLUSIONS

We cannot yet resolve the passage of single ions through neurotransmitter-gated channels. Nonetheless, many detailed mechanistic conclusions have been generated by the combined electrophysiological, molecular biological, biochemical, and pharmacological approaches outlined in this chapter. Over the next few years, much excitement will surround two fronts. First, concepts generated for ACh receptor channels will be tested and modified as appropriate for other neurotransmitter receptors as well as for channels gated by intracellular ligands. Second, these ideas will also be tested with data on three-dimensional structures at atomic resolution.

ACKNOWLEDGMENTS

I thank B. Cohen for help with Figure 1 and Table 1, M. King for help with the manuscript, and C. Jahr, N. Lim, N. McCarty, and D. Vaughn for many helpful comments. N. Davidson has been my partner on all recent studies and continues his vital contributions. Preparation of this review was supported by grants from the Muscular Dystrophy Association, the California Tobacco-Related Disease Research Program, and the National Institutes of Health (NS-11756).

Literature Cited

1. Adams, P. R. 1975. *Br. J. Pharmacol.* 53: 308
2. Adams, P. R. 1975. *J. Physiol.* 246: 61
3. Adams, P. R. 1976. *J. Physiol.* 260: 531
4. Adams, P. R. 1977. *J. Physiol.* 268: 291
5. Adams, P. R. 1981. *J. Membr. Biol.* 58: 161

290   LESTER

6. Adams, D. J., Dwyer, T. M., Hille, B. 1980. *J. Gen. Physiol.* 75: 493
7. Adams, P. R., Feltz, A. 1980. *J. Physiol.* 306: 283
8. Adams, P. R., Sakmann, B. 1978. *Proc. Natl. Acad. Sci. USA* 8: 2994
9. Adler, M., Albuquerque, E. X., Lebeda, F. J. 1978. *Mol. Pharmacol.* 14: 514
10. Adler, M., Oliviera, A. C., Albuquerque, E. X., Mansour, N. A., Eldefrawi, A. T. 1979. *J. Gen. Physiol.* 74: 129
10a. Anand, R., Conroy, W. G., Schoepfer, R., Whiting, P., Lindstrom, J. 1991. *J. Biol. Chem.* 266: 11192
11. Armstrong, D., Lester, H. A. 1979. *J. Physiol.* 294: 365
12. Ascher, P., Bregestovski, P., Nowak, L. 1988. *J. Physiol.* 399: 207
13. Ascher, P., Large, W. A., Rang, H. P. 1979. *J. Physiol.* 295: 139
14. Ascher, P., Marty, A., Neild, T. O. 1978. *J. Physiol.* 278: 177
15. Ascher, P., Marty, A., Neild, T. O. 1978. *J. Physiol.* 278: 207
16. Ascher, P., Nowak, L. 1988. *J. Physiol.* 399: 247
17. Ault, B., Evans, R. H., Francis, A. A., Oakes, D. J., Watkins, J. C. 1980. *J. Physiol.* 307: 413
18. Barnard, E. A., Henley, J. M. 1990. *Trends Neurosci.* 11: 500
19. Beam, K. G. 1976. *J. Physiol.* 258: 301
20. Benham, C. D., Tsien, R. W. 1987. *Nature* 328: 275
21. Bertrand, D., Ballivet, M., Rungger, D. 1990. *Proc. Natl. Acad. Sci. USA* 87: 1993
22. Betz, H. 1990. *Biochem.* 29: 3591
23. Bormann, J., Hamill, O. P., Sakmann, B. 1987. *J. Physiol.* 385: 243
24. Changeux, J.-P., Pinset, C., Ribera, A. B. 1986. *J. Physiol.* 378: 497
25. Charnet, P., Labarca, C., Cohen, B. N., Davidson, N., Lester, H. A., Pilar, G. 1992. *J. Physiol.* In press
26. Charnet, P., Labarca, C., Leonard, R. J., Vogelaar, N. J., Czyzyk, L., et al. 1990. *Neuron* 4: 87
27. Deleted in proof
28. Choi, D. W., Rothman, S. M. 1990. *Annu. Rev. Neurosci.* 13: 171
29. Cohen, B. N., Labarca, C., Czyzyk, L., Davidson, N., Lester, H. A. 1992. *J. Gen. Physiol.* In press
30. Cohen, B. N., Labarca, C., Davidson, N., Lester, H. 1991. *Biophys. J.* 59: 33a
31. Colquhoun, D., Sheridan, R. E. 1982. *Br. J. Pharmacol.* 75: 77
32. Cooper, E., Couturier, S., Ballivet, M. 1991. *Nature* 350: 235
33. Couturier, S., Bertrand, D., Matter, J.-M., Hernandez, M.-C., Bertrand, S., et al. 1990. *Neuron* 5: 847
34. Cull-Candy, S. G., Usowicz, M. M. 1987. *Nature* 325: 525
35. Dani, J. A. 1986. *Biophys. J.* 49: 607
36. Dani, J. A. 1989. *J. Neurosci.* 9: 884
37. Dani, J. A., Eisenman, G. 1987. *J. Gen. Physiol.* 89: 959
38. Decker, E. R., Dani, J. A. 1990. *J. Neurosci.* 10: 3413
39. Deguchi, T., Narahashi, T. 1971. *J. Pharmacol. Exp. Ther.* 176: 423
40. del Castillo, J., Katz, B. 1957. *Proc. R. Soc. London Ser. B* 146: 339
41. DiPaola, M., Kao, P. N., Karlin, A. 1990. *J. Biol. Chem.* 265: 11017
42. Dwyer, T. M., Adams, D. J., Hille, B. 1980. *J. Gen. Physiol.* 75: 469
43. Eisenman, G., Dani, J. A. 1987. *Annu. Rev. Biophys. Biophys. Chem.* 16: 205
44. Eisenman, G., Villarroel, A., Montal, M., Alvarez, O. 1990. *Prog. Cell Res.* 1: 195
45. Fairclough, R. H., Miake-Lye, R. C., Stroud, R. M., Hodgson, K. O., Doniach, S. 1986. *J. Mol. Biol.* 189: 673
46. Farley, J. M., Yeh, J. Z., Watanabe, S., Narahashi, T. 1981. *J. Gen. Physiol.* 77: 273
47. Fieber, L. A., Adams, D. J. 1991. *J. Physiol.* 434: 215
48. Finer-Moore, J., Stroud, R. M. 1984. *Proc. Natl. Acad. Sci. USA* 81: 155
49. Fong, T. M., Davidson, N., Lester, H. A. 1989. *Synapse* 4: 88
50. Friel, D. D., Bean, B. P. 1988. *J. Gen. Physiol.* 91: 1
51. Furois-Corbin, S., Pullman, A. 1989. *Biochim. Biophys. Acta* 984: 339
52. Furois-Corbin, S., Pullman, A. 1989. *FEBS Lett.* 252: 63
53. Furois-Corbin, S., Pullman, A. 1991. *Biophys. Chem.* 39: 153
54. Gage, P. W., Armstrong, C. M. 1968. *Nature* 218: 363
55. Galzi, J. L., Revah, F., Bessis, A., Changeux, J. P. 1991. *Annu. Rev. Pharmacol. Toxicol.* 31: 37
56. Giraudat, J., Dennis, M., Heidmann, T., Chang, J.-Y., Changeux, J.-P. 1986. *Proc. Natl. Acad. Sci. USA* 83: 2719
57. Giraudat, J., Dennis, M., Heidmann, T., Haumont, P., Lederer, F., et al. 1987. *Biochemistry* 26: 2410
58. Gurney, A. M., Rang, H. P. 1984. *Br. J. Pharmacol.* 82: 623
59. Guy, H. R. 1984. *Biophys. J.* 45: 249
60. Guy, H. R., Hucho, F. 1987. *Trends Neurosci.* 10: 318
61. Hamill, O. P., Sakmann, B. 1981. *Nature* 294: 462
62. Hille, B. 1991. *Ionic Channels in Excit-*

able Membranes. Sunderland, MA: Sinauer. 2nd ed. In press
63. Hollmann, M., Hartley, M., Heinemann, S. 1991. Science 252: 851
64. Horn, R., Brodwick, M., Dickey, W. D. 1979. Soc. Neurosci. Abstr. 5: 481
65. Hucho, F., Hilgenfeld, R. 1989. FEBS Lett. 257: 17
66. Huettner, J. E., Bean, B. P. 1988. Proc. Natl. Acad. Sci. USA 85: 1307
67. Hume, R. I., Dingledine, R., Heinemann, S. F. 1991. Science 253: 1028
68. Ifune, C. K., Steinbach, J. H. 1990. Biophys. J. 57: 122a
69. Imoto, K., Busch, C., Sakmann, B., Mishina, M., Konno, T., et al. 1988. Nature 335: 645
70. Imoto, K., Methfessel, C., Sakmann, B., Mishina, M., Mori, Y., et al. 1986. Nature 324: 670
71. Jahr, C. E., Stevens, C. F. 1987. Nature 325: 522
72. Jahr, C. E., Stevens, C. F. 1990. J. Neurosci. 10: 1830
73. Jahr, C. E., Stevens, C. F. 1990. J. Neurosci. 10: 3178
74. Johnson, J. W., Ascher, P. 1990. Biophys. J. 57: 1085
75. Karlin, A. 1991. Harvey Lect. Ser. 85: 71
76. Katz, B., Miledi, R. 1975. J. Physiol. 249: 269
77. Katz, B., Miledi, R. 1978. Proc. R. Soc. London 203: 119
78. Keana, J. F. W., McBurney, R. N., Sherz, M. W., Fischer, J. B., Hamilton, P. N., et al. 1989. Proc. Natl. Acad. Sci. USA 86: 5631
79. Kennedy, M. B. 1989. Trends Neurosci. 12: 417
80. Koblin, D. D., Lester, H. A. 1979. Mol. Pharmacol. 15: 559
81. Konno, T., Busch, C., von Kitzing, E., Imoto, K., Wang, F., et al. 1991. Proc. R. Soc. London Ser. B 244: 69
82. Kordas, M. 1970. J. Physiol. 65: 797
83. Krodel, E. K., Beckman, R. A., Cohen, J. B. 1979. Mol. Pharmacol. 15: 294
84. Kullberg, R., Owens, J. L., Camacho, P., Mandel, G., Brehm, P. 1990. Proc. Natl. Acad. Sci. USA 87: 2067
85. Lassignal, N. L., Martin, A. R. 1976. Science 191: 464
86. Lear, J. D., Wasserman, Z. R., DeGrado, W. F. 1988. Science 240: 1177
87. Leeson, P. D., Carling, R. W., James, K., Smith, J. D., Moore, K. W., et al. 1990. J. Med. Chem. 33: 1296
88. Leonard, R. J., Labarca, C., Charnet, P., Davidson, N., Lester, H. A. 1988. Science 242: 1578
89. Lester, H. A. 1978. J. Gen. Physiol. 72: 847
90. Lester, H. A. 1991. Annu. Rev. Physiol. 53: 477
91. Lester, H. A., Changeux, J. P., Sheridan, R. E. 1975. J. Gen. Physiol. 65: 797
92. Lester, H. A., Koblin, D. D., Sheridan, R. E. 1978. Biophys. J. 21: 181
93. Lester, H. A., Krouse, M. E., Nass, M. M., Wassermann, N. H., Erlanger, B. F. 1979. Nature 280: 509
94. Lester, H. A., Nass, M. M., Krouse, M. E., Nerbonne, J. M., Wassermann, N. H., Erlanger, B. F. 1980. Ann. N. Y. Acad. Sci. 346: 475
95. Lewis, C. A. 1979. J. Physiol. 286: 417
96. Lewis, C. A., Stevens, C. F. 1979. In Membrane Transport Processes, ed. C. F. Stevens, R. W. Tsien, 3: 89. New York: Raven
97. Lindstrom, J., Schoepfer, R., Whiting, P. 1987. Mol. Neurobiol. 1: 281
98. Lingle, C. 1983. J. Physiol. 339: 395
99. Lingle, C. 1983. J. Physiol. 339: 419
100. Lipton, S. A., Aizenman, E., Loring, R. H. 1987. Pflugers Arch. 410: 37
101. Lo, D. C., Pinkham, J. L., Stevens, C. F. 1990. Neuron 6: 31
102. Luetje, C. W., Patrick, J. 1991. J. Neurosci. 11: 837
103. Maeno, T., Edwards, C., Hashimura, S. 1971. J. Neurophysiol. 34: 32
104. Maleque, M. A., Souccar, C., Cohen, J. B., Albuquerque, E. X. 1982. Mol. Pharmacol. 22: 636
105. Marchais, D., Marty, A. 1979. J. Physiol. 297: 9
105a. Maricq, A., Peterson, A. S., Brake, A. J., Myers, R. M., Julius, D. 1991. Science 254: 432
106. Marshall, C. G., Ogden, D., Colquhoun, D. 1991. J. Physiol. 433: 73
107. Marty, A. 1978. J. Physiol. 278: 237
108. Mathie, A., Colquhoun, D., Cull-Candy, S. G. 1990. J. Physiol. 427: 625
109. Mayer, M. L., Westbrook, G. L., Guthrie, P. B. 1984. Nature 361: 261
110. Mayer, M. L., Vyklicky, L. Jr., Westbrook, G. L. 1989. J. Physiol. (London) 415: 329
111. Mayer, M. L., Westbrook, G. L. 1985. J. Physiol. (London) 361: 65
112. Mayer, M. L., Westbrook, G. L. 1987. Prog. Neurobiol. 28: 197
113. McCarthy, M. P., Stroud, R. M. 1989. J. Biol. Chem. 264: 10911
114. Mishina, M., Takai, T., Imoto, K., Noda, M., Takahashi, T., et al. 1986. Nature 321: 406
115. Montal, M., Montal, M. S., Tomich, J. M. 1990. Proc. Natl. Acad. Sci. USA 87: 6929

115a. Moriyoshi, K., Masu, M., Ishii, T., Shigemoto, R., Mizuno, N., Nakanishi, S. 1991. *Nature* 354: 31
116. Neely, A., Lingle, C. J. 1986. *Biophys. J.* 50: 981
117. Neher, E. 1983. *J. Physiol.* 339: 663
118. Neher, E., Sakmann, B. 1975. *Proc. Natl. Acad. Sci. USA* 72: 2140
119. Neher, E., Sakmann, B. 1976. *J. Physiol.* 258: 705
120. Neher, E., Steinbach, J. H. 1978. *J. Physiol.* 277: 153
121. Nowak, L., Bregestovski, P., Ascher, P., Herbet, A., Prochiantz, A. 1984. *Nature* 307: 462
122. Numann, R., Nonner, W. 1990. *Biophys. J.* 57: 124a
123. Ogden, D. C., Siegelbaum, S. A., Colquhoun, D. C. 1981. *Nature* 289: 596
124. Oiki, S., Dahno, W., Madison, V., Montal, M. 1988. *Proc. Natl. Acad. Sci. USA* 85: 8703
125. Olsen, R. W., Tobin, A. J. 1990. *FASEB J.* 4: 1469
126. Pedersen, S. E., Liu, W.-S., Cohen, J. B. 1991. *J. Biol. Chem.* Submitted
127. Rang, H. P. 1982. *Br. J. Pharmacol.* 75: 151
128. Rang H. P., Ritter, M. J. 1971. *Mol. Pharmacol.* 7: 620
129. Rang, H. P., Rylett, R. J. 1984. *Br. J. Pharmacol.* 81: 519
129a. Revah, F., Bertrand, D., Galzi, J.-L., Devillers-Thiéry, A., Mulle, C., et al. 1991. *Nature* 353: 846
130. Revah, F., Galzi, J., Giraudat, J., Haumont, P., Lederer, F., et al. 1990. *Proc. Natl. Acad. Sci. USA* 87: 4675
131. Ruff, R. L. 1977. *J. Physiol.* 264: 89
132. Ruff, R. L. 1982. *Biophys. J.* 37: 625
133. Sakmann, B., Methfessel, C., Mishina, M., Takahashi, T., Takai, T., et al. 1985. *Nature* 318: 538
134. Sanchez, J. A., Dani, J. A., Siemen, D., Hille, B. 1986. *J. Gen. Physiol.* 87: 985
135. Selyanko, A. A., Derkach, V. A., Skok, V. I. 1979. *J. Auton. Nerv. Sys.* 20: 167
136. Selyanko, A. A., Derkach, V. A., Kurennyi, D. E. 1988. *Neurophysics* 20: 122
137. Sheridan, R. E., Lester, H. A. 1975. *Proc. Natl. Acad. Sci. USA* 72: 3496
138. Sigworth, F. J. 1985. *Biophys. J.* 47: 709
139. Sigworth, F. J. 1986. *Biophys. J.* 49: 1041
140. Sine, S. M., Claudio, T., Sigworth, F. J. 1990. *J. Gen. Physiol.* 96: 395
141. Sine, S. M., Steinbach, J. H. 1984. *Biophys. J.* 46: 277
142. Skok, V. I., Selyanko, A. A., Derkach, V. A. 1989. *Neuronal Acetylcholine Receptors.* New York: Consultants Bureau
143. Steinbach, A. B. 1968. *J. Gen. Physiol.* 52: 144
144. Steinbach, A. B. 1968. *J. Gen. Physiol.* 52: 162
145. Stroud, R. M., McCarthy, M. P., Shuster, M. 1990. *Biochemistry* 29: 11009
146. Takeda, K., Trautmann, A. 1984. *J. Physiol.* 349: 353
147. Toyoshima, C., Unwin, N. 1988. *Nature* 336: 247
148. Unwin, N. 1989. *Neuron* 3: 665
149. Unwin, N., Toyoshima, C., Kubalek, E. 1988. *J. Cell Biol.* 107: 1123
150. Verdoorn, T. A., Burnashev, N., Monyer, H., Seeburg, P. H., Sakmann, B. 1991. *Science* 252: 1715
151. Verdoorn, T. A., Fraguhn, A., Ymer, S., Seeburg, P. H., Sakmann, B. 1990. *Neuron* 4: 919
152. Villarroel, A., Herlitze, S., Koenen, M., Sakmann, B. 1991. *Proc. R. Soc. London Ser. B.* 243: 69
153. White, B. H., Cohen, J. B. 1988. *Biochemistry* 27: 8741
153a. White, B. H., Cohen, J. B. 1991. *Soc. Neurosci. Abstr.* 17: 22
154. Wong, E. H. F., Kemp, J. A. 1991. *Annu. Rev. Pharmacol. Toxicol.* 31: 401
155. Woodhull, A. M. 1973. *J. Gen. Physiol.* 61: 687
156. Yakel, J. L., Shao, X. M., Jackson, M. B. 1990. *Brain Res.* 533: 46
157. Yu, L., Leonard, R. J., Davidson, N., Lester, H. A. 1991. *Mol. Brain Res.* 10: 203

Annu. Rev. Biophys. Biomol. Struct. 1992. 21:293–322

PROTEIN FOLDING IN THE CELL:
The Role of Molecular Chaperones Hsp70 and Hsp60

F. U. Hartl and J. Martin

Program of Cellular Biochemistry and Biophysics, Rockefeller Research Laboratory, Sloan-Kettering Institute, 1275 York Avenue, New York, New York 10021

W. Neupert

Institut für Physiologische Chemie, Goethestrasse 33, 8000 München 2, Germany

KEY WORDS: stress proteins, chaperonins, GroE, catalysis of protein folding

CONTENTS

293

1056–8700/92/0610–0293$02.00

PERSPECTIVES AND OVERVIEW

The fundamental discovery that the amino acid sequence of a protein contains the full information specifying its native, three-dimensional conformation marked the beginning of an era of active biophysical research on the pathways and thermodynamics of protein folding (3). Many purified proteins when denatured to random coil-like structures can refold spontaneously in vitro. This action is driven by small differences in the Gibbs free energy between the unfolded and native states (33, 38, 92, 97). Consequently, researchers assumed that in vivo folding (acquisition of tertiary structure) and assembly (acquisition of quarternary structure) of newly synthesized polypeptides also occur by an essentially spontaneous process without the help of additional components.

Over recent years, however, several proteinaceous components have been discovered that directly influence the processes by which newly made proteins attain their final conformation within the cell. With the exception of the enzymes protein disulfide isomerase and peptidyl prolyl isomerase, which catalyze specific reactions that can be rate limiting for folding (reviewed in 53, 62, 63, 64), these components have been classified as molecular chaperones (46, 48, 49) or polypeptide-chain binding proteins (168). They occur ubiquitously in prokaryotes and eukaryotes in the cytosol as well as within organelles (Table 1). Among the best characterized members of this heterogenous group of components are the constitutively expressed proteins of the Hsp70 and Hsp60 families (76). In the present context, their classification as stress- or heat-shock proteins may be somewhat misleading because these components are present in considerable amounts and fulfill essential functions under nonstressful conditions. Their expression can be induced under a great variety of cellular stresses, including heat shock, that may all have the accumulation of misfolded or partially denatured proteins in common. The term *molecular chaperone* initially referred to components such as nucleoplasmin (39, 106) and the chloroplast chaperonin Rubisco subunit binding protein (47), which assist in oligomeric assembly reactions presumably by preventing the formation of improper protein aggregates. The definition of molecular chaperone now includes the recently reported ATP-dependent functions of the various Hsp60s in actively guiding monomeric polypeptides to their native conformations.

This article summarizes the main lines of evidence that form the present view of Hsp70 and Hsp60 function in the folding and membrane translocation of newly synthesized proteins (4, 5, 8, 9, 20, 22, 27, 37, 60, 61, 68, 71, 72, 74, 94, 95, 123, 136, 143, 144, 166, 170, 177, 193, 206). The basic principle of action common to Hsp70 and Hsp60 appears to be that they

Table 1 Hsp70 and Hsp60 components as molecular chaperones

Subcellular localization	Organism	Component	Molecular mass (kDa) (monomer)	Function
Hsp70 family				
Cytosol	Prokaryotes *E. coli*	DnaK	69	Cooperates with heat-shock proteins DnaJ and GrpE in λ DNA replication and with DnaJ in activating RepA for binding to *ori*P1 DNA (43, 66, 202). Reactivates aggregated RNA polymerase (177). Facilitates protein export (154).
Cytosol	Eukaryotes Yeast	Ssa1-4p	69–72	Stabilizes precursor proteins for translocation into ER and mitochondria (22, 36, 206). Uncoates clathrin coated vesicles (19, 171, 172). Binds to nascent polypeptides (5). Binds the cellular oncogene p53 (23, 52, 155).
	Mammals	Hsc70 (Uncoating ATPase)		
ER	Yeast	Kar2p	78	Required for protein translocation into the ER and for protein assembly in the ER lumen (89, 166, 193). Association with BiP can result in retention of misfolded proteins (42, 68, 90, 95).
	Mammals	BiP/Grp78		
Mitochondria	Yeast	Ssc1p	~70	Required for membrane translocation and folding of proteins imported into mitochondria (94, 144, 145, 170).
Hsp60 family				
Cytosol	Prokaryotes *E. coli*	GroEL (Chaperonin 60)	58	Required for various phage assembly processes and for oligomeric protein assembly (49, 66, 72). Facilitate protein export of *lamB*-*lacZ* fusion proteins (154). Overexpression rescues certain temperature-sensitive lethal mutations and can stabilize normal proteins against thermal denaturation (188; A. Escher, A. A. Szalay, personal communication).
		GroES (Chaperonin 10)	10	
Mitochondria (Matrix)	Eukaryotes Fungi	Hsp60	58–64	Required for folding and oligomeric assembly of newly imported proteins in mitochondria (20, 144, 156). Cooperates with mitochondrial homologue of GroES (118).
	Mammals	Hsp58		
	Human	HuCha60		
Chloroplasts	Plants	Rubisco subunit binding protein	α-chain 61 β-chain 60	Required for oligomeric assembly of Rubisco and probably for folding and assembly of other proteins imported into chloroplasts (4, 16, 47, 82, 117, 138)

bind to segments of completely or partially unfolded polypeptides that are released upon ATP hydrolysis in an all-at-once or step-wise fashion. These chaperones can thus be involved in many cellular processes, preventing (premature) folding and aggregation, mediating correct folding, or stabilizing certain protein conformations. They may even rescue misfolded proteins by disassembling aggregates, or regulate the disposal of these proteins for degradation. Moreover, the general ability of binding and release shared by Hsp60 and Hsp70 can be utilized in various specialized processes such as clathrin uncoating and DNA replication. We discuss a model for the folding of nascent or newly translocated polypeptide chains based on their sequential and hierarchical interaction with Hsp70 and Hsp60. The function of the Hsp90 family of stress proteins in maintaining target proteins in inactive or unassembled states has been reviewed elsewhere (29, 198).

CELLULAR CONDITIONS FOR PROTEIN FOLDING

The main functional properties to be expected of factors assisting in physiological protein folding can be derived from a comparison between the conditions for folding in vitro and in vivo. Folding experiments in vitro are carried out with completely synthesized, artificially unfolded polypeptides (33, 53, 92, 97). Therefore, the same conditions apply equally to all parts of the folding polypeptide chain. The present concept of the sequence of events during refolding in vitro of an independently folding domain (usually about 100 amino acids) of a globular protein can be summarized as follows: As a result of the entropy-driven collapse of hydrophobic residues into the interior of the molecule, the multitude of random coil-like conformations present at high concentrations of denaturant converges within milliseconds towards the so-called prefolded state (23, 33, 38). Secondary structure elements may form even prior to hydrophobic collapse but become stabilized only within the compact, prefolded conformation, thereby providing the framework for further folding (33, 97). Hence, this early folding intermediate already contains considerable nonrandom structure. It is believed to be similar to the molten globule or compact intermediate states described for certain proteins at intermediate concentrations of denaturant or at acid pH (23, 102, 157). These intermediates are in rapid equilibrium with the fully unfolded state. Within the compact intermediate (33), secondary-structure elements are then thought to become arranged in a slower process (extending over seconds to minutes) via a limited number of pathways, resulting in the formation of ordered tertiary structure. This process is accompanied by a further compaction of the polypeptide as it approaches the transition state of folding described as a distorted version of the native state. Importantly, progression from the prefolded state to the native structure depends on long-range interactions between secondary structure elements that appear to require the presence of at least a complete protein domain. For example, the deletion of even a few amino acid residues from either terminus of a polypeptide chain can prevent folding in vitro that kinetically favors misfolding and aggregation (58, 169, 182, 200, 201). Independently folding domains are usually separated along the linear polypeptide chain frequently represented at the DNA level by distinct exons. However, this is not always the case; for example, the flavin adenine dinucleotide (FAD)-domain of glutathione reductase is composed of two noncontiguous parts of the chain that are 134 residues apart (173).

The fact that spontaneous folding of a protein is usually much faster than its synthesis in the cell (seconds as compared to minutes) implies that the folding of nascent chains is restricted, a characteristic of the situation in vivo (168). For example, when the synthesis of a polypeptide consisting of 100 amino acids is complete, 40 residues remain within the ribosome. Such a nascent chain will not be able to fold productively because only part of a folding domain is available. Instead, it may readily undergo intra- and intermolecular aggregation. The prefolded state of a protein is thought to be particularly sensitive to aggregation because of the exposure of hydrophobic residues (33). One should bear in mind that the concentration of nascent polypeptide chains in the cytosol of a bacterial cell such as *Escherichia coli* can reach 50 μM, the concentration of ribosomes (35). The local concentration of nascent chains in a polyribosome complex might be even higher. Aggregation usually poses problems in refolding experiments at much lower concentrations of folding chains (130). As a result, folding in vitro often proves very inefficient, while folding in the cell is generally believed to occur with efficiencies close to 100% (130). Moreover, within the cell, proteins must fold in a highly viscous 20–30% protein solution (cytosol or intraorganellar space). Whether spontaneous folding in vitro is possible under such conditions is unclear.

Thus, polypeptide chains supposedly need to be protected against misfolding and aggregation during synthesis. The folding of a single-domain protein would not occur sequentially as the amino acid residues emerge from the ribosome but only when the complete protein is available, allowing the productive engagement of its structural elements in long-range interactions. Clearly, folding as the acquisition of the native tertiary structure must be a posttranslational process. In larger proteins, of course, an amino-terminal domain may already have engaged in folding while a more carboxy-terminal one is still being synthesized (6, 11, 62, 201). For example, influenza hemeagglutinin (containing multiple folding domains) was observed to acquire some disulfide bonds cotranslationally, but its final disulfide composition and antigenic epitopes are formed post-translationally (11). With certain proteins, completion of the process of folding and assembly can take many minutes after synthesis (26, 85).

Polypeptide chains also encounter the problem of restricted folding during translocation across membranes. Proteins traverse membranes in an unfolded conformation and can only fold once translocation is complete. The following sections discuss the current concepts of how molecular chaperones mediate the formation of the native conformation by first preventing folding during synthesis or membrane translocation and then by mediating the step-wise, ATP-dependent release of poly-peptide chains that results in folding. The proposed role of these components does not violate the principles of folding derived from biophysical studies with purified proteins. Rather, molecular chaperones may provide the means to translate these principles into action under physiological conditions.

THE MEMBERS OF THE HSP70 FAMILY

It may seem a paradox that efficient folding in vivo primarily requires antifolding activity, the prevention of folding during synthesis. Three lines of evidence suggest that stress proteins of the Hsp70 class interact with nascent polypeptide chains, maintaining them in loosely folded con-formations: (*a*) Newly synthesized chains were found associated with con-stitutively expressed Hsp70 (Hsc70) in the cytosol of HeLa cells based on coimmuneprecipitation of the labeled proteins in cell extracts with antibodies directed against Hsp70 (5). (*b*) Cytosolic Hsp70 maintains pre-cursor proteins destined for translocation across the membranes of endo-plasmic reticulum (ER) or mitochondria in open, translocation-competent conformations (22, 37, 206). Overproduction of DnaK facilitates protein export to the periplasmic space in *E. coli* (154). (*c*) Organellar Hsp70 on the *trans* side of mitochondrial and ER membranes binds to the incoming polypeptides (94, 145, 170, 193). This interaction is required for efficient translocation and for correct folding.

The members of the Hsp70 family have been highly conserved through evolution (Table 1). In addition to Hsp70s strongly inducible by heat shock and other forms of cellular stress, constitutively expressed Hsp70s (Hsc70s) have essential functions under nonstressful conditions (28, 30, 114, 132, 150). These proteins include the *E. coli* DnaK (66), the yeast cytosolic proteins Ssa1p and Ssa2p (29) and the Hsc70 of mammalian cells, the so-called clathrin uncoating ATPase (19, 171). In addition, Hsp70s are found within subcellular organelles such as mitochondria (the Ssc1p of yeast)

(31, 32, 110, 131), chloroplasts (2, 122), and the endoplasmic reticulum (Kar2p in yeast and BiP in mammalian cells) (74, 133, 134, 143, 166). These organellar Hsp70s contain typical amino-terminal targeting sequences directing their sorting to the correct membrane compartment. All Hsp70s appear to have the following structural and functional features in common: (*a*) They bind ATP (19, 60, 96, 199, 207) and consist of a highly conserved amino-terminal ATP-binding domain (~450 residues) followed by a more variable carboxy-terminal substrate-binding domain (19, 54, 96, 143); (*b*) they bind to unfolded or partially denatured polypeptides (147; J. M. Flanagan, G. C. Flynn, J. Walter, J. E. Rothman & D. M. Engelman, submitted), and (*c*) they utilize the energy of ATP hydrolysis to release the bound substrates (60, 111, 112, 134).

Unfolding Is Required for Membrane Translocation of Proteins

The finding that proteins have to be unfolded for membrane translocation strongly stimulated cell biologists' interest in the mechanisms of protein folding in vivo (45, 80, 128, 160, 203). For example, stabilizing the folded conformation of an artificial mitochondrial precursor by binding methotrexate to the passenger protein dihydrofolate reductase (DHFR) rendered the fusion protein unable to traverse the mitochondrial membranes (45). The import of mitochondrial proteins from the cytosol, which is essential for the biogenesis of mitochondria, occurs at so-called translocation contact sites where outer and inner mitochondrial membranes are in close proximity (78, 80). Fusion proteins with a sufficiently long mitochondrial protein part joined to DHFR could be accumulated as membrane-spanning translocation intermediates in contact sites (162). These precursors reach into the mitochondrial matrix with their amino-terminal targeting sequence, which is proteolytically cleaved, but leave the folded DHFR outside the organelle (162, 190). Less than 50 amino acid residues were sufficient to span the 18- to 20-nm distance from outer surface of outer membrane to inner surface of inner membrane (163). The membrane-spanning sequences probably assumed a rather extended conformation. This is in agreement with the observation that urea denaturation of the precursor can speed up the translocation process considerably (44, 94, 144).

These results may explain why a loosely folded conformation of precursor proteins is a general requirement for membrane translocation. But how is this state of translocation competence achieved? Because translocation, at least with mitochondria, is predominantly posttranslational (204), noncytosolic proteins could (*a*) either fold following synthesis and become actively unfolded prior to or during translocation, or (*b*) be maintained in unfolded conformations as long as they are awaiting translocation in the cytosol. This latter mechanism applies to mitochondrial protein import and to posttranslational transport of proteins into the ER.

Cytosolic Hsp70 Stabilizes Precursor Proteins for Translocation

The presence of amino-terminal presequences retards the folding of purified precursor proteins as compared to their mature-sized counterparts (107, 160, 161). Precursor proteins may thus efficiently interact with chaperones for prolonged periods. In the bacterial cytosol, several components including SecB (25, 77, 116, 196), GroEL (8, 101, 108, 154), and the Hsp70 DnaK (154) stabilize precursor proteins, while in eukaryotes cytosolic Hsp70s (ct-Hsp70s) appear to be most important in this respect (36). SecB, probably a pentamer of 15-kilodalton (kDa) subunits, binds to the presequence and the mature part of secretory precursors (25, 77, 107, 116, 196). Because SecB, in contrast to Hsp70 and GroEL, lacks ATP-hydrolyzing activity, release from SecB appears to be accomplished by transfer of the bound protein to SecA, a peripheral ATPase of the translocation apparatus in the *E. coli* membrane (77).

Although binding of ct-Hsp70 probably also prevents folding in the case of nascent chains destined to remain in the eukaryotic cytosol (5), newly synthesized precursor proteins destined for membrane translocation provide more direct genetic and biochemical evidence for such a function (22, 36, 37, 136, 194, 206) (Figure 1, below).

The yeast *Saccharomyces cerevisiae* contains two genes coding for ct-Hsc70s (*Ssa1p* and *Ssa2p*) and two coding for inducible ct-Hsp70s (*Ssa3p* and *Ssa4p*) (28, 29). A yeast mutant in which *SSA1*, *SSA2,* and *SSA4* were disrupted was nonviable but could be rescued if transformed with a centromeric plasmid carrying the *SSA1* gene under the control of the *GAL1* promoter (37). When the cells were shifted from galactose-containing medium to glucose, the levels of ct-Hsc70s decreased, accompanied by the accumulation of precursor proteins destined to mitochondria and endoplasmic reticulum outside the organelles. The requirement of Hsp70 for protein translocation was also demonstrated in vitro using isolated microsomes and precursor proteins synthesized in a wheat germ lysate lacking functional Hsp70 (22). At least one further cytosolic activity was required, possibly for the release of the precursors from Hsp70 (136, 206). This activity could be inhibited by the sulfhydryl reagent N-ethyl maleimide (NEM) (136). The eukaryotic cytosol may contain homologues of the bacterial heat-shock proteins DnaJ and GrpE, which in *E. coli* are known to cooperate with DnaK in phage λ DNA replication (43, 66) by regulating the ATPase activity of DnaK (113). Whether DnaJ- and GrpE-like components are generally required by Hsp70s to execute their various functions remains to be seen.

Organellar Hsp70 in Protein Translocation and Folding

MITOCHONDRIA   The translocation of a folded protein domain, which has to lose at least all of its tertiary structure during membrane transport, can occur without a direct requirement for ATP or the membrane potential across the inner membrane (152). What then provides the energy for the vectorial movement of the polypeptide chain across the membranes? At low levels of ATP, the imported proteins are bound to the heat-shock proteins in the mitochondrial matrix, mt-Hsp70, and Hsp60 (94, 144) (Figure 1). Apparently, interaction with the mitochondrial Hsp70, Ssc1p, is directly required for translocation (94, 145, 170). In a temperature-sensitive yeast mutant affecting the gene coding for Ssc1p, the transfer of precursor proteins into mitochondria was defective (94). Precursor polypeptides were arrested during translocation spanning outer and inner membranes at contact sites. This block could be overcome in vitro when the precursor was first unfolded using 8 M urea and then rapidly diluted into a reaction containing the isolated mutant organelles. However, the precursor imported under these conditions remained in a highly protease-sensitive, incompletely folded conformation. Therefore, the mitochondrial Hsp70 apparently has a dual role in translocation and folding of imported proteins. Folding requires the transfer of the newly translocated poly-peptides from mt-Hsp70 to Hsp60 (see below), a step that is blocked in the Ssc1p mutant.

The energy resulting from binding of the extended amino terminus of the precursor protein to mt-Hsp70 could be utilized to successively unfold parts of the precursor still outside the organelle (141). Multiple molecules of mt-Hsp70 could bind to the traversing chain, thereby pulling it through the membrane. A typical precursor protein would be bound to cytosolic Hsp70 (22, 37). Both release from ct-Hsp70 (153, 206) and transfer of the imported polypeptide from mt-Hsp70 to Hsp60 require ATP hydrolysis (F. U. Hartl & T. Langer, unpublished data). In this model for the molecular mechanism of membrane translocation, multiple molecules of mt-Hsp70 would bind with high affinity to the extended precursor polypeptide whose folding is restricted by the membrane. Fewer molecules of ct-Hsp70 would be associated with the precursor in the cytosol that has assumed the conformation of a collapsed prefolded state during or after synthesis.

ENDOPLASMIC RETICULUM   The lumen of the ER contains an Hsp70 that was initially identified by its association with immunoglobulin heavy chains. This immunoglobulin heavy chain binding protein (BiP) (9, 74), also known as glucose-regulated protein Grp78 (134), is identical to yeast Kar2p (143, 166), which is inducible by various stress conditions including glucose restriction and the accumulation of secretory precursors. A temperature-sensitive KAR2 mutant shows a defect in translocation reminiscent of that seen in the mutation affecting the mitochondrial Hsp70 (193). At the nonpermissive temperature, precursors destined for the ER accumulated in the cytosol. Interestingly, Kar2p genetically and physically interacts with the Sec63 protein (167), a membrane component protruding into the ER lumen with a domain homologous to DnaJ. The defect in the KAR2 mutant could be reproduced using isolated microsomes of mutant cells and precursor proteins synthesized in vitro (R. Schekman & M. Rose, personal communication). Surprisingly, translocation into reconstituted microsomes was observed even in the apparent absence of BiP (142). However, very small amounts of BiP that might have escaped detection could have been sufficient to accomplish the translocation of the small quantities of radiolabeled precursor protein.

Requirement of Hsp70 for Protein Assembly in the ER

In addition to its role in protein translocation, BiP has an important function in oligomeric assembly of proteins in the ER (89). In reviewing the results of the numerous studies analyzing the interaction of BiP with secretory proteins, our discussion focuses on those observations that are more directly related to protein folding. In fact, BiP was the first Hsp70 recognized as a polypeptide-chain binding protein because of its association with immunoglobulin heavy chains in pre-B cells (74). The heavy chains remain permanently bound to BiP in these cells and await the synthesis of light chains necessary for assembly of complete immunoglobulins (9, 85). Under various conditions leading to the accumulation of incompletely folded, modified, or nonassembled proteins in the ER, these proteins are detected as complexes with BiP (42, 68, 90, 95). For example, mutated forms of the influenza virus hemeagglutinin, which cannot fold and assemble correctly, form stable complexes with BiP. In contrast, several normal proteins on the native folding pathway appear to interact only transiently (68, 89, 95, 100). The treatment of CHO cells with tunicamycin or exposure to glucose starvation causes the accumulation of undergylcosylated, misfolded proteins associated with BiP (42, 109). Under these conditions, BiP is itself induced—hence the term glucose regulated protein Grp78 (109, 134). The primary stimulus for induction seems to be the presence of malfolded proteins rather than abnormal glycosylation (100). In addition to BiP, another stress protein of the ER, Grp94, is induced when incompletely folded or assembled proteins accumulate (100, 109).

Bound proteins are released from BiP in a process requiring ATP hydrolysis (134). Metabolically poisoning cells to decrease the level of ATP prevented the trimerization of a mutant VSV G protein in the ER (41). Restoration of normal ATP levels allowed trimerization to proceed. These results indicated the existence of a pool of ATP in the lumen of the ER that had previously been unknown. The ATPase activity of purified BiP was found to be reduced in the presence of Ca^{2+} (96), raising the possibility that by modulating the level of Ca^{2+} in the ER, the capacity of BiP to retain newly made proteins could be regulated. Indeed, Ca^{2+} reportedly counteracted Mg-ATP-dependent release from BiP and secretion of variants of the T-cell antigen receptor α chain (179).

Secretory proteins must fold and assemble before leaving the ER through the secretory pathway. The main function of BiP could therefore be to retain normal proteins until assembly with other subunits is complete (84) or to prevent abnormal proteins from leaving the ER by channeling them into the ER degradation system (90, 98). However, BiP (up to 5% of lumenal ER protein) is a soluble component. It leaves the ER with the bulk flow and is retained via its carboxy-terminal KDEL signal (HDEL in the case of *S. cerevisiae* Kar2p) by a recycling mechanism between a salvage compartment and the ER (135, 151). Whether BiP-bound proteins are retained by the same mechanism is unknown. BiP may well play a general role in folding and assembly of proteins newly translocated into the ER. Data indicating that BiP is required for the physiological folding of a monomeric protein are not yet available, however.

Molecular Mechanism of Hsp70 Action

SUBSTRATE RECOGNITION   Hsp70s do not interact with defined sequence motifs. Their broad pattern of polypeptide recognition allows them to participate in many cellular processes. The affinity for certain substrates, however, may vary among the different members of the Hsp70 family. For example, clathrin cages stimulate the ATPase activity of cytosolic Hsc70 but not that of BiP (60). The principle of Hsp70 function is illustrated by the demonstration that various Hsp70s preferentially recognize short synthetic peptide sequences that may be exposed by unfolded or partially folded polypeptides. A first study using a few selected 10- to 15-residue peptides did not reveal any preference for a specific sequence or for a certain distribution of charge or hydrophobicity (60). Most peptides analyzed bound to Hsp70, but the binding affinities varied over three orders of magnitude. Recently, an extensive systematic study demonstrated that peptides of seven or eight residues optimally stimulated the ATPase of BiP (61). Consequently, the binding selectivity of BiP was tested using a mixture of randomly synthesized heptameric peptides. Sequencing the collective of bound peptides showed an enrichment of aliphatic amino acid residues (Val, Leu, Ile) and methionine at all positions of the bound peptide chains that was most pronounced within the region of the peptide core. Previously, Pelham (148, 149) proposed an interaction of Hsp70 with hydrophobic residues exposed by unfolded or partially denatured poly-peptides. While most amino acids could be tolerated, charged residues and prolines, which are preferentially surface-exposed in native proteins, were excluded from the binding site (61). Random 7-mer peptides containing an average of 1.6 aliphatic residues bound efficiently to BiP. Coating by Hsp70 of the respective segments of nascent chains (statistically occurring every 16 residues in a globular protein) (61) might thus prevent (mis)folding and aggregation during synthesis and maintain the sequences emerging from the ribosome in an extended conformation (Figure 1). However, Hsp70s could probably hold a complete polypeptide chain of up to several hundred amino acid residues in a random coil-like state within a physio-logical environment. The protein might rather be stabilized in a collapsed prefolded conformation when some of the attached Hsp70 molecules (per-haps those bound with lower affinity) fall off either spontaneously or upon ATP-dependent release; other Hsp70 molecules would remain bound more firmly (Figure 1). After completion of synthesis, the protein would thus be stabilized in an open, perhaps molten globule-like conformation, the likely equivalent of the so-called translocation-competent state (15).

In the case of proteins that have already undergone folding to the native state but expose hydrophobic peptide segments because of denaturation, the free energy of Hsp70 binding could be utilized to resolve misfolding or aggregation. Such a function may be reflected by observations made with DnaK in a model reaction containing aggregates of thermally denatured RNA polymerase (177). Dependent on ATP-hydrolysis, DnaK present in at least stoichiometric amounts to RNA polymerase can dissolve the aggregates, resulting in reactivation of the enzyme. Certain native proteins might make use of surface-accessible, extended sequences to attract the attention of Hsp70. DnaK cooperates with the heat-shock proteins DnaJ and GrpE in specific disassembly reactions; for example, this occurs in bacteriophage λ DNA replication by dissociating the DnaB protein from the λP protein, which then allows the helicase to function (40, 43, 66). Similarly, DnaK and DnaJ activate the RepA initiator protein that recognizes the origin of P1 replication by converting RepA dimers into monomers (202).

The three-dimensional structure of the carboxy-terminal domain of Hsp70, most likely responsible for specific substrate binding (19), has not yet been determined. However, molecular modeling based on a comparison of the carboxy-terminal domains of numerous Hsp70s from different sources suggested an interesting similarity with the α-1 and α-2 domains of the human major histocompatability antigen (MHC) class I protein (56, 165). One model proposes a peptide binding cleft for Hsp70 that, in contrast to that of the MHC class I molecule, would be lined predominantly by polar and charged amino acid residues (57). Another hypothesis predicts a peptide binding cleft containing both polar and apolar residues (165). This prediction seems plausible given that Hsp70 can accommodate both polar and apolar residues, possibly via interaction with the polypeptide backbone.

ATP HYDROLYSIS REQUIRED FOR RELEASE   Although the binding of unfolded proteins or peptides to Hsp70 likely is independent of ATP, their release requires ATP hydrolysis by Hsp70 (24, 60, 61, 84, 111, 134, 207) and probably cooperation with additional factors such as DnaJ and GrpE or perhaps their homologues (66, 136, 206). These heat-shock proteins stimulate the ATPase activity of DnaK (113). ATP hydrolysis, at least in the case of BiP, may be regulated by Ca^{2+} (96, 179). The binding of nucleotides can modulate the conformation of Hsp70 as revealed by changes in its sensitivity towards proteases (96). While ATP stabilizes Hsc70 in monomeric form, the presence of ADP favors the formation of dimers (172). The affinity of Hsp70 for ADP was found to be approximately sixfold higher than that for ATP. The ADP-bound form of Hsp70 also appears to associate with unfolded polypeptides more avidly. The release of the bound substrate could thus involve the exchange of ADP by ATP and its concurrent or subsequent hydrolysis (147). It is assumed that a conformational change of the amino-terminal ATP-binding domain of Hsp70 may be transferred to the carboxy-terminal substrate-binding domain, resulting in a decrease of binding affinity. Correspondingly, substrate binding stimulates the ATPase activity of Hsp70 (60, 61).

The ATP binding and hydrolytic activity is contained in the approximately 44-kDa amino-terminal domain of Hsp70 that is preserved upon limited proteolysis of the intact molecule (19, 96, 143). The recent resolution to 2.2 Å of the three-dimensional structure of the ATP binding domain of Hsc70 (54) revealed that its fold is almost identical to that of the globular monomer of actin (55). This observation is quite surprising because Hsc70 and actin share no sequence similarity. The structure of the nucleotide-binding site of Hsp70 is also similar to that of hexokinase (54).

The ATP requirement for release from Hsp70 is probably reflected in the dependence of protein translocation across subcellular membranes on cytosolic ATP (80, 128, 189). The absence of ATP renders precursor proteins destined for mitochondria (153) and the ER (206) incompetent for membrane translocation. On the other hand, studies of the import of artificial precursor proteins into mitochondria that do not (or only weakly) interact with Hsp70 showed that translocation was independent of ATP (Figure 1) (152).

THE MEMBERS OF THE HSP60 FAMILY

Evidence indicates an active role in mediating protein folding for the members of the Hsp60 family of stress proteins (12, 20, 71, 72, 123, 127, 144). The Hsp60 components have been defined as a subclass of molecular chaperones termed *chaperonins* (83) (Table 1). They are found in the bacterial cytosol and in the inner compartment of chloroplasts (stroma) and mitochondria (matrix) (49, 76). Like certain Hsp70s, these proteins are constitutively expressed. While GroEL can be induced severalfold under heat-shock conditions, expression of mitochondrial Hsp60 is stimu-lated by heat stress only two- to threefold (20). The chaperonins also exhibit a weak ATPase activity (18, 123, 192) but are structurally unrelated to the Hsp70s (except for a carboxy-terminal methionine-rich sequence of unknown function) (10). They form large tetradecameric complexes consisting of two stacked rings of seven 60-kDa subunits each (86, 87, 91, 159).

The chloroplast chaperonin Rubisco subunit-binding protein was initially found associated with the newly imported small subunits and the chloroplast-encoded large subunits of ribulose bisphosphate carboxylase oxygenase (Rubisco) but not with the completely assembled enzyme (4, 16, 47, 137, 138). This association was noncovalent and required ATP hydrolysis for dissociation. The Rubisco binding protein consists of dis-tinct but sequence-related α and β subunits that form mixed 14-mer com-plexes (82). The 61-kDa α subunit is 46% identical to the product of the *groEL* gene of *E. coli* (83).

The *groEL* gene is part of the *groE* operon that also contains the information for a smaller protein, GroES (also known as chaperonin 10). In its functional state, GroES exists as an oligomer (probably a heptamer) of 10-kDa subunits (18, 66). Various mutations in *groEL* and *groES* affect the assembly of λ phage capsids but not cell growth of the host (67, 178, 180, 183). However, gene deletion experiments showed that both genes are essential for growth at all temperatures (51). The GroE proteins are the major heat-shock proteins of *E. coli*. The synthesis of GroEL can increase from a basal level of about 2% of total cellular protein at 37°C to about 12% at 46°C (140). Ample evidence suggests a physical interaction of GroEL and GroES as well as their involvement in folding and assembly of authentic and foreign proteins (66). Overexpression of the *groE* operon suppressed several heat-sensitive mutations, probably by maintaining the

A

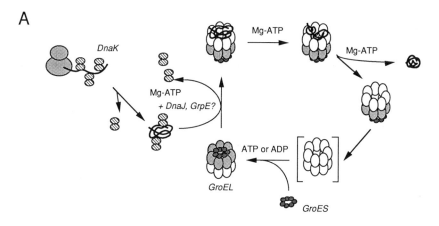

B

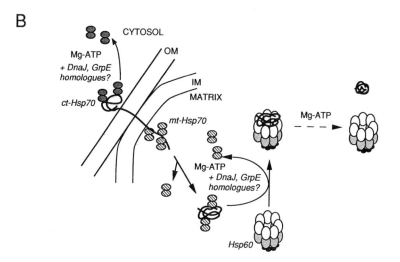

Figure 1 Hypothetical model for the differential function of Hsp70 and GroEL (Hsp60) in protein folding. (*A*) Folding in the bacterial cytosol. Nascent polypeptides interact with DnaK before reaching GroEL. Release of tightly bound DnaK may require the cooperation of heat-shock proteins DnaJ and GrpE. A single cycle of GroEL/GroES dependent folding is shown. Association with GroES may inhibit one of the 7-mer rings of GroEL for substrate binding (35). Whether top and bottom surfaces of GroEL are initially equivalent is unclear. Folding is assumed to occur by a surface-mediated process. Mg-ATP indicates the requirement for ATP hydrolysis. See text for details. (*B*) Folding in the mitochondrial matrix. Newly synthesized precursor proteins are stabilized in a loosely folded conformation by cytosolic Hsp70 (ct-Hsp70). During and after membrane translocation, the polypeptides interact with mitochondrial Hsp70 (mt-Hsp70). Release from Hsp70 and transfer to Hsp60 for folding may require putative homologues of DnaJ and GrpE. See text for details. Abbreviations are: OM, outer mitochondrial membrane; IM, inner mitochondrial membrane.

affected proteins in a functional conformation at the nonpermissive temperature (188). Increasing the levels of GroEL and GroES allowed the efficient assembly of heterologously expressed prokaryotic Rubisco (72). At wild-type levels of GroE, similar amounts of Rubisco were synthesized, but the newly made subunits could not assemble into the functional complexes. Overexpression of GroEL and GroES was also required for the functional expression of a thermolabile, heterodimeric luciferase at elevated temperatures (A. Escher & A. A. Szalay, personal communication). GroE overproducers could become useful in the future to facilitate the biotechnological production of large amounts of foreign proteins in bacteria that often results in the formation of inclusion bodies (88, 130).

More recently, an Hsp60 was identified in mitochondria of *Tetrahymena thermophila* (125, 126) and in the mitochondria of various other species including humans (93, 131, 164, 195). The protein is synthesized constitutively as a cytosolic precursor and is assembled within the organelles. Hsp60 is coded for by an essential gene and constitutes roughly 1% of the total mitochondrial protein in yeast or *Neurospora crassa* under non-heat-shock conditions (20, 91, 164). A homologue of the GroES protein exhibiting significant sequence similarity has been discovered in mitochondria (118) and is probably present in chloroplasts as well (A. Gatenby, personal communication). The chaperonins seem to be restricted to archaebacteria, eubacteria, and to organelles of endosymbiotic origin. However, a recent report states that a component of the eukaryotic cytosol, the TCP-1 protein complex, is remotely related to Hsp60 (1) (see below).

Multiple Functions of Mitochondrial Hsp60

Mitochondria are a particularly suitable system for studying processes of physiological protein folding and assembly (76). In order to multiply by growth and division, these organelles have to import most of their proteins from the cytosol in an unfolded conformation (78, 80). Protein import and subsequent folding can be faithfully reproduced with isolated mitochondria and precursor proteins synthesized in vitro. Protein synthesis and physiological folding can be separated experimentally because of the posttranslational nature of the uptake reaction, a unique advantage of this system.

MONOMERIC CHAIN FOLDING AND OLIGOMERIC ASSEMBLY   Evidence for a function of Hsp60 in protein assembly came from the analysis of the temperature-sensitive lethal yeast mutant *mif4,* which is defective in the *MIF4* gene coding for Hsp60 (20, 21, 121; H. Koll, B. Guiard, J. Rassow, J. Ostermann, A. L. Horwich, et al, submitted). Because of a single amino acid substitution (A. Horwich, unpublished data), the altered Hsp60 undergoes a conformational change at the nonpermissive temperature that results in the loss of function. Proteins such as the precursor of the β subunit of the F_1-ATPase or the trimeric matrix enzyme ornithine transcarbamylase are imported normally by the mutant mitochondria and are proteolytically processed, but cannot assemble into oligomeric complexes (20). The unassembled subunits have a tendency to aggregate in the matrix compartment.

The Hsp60 14-mer is also required for its own assembly (21). When wild-type Hsp60 monomers were expressed in *mif4* mutant cells, they could not form a functional Hsp60 14-mer complex at the nonpermissive temperature. Thus, the machinery necessary for the folding and assembly of many if not most mitochondrial proteins cannot undergo self-assembly in vivo (21). On the other hand, a study of the (re)assembly of urea-denatured GroEL in vitro concluded that 14-mers are first formed spontaneously and then catalyze further assembly in a Mg-ATP dependent reaction (115). Self-assembly is also possible for GroES, at least under appropriate conditions in vitro (124).

A biochemical analysis of the interaction between imported proteins and mitochondrial Hsp60 revealed that the basic role of this chaperonin probably lies in mediating the folding of monomeric polypeptide chains (144). When the cytosolic protein mouse dihydrofolate reductase (DHFR) was imported into mitochondria as a fusion protein carrying a cleavable amino-terminal targeting sequence, its folding into the protease-resistant, native conformation occurred with a half-time of about 3 min. This was much slower than import into mitochondria of the urea-denatured precursor. On the other hand, DHFR is known to fold rapidly in vitro (123, 184). This retardation of folding in mitochondria results from complex formation with Hsp60 (144). When the mitochondria used in the import reaction were depleted of ATP, the complex between DHFR and Hsp60 was stable and could be isolated from mitochondrial extracts. The Hsp60-bound DHFR was highly sensitive towards digestion by proteinase K, indicating that it was in an unfolded or incompletely folded conformation. ATP hydrolysis and an additional factor were necessary to allow folding of the Hsp60-associated protein. *E. coli* GroES can be substituted for this factor (118; F. U. Hartl & A. L. Horwich, unpublished data). In the absence of the mitochondrial GroES, the ATP-dependent folding reaction slowed down, allowing the detection of a partially folded form of DHFR that was still associated with Hsp60 (144). Folding of DHFR in mitochondria could also be blocked by pretreatment of the organelles with NEM. Under these conditions, the DHFR fusion protein transiently associated with Hsp60 but then formed incorrectly folded aggregates. These results suggested an active function of Hsp60 in protein folding that is not simply explained by binding and release of the incompletely folded polypeptide (144) (Figure 1). The Rubisco subunit-binding protein probably has a similar role in the folding of proteins imported into chloroplasts or synthesized within the organelles (117, 156).

ANTIFOLDING IN PROTEIN EXPORT   In addition to the functions in folding and assembly, Hsp60 is required for the export of certain proteins from the matrix to the intermembrane space of mitochondria (20, 78; H. Koll, B. Guiard, J. Rassow, J. Ostermann, A. L. Horwich, et al, submitted). For example, the cytosolic precursor of cytochrome b_2 is first imported completely and is then transported back across the inner membrane following a bacterial-type export pathway (79). This mechanism of intra-mitochondrial sorting is thought to reflect the endosymbiotic origin of mitochondria from prokaryotic ancestors (78). The information for export of cytochrome b_2 is contained in a hydrophobic amino-terminal signal sequence. Evidence that Hsp60 is involved in protein sorting to the intermembrane space again came from analyzing the Hsp60-deficient mutant *mif4* (20). The mutant mitochondria accumulated incompletely processed forms of cytochrome b_2 and of the Rieske Fe/S protein, which follows a similar route to the intermembrane space (81). These findings suggested a role for Hsp60 in maintaining precursor proteins imported into the matrix in an open conformation competent for export across the inner membrane. A similar function in bacterial protein export has been observed with *E. coli* GroEL for a very limited subset of secretory precursors (8, 101, 154), while the main chaperone for bacterial export appears to be SecB (25, 77, 116, 160, 161, 196).

How is the antifolding function of Hsp60 related to its role in mediating folding? A fusion protein consisting of the presequence of the intermembrane-space protein cytochrome b_2 and DHFR was imported into ATP-depleted mitochondria. A stable complex with Hsp60 formed in which DHFR was unfolded. Strikingly, the DHFR moiety could not fold when ATP was added. Folding occurred only after translocation to the intermembrane space had taken place (H. Koll, B. Guiard, J. Rassow, J. Ostermann, A. L. Horwich, et al, submitted). The hydrophobic export sequence may retard the folding of the mature protein part as demonstrated for certain bacterial secretory proteins such as the precursor of maltose binding protein (160, 161). Rebinding to Hsp60 following ATP-dependent release could be more rapid than folding, thus preserving an unfolded conformation of the protein. This possibility would be in agreement with results obtained by analyzing the interaction between pre-β-lactamase and GroEL in vitro (8, 103). A model of kinetic partitioning has been proposed to interpret the binding properties of secretory precursor proteins to SecB (75). In contrast to the chaperonins, SecB does not hydrolyze ATP.

Molecular Mechanism of Chaperonin Action

To understand the molecular details of the mechanism by which the chaperonins mediate folding and assembly, one must reproduce their function in vitro using the purified components. The first important information came from studies reconstituting the GroEL- and GroES-dependent homooligomeric assembly of prokaryotic Rubisco (71). Rubisco subunits completely unfolded in 6 M guanidinium chloride or denatured at acid pH were found to form stable binary complexes with GroEL, presumably as partially folded intermediates. This interaction prevented the aggregation of the protomers otherwise observed upon dilution from denaturant. ATP hydrolysis and the cooperating component GroES proved to be necessary for the formation of the assembled, biologically active enzyme (71). As discussed below, the Rubisco protomers likely underwent partial folding at GroEL and were ultimately discharged in a conformation competent for assembly with another subunit. Similar results were reported for the chaperonin-dependent assembly of dimeric citrate synthase (12), a protein whose refolding from denaturant had been unsuccessful so far. Recently, studies on the GroE-mediated refolding of monomeric dihydrofolate reductase (123, 191) and rhodanese (123, 127) shed new light on the mechanism of GroE action. Notably, all the in vitro studies consistently failed to provide evidence for a function of GroEL in refolding protein aggregates.

STABILIZATION OF AN EARLY FOLDING INTERMEDIATE   The GroEL 14-mer complex appears to bind only one or perhaps two protein molecules, as demonstrated using various substrate proteins ranging in size between ~20–50 kDa (71, 103, 108, 123, 191). The stoichiometry of bound polypeptides per GroEL oligomer may increase with smaller substrates. One approach towards understanding chaperonin-mediated folding relies on (a) defining the conformation in which a protein substrate is stably bound by GroEL and (b) characterizing intermediates associated with the chaperonin during the folding process. The conformation of GroEL-bound DHFR from chicken and of bovine rhodanese were examined using fluorescence spectroscopy (123). Binding was performed by adding the substrate proteins from 6 M guanidinium chloride to GroEL containing buffer in the absence of ATP hydrolysis. The intrinsic tryptophanyl fluorescence of the bound polypeptides was used to probe their tertiary structure. This approach was possible because both the sequences of GroEL and GroES lack tryptophans (83, 87). In both cases, the maximum wavelength of emission was at an intermediate position between that of the native and fully unfolded conformations (123). A marked increase in the fluorescence intensity, probably resulting from dequenching of Trp24, accompanied unfolding of DHFR. The GroEL-associated DHFR showed a fluorescence intensity nearly as high as DHFR unfolded in 6 M guanidinium chloride, indicating that the conformation stabilized by GroEL lacked the specific tertiary structure present in the native protein. This observation was in agreement with the very high protease sensitivity of the GroEL-bound species (123, 191). Fluorescence quenching experiments showed that the tryptophans in GroEL-bound DHFR and rhodanese were better protected from solvent than in the fully unfolded conformations but significantly more accessible than in the native structures (123). These findings suggested that the GroEL-associated polypeptides were in a partially folded conformation perhaps similar to the molten globule (23, 34, 102, 158) or compact intermediate (33) states. An analysis of the binding of the fluorescent probe anilino-naphthalene sulfonate (ANS), whose fluorescence depends on the hydrophobicity of its environment, corroborated these results. Adsorption of ANS is typically observed with loosely folded protein conformations such as the molten globule (23, 157, 158, 175). Both GroEL-bound DHFR and rhodanese showed strong ANS fluorescence that was observed neither with the fully unfolded nor with the native proteins (123).

The nature of the structural elements recognized by GroEL is still unknown. Available evidence suggests that these elements are present in practically every protein whose interaction with GroEL has been tested so far. They could be extended peptide sequences, certain secondary structure elements, or conformational arrangements such as hydrophobic clusters or patches that would be transiently exposed by early folding intermediates resembling the molten globule. Using transferred nuclear Overhauser effect (NOE) measurements, Landry & Gierasch (104) recently showed that a 13-amino acid residue peptide representing the amino-terminal α-helix of rhodanese binds to GroEL in an α-helical conformation, albeit with low affinity. These investigators proposed that GroEL may recognize the hydrophobic face of amphiphilic α-helices occurring at the amino terminus of nascent polypeptide chains (105). Assuming that the reported interaction was specific, these findings will be very important for eventually understanding the functional principle of GroEL in facilitating protein folding. The binding of secondary structure elements suggests a mechanism of action distinct from that proposed for the members of the Hsp70 family of molecular chaperones (see above).

FOLDING AT GroEL   A molten globule-like conformation may represent the likely conformation of a polypeptide competent for translocation across membranes (15). The molten globule may also be the global conformation of newly synthesized proteins in which they enter the pathway of chaperonin-mediated folding. Initiation of folding by Mg-ATP and GroES resulted in the progression of GroEL-associated rhodanese to a more compact folding intermediate (123). This process was accompanied by a decrease in ANS fluorescence and an increase in intrinsic protease resistance. Similar results were obtained with folding of DHFR (123). These more compact intermediates were still bound to the GroEL double ring, suggesting that at least a partial folding reaction took place in very close association with the chaperonin.

The process of folding at the surface of GroEL depends critically on the presence of GroES. In the absence of GroES, ATP hydrolysis by GroEL appears to result in the complete release of the bound protein (123, 191). In DHFR, which folds spontaneously in vitro, this release was sufficient to allow the formation of the native structure. However, following complete release, DHFR could rebind to GroEL before completing folding, thus explaining why GroEL retarded the reactivation of DHFR as compared to the rate of spontaneous folding (123). In contrast, complete release in the absence of GroES did not lead to reactivation of rhodanese but rather to efficient cycling between the GroEL-bound and free states. Unlike DHFR, rhodanese cannot fold efficiently in vitro. Upon dilution from denaturant, the protein forms a collapsed intermediate that aggregates rapidly (181). This aggregation is prevented by binding of the rhodanese intermediate to GroEL (123, 127). The fact that complete release from GroEL in the absence of GroES did in fact occur could be proven using the pseudo-unfolded protein casein (146, 197) as a competitor for binding to GroEL. In the presence of Mg-ATP, casein displaced GroEL-bound DHFR or rhodanese (123). The released DHFR then folded spontaneously, while the fate of rhodanese was aggregation. Polypeptides folding at GroEL were protected from displacement by casein when GroES was present. Apparently during folding, the proteins were isolated from the bulk phase of the solution. According to these results, GroEL would have to interact with more than one segment of the protein substrate. Folding could occur by releasing these segments in a step-wise or sequential manner, a process that requires regulation by GroES (123). The substrate-binding region of GroEL has not yet been identified. Binding to GroEL may occur at the central area of one of the 7-mer rings where all of its subunits could contribute binding sites for segments of the polypeptide chain, perhaps forming a kind of channel. Only one of the 7-mer rings may be active at a time for binding dependent on regulation by GroES (34).

The molten globule state during folding presumably adopts a progressively more compact packing of its secondary structure elements, resulting in the formation of ordered tertiary structure (102). We propose that this reaction occurs by a mechanism of partial release while the protein remains in close association with GroEL. Unproductive interactions could be reversed, utilizing the energy of rebinding to GroEL, since these interactions would not allow the successful internalization of structural elements recognized by GroEL. Eventually, the protein would be set free in a conformation still before or already past the transition state of the folding pathway. In the case of oligomeric proteins such as Rubisco (71, 72), the monomers associated with GroEL are likely to assume the conformation of a folding intermediate able to associate with other subunits. Stabilization by GroEL would increase the concentration of this type of rate-limiting intermediate for the assembly reaction. It seems reasonable to assume that oligomerization takes place upon ATP-dependent release of the GroEL-bound monomers. Molecules that were unsuccessful in finding the proper partner to associate with could rebind to GroEL, thereby avoiding unwanted interactions.

Although how the chaperonins could increase the rate of an assembly reaction is evident, whether they actually catalyze the folding of monomeric polypeptide chains is unclear. Do the chaperonins mediate folding by lowering the activation energy of the productive folding pathway, or do they do so exclusively by raising energy barriers blocking pathways that lead to misfolding and aggregation?

ATP REQUIREMENT OF FOLDING   Research has not formally shown that GroES may not interact directly with the polypeptide substrate folding at GroEL. According to the present view, however, the key to the function of GroES lies in its regulatory influence on the ATP-hydrolytic activity of GroEL (18, 123, 192). The GroEL 14-mer probably has 14 ATP binding sites. In the absence of substrate, the GroEL complex exhibits a low but significant ATPase activity with a K_m for ATP of 7 μM (192). This activity is almost completely suppressed by interaction with GroES at a 1:1 molar ratio of GroES 7-mer to GroEL 14-mer (123, 192). GroES and GroEL form an isolatable complex in the presence of Mg-ATP or ADP (18, 192; A. Girshovich, unpublished data; J. Martin, unpublished data). Under the influence of GroES, the GroEL ATPase becomes strictly substrate dependent (123). In the case of rhodanese, approximately 100 molecules of ATP were hydrolyzed per protein molecule folded, suggesting that the GroEL 14-mer went through several cycles of ATP hydrolysis (123). The amount of ATP required for folding in vivo is unknown; one should keep in mind that the synthesis of a single molecule of rhodanese (293 residues) consumes roughly 1200 molecules of ATP, i.e. the ATP requirement for chaperonin-mediated folding will probably be a comparatively minor expense.

A HYPOTHESIS FOR THE FOLDING OF NEWLY SYNTHESIZED POLYPEPTIDES

Recent findings for protein folding in mitochondria may suggest a principle mechanism for the acquisition of tertiary structure in vivo. Division of labor between molecular chaperones of the Hsp70 and Hsp60 families appears to be an integral element (76, 141). Although members of both groups of stress proteins interact with unfolded or incompletely folded polypeptides and utilize the energy of ATP hydrolysis for releasing the bound substrates, important functional differences are becoming apparent. Physiological folding of a newly synthesized polypeptide may occur by the following three-step reaction consisting of (a) protection and maintenance of folding competence by Hsp70, (b) ATP-dependent transfer from Hsp70 to Hsp60, and (c) ATP-dependent folding at Hsp60 (Figure 1).

Maintenance of Folding Competence by Hsp70

Components of the Hsp70 family can associate with the folding poly-peptide before those of the Hsp60 family, suggesting a hierarchy of inter-action with molecular chaperones. For example, the mitochondrial Hsp70 binds to the extended protein sequences reaching into the matrix while they are still in the process of membrane translocation (94, 145, 170). Similarly, cytosolic Hsp70 is thought to interact with nascent polypeptides emerging from the ribosome (5). Hsp70 binds unfolded peptide sequences (60, 61) and exhibits the highest binding affinities with mutant polypeptides that have little stable secondary structure (147; J. M. Flanagan, G. C. Flynn, J. Walter, J. E. Rothman & D. M. Engelman, submitted).

The main purpose of the interaction of a nascent polypeptide chain with Hsp70 would be to prevent premature (mis)folding and aggregation of proteins (or their independently folding domains) during synthesis. It is unknown how many Hsp70 molecules could bind to a sequence of, say, 100 amino acids emerging from a ribosome (statistically containing perhaps up to 5 binding sites) (61). Binding of Hsp70 could prevent or retard the hydrophobic collapse of the molecule, and the emerging chain would transiently be held in a relatively extended conformation with little stable secondary structure. The initial binding may require the cooperation between Hsp70 and a DnaJ-homologous component. Because of its slow, ATP-dependent release activity, bound Hsp70 would fall off the substrate perhaps with kinetics adjusted to the speed of protein synthesis (60). This would allow the internalization of hydrophobic regions to a molten globule-like state now stabilized by fewer Hsp70 molecules.

The interaction with Hsp70 alone appears not to be sufficient to promote the formation of ordered tertiary structure, at least in the case of proteins imported into the mitochondrial matrix (94). The role of Hsp70 in protein folding could mainly consist of stabilizing the newly synthesized chains in loose conformations competent for the folding process mediated by a further component(s) or for membrane translocation (so-called "folding-competent" and "translocation-competent" states). Alternatively, the stabilization of nascent chains followed by cycles of ATP-dependent release and rebinding of Hsp70 may be sufficient for the folding of a subset of total soluble proteins that might contain sequence elements supporting the productive interaction with Hsp70. In fact, the existence of sequence information that ensures that a newly synthesized protein forms the correct intermediate conformations on the folding pathway was demonstrated by the mutational analysis of the in vivo folding of P22 tailspike polypeptide (69, 70, 129). This information is not required to stabilize the native state of the protein. Because of coevolution with molecular chaperones, proteins may contain structural elements directing the programmed interaction with these components.

Transfer from Hsp70 to Hsp60

Folding in mitochondria appears to depend on the newly imported proteins being transferred from Hsp70 to Hsp60 (94, 144). Very little is known about this transfer reaction. In light of the finding that binding of Hsp70 is necessary for membrane translocation, while Hsp60 function appears to be of little importance at this stage (94, 144), transfer to Hsp60 should occur when import of the protein (or its domains in case of larger polypeptides) is complete. Other mitochondrial components, perhaps similar to the NEM-sensitive factor contained in reticulocyte lysates (136), may have to cooperate with Hsp70 to ultimately allow its complete release from the imported protein. Natural candidates could be mitochondrial homologues of E. coli DnaJ and GrpE that are known to physically interact with the Hsp70 DnaK (66). Homologues of DnaJ have been reported for mitochondria (7), for the yeast nucleus (17), and for the cytosol (17, 119). In addition to their roles in DNA replication (43, 66, 202), DnaJ, DnaK, and GrpE have as yet undefined functions of general importance for normal growth of E. coli (13, 14, 66, 174) that may include protein folding (65). DnaK is dispensable at intermediate growth temperatures around 30°C (although the cells grow very poorly) and becomes essential for growth at temperatures below and above 30°C (13, 14). At present, all results would be compatible with DnaK having a critical buffer function in protein folding, holding and protecting nascent chains until they can be taken over by GroEL. Under non-heat-shock conditions, cells would contain fewer GroEL molecules than nascent chains; the basal level of the GroEL 14-mer is about 15 μM, while the concentration of nascent chains is 30–50 μM and that of DnaK is 100 μM (calculated according to refs. 35, 73, 139). Furthermore, GroEL may bind nascent chains only at a later stage of synthesis than DnaK and would therefore be unable to efficiently prevent their aggregation. This lack of protection would become more critical at higher growth temperatures. We propose that DnaK, DnaJ, and GrpE cooperate with GroE/GroES in the de novo folding of proteins.

Hsp60-Mediated Folding

Evidently, Hsp70 cannot assume some specific functions of Hsp60 in protein folding. The chaperonins appear to mediate folding by a process of step-wise release while the folding polypeptide remains sequestered at their surface (123, 144). Surface-mediated folding may critically depend on an oligomeric machinery in which the individual Hsp60 monomers contribute binding sites for polypeptide segments whose action would be coordinated in the oligomeric chaperonin complex.

Although both mitochondrial Hsp60 and *E. coli* GroEL/GroES fulfill essential functions under all growth conditions (51), it is unclear what percentage of total proteins depend on chaperonins for folding. Given the importance for protein folding we assign to Hsp60, one would expect that chaperonin-like components were present in every cellular compartment capable of de novo folding. A functional equivalent of Hsp60 in the eukaryotic cytosol has not been found so far, but a remote structural homology to GroEL and mitochondrial Hsp60 has been reported for the TCP-1 protein complex (1), which led to the proposal of a molecular chaperone function for TCP-1 (49), a high-molecular-weight complex similar in size to that of the chaperonins (V. Lewis & K. Willison, personal communication). TCP-1 was originally described as involved in the phenomenon of male-specific transmission ratio distortion in mice (120, 176). The protein is abundantly expressed in developing sperm, but a more general function is suggested by the detection of TCP-1 in the cytosol of all other cell types analyzed to date (186, 205). A cold-sensitive mutation in yeast affecting TCP-1 impairs mitotic spindle formation (187). The recent discovery of the thermoprotection factor TF55 of the thermophilic archaebacterium *Sulfolobus shibatae* makes TCP-1 a very attractive candidate for an Hsp60-like function in the cytosol (185). TF55, the major heat-shock protein of *S. shibatae*, appears to be an 18-mer complex of 55-kDa subunits with ~40% sequence identity to TCP-1 of mouse and yeast (185). These findings may support speculations on the existence of two evolutionary lines of chaperonins, one leading from eubacteria to mitochondria and chloroplasts and the other leading from archaebacteria to the eukaryotic cytosol.

FUTURE ASPECTS

It is now generally accepted that protein folding in the cell needs mediation by molecular chaperone components. Despite considerable advances towards understanding the function of Hsp70 and Hsp60, many aspects of their molecular mechanisms of action are still unclear. We are just beginning to understand how unfolded proteins are recognized and how their folding is prevented or promoted. In no case is the structural basis for binding fully established. While at least a partial crystal structure of Hsp70 is available, such information is completely lacking for the Hsp60 components. Remaining questions include: How is ATP hydrolysis transformed into conformational changes of the chaperone, ultimately resulting in folding of the protein substrate? Or, from a more cell-biological point of view, what is the exact sequence of interactions with chaperones during and following synthesis of a polypeptide chain? Can these processes, for example the functional cooperation between Hsp70 and Hsp60, faithfully be reproduced in vitro? Given the significance and the current interest in aspects of protein folding in vivo, we will probably not have to wait long for the answers to many of these questions.

ACKNOWLEDGMENTS

We thank D. Engelman, J. Flanagan, A. Gatenby, A. Girshovich, A. Horwich, V. Lewis, G. Lorimer, J. King, M. Rose, J. Rothman, R. Schekman, A. Szalay, and K. Willison for sharing unpublished information, and A. Horwich for stimulating discussion. Work in the authors' laboratories was supported by the Deutsche Forschungsgemeinschaft.

Literature Cited

1. Ahmad, S., Gupta, R. S. 1990. *Biochim. Biophys. Acta* 1087: 253–55
2. Amir-Shapira, D., Leustek, T., Dalie, B., Weissbach, H., Brot, N. 1990. *Proc. Natl. Acad. Sci. USA* 87: 1749–52
3. Anfinsen, C. B. 1973. *Science* 181: 223–30
4. Barraclough, R., Ellis, R. J. 1980. *Biochim. Biophys. Acta* 608: 19–31
5. Beckmann, R. P., Mizzen, L. A., Welch, W. J. 1990. *Science* 248: 850–54
6. Bergman, L. W., Kuehl, W. M. 1979. *J. Supramol. Struct.* 11: 9–24
7. Blumberg, H., Silver, P. A. 1991. *Nature* 349: 627–30
8. Bochkareva, E. S., Lissin N. M., Girshovich, A. S. 1988. *Nature* 336: 254–57
9. Bole, D. G., Hendershot, L. M., Kearney, J. F. 1986. *J. Cell Biol.* 102: 1558–66
10. Bosch, T. C. G. 1991. In *Heatshock*, ed. S. Lindquist, B. Mareska. Heidelberg: Springer Verlag. In press
11. Brackman, I., Hoover-Lefty, H., Wagner, K. R., Helenius, A. 1991. *J. Cell Biol.* 114: 401–12
12. Buchner, J., Schmidt, M., Fuchs, M., Jaenicke, R., Rudolph, R., et al. 1991. *Biochemistry* 30: 1586–91
13. Bukau, B., Walker, G. C. 1989. *J. Bacteriol.* 171: 2337–46
14. Bukau, B., Walker, G. C. 1990. *EMBO J.* 9: 4027–36
15. Bychkova, V. E., Pain, R. H., Ptitsyn, O. B. 1988. *FEBS Lett.* 238: 231–34

16. Cannon, S., Wang, P., Roy, H. 1986. *J. Cell Biol.* 103: 1327–35
17. Caplan, J., Douglas, M. G. 1991. *J. Cell Biol.* 114: 609–21
18. Chandrasekhar, G. N., Tilly, K., Woolford, C., Hendrix, R., Georgopoulos, C. 1986. *J. Biol. Chem.* 261: 12414–19
19. Chappell, T. G., Konforti, B. B., Schmid, S. L., Rothman, J. E. 1987. *J. Biol. Chem.* 262: 746–51
20. Cheng, M. Y., Hartl, F. U., Martin J., Pollock R. A., Kalousek F., et al. 1989. *Nature* 337: 620–25
21. Cheng, M. Y., Hartl, F. U., Horwich, A. L. 1990. *Nature* 348: 455–58
22. Chirico, W. J., Waters, G. M., Blobel, G. 1988. *Nature* 332: 805–10
23. Christensen, H., Pain, R. H. 1991. *Eur. Biophys. J.* 19: 221–29
24. Clarke, C. F., Cheng, K., Frey, A. B., Stein, R., Hinds, W., Levine, A. J. 1988. *Mol. Cell. Biol.* 8: 1206–15
25. Collier, D. N., Bankaitis, V. A., Weiss, J. B., Bassford, P. J. 1988. *Cell* 53: 273–83
26. Colman, A., Besley, J., Valle, G. 1982. *J. Mol. Biol.* 160: 459–72
27. Copeland, C. S., Doms, R. W., Bolzau, E. M., Webster, R. G., Helenius, A. 1986. *J. Cell Biol.* 103: 1179–91
28. Craig, E. A. 1988. *Annu. Rev. Genet.* 22: 631–77
29. Craig, E. A. 1990. See Ref. 132a, pp. 301–22
30. Craig, E. A., Gross, C. A. 1991. *Trends Biochem. Sci.* 16: 135–40
31. Craig, E. A., Kramer, J., Kosic-Smithers, J. 1987. *Proc. Natl. Acad. Sci. USA* 84: 4156–60
32. Craig, E. A., Kramer, J., Shilling, J., Werner-Washburne, M., Holmes, S., et al. 1989. *Mol. Cell Biol.* 9: 3000–8
33. Creighton, T. E. 1990. *Biochem. J.* 270: 1–16
34. Creighton, T. E. 1991. *Nature* 352: 17–18
35. Darnell, J., Lodish, H., Baltimore, D. 1986. *Molecular Cell Biology*, p. 137. New York: Freeman
36. Deshaies, R. J., Koch, B. D., Schekman, R. 1988. *Trends Biochem. Sci.* 13: 384–88
37. Deshaies, R. J., Koch, B. D., Werner-Washburne, M., Craig, E. A., Schekman, R. 1988. *Nature* 332: 800–5
38. Dill, K. A. 1990. *Biochemistry* 29: 7135–55
39. Dingwall, C., Laskey, R. A. 1990. *Sem. Cell Biol.* 1: 11–17
40. Dodson, M., McMacken, R., Echols, H. 1989. *J. Biol. Chem.* 264: 10719–25
41. Doms, R., Keller, D., Helenius, A., Balch, W. 1987. *J. Cell Biol.* 105: 1957–69
42. Dorner, A. J., Bole, D. G., Kaufman, R. J. 1987. *J. Cell Biol.* 105: 2665–74
43. Echols, H. 1990. *J. Biol. Chem.* 265: 14697–14700
44. Eilers, M., Oppliger, W., Schatz, G. 1987. *EMBO J.* 6: 1073–77
45. Eilers, M., Schatz, G. 1986. *Nature* 322: 228–32
46. Ellis, R. J. 1987. *Nature* 328: 378–79
47. Ellis, R. J. 1990. *Science* 250: 954–59
48. Ellis, R. J. 1990. *Sem. Cell Biol.* 1: 1–9
49. Ellis, R. J., Van der Vies, A. 1991. *Annu. Rev. Biochem.* 60: 327–47
50. Deleted in proof
51. Fayet, O., Ziegelhoffer, T., Georgopoulos, C. 1989. *J. Bacteriol.* 171: 1379–85
52. Findlay, C. A., Hinds, P. W., Tan, T. H., Eliyahu, D., Oren, M., Levien, A. J. 1988. *Mol. Cell. Biol.* 8: 531–39
53. Fischer, G., Schmid, F. X. 1990. *Biochemistry* 29: 2206–12
54. Flaherty, K. M., DeLuca-Flaherty C., McKay D. B. 1990. *Nature* 346: 623–28
55. Flaherty, K. M., McKay, D. B., Kabsch, W., Holmes, K. C. 1991. *Proc. Natl. Acad. Sci. USA* 88: 5041–45
56. Flajnik, M. E., Canel, C., Kramer, J., Kasahara, M. 1991. *Proc. Natl. Acad. Sci. USA* 88: 537–41
57. Flajnik, M. E., Canel, C., Kramer, J., Kasahara, M. 1991. *Immunogenetics.* In press
58. Flanagan, J. M., Kataoka, M., Sortie, D., Engelman, D. M. 1991. *Proc. Natl. Acad. Sci. USA.* In press
59. Deleted in proof
60. Flynn, G. C., Chappell, T. G., Rothman, J. E. 1989. *Science* 245: 385–90
61. Flynn, G. C., Rohl, J., Flocco, M. T., Rothman, J. E. 1991. *Nature* 353: 726–30
62. Freedman, R. B. 1984. *Trends. Biochem. Sci.* 9: 438–41
63. Freedman, R. B. 1989. *Cell* 57: 1069–72
64. Freedman, R. B., Bulleid, N. J., Hawkins, H. C. Paver, J. K. 1989. *Biochem. Soc. Symp.* 55: 167–92
65. Gaitanaris, G. A., Papavassiliou, A. G., Rubock, P., Silverstein, S. J., Gottesman, M. E. 1990. *Cell* 61: 1013–20
66. Georgopoulos, C., Ang, D., Liberek, K., Zylicz, M. 1990. See Ref. 132a, pp.191–222
67. Georgopoulos, C. P., Hendrix, R. W., Casjens, S. R. Kaiser, A. D. 1973. *J. Mol. Biol.* 76: 45–60

68. Gething, M. J., McCommon, K., Sambrook, J. 1986. *Cell* 46: 939–50
69. Goldenberg, D. P., King, J. 1981. *J. Mol. Biol.* 145: 633–51
70. Goldenberg, D. P., Smith, D. H., King, J. 1983. *Proc. Natl. Acad. Sci. USA* 80: 7060–64
71. Goloubinoff, P., Christeller, J. T., Gatenby, A. A., Lorimer, G. H. 1989. *Nature* 342: 884–89
72. Goloubinoff, P., Gatenby, A. A., Lorimer, G. H. 1989. *Nature* 337: 44–47
73. Goodsell, D. S. 1991. *Trends Biochem. Sci.* 16: 203–6
74. Haas, I. G., Wabl, M. 1983. *Nature* 306: 387–89
75. Hardy, S. J., Randall, L. L. 1991. *Science* 251: 439–43
76. Hartl, F.-U. 1991. *Sem. Immunol.* 3: 5–16
77. Hartl, F. U., Lecker, S., Schiebel, E., Hendrick, J. P., Wickner, W. 1990. *Cell* 63: 269–79
78. Hartl, F. U., Neupert W. 1990. *Science* 247: 930–38
79. Hartl, F. U., Ostermann, J., Guiard, B., Neupert, W. 1987. *Cell* 51: 1027–37
80. Hartl, F. U., Pfanner, N., Nicholson, D., Neupert, W. 1989. *Biochim. Biophys. Acta* 998: 1–45
81. Hartl, F. U., Schmidt, B., Wachter, E., Weiss, H., Neupert, W. 1986. *Cell* 47: 939–51
82. Hemmingsen, S. M., Ellis, R. J. 1986. *Plant Physiol.* 80: 269–76
83. Hemmingsen, S. M., Woolford, C., Van der Vies, S. M., Tilly, K., Dennis, D. T., et al. 1988. *Nature* 333: 330–34
84. Hendershot, L., Bole, D., Köhler, G., Kearney, J. F. 1987. *J. Cell Biol.* 104: 761–67
85. Hendershot, L. M. 1990. *J. Cell Biol.* 111: 829–37
86. Hendrix, R. W. 1979. *J. Mol.Biol.* 129: 375–92
87. Hohn, T., Hohn, B., Engel, A., Wurtz, M. 1979. *J. Mol. Biol.* 129: 359–73
88. Horwich, A. L., Neupert, W., Hartl, F. U. 1990. *Trends Biotechnol.* 8: 126–31
89. Hurtley, S. M., Helenius, A. 1989. *Annu. Rev. Cell Biol.* 5: 277–307
90. Hurtley, S. M., Bole, D. G., Hoover-Litty, H., Helenius, A., Copeland, C. S. 1989. *J. Cell Biol.* 108: 2117–26
91. Hutchinson, E. G., Tichelaar, W., Hofhaus, G., Weiss, H., Leonard, K. R. 1989. *EMBO J.* 8: 1485–90
92. Jaenicke, R. 1987. *Prog. Biophys. Mol. Biol.* 49: 117–237
93. Jindahl, S., Dudani, A. K., Singh, B., Harley, C. B., Gupta, R. S. 1989. *Mol. Cell Biol.* 9: 2279–83
94. Kang, P. J., Ostermann, J., Shilling, J., Neupert, W., Craig, E. A., Pfanner, N. 1990. *Nature* 348: 137–43
95. Kassenbrock, C. K., Garcia, P. D., Walter, P., Kelly, R. B. 1988. *Nature* 333: 90–93
96. Kassenbrock, C. K., Kelly, R. B. 1989. *EMBO J.* 8: 1461–67
97. Kim, P. S., Baldwin, R. L. 1990. *Annu. Rev. Biochem.* 59: 631–60
98. Klausner, R. D., Lippincott-Schwartz, J., Bonifacino, J. S. 1990. *Annu. Rev. Cell Biol.* 6: 403–31
99. Deleted in proof
100. Kozutsumi, Y., Segal, M., Normington, K., Gething, M. J., Sambrook, J. 1988. *Nature* 332: 462–64
101. Kusukawa, N., Yura, T., Ueguchi, C., Akiyama, Y., Ito, K. 1989. *EMBO J* 8: 3517–21
102. Kuwajima, K. 1989. *Proteins Struct. Funct. Genet.* 6: 87–103
103. Laminet, A. A., Ziegelhoffer, T., Georgopoulos, C., Plückthun, A. 1990. *EMBO J.* 9: 2315–19
104. Landry, S. J., Gierasch, L. M. 1991. *Biochemistry* 30: 7359–62
105. Landry, S. J., Gierasch, L. M. 1991. *Trends Biochem. Sci.* 16: 159–63
106. Laskey, R. A., Honda, B. M., Mills, A. D., Finch, J. T. 1978. *Nature* 275: 416–20
107. Lecker, S., Driessen, A. J. M., Wickner, W. 1990. *EMBO J.* 9: 2309–14
108. Lecker, S., Lill, R., Ziegelhoffer, T., Georgopoulos, C., Bassford, P. J., et al. 1989. *EMBO J.* 8: 2703–9
109. Lee, A. S. 1987. *Trends Biochem. Sci.* 12: 20–23
110. Leustek, T., Dalie, B., Amir-Shapira, D., Brot, N., Weissbach, H. 1989. *Proc. Natl. Acad. Sci. USA* 86: 7805–8
111. Lewis, M. J., Pelham, H. R. B. 1985. *EMBO J.* 4: 3137–43
112. Liberek, K., Georgopoulos, C., Zylicz, M. 1988. *Proc. Natl. Acad. Sci. USA* 18: 6632–36
113. Liberek, K., Marzzalek, J., Ang, D., Georgopoulos, C., Zylicz, M. 1991. *Proc. Natl. Acad. Sci. USA* 88: 2874–78
114. Lindquist, S., Craig, E. A. 1988. *Annu. Rev. Genet.* 22: 631–77
115. Lissin, N. M., Venyaminov, S. Yu., Girshovich, A. S. 1990. *Nature* 348: 339–42
116. Liu, G., Topping, T. B., Randall, L. L. 1989. *Proc. Natl. Acad. Sci. USA* 86: 9213–17
117. Lubben, T. H., Donaldson, G. K., Viitanen, P. V., Gatenby, A. A. 1989. *Plant Cell* 1: 1223–30
118. Lubben, T. H., Gatenby, A. A., Don-

aldson, G. K., Lorimer, G. H., Viitanen, P. V. 1990. *Proc. Natl. Acad. Sci. USA* 87: 7683–87

119. Luke, M. M., Sutton, A., Arndt, K. T. 1991. *J. Cell Biol.* 114: 623–38
120. Lyon, M. F. 1984. *Cell* 37: 621–28
121. Mahlke, K., Pfanner, N., Martin, J., Horwich, A. L., Hartl, F. U., Neupert, W. 1990. *Eur. J. Biochem.* 192: 551–55
122. Marshall, J. S., DeRocher, A. E., Keegstra, K., Vierling, E. 1990. *Proc. Natl. Acad. Sci. USA* 87: 374–78
123. Martin, J., Langer, T., Boteva, R., Schramel, A., Horwich, A. L., Hartl, F.-U. 1991. *Nature* 352: 36–42
124. Mascagni, P., Tonolo, M., Ball, H., Lim, M., Ellis, R. J., Coates, A. 1991. *FEBS Lett.* 286: 201–3
125. McMullin, T. W., Hallberg, R. L. 1987. *Mol. Cell. Biol.* 7: 4414–23
126. McMullin, T. W., Hallberg, R. L. 1988. *Mol. Cell. Biol.* 8: 371–80
127. Mendoza, J. A., Rogers, E., Lorimer, G. H., Horowitz, P. M. 1991. *J. Biol. Chem.* 266: 13044–49
128. Meyer, D. I. 1988. *Trends Biochem. Sci.* 13: 471–74
129. Mitraki, A., Fane, B., Haase-Pettingell, C., Sturtevant, J., King, J. 1991. *Science* 253: 54–58
130. Mitraki, A., King, J. 1989. *Bio/Technology* 7: 690–97
131. Mizzen, L. A., Chang, C., Garrels, J. I., Welch, W. J. 1989. *J. Biol. Chem.* 264: 20664–75
132. Morimoto, R. J., Milarski, K. L. 1990. See Ref. 132a, pp. 323–60
132a. Morimoto, R., Tissieres, A., Georgopoulos, C. eds. 1990. *Stress Proteins in Biology and Medicine.* Cold Spring Harbor, New York: Cold Spring Harbor Lab.
133. Morrison, S. L., Scharff, M. D. 1975. *J. Immunol.* 114: 655–59
134. Munro, S., Pelham, H. R. B. 1986. *Cell* 46: 291–300
135. Munro, S., Pelham, H. R. B. 1987. *Cell* 48: 899–907
136. Murakami, H., Pain, D., Blobel, G. 1988. *J. Cell Biol.* 107: 2051–57
137. Musgrove, J. E., Ellis, R. J. 1986. *Philos. Trans. R. Soc. London Ser. B* 313: 419–28
138. Musgrove, J. E., Johnson, R. A., Ellis, R. J. 1987. *Eur. J. Biochem.* 163: 529–34
139. Neidhardt, F. C., van Bogelen, R. A. 1987. In Escherichia coli *and* Salmonella typhimurium. *Cellular and Molecular Biology*, ed. F. C. Neidhardt, J. L. Ingraham, K. B. Low, B. Magasanik, M. Schaechter, H. E. Umbarger, 2: 1334–45. Washington, DC: Am. Soc.

Microbiol.
140. Neidhardt, J. E., Phillips, T. A., van Bogelen, P. A., Smith, M. W., Georgalis, Y., Subramanian, A. R. 1981. *J. Bacteriol.* 145: 513–20
141. Neupert, W., Hartl, F. U., Craig, E., Pfanner, N. 1990. *Cell* 63: 447–50
142. Nicchitta, C. V., Blobel, G. 1990. *Cell* 60: 259–69
143. Normington, K., Kohno, K., Kozutsumi, Y., Gething, M. J., Sambrook, J. 1989. *Cell* 57: 1223–36
144. Ostermann, J., Horwich, A. L., Neupert, W., Hartl, F. U. 1989. *Nature* 341: 125–30
145. Ostermann, J., Voos, W., Kang, P. J., Craig, E. A., Neupert, W., Pfanner, N. 1991. *FEBS Lett.* 277: 281–84
146. Ostoa-Saloma, P., Ramirez, J., Perez-Montfort, R. 1990. *Biochim. Biophys. Acta* 1041: 140–52
147. Palleros, D. R., Welch, W. J., Fink, A. L. 1991. *Proc. Natl. Acad. Sci. USA* 88: 5719–23
148. Pelham, H. R. B. 1986. *Cell* 46: 959–61
149. Pelham, H. R. B. 1988. *Nature* 332: 776–77
150. Pelham, H. R. B. 1990. See Ref. 132a, pp. 287–300
151. Pelham, H. R. B., Hardwick, K. G. Lewis, M. J. 1988. *EMBO J.* 7: 1757–62
152. Pfanner, N., Rassow, J., Guiard, B., Sollner, T., Hartl, F. U., Neupert W. 1990. *J. Biol. Chem.* 265: 16324–29
153. Pfanner, N., Tropschug, M., Neupert, W. 1987. *Cell* 49: 815–23
154. Phillips, G. J., Silhavy, T. J. 1990. *Nature* 344: 882–84
155. Pinhashi-Kimhi, O., Michalovitz, D., Ben-Zeev, A., Oren, M. 1986. *Nature* 320: 182–84
156. Prasad, T. K., Hack, E., Hallberg, R. L. 1990. *Mol. Cell. Biol.* 10: 3979–86
157. Ptytsin, O. B. 1991. *J. Protein Chem.* 6: 272–93
158. Ptitsyn, O. B., Pain, R. H., Semisotnov, G. V., Zerownik, E. Razgulyaev, O. I. 1990. *FEBS Lett.* 262: 20–24
159. Pushkin, A. V., Tsuprun, V. L., Solovjeva Shubin, V. V., Evstigneeva, Z. G., Kretovich, W. L. 1982. *Biochim. Biophys. Acta* 704: 379–84
160. Randall, L. L., Hardy, S. J. S. 1986. *Cell* 46: 921–28
161. Randall, L. L., Hardy, S. J. S. 1989. *Science* 243: 1156–59
162. Rassow, J., Guiard, B., Wienhues, U., Herzog, V., Hartl, F. U., Neupert, W. 1989. *J. Cell Biol.* 109: 1421–28
163. Rassow, J., Hartl, F. U., Guiard, B., Pfanner, N., Neupert, W. 1990. *FEBS Lett.* 275: 190–94

164. Reading, D. S., Hallberg, R. L., Myers, A. M. 1989. *Nature* 337: 655–59
165. Rippmann, F., Taylor, W. R., Rothbard, J. B., Green, N. M. 1991. *EMBO J.* 10: 1053–59
166. Rose, M. D., Misra, L. M., Vogel, J. P. 1989. *Cell* 57: 1211–21
167. Rothblatt, J. A., Deshaies, R. J., Sanders, S. L., Daum, G., Schekman, R. 1989. *J. Cell Biol.* 109: 2641–52
168. Rothman, J. E. 1989. *Cell* 59: 591–601
169. Sachs, D. H., Schechter, A. N., Eastlake, A., Anfinsen, C. B. 1974. *Nature* 251: 242–44
170. Scherer, P. E., Krieg, U. C., Hwang, S. T., Vesteweber, D., Schatz, G. 1990. *EMBO J.* 9: 4315–22
171. Schlossman, D. M., Schmid, S. L., Braell, W. A., Rothman, J. E. 1984. *J. Cell Biol.* 99: 723–33
172. Schmid, S. L., Braell, W. A., Rothman, J. E. 1985. *J. Biol. Chem.* 260: 10057–62
173. Schulz, G. E., Schirmer, R. H., Sachsenheimer, W., Pai, E. F. 1978. *Nature* 273: 120–24
174. Sell, S. M., Eisen, C., Ang, D., Zylicz, M., Georgopoulos, C. 1990. *J. Bacteriol.* 172: 4827–35
175. Semisotnov, G. V., Rodionova, N. A., Kutyshenko, V. P., Ebert, B., Blanck, J., Ptitsyn, O. B. 1987. *FEBS Lett.* 224: 9–13
176. Silver, L. M., Artzt, K., Bennett, D. 1979. *Cell* 17: 275–84
177. Skowyra, D., Georgopoulos, C., Zylicz, M. 1990. *Cell* 62: 939–44
178. Sternberg, N. 1973. *J. Mol. Biol.* 76: 25–44
179. Suzuki, C. K., Bonifacino, J. S., Lin, A. Y., Davis, M. M., Klausner, R. D. 1991. *J. Cell Biol.* 114: 189–205
180. Takano, T., Kakefuda, T. 1972. *Nat. New Biol.* 239: 34–37
181. Tandon, S., Horwitz, P. M. 1986. *J. Biol. Chem.* 261: 15615–81
182. Taniuchi, H. 1970. *J. Biol. Chem.* 245: 5459–68
183. Tilly, K., Murialdo, H., Georgopoulos, C. 1983. *Proc. Natl. Acad. Sci. USA* 78: 1629–33
184. Touchette, N. A., Perry, K. M., Matthews, C. R. 1986. *Biochemistry* 25: 5445–52
185. Trent, J., Nimmesgern, E., Wall, J. S., Hartl, F. U., Horwich, A. L. 1991. *Nature.* In press
186. Ursic, D., Ganetzky, B. 1988. *Gene* 68: 267–74
187. Ursic, D., Culbertson, M. R. 1991. *Mol. Cell. Biol.* 11: 2629–40
188. Van Dyk, T. K., Gatenby, A. A., LaRossa, R. A. 1989. *Nature* 324: 451–53
189. Verner, K., Schatz, G. 1988. *Science* 241: 1307–13
190. Vestweber, D., Schatz, G. 1988. *J. Cell Biol.* 107: 2037–43
191. Viitanen, P. V., Donaldson, G. K., Lorimer, G. H., Lubben, T. H., Gatenby, A. A. 1991. *Biochemistry* 30: 9716–23
192. Viitanen, P. V., Lubben, T. H., Reed, J., Galoubinoff, P., O'Keefe, D. P., Lorimer, G. 1990. *Biochemistry* 29: 5665–71
193. Vogel, J. P., Misra, L. M., Rose, M. D. 1990. *J. Cell Biol.* 110: 1885–95
194. Waegemann, K., Paulsen, H., Soll, J. 1990. *FEBS Lett.* 261: 89–92
195. Wardinger, D., Eckerskorn, C., Lottspeich, F., Cleve, H. 1988. *Biol. Chem. Hoppe-Seyler* 369: 1185–89
196. Watanabe, M., Blobel, G. 1989. *Cell* 58: 695–705
197. Waxman, L., Goldberg, A. L. 1986. *Science* 232: 500–3
198. Welch, W. J. 1990. See Ref 132a, pp. 223–78
199. Welch, W. J., Feramisco, J. R. 1985. *Mol. Cell Biol.* 5: 1229–37
200. Wetlaufer, D. 1981. *Adv. Protein Chem.* 34: 61–92
201. Wetlaufer, D. B., Ristow, S. 1973. *Annu. Rev. Biochem.* 42: 135–58
202. Wickner, S., Hoskins, J., McKennly, K. 1991. *Nature* 350: 165–67
203. Wickner, W. T., Driessen, A., Hartl, F. U. 1990. *Annu. Rev. Biochem.* 60: 101–24
204. Wienhues, U., Becker, K., Schleyer, M., Guiard, B., Tropschug, M., et al. 1991. *J. Cell Biol.* In press
205. Willson, K., Lewis, V., Zuckerman, K. S., Cordell, J., Dean, C., et al. 1989. *Cell* 57: 621–32
206. Zimmermann, R., Sagstetter, M., Lewis, M. J., Pelham, H. R. B. 1988. *EMBO J.* 7: 2875–80
207. Zylicz, M., LeBowitz, J. H., McMacken, R., Georgopoulos, C. 1983. *Proc. Natl. Acad. Sci. USA* 80: 6431–35

Annu. Rev. Biophys. Biomol. Struct. 1992. 21:323–48

SOLUBILIZATION AND FUNCTIONAL RECONSTITUTION OF BIOMEMBRANE COMPONENTS

John R. Silvius

Department of Biochemistry, McGill University, Montréal, Québec, Canada H3G 1Y6

KEY WORDS: membrane proteins, detergents, membrane solubilization, membrane reconstitution, proteoliposomes

CONTENTS

OVERVIEW

Although reconstitution of membrane proteins has long been an important tool of membrane biophysics, the nature of the reconstitution process itself remains in many ways surprisingly ill defined. This is understandable, as our comprehension of the native structures and the interactions of membrane components is still limited, yet efforts to attain a systematic understanding of the reconstitution process are neither futile nor

323

1056–8700/92/0610–0323$02.00

misguided. We have, in fact, progressed substantially toward this goal, and while most practical reconstitution procedures are still developed using a sizeable measure of trial and error, they nonetheless build on a set of established basic principles that usefully limits the number and the range of experimental variables that must be explored.

A successful membrane reconstitution strategy comprises three principal aspects: the partial or complete solubilization of membrane protein and lipid components, the preservation of recoverable activity of membrane proteins in the solubilized state, and the reassembly of solubilized proteins and lipids to form a reconstituted membrane. This review discusses these three issues in turn and focuses on reconstitution strategies entailing the use of detergents, which have proven most widely useful for membrane proteins. Excellent previous reviews offer overviews of the reconstitution process from different perspectives (65, 86, 90, 99, 111, 112, 156, 179, 232), discussions of methods for characterizing and separating solubilized membrane proteins (45, 111, 156, 183, 224, 232), and descriptions of the reconstitution of specific classes of membrane proteins, including receptors (111, 112, 122, 127), transport proteins (14, 100), and energy-transducing proteins (34, 65, 179).

DETERGENT SOLUBILIZATION OF MEMBRANES

Basic Properties of Detergents

Several excellent reviews of the detergents commonly used in membrane solubilization, including compendia of their physical properties, have appeared (84, 86, 89, 131). The following discussion underscores some key properties of detergents that must be considered in designing practical, well-controlled procedures for membrane solubilization.

Although detergent preparations of ever-greater purity and homogeneity are becoming widely available, potential effects of detergent contaminants must still be considered in any reconstitution procedure. Peroxidized contaminants of alkyl polyoxyethylene detergents (15, 37), and long-chain alcohols derived from alkyl glycoside detergents (136), can form in aqueous stock solutions of these species even when the original detergent preparation is of high purity. Many detergent preparations [including most bile salts and alkyl poly(oxyethylene) and poly(oxyethylene) sorbitol ester detergents] are contaminated with homologues or other compounds that are structurally related to the principal component(s) but that may have considerably lower critical micelle concentrations. Low levels of such contaminants may not greatly affect the solubilizing properties of the detergent but may remain more tenaciously associated with the reconstituted membrane than does the major species in the final stages of detergent removal.

The thermodynamics of micelle formation by single amphiphiles and by mixtures of amphiphiles has been well described elsewhere (39, 155, 223) and is not discussed in detail here. Although a population of micelles constitutes a collection of molecular aggregates and not a true phase, calculations of the extent of micelle formation in a given amphiphile-water system can often be considerably simplified by treating the formation of micelles as analogous to a phase-separation process. This picture has given rise to the familiar but approximate concept of a unique critical micelle concentration (cmc), the amphiphile concentration at which the solution is effectively saturated with the monomeric species and above which micelles appear in coexistence with monomers. As Tanford (223) has pointed out, the phase-separation approximation permits accurate quantitative descriptions of the monomer-micellar equilibria of detergents that form large micelles but is less appropriate for surfactants with low aggregation numbers (e.g. bile salts).

The distribution of detergent molecules between the monomeric and other associated states is influenced by numerous experimentally relevant physical variables. The first of these is temperature, which can affect the micelle-forming properties of a detergent in several ways. The critical micellar concentrations and the bilayer-partitioning properties of nonionic detergents are often appreciably temperature-dependent (46, 132, 203). Some widely used detergents, including alkylsulfates (22) and alkyl N-methylglucamides (81, 238), form precipitates rather than micellar dispersions at the low temperatures at which biochemical manipulations are often performed. By contrast, solutions of many nonionic detergents separate macroscopically into detergent-rich and detergent-depleted aqueous phases above their so-called cloud-point temperature (160). This temperature lies above 37°C for most biochemically useful detergents, with the noteworthy exception of Triton X-114, whose cloud-point temperature of approximately 28°C provides the basis for a useful [though not infallible (2, 140, 234)] test for identifying integral membrane proteins by their preferential partitioning into the detergent-rich phase (25). However, certain other commonly used detergents, including octyl glucoside and Triton X-100, can also exhibit cloud points at relatively low temperatures when combined with membrane lipids (6, 132, 170, 184, 202), and such phenomena may play an important role in certain reconstitution processes (202). Pure and mixed micelles containing nonionic detergents can also show a marked increase in aggregation number with increasing temperature even below the cloud point (132, 160).

Several factors other than temperature can also modulate the micelle-forming (and membrane-solubilizing) properties of detergents. Among these are ionic strength (for charged detergents), pH (for titratable detergents such as bile salts and alkylbetaines), the presence of divalent cations (for certain anionic detergents, notably bile salts), the absolute concentrations of lipids and detergents [if processes of superaggregation and/or macroscopic phase separation are possible (181)], and the presence of cosolvents, chaotropes, or other solutes that alter water structure and/or activity. In fact, the micellar-bilayer equilibrium can be shifted dramatically in some detergent-lipid systems by varying one or more of the above parameters. This potential may be useful in some experimental applications [e.g. to initiate bilayer formation from solubilized components by abruptly changing the temperature or the ionic strength (46, 222)] but may complicate others when one must change one or more of the above variables without perturbing the micellar-bilayer equilibrium.

Solubilization of Lipid Bilayers

When a particular detergent and membrane preparation are combined, a key determinant of the final extent of membrane solubilization is the ratio of nonmonomeric detergent to the membrane lipid and protein components, where the designation *nonmonomeric detergent* includes both bilayer-intercalated and micellar detergent molecules (97, 130, 131, 209, 218, 219). As the discussion below illustrates, proper control of this variable is crucial to the design of an effective and reproducible membrane solubilization protocol.

The picture of micelles as a pseudophase provides the basis for an approximate but frequently useful description of the thermodynamics of solubilization of lipid bilayers by detergents (4, 6, 46, 58, 97, 129, 170, 173, 218). Consider a simple mixture of a homogeneous detergent and a single bilayer-forming membrane lipid. Because the lipid is essentially insoluble in monomeric form, its distribution in this system is defined by its mole fractions in lamellar structures (x_L[lam]) and/or in mixed micelles (x_L[mic]), whichever is/are present. If both bilayers and micelles can be treated as phases, their coexistence at equilibrium is equivalent to a phase separation and occurs (at a given temperature, ionic strength, etc) only for unique values of x_L[lam] and x_L[mic], and hence for unique values of the corresponding detergent mole fractions x_D[lam] and x_D[mic].

When the above conclusions are combined with considerations of mass balance, the progress of solubilization of a single-component lipid bilayer by a detergent is predicted to follow the idealized profile shown in Figure 1 so long as nonideality in lipid-detergent mixing is not excessive (130, 131). In the region designated I, an increase in the total detergent concentration increases both the concentration of monomeric detergent and the mole

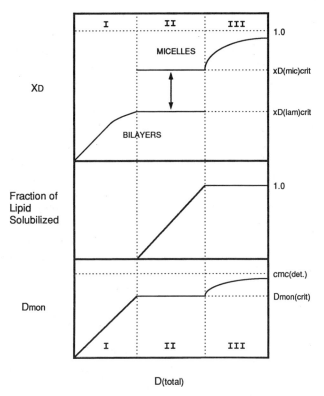

Figure 1 Stages in the solubilization of a homogeneous lipid bilayer by increasing concentrations of a detergent [D(total)], as predicted using the phase-separation approximation described in the text. The regions designated I, II, and III correspond respectively to ranges of total detergent concentration in which bilayers only, bilayers and micelles, or micelles only are present. (*Top panel*) Mole fraction(s) of detergent in bilayers and/or micelles. (*Middle panel*) Fraction of total lipid incorporated into mixed micelles. (*Bottom panel*) Concentration of monomeric detergent (D_{mon}). For simplicity, the variation of the monomeric detergent concentration with the total detergent concentration in region I is shown as linear but may also be nonlinear, particularly at higher detergent levels.

fraction of detergent in the bilayer (x_D[lam]), but no coexisting mixed micelles are formed. The incorporation of low mole fractions of detergent into the lipid bilayers can be described as a straightforward partitioning equilibrium with a well-defined partition coefficient (97, 130, 170, 204, 218), although this picture may not remain valid at high mole fractions of bilayer-intercalated detergent. While bilayer solubilization does not occur in this region, the detergent-doped bilayers typically show evidence of local structural perturbation [notably, increased permeability (19, 119, 178, 198,

200, 226, 227, 247) and in some cases a change in vesicle size (6, 7, 95, 119, 173, 228, 233)].

In the region designated II in Figure 1, the mole fraction of detergent in the bilayer plateaus at its saturation level $x_D[\text{lam}]^{\text{crit}}$, and solubilization begins with the appearance of a coexisting population of mixed micelles containing a different mole fraction of detergent $x_D[\text{mic}]^{\text{crit}}$. In this region, the fraction of lipid solubilized rises linearly with increasing total detergent concentration, while the concentration of monomeric detergent is predicted to attain a constant value, $D_{\text{mon}}^{\text{crit}}$. Finally, in region III, the lipid is completely solubilized into mixed micelles. As the total concentration of detergent increases in this range, the mole fraction of detergent in the micelles rises further; the average micelle molecular weight typically decreases (58, 145, 194, 209); and the concentration of detergent monomers asymptotically approaches the cmc of the pure detergent.

The process of bilayer solubilization in some representative detergent-lipid systems can be described, to a first order approximation, by the "phase-separation" model outlined above. One can use various experimental methods, including turbidometry (6, 129, 173), 90° and quasielastic light-scattering (4, 57, 145, 215, 233), fluorescence resonance energy transfer (46, 58, 170, 233, 238, 239), electron spin resonance (246), and ^{31}P-NMR (77, 97, 119, 129) as well as centrifugation, to measure the progress of lipid-bilayer solubilization. One can also estimate the parameters $D_{\text{mon}}^{\text{crit}}$, $x_D[\text{lam}]^{\text{crit}}$, and $x_D[\text{mic}]^{\text{crit}}$ from such measurements when different concentrations of lipid are titrated with increasing amounts of detergent (6, 129, 170, 173). Interestingly, the values of $x_D[\text{lam}]^{\text{crit}}$ and $x_D[\text{mic}]^{\text{crit}}$ can vary substantially for different detergents in combination with the same phospholipid. For solubilization of egg lecithin, for example, the values of these parameters are approximately 0.22 and 0.40–0.45, respectively, using sodium cholate (173, 200, 239); 0.60–0.65 and 0.75 using octyl glucoside (6, 97, 170, 173); 0.40 and 0.69 using $C_{12}E_8$ (129); and 0.39 and 0.71 using Triton X-100 (52, 173). These findings are consistent with the predictions of models that stress the importance of molecular geometries (expressed as effective shapes) in determining the equilibrium compositions and relative stabilities of micellar vs lamellar structures (93).

The above (idealized) model of bilayer solubilization leads to a further prediction that proves useful in practice: to achieve a consistent degree of bilayer solubilization when adding a given detergent to samples of varying lipid content or concentration, it is sufficient to adjust the amount of detergent in each sample to attain a constant value of the parameter:

$$([\text{Detergent}]_{\text{total}} - D_{\text{mon}}^{\text{crit}})/[\text{Lipid}]_{\text{total}}$$

(for related treatments, see 95, 131, 187). The relevant value of $D_{\text{mon}}^{\text{crit}}$ is

best determined by experiment (see above) but if necessary may be estimated using the following formula when mixing of lipid and detergent in
micelles is near-ideal (39, 86, 223):

$$D_{mon}{}^{crit}(\text{estimated}) = \text{cmc(Detergent)} \cdot x_D[\text{mic}]^{crit}$$

where cmc(Detergent) is the cmc value for the pure detergent and $x_D[\text{mic}]^{crit}$
typically has a value of ~ 0.7–0.75 for nonionic detergents, for which the
assumptions needed to derive the above formula are reasonable ones (6,
52, 97, 129, 170, 173).

Can the above conclusions readily be extrapolated to describe the solubilization of multicomponent lipid and lipid-protein bilayers? For mixed-
lipid bilayers, the answer is yes so long as the thermodynamics of detergent
interactions with the different lipid components are similar. In principle
this result is not assured because the lipids found in a typical membrane
vary in a number of properties, including hydrocarbon chain length, head-
group charge, hydration, and overall effective shape, that could affect their
partitioning between lipid-saturated mixed micelles and detergent-saturated
bilayers. Indeed, dispersions of different phospholipids in pure form appear
to differ significantly in their susceptibilities to solubilization by detergents
such as Triton X-100 (52, 87) and bile salts (201). Different lipids may also
be distributed differently between mixed micelles and coexisting bilayers
when a mixture of membrane lipids is partially solubilized with detergent
(21, 139, 229). However, in such partially solubilized systems, the ratios
($x_L[\text{mic}]/x_L[\text{lam}]$) for different lipid species typically vary over no more
than a twofold range. In general, the solubilization of a multicomponent
lipid bilayer by a detergent follows the overall scheme described above,
typically proceeding from initiation to completion over a range of deter-
gent/lipid ratios only slightly broader than that observed for solubilization
of a single-component lipid bilayer under similar conditions. Nonetheless,
some level of differential solubilization of particular lipids from membranes may be observed even when such lipids do not interact specifically
with other membrane components, such as membrane proteins (139).

Although the above discussion has focused on the thermodynamic
aspects of lipid bilayer solubilization, one should note that for some detergents and types of lipid dispersions the kinetics of solubilization are slow
enough to be an important factor in experimental design. Multilamellar
vesicles equilibrate slowly ($>$ hours) with many detergents, particularly at
low to moderate detergent/lipid ratios (8, 133, 159). Solubilization of
unilamellar structures by detergents is usually much faster ($<$ minutes) at
room temperature but may be markedly slower at low temperatures.
Finally, some membranes, such as the purple membrane of *Halobacterium
halobium*, are solubilized much more slowly than are simple lipid bilayers

even in the presence of high detergent concentrations (51). Therefore one must include time among the variables examined in optimizing the solubilization conditions for a given membrane protein.

Solubilization of Lipid-Protein Bilayers

Given that the fundamental structural unit of biological membranes is a lipid bilayer, we might anticipate that the solubilization of integral membrane proteins by detergents would simply follow the disruption of the lipid bilayer, resulting in essentially parallel solubilization of different protein and lipid species. This is indeed the case for some membrane systems such as the sarcoplasmic reticulum (178, 197) and may be observed for other membrane systems under conditions (low membrane concentrations, high cmc detergents, etc) where small variations in the total detergent concentration lead to large changes in the ratio of nonmonomeric detergent to lipid. In other cases, however, the progress of solubilization of different membrane components does not simply follow that of overall membrane disruption, and selective extraction of particular subsets of membrane proteins is sometimes possible under carefully controlled conditions (43, 102, 117, 131, 137, 182). As a result, the optimum conditions for solubilization of a given protein from a membrane should be determined by titration with the detergent(s) to be tested (90), a procedure that avoids the use of excessive levels of detergent and that often allows some degree of fractionation of the total membrane protein population.

Although the differential solubilization of various membrane proteins by detergents has to date been investigated mainly on an empirical basis, we can nonethless identify some potentially important determinants of such behavior. First (and most obviously), different proteins will dictate different optimal dimensions and organizations, and hence different overall free energies of formation, for the micelles into which they become incorporated. Second, membrane proteins may vary in the ease with which detergent molecules can compete with endogenous lipid molecules for solvation of the protein-lipid interface. While displacement of endogenous lipids by detergents from the protein surface is not essential for protein solubilization, the ease and extent of such substitution may significantly influence the optimal geometry and the overall free energy of formation of a protein-containing mixed micelle. Finally, the solubilization of many membrane proteins may entail perturbations of intra- and/or intermolecular protein-protein interactions, the magnitude of which will obviously influence the overall free energy of solubilization. For example, proteins that are normally anchored to a membrane-associated cytoskeleton (23, 151, 248), or that normally exist as oligomers too large to be accomodated as such in mixed micelles (116, 117), should be relatively resistant to solubilization from the membrane by detergents. Future experimental studies will hopefully provide more information to assess the relative importance of these and other factors in determining the differential detergent extractibility of different membrane proteins.

THE SOLUBILIZED STATE OF MEMBRANE PROTEINS

The development of a rational approach to the solubilization of functional membrane proteins requires consideration of detergent-protein as well as detergent-lipid interactions. The section below considers from a structural and physical perspective the interactions of membrane-solubilizing amphiphiles with membrane proteins, and those that follow consider the functional consequences of such interactions and some practical implications for membrane protein solubilization.

Interactions of Membrane Proteins with Solubilizing Amphiphiles

A first and obvious site for detergents to interact with membrane proteins is the lipid-protein interface. Detergents often compete with endogenous lipids for occupancy of the hydrophobic surfaces of integral membrane proteins, although this competition is often relatively inefficient. The most rudimentary evidence to support the latter conclusion is the common observation that cosolubilized samples of lipid, detergent, and various membrane proteins, when fractionated into protein-free and protein-containing micelles, typically show a greater ratio of lipid to detergent in the latter structures (29, 123, 125, 218). Direct studies of lipid-detergent competition at the protein-lipid interface (48, 63, 138, 235) have typically found that a very large molar excess of detergent over lipid is required to displace lipids extensively from the protein surface. This fact contrasts strikingly with the observation that phospholipids with different acyl chain and headgroup structures typically compete with similar affinities for association with most of the lipid-contacting sites on the surface of an integral membrane protein (53, 134). The relative inefficiency of some commonly used detergents in displacing membrane lipids from the lipid-protein interface suggests that the detergent molecules are a rather poor replacement for lipids, in terms of their fit to the hydrophobic protein surface. It remains to define clearly what structural differences between membrane lipids and common detergents (e.g. differences in polar groups, in hydrocarbon moieties, etc) are most important in determining the comparative inefficiency of binding of detergents to membrane proteins. Fortunately, the above results also indicate that a solubilized membrane protein can retain much of its complement of surface-associated lipids (which often stabilize the protein considerably) if excessive ratios of non-monomeric detergent to lipid are avoided. This fact is effectively exploited in some mild and very useful lipid-substitution procedures for membrane proteins (101, 240, 241).

Although a substantial body of evidence indicates that even "benign" detergents can perturb protein-protein as well as protein-lipid interactions, we are only beginning to elucidate the detailed nature and mechanisms of the former perturbations. Purely hydrophobic transmembrane α-helices are highly stable structural elements (168, 176), but certain other features of membrane protein structure may be considerably more sensitive to detergent disruption. A particularly acute (and largely unexplored) question is the degree to which detergents can perturb structurally important polar interactions within the membrane-embedded portions of membrane proteins (176). Ionic detergents, for example, by acting as lipophilic counterions, could in principle destabilize pairing of charged amino acids that may stabilize contacts between transmembrane α-helices in some membrane proteins (41, 78, 176). Transmembrane helices containing buried polar residues, and particularly membrane-traversing amphiphilic helices, may be generally more likely than purely hydrophobic helices to adopt an altered (e.g. interfacial) disposition when a protein is solubilized into micelles. The potential for these or other conformational changes in micellar environments is illustrated by demonstrations that various integral membrane proteins can undergo dramatic changes of conformation and/or state of association in different environments (44, 175, 195, 214).

While much fundamental information is still needed to predict and to characterize the effects of detergents on basic features of membrane protein structure, two emerging experimental approaches seem especially promising. The first is the three-dimensional crystallization of integral membrane proteins in the presence of detergents (118, 152, 196), which requires systematic evaluation of the details of detergent-protein interactions (71, 72, 152) and which in the case of the reaction center complexes of *Rhodopseudomonas viridis* and *Rhodobacter sphaeroides* has permitted direct visualization of the disposition of detergent around the crystallized protein molecules (195a, 196). A second promising approach to examining basic features of protein-protein interactions within membranes is through physical studies of the interactions between polypeptides or proteins with simple and well-characterized membrane-penetrating domains (26, 142, 176; M. A. Lemmon, B. Adair, B.-J. Bormann, C. E. Dempsey, J. M. Flanagan, et al, submitted). Such studies can provide much-needed basic information to describe, at both the thermodynamic and the structural level, the nature of intra- and intermolecular protein-protein interactions within the membrane interior and the effects of detergents (and other potential perturbants) on such interactions.

Stability of Detergent-Solubilized Proteins

The most perilous step in a reconstitution procedure is usually the passage of the protein through the solubilized state, which almost invariably entails a significant loss of recoverable protein activity. A few membrane proteins, of which bacteriorhodopsin is a classic example (135), can readily recover their native structures and functional properties when reconstituted even after apparently complete denaturation. Most membrane proteins, however, undergo irreversible inactivation at a finite rate, through denaturation and/or aggregation, when solubilized into detergent or detergent-lipid mixed micelles. The rate of inactivation typically increases with increases in either the experimental temperature (17, 49, 62, 109, 157, 219) or the ratio of detergent to lipid in the protein-containing micelles (1, 123, 138, 219). While the inactivated proteins themselves are sometimes characterized experimentally, the primary cause of the inactivation is often more difficult to identify. Nonetheless, some insights are emerging to define potential mechanisms of detergent inactivation of membrane proteins.

A first, very general way in which detergents may affect the stability of solubilized proteins is through perturbations of the physical properties of the protein environment. The extent of such perturbations depends not only on the physical properties of the detergent but also on the detergent/lipid ratio in the protein-containing micelles and on the intramicellar distribution of detergent molecules, which for some detergents may be highly nonrandom vis-à-vis the lipids (145, 158, 166). The fluidity of a micellar interior is often suggested to influence the rates and the amplitudes of conformational fluctuations within membrane proteins (153, 199), including those that may lead to irreversible loss of activity. The rate of denaturation of bleached rhodopsin, for example, is markedly different in micelles of different detergents and may reflect the fluidity of the micelle interior (49, 92), although other explanations for this apparent correlation have been suggested (16). Another general physical property of a micelle that may influence the stability of an incorporated protein is the surface charge, which may affect directly the conformational stability of a protein or modulate the binding to the protein of charged molecules that influence its stability. In practice, however, such generalized effects of micellar physical properties on the stability of a solubilized protein are often difficult to distinguish from the consequences of more direct detergent-protein interactions. The most readily identifiable perturbations of the latter type are those that lead to changes in the state of membrane protein oligomerization; some well-studied examples of these are discussed below.

The plasma membrane (Na,K)-ATPase from several vertebrate sources is generally thought to exist as an $\alpha_2\beta_2$ tetramer in its native state and can be solubilized in this form at moderate detergent/lipid ratios (14, 42, 82). However, in the presence of a large excess of alkyl poly(oxyethylene) detergents such as $C_{12}E_8$, an appreciable fraction of the protein behaves as an $\alpha\beta$ dimer in sedimentation or gel-filtration analyses (14, 42, 60–63, 83, 103). The putative dimeric ("protomeric") form of the dogfish rectal gland enzyme in these detergents is apparently capable of both ATP hydrolysis and occlusion of Rb^+ (61) but nonetheless appears to inactivate much more rapidly than the tetrameric form. Interestingly, it has been suggested that both the stabilizing effects of glycerol on the $C_{12}E_8$-solubilized (Na,K)-ATPase (60) and differences in the detergent stability of the enzyme from different sources (29, 60, 62, 103, 177) may be related to the ease of formation of the comparatively labile $\alpha\beta$ form.

Detergent-induced deoligomerization of several other membrane proteins may be responsible for the destabilization of these species in the solubilized state. Immunoprecipitation experiments have demonstrated a progressive (and not readily reversible) dissociation of the heterotetrameric basophil IgE receptor, the rate of which depends on both the detergent/lipid ratio and the nature of the detergent (109, 188). *Escherichia coli* phosphatidylserine decarboxylase is gradually dissociated, apparently irreversibly, from an active oligomer to an inactive monomer when exposed to high levels of certain detergents (e.g. bile salts) but not of others (such as Triton X-100). Interestingly, cross-linking of the functional oligomer reportedly stabilized the enzyme against the inactivating effects of detergents of the latter type (189). Various other membrane proteins, such as mitochondrial cytochrome *c* oxidase (192), cytochrome P-450 (47, 236, 237), and the sarcoplasmic reticulum Ca^{2+}-ATPase (10, 11, 123, 125, 157), also exhibit progressive deoligomerization at increasing detergent concentrations or detergent/lipid ratios. In these latter cases, however, deoligomerization has not been causally linked to decreased stability of the solubilized protein.

Increasing levels of detergent need not inherently favor the deoligomerization of membrane proteins. A trivial illustration of this statement is that detergent-promoted denaturation of a solubilized protein may favor subsequent (artifactual) protein aggregation (11, 90, 103, 143). In a more subtle example, a detergent that interacts efficiently with membrane lipids but less so with a membrane protein may promote self-association of the protein [including unphysiological aggregation (144)], without necessarily inducing denaturation. This effect can arise if the detergent reduces the thermodynamic activity of the lipids that normally solvate the protein's hydrophobic surface, yet fails to stabilize the surface with comparable effectiveness.

The structural bases of detergent-induced inactivation of membrane proteins are more difficult to assign when the critical perturbations occur within rather than between individual polypeptide chains. The detergent inactivation of some membrane proteins is accompanied by substantial and readily detectable changes in conformation (123, 146, 210). However, such changes need not occur inherently upon protein activation, and it is often difficult to prove that any specific structural change detected in an inactivated membrane protein represents the primary inactivation event rather than a subsequent structural transformation. Moreover, detergents may in principle perturb the conformational stability of membrane proteins by several distinct mechanisms, including modulation of environmental fluidity (see above), displacement from the protein surface of lipids needed to stabilize the protein structure (191, 219), or binding of detergent to the protein at sites not normally occupied by lipid (212). In the face of such complexities, it may be as useful to analyze the detergent inactivation of many membrane proteins from a thermodynamic perspective [e.g. as a detergent-induced exacerbation of the inherent thermolability of the protein of interest (79)] as from a mechanistic one.

Choice of Detergent and Solubilization Conditions

Although various detergents are now available in purities adequate for use in membrane protein solubilization and reconstitution, we still have no wholly rational basis for identifying a particular detergent or class of detergents a priori as optimal candidates for a given application. While in some cases various homologous membrane proteins [e.g. the β_2-adrenergic receptor and its homologues (127, 167, 181)] can be successfully solubilized using similar experimental conditions, in other cases different proteins from a homologous family, or even preparations of the same protein from different sources, can show sharply different patterns of stability in various detergents (29, 30, 62, 177). We therefore must consider efficient empirical strategies for identifying the most suitable detergent(s) for a given membrane-biochemical application, even as we seek to use physical principles like those discussed above to refine and focus such strategies.

The development of an effective solubilization-reconstitution protocol for a new membrane protein must begin (once a suitable functional assay is established) by screening multiple detergents with diverse structures and physical properties. Hjelmeland & Chrambach (90) present detailed practical suggestions for the design of an efficient screening procedure. Various short lists of detergents for such initial screenings have been suggested previously (e.g. 90); a minimal one would include CHAPS, cholate, digitonin, $C_{12}E_8$, and at least one alkyl glucoside [for many applications, decyl or lauryl maltoside is preferable to the more commonly used octyl glucoside (49, 190, 231)]. Charged and zwitterionic detergents with linear alkyl chains, and detergents with alkyl chains much shorter than those of normal membrane phospholipids (e.g. octyl glucoside) should generally be used with great caution, because for many proteins these species produce irreversible inactivation at concentrations very close to solubilizing levels (18, 113, 138, 180, 190). Detergents with relatively rigid apolar portions, such as the bile salts, CHAPS, and digitonin, have been suggested (with some supportive but not conclusive evidence) to be inherently more benign toward membrane proteins than are detergents with similar polar groups but flexible hydrocarbon chains, either because the former species promote a more ordered micellar environment (68, 92) or because such species associate less readily with protein surfaces (211, 240) and hence less readily disrupt critical lipid-protein or protein-protein interactions (16). Mixtures of detergents are frequently more effective in solubilizing functional proteins than are single detergents. Although possible combinations are limitless, in practice mixtures of nonionic detergents with bile salts (10, 106, 163, 174, 180, 211), and of digitonin [itself a mixture (89, 182)] with other nonionic detergents (217), have proven particularly advantageous for the solubilization and/or reconstitution of several membrane proteins.

The identification and optimization of other important experimental variables must of course accompany the selection of an effective detergent for solubilization of a membrane protein in order to maximize the stability of the solubilized protein. Such factors include: maintenance of moderate rather than high ratios of nonmonomeric detergent to lipid throughout the experimental protocol (see below); use of the lowest temperature compatible with efficient solubilization; maintenance throughout the protocol of adequate levels of detergent and/or lipid to avoid irreversible aggregation of the protein (24, 115, 230); the addition or the scrupulous removal of factors such as divalent cations or soluble ligands that interact specifically with the molecule of interest (36, 115, 157, 162, 172, 220, 221); the possible addition of soluble molecules that nonspecifically modulate protein stability, such as ethylene glycol, glycerol, or polyethylene glycol (73, 74, 157, 242); and maintenance of an adequate reducing potential (242). The ratio of nonmonomeric detergent to lipid can be particularly difficult to control properly, particularly when the experimental protocol involves dilute samples, high cmc detergents, or procedures such as chromatography or gradient centrifugation in detergent-containing media. A useful practice in such cases is to incorporate directly into the detergent stocks a defined mole fraction of cosolubilized phospholipid and/or sterol in order to buffer the system against excessive displacement of these components from the protein surface by detergent (1, 13, 17, 20, 28, 36, 55, 64, 127, 150, 161, 164, 187, 225, 245). Extensive replacement of the native lipid environment of a membrane protein by heterologous lipids is usually better accomplished by detergent-mediated lipid exchange (101, 241) rather than by extensive delipidation of the protein and subsequent readdition of lipids, which often leads to extensive protein inactivation.

REFORMATION OF LIPID-PROTEIN VESICLES

In the simplest case, the gradual and selective removal of detergent from a detergent-lipid-protein mixture should lead to reassociation of lipids and proteins in a sequence that is the mirror image of the solubilization process. This seldom occurs in practice. Equilibration in detergent-lipid-(protein) systems can be a relatively slow process, particularly as the mole fraction of detergent decreases to low levels. This fact can complicate efforts to achieve homogeneous reconstitutions of membrane proteins with lipids, but it also can permit the reconstitution of a given protein-lipid mixture into varied final states by judicious adjustment of experimental conditions.

Methods of Detergent Removal

Several methods have been employed for complete or partial removal of detergent from detergent-lipid-(protein) mixtures (69, 70). Most of these, such as simple dilution (96, 104, 180, 225), dialysis (10, 13, 36, 76, 95, 154, 187), gel filtration (31, 33, 113, 148, 154, 216), ultracentrifugation (101, 241), selective precipitation (176a), and ultrafiltration (70), remove amphiphiles in the form of monomers (or small aggregates) and hence are useful only for detergents with higher (mM) cmc values. In some cases, a low cmc detergent can be exchanged for a higher cmc detergent [e.g. through gel filtration (70), centrifugation (85), or hydrophobic exchange chromatography (69, 193)]. The higher cmc detergent can subsequently be removed using the methods described above. However, such procedures require optimization of several experimental parameters and prolong the total time that the protein is exposed to detergents. A more widely used method for the removal of low cmc detergents is the selective adsorption of the detergent on hydrophobic resins (29, 40, 80, 91, 128). Ideally, this method also selectively removes the detergent in its monomeric form, which is rapidly and efficiently sequestered by the hydrophobic beads when they are placed in direct contact with the detergent-lipid-(protein) sample. In practice, however, a significant amount of lipid and/or protein may also become adsorbed to the beads during reconstitution. This problem may sometimes be reduced by careful adjustment of the ratios of beads, detergent, and lipid employed (114, 128, 186); by preincubating the beads with phospholipids (115); or by exposing the sample to the beads repeatedly but for short times (114, 227).

Formation of Vesicles from Solubilized Components

The formation of lipid or lipid-protein vesicles upon detergent removal comprises three distinct aspects: the coalescence of mixed micelles of detergents, lipids, and proteins into larger structures as the proportion of detergent is reduced; the appearance at some stage of closed vesicular structures; and the subsequent (typically incomplete) equilibration of vesicle size and composition, through various mass-transfer processes, as detergent removal continues.

Even a simple solubilized lipid-protein-detergent dispersion represents a heterogeneous sample in which protein-containing micelles typically coexist with protein-free micelles, and neither micelle population is entirely homogeneous in size and composition. This heterogeneity is often reflected in the reconstitution process, in which different structures may coalesce at quite different stages of detergent removal or on quite different time scales. In practice, a major challenge in developing a successful reconstitution procedure is to identify conditions that yield a preparation of lipid-protein vesicles that is acceptably homogeneous in size and/or lipid/protein ratio (12, 65, 85, 95, 96).

How do small detergent-lipid-(protein) micelles coalesce during detergent removal to yield structures large enough to form lipid vesicles? In the simplest picture, oblate mixed micelles would grow in size and increase in axial ratio as their detergent/lipid ratio decreased, ultimately attaining an average size and composition that can support the formation of closed (vesicular) structures of comparable energy (120, 121, 244). At least two findings may complicate this simple picture for at least some lipid/detergent systems, however. First, the observation that distinct populations of mixed micelles and extended bilayers, with quite different compositions, can coexist in detergent-lipid mixtures suggests an element of critical behavior in the interconversions of these structures. Second, recent electron-microscopic and small-angle neutron-scattering studies suggest the formation of extended rod-like structures at intermediate detergent/lipid ratios in mixtures of egg phosphatidylcholine (egg PC) with octyl glucoside (232) or with cholate (88, 239), although no such structures have been observed in mixtures of egg PC with Triton X-100 (57). The potential importance (if any) of these or other structures as intermediates between mixed micelles and extended bilayers in these systems must be assessed, because detergent-lipid-protein mixed micelles may differ greatly from detergent-lipid micelles in their ability to integrate into such structures (202).

A second key step in the reconstitution process is the initial formation of closed (though typically somewhat leaky) lipid (protein) vesicles. Although the mechanisms of this process are not fully understood and may differ considerably for different detergent-lipid-protein systems, two general points are well-established. First, the formation of vesicles, particularly in heterogeneous (e.g. protein-containing) systems is seldom a truly concerted process. Not only does vesicle formation typically progress over a finite range of total detergent/lipid ratios, but membrane proteins may often incorporate into lipid vesicles after rather than during the initial formation of vesicles (32, 65, 66, 85, 95). Second, the vesicles first formed upon detergent removal are typically rather plastic structures that can undergo substantial further changes in their dimensions and/or composition, depending on the experimental conditions they encounter before they attain their final (meta)stable state. The practical importance of these two factors in the overall reconstitution process is discussed below.

The vesicular structures initially formed upon detergent removal from a micellar detergent-lipid (protein) sample can often equilibrate reasonably rapidly by intervesicular mass transfer (4, 6, 165, 249) so long as the level of residual detergent remains high. However, reduction of the level of vesicle-bound detergent usually strongly decreases the rates of such equilibration processes (4, 6) while simultaneously shifting the equilibrium dimensions and organization of the vesicles (5, 6, 94, 204, 215). In a practical reconstitution procedure, one often cannot reduce the detergent concentration slowly enough to follow faithfully this and other shifting equilibria (e.g. for vesicle-protein association) throughout the course of detergent removal. As a result, a final reconstituted membrane preparation seldom exists in a true equilibrium state. Instead, the character of the preparation will depend strongly on the rate and other conditions of sample passage through the range of detergent/lipid ratios where formation of closed vesicles is favored yet equilibration of materials between vesicles remains reasonably efficient. Variations in the conditions of this critical step can lead to major variations in vesicle size (4, 6, 154), heterogeneity (66, 95, 96), and asymmetry of protein orientation (32, 35, 65, 85) in the final reconstituted preparation.

Two well-studied examples illustrate the above points. The first is the generation of lipid vesicles by dilution of micellar cholate-lipid solutions. Rapid dilution of such solutions to very low cholate concentrations yields a stable population of relatively small vesicles. By contrast, less extensive dilution of similar cholate-lipid solutions leads to the formation of vesicles that subsequently grow, apparently through detergent-promoted intervesicle lipid exchange (4, 165), to yield relatively large vesicles that can then be freed of residual cholate without further change in size (4). A second illustrative example is that of the reconstitution of octyl glucoside-solubilized rhodopsin and lipid. Gradual dialysis of a micellar octyl glucoside-phospholipid-rhodopsin dispersion leads to the formation of vesicles with a very heterogeneous distribution of lipid/protein ratios (95), while rapid dilution of a similar sample leads to the formation of vesicles with a much more uniform distribution of protein (96). It has been suggested that the rapid removal of octyl glucoside by dilution may cause rhodopsin-containing and rhodopsin-free micelles to destabilize essentially simultaneously, and hence to assemble homogeneously into vesicles, while gradual removal of detergent allows the components of protein-containing and protein-free micelles to assemble into vesicles at different stages, yielding a more heterogeneous end-product (96). This second example [and others like it (65, 100)] points out that a more gradual removal of detergent from a solubilized lipid-protein system need not inherently favor formation of more homogeneous samples. In optimizing a new reconstitution protocol, the effects of varying rates of detergent removal on the character of the final preparation should be explored.

In many cases, it may be difficult to obtain reconstituted lipid-protein vesicles of adequate size and/or homogeneity simply by adjusting the experimental variables discussed above. One can often improve these characteristics of a reconstituted preparation by subjecting the sample to one or more freeze-thawing steps during or after detergent removal. Such treatments can be particularly advantageous in applications such as reconstitution of transport, where small vesicle size often limits the apparent activity of the final preparation (12, 17, 33, 108, 115, 147, 148, 243). Intervesicle fusion is the most easily identifiable consequence of freeze-thawing (169), but the process also clearly produces other, more subtle changes in the organization of protein-lipid mixtures. Although these may often be beneficial, the possibility of unfavorable perturbations of membrane protein structure (e.g. aggregation) by freeze-thawing should not be ignored.

A final aspect of most reconstitution protocols is the removal of residual detergent. Removal of all traces of detergent can be very difficult (particularly for low cmc detergents), and reconstituted preparations commonly contain some low but finite level of residual detergent that, one hopes, does not impair the functions or properties to be assayed. For some reconstitutions, an upper bound for the tolerable content of residual detergent may be estimated by determining the lowest mole fraction of bilayer-intercalated detergent (relative to membrane lipid) that detectably perturbs the function of interest in the native membrane. Bilayer-intercalated detergent molecules can affect the behavior of many membrane proteins at concentrations well below those producing solubilization (9, 27, 54, 141, 149), and even very low mole fractions of residual detergent can strongly influence some important physical properties of the lipid bilayer [e.g. permeability toward small molecules (19, 198, 226, 227, 247)]. An important question that arises in such cases is whether detergent removal becomes progressively more difficult, either for kinetic (226, 227) or for thermodynamic reasons (3), as the detergent content of the sample is reduced to low levels. Although the evidence on this point is mixed for pure lipid vesicles (3, 124, 128, 227), in principle, small amounts of detergent molecules can remain tenaciously associated with a reconstituted sample by binding strongly to a membrane protein.

Incorporation of Solubilized Proteins into Preformed Vesicles

Given the numerous factors that can affect the size and homogeneity of lipid-protein vesicles reconstituted from micellar dispersions, we should not be surprised that a variety of approaches have been explored to incorporate membrane proteins into preformed lipid vesicles. In early variations of this approach, a detergent-solubilized protein was combined with unilamellar lipid vesicles, then subjected to mechanical stress (freeze-thaw and/or sonication) before removal of the detergent (80, 107, 108, 115, 150). The mechanics of this process at the molecular level are actually quite complex. Upon mixing of solubilized protein with lipid vesicles, the protein-associated detergent redistributes to some extent into the lipid bilayers, modifying their ability to incorporate the protein (see below). Concomitantly, the partial removal of detergent from the protein may affect the protein's folding, aggregation state, or other properties that can influence its association with lipid bilayers. The reproducible success of such reconstitution procedures thus requires careful definition of several variables, including the relative concentrations of protein, detergent, and lipid in the solubilized protein preparation and in the protein-vesicle mixture; the oligomeric state(s) of the solubilized protein; and the conditions (time, temperature, etc) of protein-vesicle incubation and subsequent mechanical perturbation.

A recent variation of the above procedures is the spontaneous incorporation of solubilized membrane proteins into preformed lipid bilayers. Such incorporation, which has been reported for several membrane proteins, is often relatively inefficient when large liquid-crystalline phospholipid vesicles are used but is markedly enhanced when one uses small unilamellar vesicles or vesicles doped with amphipathic contaminants such as cholesterol, short-chain lecithins, detergents, lysolipids, fatty acids, or even previously incorporated proteins (38, 50, 56, 66, 67, 110, 185, 186,

195, 205–208, 213). The features of vesicle organization that promote incorporation of solubilized membrane proteins are sometimes described generically as "defects," a term that probably encompasses a variety of types of static instabilities and temporal fluctuations in lipid packing and bilayer curvature. Monomers and small aggregates of membrane proteins typically appear to associate with lipid vesicles more efficiently than do large aggregates.

Elucidation of the mechanisms of protein incorporation into preformed vesicles is important for an understanding of not only reconstitution procedures like the above but also reconstitutions of lipid-protein vesicles from initially micellar dispersions, in the course of which lipid vesicle formation may sometimes precede protein insertion (see above). The mechanisms of these processes remain to be characterized in detail and may differ considerably for different protein-lipid-detergent systems. One should first distinguish integration events in which large protein-lipid aggregates or protein-rich vesicles combine with lipid vesicles, in a process best analyzed as a fusion event (147), from those in which proteins insert into lipid (detergent) bilayers as monomers or small aggregates (67, 99). In the latter case, we may distinguish three possible stages of protein-bilayer association (75, 98, 105, 171): simple surface adsorption of individual proteins or protein aggregates, interfacial penetration by the adsorbed proteins, and transbilayer integration of the protein. Differentiating and quantitating the relative proportions of these three states for a given vesicle-associated protein preparation is experimentally demanding. Nonetheless, such information is essential for the further definition of the mechanisms of protein integration into bilayers and of the effects of variables such as vesicle composition and morphology, and the state of protein dispersal, on individual steps of the integration process (38, 59, 99). An important practical question is whether conditions that favor a high extent of stable protein association with vesicles are the same as (or at least compatible with) those that favor an optimal extent of proper transbilayer integration of the associated protein molecules.

Novel reconstitution strategies like the above inevitably raise the question of whether the reconstituted proteins achieve a native disposition in the vesicle membrane. Such questions are quite legitimate [and the answers are reassuring in some cases (38, 50, 185, 195, 207, 208, 213), though not in all (59)]. However, a similar healthy skepticism (and thorough experimental characterization) should be applied to evaluate the degree to which any reconstituted membrane protein approaches its native counterpart in situ (32). Numerous experimental tests may be required to verify what fraction of the protein molecules in a reconstituted preparation is native in terms of, for example, biochemical function(s), secondary and tertiary structure, the transmembrane topology of all protein segments, and the state of oligomeric assembly (subunits may become lost, scrambled, or even added during solubilization and reconstitution). Although a "perfect" reconstitution may not be required in many applications, one must never forget that most reconstituted preparations contain very significant fractions of nonnative protein molecules, whose potential effects on the behavior of the preparation must be carefully considered.

CONCLUDING REMARKS

A basic understanding of the interactions between membrane proteins, lipids, and detergents provides an indispensable basis to seek efficiently the optimal conditions for solubilization and reconstitution of a given membrane protein. Some important questions in this area are just beginning to be explored in detail, including: the microscopic structures of protein-(lipid)-detergent micelles, the intra- and interchain interactions that stabilize the membrane-penetrating portions of membrane proteins, the fundamental mechanisms by which lipid molecules reassemble with each other and with proteins during vesicle reconstitution, and the possibly extensive plasticity of the conformations and interactions of integral membrane proteins in nonmembraneous environments. New information from these areas may considerably refine the art of membrane protein reconstitution.

What is the future of classical membrane reconstitution when a variety of membrane proteins can be expressed in novel membrane contexts using molecular-biological methods? The latter approach clearly offers a powerful alternative to reconstitution for assigning particular biochemical and biological functions to individual protein species. However, by its ability to simplify and to control almost arbitrarily the environment in which a membrane protein is incorporated, the reconstitution approach offers unique advantages for studies of membrane protein structure, of modulatory effects of the membrane environment on membrane protein behavior, and of the sometimes complex interactions between membrane components that effect or regulate many membrane functions. As the known repertoire (and, through genetic engineering, the availability) of natural and mutated membrane proteins steadily expands, so will our need for efficient, reliable methods for manipulating and reconstituting them.

ACKNOWLEDGMENTS

I thank Drs. Dov Lichtenberg, Burton Litman, Anthony Scotto, and Anne Walter for useful discussions, Donald Engelman and Anne Walter for providing relevant manuscripts prior to publication, and Anne Walter and Anthony Scotto for critically reading the manuscript. This work was supported in part by a Scientist award to the author from the Medical Research Council of Canada, which is gratefully acknowledged.

Literature Cited

1. Agnew, W. S., Raftery, M. A. 1979. *Biochemistry* 18: 1912
2. Alcaraz, G., Kinet, J.-P., Kumar, N., Wank, S. A., Metzger, H. 1984. *J. Biol. Chem.* 259: 14922
3. Allen, T. M., Romans, A. Y., Kercret, H., Segrest, J. P. 1980. *Biochim. Biophys. Acta* 601: 328
4. Almog, S., Kushnir, T., Nir, S., Lichtenberg, D. 1986. *Biochemistry* 25: 2597
5. Almog, S., Lichtenberg, D. 1988. *Biochemistry* 27: 873
6. Almog, S., Litman, B. J., Wimley, W., Cohen, J., Wachtel, E. J., et al. 1990. *Biochemistry* 29: 4582
7. Alonso, A., Sáez, R., Villena, A., Goñi, F. M. 1982. *J. Membrane Biol.* 67: 55
8. Alonso, A., Urbaneja, M.-A., Goñi, F. M., Carmona, F. G., Cánovas, F. G., Gómez-Fernández, J. C. 1987. *Biochim. Biophys. Acta* 902: 237
9. Andersen, J. P., le Maire, M., Kragh-Hansen, U., Champeil, P., Moller, J. V. 1983. *Eur. J. Biochem.* 134: 205
10. Andersen, J. P., Skriver, E., Mahrous, T. S., Moller, J. V. 1983. *Biochim. Biophys. Acta* 728: 1
11. Andersen, J. P., Vilsen, B., Nielsen, H., Moller, J. V. 1986. *Biochemistry* 25: 6439
12. Anholt, R., Fredkin, D. R., Deerinck, T., Ellisman, M., Montal, M., Lindstrom, J. 1982. *J. Biol. Chem.* 257: 7122
13. Anholt, R., Lindstrom, J., Montal, M. 1981. *J. Biol. Chem.* 256: 4377
14. Anner, B. M. 1985. *Biochim. Biophys. Acta* 822: 319
15. Ashani, Y., Catravas, G. N. 1980. *Anal. Biochem.* 109: 55
16. Baker, B. N., Donovan, W. J., Williams, T. P. 1977. *Vision Res.* 17: 1157
17. Baldwin, S. A., Baldwin, J. M., Lienhard, G. E. 1982. *Biochemistry* 21: 3836
18. Banerjee, R., Epstein, M., Kandrach, M., Zimniak, P., Racker, E. 1979. *Membr. Biochem.* 2: 283
19. Bangham, J. A., Lea, E. J. A. 1978. *Biochim. Biophys. Acta* 511: 388
20. Barchi, R. L., Cohen, S. A., Murphy, L. E. 1980. *Proc. Natl. Acad. Sci. USA* 77: 1306
21. Bayerl, T., Klose, G., Blanck, J., Ruck-

paul, K. 1986. *Biochim. Biophys. Acta* 858: 285
22. Becker, R., Helenius, A., Simons, K. 1975. *Biochemistry* 14: 1835
23. Ben-Ze'ev, A., Duerr, A., Solomon, F., Penman, S. 1979. *Cell* 17: 859
24. Beyer, K., Klingenberg, M. 1983. *Biochemistry* 22: 639
25. Bordier, C. 1981. *J. Biol. Chem.* 256: 160
26. Bormann, B.-J., Knowles, W. J., Marchesi, V. T. 1989. *J. Biol. Chem.* 264: 4033
27. Briley, M. S., Changeux, J.-P. 1978. *Eur. J. Biochem.* 84: 429
28. Bristow, D. R., Martin, I. L. 1987. *J. Neurochem.* 49: 1386
29. Brotherus, J. R., Jacobsen, L., Jorgensen, P. L. 1983. *Biochim. Biophys. Acta* 731: 290
30. Brotherus, J. R., Jost, P. C., Griffith, O. H., Hokin, L. E. 1979. *Biochemistry* 18: 5043
31. Brunner, J., Skrabal, P., Hauser, H. 1976. *Biochim. Biophys. Acta* 455: 322
32. Cardoza, J. D., Kleinfeld, A. M., Stallcup, K. C., Mescher, M. F. 1984. *Biochemistry* 23: 4401
33. Carter-Su, C., Pillion, D. J., Czech, M. P. 1980. *Biochemistry* 19: 2374
34. Casey, R. P. 1984. *Biochim. Biophys. Acta* 768: 319
35. Casey, R. P., Ariano, B. H., Azzi, A. 1982. *Eur. J. Biochem.* 122: 313
36. Catterall, W. A., Morrow, L. C., Hartshorne, R. P. 1979. *J. Biol. Chem.* 254: 11379
37. Chang, H. W., Bock, E. 1980. *Anal. Biochem.* 104: 112
38. Christiansen, K., Carlsen, J. 1985. *Biochim. Biophys. Acta* 815: 215
39. Clint, J. H. 1975. *J. Chem. Soc. Far. Trans* 71: 1327
40. Cornelius, F., Skou, J. C. 1984. *Biochim. Biophys. Acta* 772: 357
41. Cosson, P., Lankford, S. P., Bonifacino, J. S., Klausner, R. D. 1991. *Nature* 351: 414
42. Craig, W. S. 1982. *Biochemistry* 21: 2667
43. Cunningham, K., Wickner, W. T. 1989. *Proc. Natl. Acad. Sci. USA* 86: 8673

44. Curman, B., Klareskog, L., Peterson, P. A. 1980. *J. Biol. Chem.* 255: 7820
45. Davis, A. 1984. See Ref 231a, p. 161
46. deGraça Miguel, M., Eidelman, O., Ollivon, M., Walter, A. 1989. *Biochemistry* 28: 8921
47. Dean, W. L., Gray, R. D. 1982. *J. Biol. Chem.* 257: 14679
48. de Foresta, B., le Maire, M., Orlowski, S., Champeil, P., Lund, S., et al. 1989. *Biochemistry* 28: 2558
49. de Grip, W. 1982. *Methods Enzymol.* 81: 256
50. Dencher, N. A. 1986. *Biochemistry* 25: 1195
51. Dencher, N. A., Heyn, M. P. 1978. *FEBS Lett.* 96: 322
52. Dennis, E. A. 1974. *Arch. Biochem. Biophys.* 165: 764
53. Devaux, P. F., Seigneuret, M. 1985. *Biochim. Biophys. Acta* 822: 63
54. Dhariwal, M. S., Jefcoate, C. R. 1989. *Biochemistry* 28: 8397
55. Driessen, A. J. M., Wickner, W. T. 1990. *Proc. Natl. Acad. Sci. USA* 87: 3107
56. Dufour, J.-P., Nunnally, R., Buhle, L. Jr., Tsong, T. Y. 1981. *Biochemistry* 20: 5576
57. Edwards, K., Almgren, M., Bellare, J., Brown, W. 1989. *Langmuir* 5: 473
58. Eidelman, O., Blumenthal, R., Walter, A. 1988. *Biochemistry* 27: 2839
59. Enoch, H. G., Fleming, P. J., Strittmatter, P. 1979. *J. Biol. Chem.* 254: 6483
60. Esmann, M. 1984. *Biochim. Biophys. Acta* 787: 81
61. Esmann, M. 1985. *Biochim. Biophys. Acta* 815: 196
62. Esmann, M. 1986. *Biochim. Biophys. Acta* 857: 38
63. Esmann, M., Skou, J. C. 1984. *Biochim. Biophys. Acta* 787: 71
64. Evans, E. A., Gilmore, R., Blobel, G. 1986. *Proc. Natl. Acad. Sci. USA* 83: 581
65. Eytan, G. D. 1982. *Biochim. Biophys. Acta* 694: 185
66. Eytan, G. D., Broza, R. 1978. *FEBS Lett.* 85: 175
67. Eytan, G., Matheson, M. J., Racker, E. 1975. *FEBS Lett.* 57: 121
68. Fisher, L., Oakenfull, D. 1979. *Aust. J. Chem.* 32: 31
69. Furth, A. J. 1980. *Anal. Biochem.* 109: 205
70. Furth, A. J., Bolton, H., Potter, J., Priddle, J. D. 1984. *Methods Enzymol.* 104: 318
71. Garavito, R. M., Hinz, U., Neuhaus, J.-M. 1984. *J. Biol. Chem.* 259: 42
72. Garavito, R. M., Jenkins, J., Jansonius, J. N., Karlsson, R., Rosenbusch, J. P.

1983. *J. Mol Biol.* 164: 313
73. Gekko, K., Timasheff, S. 1981. *Biochemistry* 20: 4667
74. Gekko, K., Timasheff, S. 1981. *Biochemistry* 20: 4677
75. Gennis, R. B. 1989. *Biomembranes: Molecular Structure and Function.* New York: Springer-Verlag
76. Goldin, S. M. 1977. *J. Biol. Chem.* 252: 5630
77. Goñi, F. M., Urbaneja, M.-A., Arrondo, J. L. R., Alonso, A., Durrani, A. A., Chapman, D. 1986. *Eur. J. Biochem.* 160: 659
78. Green, N. M. 1991. *Nature* 351: 349
79. Gruber, H. J., Low, P. S. 1988. *Biochim. Biophys. Acta* 944: 414
80. Haaker, H., Racker, E. 1979. *J. Biol. Chem.* 254: 6598
81. Hanatani, M., Nishifuji, K., Futai, M., Tsuchiya, T. 1984. *J. Biochem.* 95: 1349
82. Hastings, D. F., Reynolds, J. A. 1979. *Biochemistry* 18: 817
83. Hayashi, Y., Takagi, T., Maezawa, S., Matsui, H. 1983. *Biochim. Biophys. Acta* 748: 153
84. Helenius, A., McCaslin, D. R., Fries, E., Tanford, C. 1979. *Methods Enzymol.* 56: 734
85. Helenius, A., Sarvas, M., Simons, K. 1981. *Eur. J. Biochem.* 116: 27
86. Helenius, A., Simons, K. 1975. *Biochim. Biophys. Acta* 415: 29
87. Hertz, R., Barenholz, Y. 1977. *J. Colloid Interface Sci.* 60: 188
88. Hjelm, R. P., Alkan, M. H., Thiyagarajan, P. 1990. *Mol. Cryst. Liq. Cryst.* 180A: 155
89. Hjelmeland, L. M. 1986. *Methods Enzymol.* 124: 135
90. Hjelmeland, L. M., Chrambach, A. 1984. *Methods Enzymol.* 104: 305
91. Holloway, P. W. 1973. *Anal. Biochem.* 53: 301
92. Hong, K., Hubbell, W. L. 1973. *Biochemistry* 12: 4517
93. Israelachvili, J. N., Mitchell, D. J., Ninham, B. W. 1976. *J. Chem. Soc. Faraday Trans.* II 72: 1525
94. Israelachvili, J. N., Mitchell, D. J., Ninham, B. W. 1977. *Biochim. Biophys. Acta* 470: 185
95. Jackson, M. L., Litman, B. J. 1982. *Biochemistry* 21: 5601
96. Jackson, M. L., Litman, B. J. 1985. *Biochim. Biophys. Acta* 812: 369
97. Jackson, M. L., Schmidt, C. F., Lichtenberg, D., Litman, B. J., Albert, A. D. 1982. *Biochemistry* 21: 4576
98. Jacobs, R. E., White, S. H. 1989. *Biochemistry* 28: 3421
99. Jain, M. K., Zakim, D. 1987. *Biochim. Biophys. Acta* 906: 33

100. Jones, O. T., Earnest, J. P., McNamee, M. G. 1987. In *Biological Membranes*: *A Practical Approach*, ed. J. B. C. Findlay, W. H. Evans, p. 197. London: IRL
101. Jones, O. T., Eubanks, J. H., Earnest, J. P., McNamee, M. G. 1988. *Biochim. Biophys. Acta* 944: 359
102. Jorgensen, P. L. 1974. *Biochim. Biophys. Acta* 356: 36
103. Jorgensen, P. L., Andersen, J. P. 1986. *Biochemistry* 25: 2889
104. Kagawa, Y., Racker, E. 1971. *J. Biol. Chem.* 246: 5477
105. Kaiser, E. T., Kezdy, F. J. 1987. *Annu. Rev. Biophys. Biophys. Chem.* 16: 561
106. Kanner, B. I. 1978. *FEBS Lett.* 89: 47
107. Karlish, S. J. D., Pick, U. 1981. *J. Physiol. London* 312: 505
108. Kasahara, M., Hinkle, P. C. 1977. *J. Biol. Chem.* 252: 7384
109. Kinet, J.-P., Alcaraz, G., Leonard, A., Wank, S., Metzger, H. 1985. *Biochemistry* 24: 4117
110. Klausner, R. D., Bridges, K., Tsunoo, H., Blumenthal, R., Weinstein, J. N., Ashwell, G. 1980. *Proc. Natl. Acad. Sci. USA* 77: 5087
111. Klausner, R. D., van Renswoude, J., Blumenthal, R., Rivnay, B. 1984. See Ref. 231a, p. 209
112. Klausner, R. D., van Renswoude, J., Rivnay, B. 1984. *Methods Enzymol.* 104: 340
113. Konigsberg, P. J. 1982. *Biochim. Biophys. Acta* 685: 355
114. Krämer, R., Heberger, C. 1986. *Biochim. Biophys. Acta* 863: 289
115. Krämer, R., Klingenberg, M. 1979. *Biochemistry* 18: 4209
116. Kreibich, G., Ojakian, G., Rodriguez-Boulan, E., Sabatini, D. D. 1982. *J. Cell. Biol.* 93: 111
117. Kreibich, G., Ulrich, B. L., Sabatini, D. D. 1978. *J. Cell Biol.* 77: 464
118. Kühlbrandt, W. 1988. *Q. Rev. Biophys.* 21: 429
119. Lasch, J., Hoffmann, J., Omelyanenko, W. G., Klibanov, A. A., Torchilin, V. P., et al. 1990. *Biochim. Biophys. Acta* 1022: 171
120. Lasic, D. D. 1982. *Biochim. Biophys. Acta* 692: 501
121. Lasic, D. D. 1988. *Biochem. J.* 256: 1
122. Lefkowitz, R. J., Cerione, R. A., Codina, J., Birnbaumer, L., Caron, M. G. 1985. *J. Membr. Biol.* 87: 1
123. le Maire, M., Lind, K. E., Jorgensen, K. A., Roigaard, H., Moller, J. V. 1978. *J. Biol. Chem.* 253: 7051
124. le Maire, M., Moller, J. V., Champeil, P. 1987. *Biochemistry* 26: 4803
125. le Maire, M., Moller, J. V., Tanford, C. 1976. *Biochemistry* 15: 2336
126. Deleted in proof
127. Levitzki, A. 1985. *Biochim. Biophys. Acta* 822: 127
128. Lévy, D., Bluzat, A., Seigneuret, M., Rigaud, J.-L. 1990. *Biochim. Biophys. Acta* 1025: 179
129. Lévy, D., Gulik, A., Seigneuret, M., Rigaud, J.-L. 1990. *Biochemistry* 29: 9480
130. Lichtenberg, D. 1985. *Biochim. Biophys. Acta* 821: 470
131. Lichtenberg, D., Robson, R. J., Dennis, E. A. 1983. *Biochim. Biophys. Acta* 737: 285
132. Lichtenberg, D., Yedgar, S., Cooper, G., Gatt, S. 1979. *Biochemistry* 18: 2574
133. Lichtenberg, D., Zilberman, Y., Greenzaid, P., Zamir, S. 1979. *Biochemistry* 18: 3517
134. London, E., Feigenson, G. W. 1981. *Biochemistry* 20: 1939
135. London, E., Khorana, H. G. 1982. *J. Biol. Chem.* 257: 7003
136. Lorber, B., Bishop, J. B., DeLucas, L. J. 1990. *Biochim. Biophys. Acta* 1023: 254
137. Lund, H. 1987. *Biochim. Biophys. Acta* 918: 67
138. Lund, S., Orlowski, S., de Foresta, B., Champeil, P., le Maire, M., Moller, J. V. 1989. *J. Biol. Chem.* 264: 4907
139. MacDonald, R. I. 1980. *Biochemistry* 19: 1916
140. Maher, P. A, Singer, S. J. 1985. *Proc. Natl. Acad. Sci. USA* 82: 958
141. Mandersloot, J. G., Roelofsen, B., de Gier, J. 1978. *Biochim. Biophys. Acta* 508: 478
142. Maniolos, N., Bonifacino, J. S., Klausner, R. D. 1990. *Science* 249: 274
143. Martin, D. W. 1983. *Biochemistry* 22: 2276
144. Mascher, E., Lundahl, P. 1987. *J. Chromatogr.* 397: 175
145. Mazer, N. A., Benedek, G. B., Carey, M. C. 1980. *Biochemistry* 19: 601
146. McCaslin, D. R., Tanford, C. 1981. *Biochemistry* 20: 5212
147. McCormick, J. I., Silvius, J. R., Johnstone, R. M. 1985. *J. Biol. Chem.* 260: 5706
148. McCormick, J. I., Tsang, D., Johnstone, R. M. 1984. *Arch. Biochem. Biophys.* 231: 355
149. McIntosh, D. B., Davidson, G. A. 1984. *Biochemistry* 23: 1959
150. Mende, P., Kolbe, H. V. J., Kadenbach, B., Stipani, I., Palmieri, F. 1982. *Eur. J. Biochem.* 128: 91
151. Mescher, M. F., Jose, M. J. L., Balle, S. P. 1981. *Nature* 289: 139

152. Michel, H. 1983. *Trends Biochem. Sci.* 8: 56
153. Milder, S. J., Thorgeirsson, T. E., Miercke, L. J. W., Stroud, R. M., Kliger, D. S. 1991. *Biochemistry* 30: 1751
154. Mimms, L. T., Zampighi, G., Nozaki, Y., Tanford, C., Reynolds, J. A. 1981. *Biochemistry* 20: 833
155. Mittal, K. L., ed. 1977. *Micellization, Solubilization and Microemulsions*, Vols. 1, 2. New York: Plenum
156. Moller, J. V., le Maire, M., Andersen, J. P. 1986. In *Progress in Lipid-Protein Interactions*, ed. A. Watts, J. J. H. H. M. de Pont, 2: 147. Amsterdam: Elsevier
157. Moller, J. V., Lind, K. E., Andersen, J. P. 1980. *J. Biol. Chem.* 255: 1912
158. Müller, K. 1981. *Biochemistry* 20: 404
159. Müller, K., Schuster, A. 1990. *Chem. Phys. Lipids* 52: 111
160. Nakagawa, T. 1967. In *Non-Ionic Surfactants*, ed. J. J. Schick, p. 558. New York: Marcel Dekker
161. Naldini, L., Cirillo, D., Moody, T. W., Comoglio, P. M., Schlessinger, J., Kris, R. 1990. *Biochemistry* 29: 5153
162. Nedivi, E., Schramm, M. 1984. *J. Biol. Chem.* 259: 5803
163. Newby, A. C., Crambach, A. 1979. *Biochem. J.* 177: 623
164. Newman, M. J., Wilson, T. H. 1980. *J. Biol. Chem.* 255: 10583
165. Nichols, J. W. 1986. *Biochemistry* 25: 4596
166. Nichols, J. W., Ozarowski, J. 1990. *Biochemistry* 29: 4600
167. Niznik, H. B., Otsuka, N. Y., Dumbrille-Ross, A., Grigoriadis, D., Tirpak, A., Seeman, P. 1986. *J. Biol. Chem.* 261: 8397
168. Nozawa, T., Ohta, M., Hatano, M., Hayashi, H., Shimada, K. 1986. *Biochim. Biophys. Acta* 850: 343
169. Oku, N., MacDonald, R. C. 1983. *Biochemistry* 22: 855
170. Ollivon, M., Eidelman, O., Blumenthal, R., Walter, A. 1988. *Biochemistry* 27: 1695
171. Papahadjopoulos, D., Moscarello, M., Eylar, E. H., Isac, T. 1975. *Biochim. Biophys. Acta* 401: 317
172. Parries, G. S., Hokin-Neaverson, M. 1984. *Biochemistry* 23: 4785
173. Paternostre, M.-T., Roux, M., Rigaud, J.-L. 1988. *Biochemistry* 27: 2668
174. Peterson, G. L., Schimerlik, M. I. 1984. *Prep. Biochem.* 14: 33
175. Petri, W. A. Jr., Wagner, R. R. 1979. *J. Biol. Chem.* 254: 4313
176. Popot, J.-L., Engelman, D. M. 1990. *Biochemistry* 29: 4031
176a. Popot, J.-L., Gerchman, S.-E., Engel-man, D. E. 1987. *J. Mol. Biol.* 198: 655
177. Powell, L. D., Cantley, L. C. 1980. *Biochim. Biophys. Acta* 599: 436
178. Prado, A., Arrondo, J. L. R., Villena, A., Goñi, F. M., Macarulla, J. M. 1983. *Biochim. Biophys. Acta* 733: 163
179. Racker, E. 1979. *Methods Enzymol.* 55: 699
180. Racker, E., Violand, B., O'Neal, S., Alfonzo, M., Telford, J. 1979. *Arch. Biochem. Biophys.* 198: 470
181. Regan, J. W., Nakata, H., DeMarinis, R. M., Caron, M. G., Lefkowitz, R. J. 1986. *J. Biol. Chem.* 261: 3894
182. Repke, H. 1987. *Biochim. Biophys. Acta* 929: 47
183. Reynolds, J. A., McCaslin, D. R. 1985. *Methods Enzymol.* 117: 41
184. Ribeiro, A. A., Dennis, E. A. 1974. *Chem. Phys. Lipids* 12: 31
185. Richard, P., Rigaud, J.-L., Gräber, P. 1990. *Eur. J. Biochem.* 193: 921
186. Rigaud, J.-L., Paternostre, M.-T., Bluzat, A. 1988. *Biochemistry* 27: 2677
187. Rivnay, B., Metzger, H. 1982. *J. Biol. Chem.* 257: 12800
188. Rivnay, B., Wank, S. A., Poy, G., Metzger, H. 1982. *Biochemistry* 21: 6922
189. Rizzolo, L. J. 1981. *Biochemistry* 20: 868
190. Robinson, N. C., Neumann, J., Wiginton, D. 1985. *Biochemistry* 24: 6298
191. Robinson, N. C., Strey, F., Talbert, L. 1980. *Biochemistry* 19: 3656
192. Robinson, N. C., Talbert, L. 1986. *Biochemistry* 25: 2328
193. Robinson, N. C., Wiginton, D., Talbert, L. 1984. *Biochemistry* 23: 6121
194. Robson, R. J., Dennis, E. A. 1978. *Biochim. Biophys. Acta* 508: 513
195. Roepe, P. D., Kaback, H. R. 1990. *Biochemistry* 29: 2572
195a. Roth, M., Arnoux, B., Ducruix, A., Reiss-Husson, F. 1991. *Biochemistry* 30: 9403
196. Roth, M., Lewit-Bentley, A., Michel, H., Deisenhofer, J., Huber, R., Oesterhelt, D. 1989. *Nature* 340: 659
197. Roux, M., Champeil, P. 1984. *FEBS Lett.* 171: 169
198. Ruiz, J., Goñi, F. M., Alonso, A. 1988. *Biochim. Biophys. Acta* 937: 127
199. Schleicher, A., Franke, R., Hofmann, K. P., Finkelmann, H., Welte, W. 1987. *Biochemistry* 26: 5908
200. Schubert, R., Beyer, K., Wolburg, H., Schmidt, K.-H. 1986. *Biochemistry* 25: 5263
201. Schubert, R., Schmidt, K.-H. 1988. *Biochemistry* 27: 8787
202. Schürholz, T., Gieselmann, A., Neu-

mann, E. 1989. *Biochim. Biophys. Acta*
986: 225

203. Schurtenberger, P., Bertani, R.,
Känzig, W. 1986. *J. Colloid Interface
Sci.* 114: 82

204. Schurtenberger, P., Mazer, N., Känzig,
W. 1985. *J. Phys. Chem.* 89: 1042

205. Scotto, A. W., Gompper, M. E. 1990.
Biochemistry 29: 7244

206. Scotto, A. W., Goodwyn, D., Zakim,
D. 1987. *Biochemistry* 26: 833

207. Scotto, A. W., Zakim, D. 1985. *Biochemistry* 24: 4066

208. Scotto, A. W., Zakim, D. 1986. *Biochemistry* 25: 1555

209. Shankland, W. 1970. *Chem. Phys.
Lipids* 4: 109

210. Shichi, H., Lewis, M. S., Irreverre, F.,
Stone, A. L. 1969. *J. Biol. Chem.* 244:
529

211. Silvius, J. R., McMillen, D. A., Saley,
N. D., Jost, P. C., Griffith, O. H. 1984.
Biochemistry 23: 538

212. Simmonds, A. C., East, J. M., Jones,
O. T., Rooney, E. K., McWhirter, J.,
Lee, A. G. 1982. *Biochim. Biophys. Acta*
693: 398

213. Simon-Plas, F., Venema, K., Grouzis,
J.-P., Gibrat, R., Rigaud, J., Grignon,
C. 1991. *J. Membr. Biol.* 120: 51

214. Simons, K., Helenius, A., Leonard, K.,
Sarvas, M., Gething, M. J. 1978. *Proc.
Natl. Acad. Sci USA* 75: 5306

215. Stark, R. E., Gosselin, G. J., Donovan,
J. M., Carey, M. C., Roberts, M. F.
1985. *Biochemistry* 24: 5599

216. Stoffel, W., Zierenberg, O., Scheefers,
M. 1977. *Hoppe-Seyler's Z. Phys.
Chem.* 358: 865

217. Strauss, W. L., Ghai, G., Fraser, C.
M., Venter, J. C. 1979. *Arch. Biochem.
Biophys.* 196: 566

218. Stubbs, G. W., Litman, B. J. 1978. *Biochemistry* 17: 215

219. Stubbs, G. W., Litman, B. J. 1978. *Biochemistry* 17: 220

220. Sussman, M. L., Hays, J. B. 1977.
Biochim. Biophys. Acta 465: 559

221. Swoboda, G., Hasselbach, W. 1988.
Eur. J. Biochem. 172: 325

222. Taguchi, T., Kasai, M. 1983. *Biochim.
Biophys. Acta* 729: 229

223. Tanford, C. 1980. *The Hydrophobic
Effect: Formation of Micelles and Bio-
logical Membranes.* New York: Wiley-
Interscience. 2nd ed.

224. Tanford, C., Reynolds, J. A. 1976.
Biochim. Biophys. Acta 457: 133

225. Tokuda, H., Shiozuka, K., Mizushima,
S. 1990. *Eur. J. Biochem.* 192: 583

226. Ueno, M. 1987. *Biochim. Biophys. Acta*
904: 140

227. Ueno, M., Tanford, C., Reynolds, J. A.
1984. *Biochemistry* 23: 3070

228. Urbaneja, M.-A., Goñi, F. M., Alonso,
A. 1988. *Eur. J. Biochem.* 173: 585

229. Urbaneja, M. A., Nieva, J. L., Goñi, F.
M., Alonso, A. 1987. *Biochim. Biophys.
Acta* 904: 337

230. Valpuesta, J. M., Arrondo, J.-L. R.,
Barbero, M. C., Pons, M., Goñi, F. M.
1986. *J. Biol. Chem.* 261: 6578

231. VanAken, T., Foxall-VanAken, S.,
Castleman, S., Ferguson-Miller, S.
1986. *Methods Enzymol.* 125: 27

231a. Venter, J. C., Harrison, L. C. eds.
1984. *Molecular and Chemical Characterization of Membrane Receptors.*
New York: Liss

232. Vinson, P. K., Talmon, Y., Walter, A.
1989. *Biophys. J.* 56: 669

233. van Renswoude, J., Kempf, C. 1984.
Methods Enzymol. 104: 329

234. Volk, T., Geiger, B. 1986. *J. Cell Biol.*
103: 1441

235. Volwerk, J. J., Mrsny, R. J., Patapoff,
T. W., Jost, P. C., Griffith, O. H. 1987.
Biochemistry 26: 466

236. Wagner, S. L., Dean, W. L., Gray, R.
D. 1984. *J. Biol. Chem.* 259: 2390

237. Wagner, S. L., Gray, R. D. 1985. *Biochemistry* 24: 3809

238. Walter, A., Suchy, S. E., Vinson, P. K.
1990. *Biochim. Biophys. Acta* 1029: 67

239. Walter, A., Vinson, P. K., Kaplan, A.,
Talmon, Y. 1991. *Biophys. J.* 60: 1315–
25

240. Warren, G. B., Houslay, M. D., Metcalfe, J. C., Birdsall, N. J. M. 1975.
Nature 255: 684

241. Warren, G. B., Toon, P. A., Birdsall,
N. J. M., Lee, A. G., Metcalfe, J. C.
1974. *Proc. Natl. Acad. Sci. USA* 71:
622

242. Welte, W., Leonhard, M., Diederichs,
K., Weltzien, H.-U., Restall, C., Hall,
C., Chapman, D. 1989. *Biochim.
Biophys. Acta* 984: 193

243. Wright, J. K., Schwarz, H., Straub, E.,
Overath, P., Bieseler, B., Beyreuther,
K. 1982. *Eur. J. Biochem.* 124: 545

244. Wrigglesworth, J. M., Wooster, M. S.,
Elsden, J., Danneel, H.-J. 1987.
Biochem. J. 246: 737

245. YaDeau, J. T., Blobel, G. 1989. *J. Biol.
Chem.* 264: 2928

246. Yoshioka, H. 1987. *J. Colloid Interface
Sci.* 119: 371

247. Young, M., Dinda, M., Singer, M.
1983. *Biochim. Biophys. Acta* 735: 429

248. Yu, J., Fischman, D. A., Steck, T. L.
1973. *J. Supramol. Struct.* 1: 233

249. Zwizinski, C., Wickner, W. 1977.
Biochim. Biophys. Acta 471: 169

Annu. Rev. Biophys. Biomol. Struct. 1992. 21:349–77

PATHWAY ANALYSIS OF PROTEIN ELECTRON-TRANSFER REACTIONS

José Nelson Onuchic[1]

Department of Physics, University of California, San Diego, La Jolla, California 92093

David N. Beratan[2]

Jet Propulsion Laboratory, California Institute of Technology, Pasadena, California 91109, and Beckman Institute, California Institute of Technology, Pasadena, California 91125

Jay R. Winkler and Harry B. Gray

Beckman Institute, California Institute of Technology, Pasadena, California 91125

KEY WORDS: electron-tunneling pathways, electron coupling, ruthenium-modified proteins, cytochrome *c*, myoglobin

CONTENTS

[1] This review was begun when JNO was in residence at the Instituto de Física e Química de São Carlos, Universidade de São Paulo, 13560 São Carlos, S.P., Brazil.
[2] Present address: Department of Chemistry, University of Pittsburgh, Pittsburgh, Pennsylvania 15260.

1056–8700/92/0610–0349$02.00

PERSPECTIVES AND OVERVIEW

One of the central challenges in molecular biophysics is to understand how proteins control biochemical reactions in living organisms. In their folded states, proteins exhibit a variety of structural fluctuations. The question before us is; how do protein structure and dynamics control biological function? Our goal is to develop tools that allow us to simulate and understand those aspects of biomolecular structure and dynamics that establish the unique capabilities of these molecules. Our hope is to arrive at a deeper understanding of the mechanisms that control biochemical reactions and to establish design criteria for new proteins that will perform specific tasks.

With these issues in mind, this review focuses on electron transfer reactions. These reactions are extremely important in biology, particularly in bioenergetic reaction pathways (23, 32, 72). For example, in the early steps of photosynthesis, high efficiency solar-energy conversion is achieved with a complex of protein-bound electron donors and acceptors. Control of charge separation and recombination rates is required to insure that productive forward electron-transfer reactions within this complex occur rapidly, while wasteful back reactions occur orders of magnitude more slowly. Initial light-driven transfer steps are complete within 3 ps, and charge separation is subsequently stabilized for tens of milliseconds with a quantum efficiency near 100%. A comparable selective acceleration of electron transfer reactions has not been achieved in any artificial system.

Our goal in this paper is to present the results of a collaboration between theory and experiment aimed at developing a computational design capability for electron-transfer proteins. The theoretical methods we describe contain the minimal description that is needed to model adequately the fundamental mechanisms of protein-mediated electron tunneling. Although the description does not include every detail of the protein electronic structure, the model makes concrete, testable predictions about primary, secondary, tertiary, and quaternary structural effects on electron-transfer rates. Measurements of electron transfer rates in ruthenium-modified (ruthenated) proteins test the method's reliability. We find that inclusion of protein features neglected in structureless barrier models is essential for understanding the observed transfer rates in these systems.

ELECTRON TUNNELING MATRIX ELEMENTS

This review focuses on the calculation of tunneling matrix elements (T_{DA}) and the comparison of these couplings with those derived from experiment (28, 38, 42, 51, 60). The tunneling matrix element is associated with the weak long-distance electronic coupling between donor (D) and acceptor (A) mediated by the protein. Electron-transfer rates in the proteins discussed here are in the nonadiabatic limit and are therefore proportional to T_{DA}^2. In this section, we present a short discussion of the dynamical limits associated with the nonadiabatic electron-transfer rate formulation. Special attention is given to the Hamiltonian that we use to describe our problem and why the nonadiabatic limit is appropriate for long-distance electron transfer in proteins.

We begin our discussion by presenting the Hamiltonian that has been used extensively for the generic electron transfer problem (12, 34, 52, 65, 67):

$$\mathcal{H}_{ET} = T_{DA}(\mathbf{Q})\sigma_x + \tfrac{1}{2}[\alpha_D^{eff}(\mathbf{Q})+\alpha_A^{eff}(\mathbf{Q})] + \tfrac{1}{2}[\alpha_D^{eff}(\mathbf{Q})-\alpha_A^{eff}(\mathbf{Q})]\sigma_z + \mathcal{H}_{\mathbf{Q}}. \qquad 1.$$

The terms σ_x and σ_z are the Pauli matrices, where the expression $\sigma_z = 1$ or -1 is associated with the donor- or acceptor-localized state, respectively. $\mathcal{H}_{\mathbf{Q}}$ supplies the dynamics for the nuclear coordinates ($\mathbf{Q}$), and $\alpha_D^{eff}(\mathbf{Q})$ [$\alpha_A^{eff}(\mathbf{Q})$] is the instantaneous energy for the reactants (products) state.

Two major aspects of this Hamiltonian should be considered. First, it is necessary to describe why a multisite many-electron Hamiltonian can be reduced [renormalized to an effective two-level one-electron system (Equation 1)]. Second, if this renormalization is valid, we must present the conditions for the electron transfer rate to fall in the nonadiabatic limit (28, 51), i.e.

$$k_{ET} = \frac{2\pi}{\hbar} T_{DA}^2(FC), \qquad 2.$$

where (FC) is the nuclear (or Franck–Condon) factor. The analysis of experiments presented in this review relies on the separability of the rate expression.

Ideally, we would describe the molecular system from first principles including the motion of all the electrons and nuclei. Because this task is impossible, our strategy is to break the problem into pieces that can be

understood. To be successful, such a simplification relies on the identification of the relevant energy scales of the problem.

Before addressing the details of the molecular electronic structure, we
assume that the Born-Oppenheimer approximation is valid. This assumption is appropriate if the energies for nuclear excitations are much smaller
than those for electronic excitations. We comment later about the important excitations in the electron-tunneling problem and why we believe this
assumption is valid. The electronic energies of chemical bonds are much
smaller than the electronic excitation energies of core electrons. We can
therefore describe our problem as valence electrons moving in a pseudo-
potential provided by the core electrons and nuclei. Actually, we can
expand this picture by assuming that the energy associated with electronic
coupling between atoms (or bonds) is small compared to the energy of
excited states on isolated atoms, leading to a tight-binding or extended-
Hückel picture (for details, see 6, 10, 12, 58).

The initial tight-binding electronic Hamiltonian for D, A, and their
bridge is written (4, 6, 12, 27, 47, 48, 58, 59, 63, 64, 66, 70, 71):

$$\mathcal{H}_{el} = \alpha_D a_D^\dagger a_D + \alpha_A a_A^\dagger a_A + \sum_{i_D} v_{D,i_D}(a_D^\dagger a_{i_D} + a_{i_D}^\dagger a_D) +$$

$$\sum_{i_A} v_{A,i_A}(a_A^\dagger a_{i_A} + a_{i_A}^\dagger a_A) + \sum_i \alpha_i a_i^\dagger a_i + \sum_{i,j>i} v_{ij}(a_i^\dagger a_j + a_j^\dagger a_i), \quad 3.$$

where the $a_\mu^\dagger$ (a_μ) creates (destroys) an electron on the μth orbital. The first
two terms in the Hamiltonian represent the donor and acceptor sites.
The third and fourth terms contain the coupling between the donor and
acceptor, respectively, and the bridge. Bridge orbitals coupled to the donor
and acceptor are labeled i_D and i_A, respectively. The last two terms are
the bridge Hamiltonian. Because we are using the Born-Oppenheimer
approximation, all the electronic energies (α and v) are a function of the
nuclear configuration $\mathbf{Q}$.

How do we reduce the above Hamiltonian (Equation 3) to a two-level
system (reactants and products)? One way is to use the Löwdin partitioning
technique (47, 59). With this method, one maps an eigenvalue problem of
high dimension onto an equivalent problem of lower dimension. The
Hamiltonian or Equation 3 in matrix notation is:

$$\begin{pmatrix} \mathcal{H}_{DA} & \mathcal{H}_{DA,B} \\ \mathcal{H}_{B,DA} & \mathcal{H}_{bridge} \end{pmatrix}, \quad 4.$$

where $\mathcal{H}_{DA}$ is the matrix Hamiltonian that only includes the donor and
acceptor sites. The direct coupling between D and A in the case of long-
distance transfer is negligible. $\mathcal{H}_{bridge}$ is the Hamiltonian matrix for the

bridge, and $\mathscr{H}_{B,DA}$ is the matrix that couples the donor and acceptor to the bridge. Löwdin diagonalization yields a reduced 2×2 matrix

$$\bar{\mathscr{H}}_{DA} = \mathscr{H}_{DA} - \mathscr{H}_{DA,B}\mathscr{H}_{bridge}^{-1}\mathscr{H}_{B,DA}. \qquad 5.$$

The effective matrix one obtains is

$$\bar{\mathscr{H}}_{DA} = \begin{bmatrix} \alpha_D^{eff}(E) & T_{DA}(E) \\ T_{AD}(E) & \alpha_A^{eff}(E) \end{bmatrix}, \qquad 6a.$$

where

$$\alpha_{D(A)}^{eff}(E) = \alpha_{D(A)} + \Delta_{D(A)}(E), \qquad 6b.$$

$$\Delta_{D(A)} = \sum_{i,j} v_{D(A)i}G_{ij}(E)v_{jD(A)}, \qquad 6c.$$

and

$$T_{DA} = \sum_{i,j} v_{Di}G_{ij}(E)v_{jA}. \qquad 6d.$$

The is and js in the sums run over the bridge orbitals. G is the Green's function for the bridge, i.e. the Green's function (7, 25, 26, 35, 50, 52, 66, 67a) associated with $\mathscr{H}_{el}$ without the donor and acceptor terms, $G = (\mathscr{H}_{bridge} - E)^{-1}$.

Equation 6 is equivalent to Equation 5, i.e. the eigenvalues for the two equations are the same. However, we are only interested in the two states that define the two-level system. The first step in analyzing these states is to determine the tunneling energy. The effective donor energy can be obtained from Equation 6 by solving

$$\bar{\alpha}_D = \alpha_D^{eff}(\bar{\alpha}_D). \qquad 7.$$

The root of this equation closest to α_D is the effective donor energy. This result is equivalent to the one used in our laboratory (see 4, 65, for example) when considering the isolated donor-plus-bridge system. A similar calculation can be performed for the acceptor. The tunneling energy, E_T, is obtained for the nuclear configuration $\mathbf{Q}$ where

$$E_T = \bar{\alpha}_D = \bar{\alpha}_A. \qquad 8.$$

After calculating the tunneling energy, we can finally obtain the two-level system by fixing the value of E in Equation 6 equal to E_T. How good is this approximation? Let us refer to the symmetric and antisymmetric state energies that define the two-level system as E_1 and E_2, respectively. $E_2 - E_1$ is twice the tunneling matrix element. E_T is exactly midway between E_2 and E_1. Therefore, if we compare E_2 and E_1 as the eigenvalues of

Equation 6, setting $E = E_T$, we introduce errors of the order $E_2 - E_1$. Because E in Equation 6 only appears in terms like $\alpha_i - E$, the error introduced is approximately $(T_{DA}/|\alpha_{bridge} - E_T|)$. This error is of the order of the overlap between the effective donor and the acceptor states.

In order for the two-level approximation to hold, the separation between levels one and two, $2T_{DA}$, must be small compared to the energy separation between these states and the bridge. Actually, the ratio of these two quantities determines the precision of the approximation. Also, for the Born-Oppenheimer approximation to hold, these energy separations must be large compared to any relevant nuclear excitation energies. Finally, for this approximation to be valid, the investigator must consider one more time (energy) scale. As the electron tunnels from the donor to the acceptor, it spends a certain time in the classically forbidden region (12, 18). If this time is much shorter than the period of the vibrational modes, the atoms stay fixed as the electron tunnels; in other words, the Born-Oppenheimer approximation works. These approximations are reasonably good for electron transfer in proteins, and the reader is referred elsewhere (5, 12, 65) for further details.

To conclude this section, we comment on the nonadiabatic approximation that leads to an electron-transfer rate given by Equation 2. In order for this limit to be valid, the electronic frequency, $T_{DA}/\hbar$, must be low compared to that of the relevant nuclear motion. In the past six years, many papers have addressed this subject (see 67 and references therein for details). In long-distance electron transfer, the tunneling matrix elements are so small that this approximation most likely is adequate.

THE PATHWAY MODEL

The pathway model of electronic coupling in proteins (3, 6, 7, 8, 11) was developed based on earlier studies of electronic coupling in model compounds (4, 7, 63). Tunneling is much more efficient (decays more slowly) through bonded orbitals than through space, because the potential barrier is effectively lower. In proteins, the bonded-path connection length between D and A can be extremely long compared with the direct through-space distance. Our pathway method searches for the combination of bonded and nonbonded interactions that maximizes the total D-A interaction mediated by a combination of through-bond and through-space coupling through the protein. The tunneling pathways obtained contain mostly bonded interactions (with occasional through-space connections).

The intervening protein could provide two distinct mediation mechanisms to couple D and A. One mechanism mediates the interaction by a few very specific combinations of interacting bonds (fragments of amino acids) between D and A. The bonds would couple D and A through a sequence of directly connected covalent bonds, hydrogen bonds, and noncovalent contacts. Each of these combinations is called a *physical tunneling pathway* and plays a role in the D-A coupling (8). The other distinct way that the protein might couple D and A involves a sufficiently large number of pathways such that modifying a single pathway in this network will have a very small effect on the net coupling and the rate. In this case, no particular detail of the protein will greatly affect the rate.

An elaboration of the discussion of a physical tunneling pathway can help us focus the discussion of the D-A coupling mechanism. For a single physical pathway, one can use exact and perturbation theory methods for calculating the coupling arising from that physical pathway. Numerical strategies (for both exact and perturbation methods) usually write the decay of the wave function as a product of decays per bond [or delocalized group (63, 64)]. Within a lowest-order perturbation theory calculation, the per-bond decay depends only on the tunneling energy and on the nature of the particular bonds in the pathway. This method (applied to lowest order) neglects scattering corrections to the wave function propagation in the protein bridge. The scattering corrections (equivalent to higher-order perturbation-theory corrections) for a given pathway arise from enumerations of bonds in the tunneling pathway longer than the shortest path from D to A. For example, a physical pathway consisting of bonds 1, 2, 3, 4, . . . has the direct pathway 1-2-3-4 . . . and the scattering pathways 1-2-3-2-3-4 . . . , etc. We now discuss how one can exactly account for the scattering pathways in the electronic-coupling calculation for a one-dimensional physical pathway by correcting the self energy of each orbital on the path. Exact methods, particularly Green's function approaches, often write the coupling as a product as well. In this case, the terms in the product explicitly include these scattering corrections. In the same way, the effect of side groups appended to the physical pathway can also be included.

For a single physical pathway, the tunneling matrix element can be written (7, 53)

$$t_{\mathrm{DA}} = \mathrm{prefactor} \prod_{i=1}^{N} \varepsilon_i. \qquad\qquad 9.$$

Neglecting interactions between pathways within the protein bridge, T_{DA} is a sum over t_{DA}s for all physical pathways. For a pathway, ε_i for each block in the path (66) may be calculated approximately or exactly as discussed above. The prefactor depends on details of the interaction between the D or A with the first or last, respectively, bond of the tunneling pathway. When experimental systems with similar (or properly scaled) prefactors and *FC* factors are compared, differences in electron-transfer rates are expected to result from differences in the coupling via the physical pathways of the systems. The challenge in proteins, then, is to identify the chains of orbitals that define dominant pathways. The dominant tunneling pathways correspond to the combinations of bonds in the protein that maximize the products in Equation 9.

As an example of how to compute ε_i, we consider a linear chain of identical (Figure 1*a*) orbitals coupling the donor and the acceptor. (The orbital energy is α_B and the coupling between neighbors is v.) If back-scattering is neglected, the decay per orbital is

$$\varepsilon = v/(E_T - \alpha_B), \qquad \qquad 10.$$

where v is the coupling between neighboring bridge orbitals, and α is the orbital energy. The exact result, including backscattering, can also be written as the product given by Equation 9. The decay ε_i between bonds i and $i+1$ is:

$$\varepsilon_i(E_T) = \frac{G_{1,i+1}^{i+1}}{G_{1,i}^i} = \frac{v}{E_T - (\alpha_B + \delta_i^{bs})}, \qquad \qquad 11.$$

where δ_i^{bs} is the site self-energy correction due to backscattering. G^j is the Green's function for a linear bridge of j orbitals. In the long chain limit $(i \gg 1)$, this result converges to the infinite-chain limit

$$\varepsilon_{exact}^\infty(E) + \frac{1}{\varepsilon_{exact}^\infty(E)} = \frac{E - \alpha_B}{v}. \qquad \qquad 12.$$

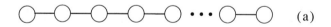 (a)

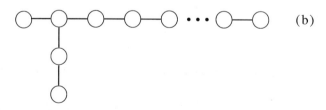 (b)

Figure 1   (*a*) Schematic representation of a linear bridge. Only nearest neighbors are coupled. (*b*) Schematic representation of a side group coupled to an orbital in the pathway.

We refer the reader elsewhere (66) for details about how these Green's functions can be calculated and for a description of our stepwise Green's function method.

The effect of pendant (side) groups can also be included without destroying the pathway concept. This concept is associated with the possibility of writing t_{DA} as a product of εs. Figure 1b suggests that pathways can include the effects of side groups attached to a single site by modifying the self energy of the orbital that the pendant group is attached to. Assuming that the side chain is coupled to pathway orbital i via orbital $s1$, the side chain can be eliminated by renormalizing the orbital i energy:

$$\alpha_i^{\text{eff}} = \alpha_i + v_{i,s1} G_{s1,s1}^{\text{sc}} v_{s1,i}. \qquad\qquad 13.$$

$G_{s1,s1}^{\text{sc}}$ is the diagonal matrix element of the Green's function for site $s1$ when only the side chain is included in the Hamiltonian. Using this procedure, many side chains can be immediately eliminated at the early stages of the calculation, greatly simplifying the problem.

The validity of the pathway approximation only becomes suspect when loops involving several paths appear. If interference between pathways is considerable, contributions from independent pathways enter T_{DA} in a rather complex manner. To address this issue, we developed a stepwise Green's function technique, and research is underway to understand the general applicability of the pathway concept. The simple pathway concept without the inclusion of effects like those discussed above can still teach us much about the mediation of electron tunneling in proteins.

Our strategy for mapping tunneling pathways in proteins involves making approximations to the decay factors ε_i and performing computer searches for the combination of interacting bonds with decay factors that maximize the product in Equation 9.

PATHWAY SEARCH STRATEGIES

The Conceptual Basis of the Calculations

The single maximum coupling pathway between two points in a protein indicates, at the very least, the coupling strength between those regions of the molecule. This section describes our simple approximations (based on intuition gained from model compound studies) used to produce a computationally tractable approximation to the coupling given in Equation 9 in which a product of decay factors give the contribution to T_{DA} from a single pathway. Our ansatz partitions electronic mediation through protein into three types of interactions: covalent, hydrogen-bonded, and through-space. This division was based on the fact that bond-mediated interactions are much longer range than through-space interactions (7).

The barrier to tunneling through a bonded medium is considerably lower than tunneling through vacuum (6, 10, 11) so the exponential decay of bond-mediated coupling is slower than through-space tunneling. Hydrogen bonds are weaker than covalent bonds, so it was not immediately apparent that they would be key mediators of tunneling. However, because hydrogen bonds bring lone-pair and bonding orbitals into close proximity, we expect their mediation properties to be substantial (8, 64).

Bonded and nonbonded interaction energies are obviously a function of atom type, hybridization, and orientation. However, the distinction between bonded and nonbonded interactions is so strong that a preliminary understanding of coupling pathways arises from determining the mix of these interactions on the dominant routes. For a single pathway consisting of covalent (C), hydrogen-bonded (H), and through-space (S) interactions, Equation 9 can be rewritten:

$$T_{DA} \propto \prod_i \varepsilon_C(i) \prod_j \varepsilon_S(j) \prod_k \varepsilon_H(k). \qquad 14.$$

Because the rate of electron transfer (Equation 2) is proportional to T_{DA}^2, we can estimate relative rates from Equation 14 for a given nuclear FC factor. By writing the T_{DA} expression with a proportionality, we have suppressed prefactors associated with D-bridge and bridge-A coupling. These factors have been discussed elsewhere (22, 64) and for the purposes of this discussion are assumed to be the same for all pathways. Simpler models for electron tunneling in proteins would write T_{DA} (and the transfer rate) as proportional to an exponentially decaying factor arising from a simple one-dimensional square barrier (28):

$$k_{ET}(\text{square}) = A \exp(-\beta R)(FC). \qquad 15.$$

The goal of the algorithm described in the next section is to find the combination of bonds between D and A that maximizes the product in Equation 14 given simple rules for approximating the decay factors ε. Other theoretical strategies for calculating the tunneling matrix element are also being developed (14, 19, 46).

Coupling Decay Factors

We now consider the range of decay parameters that are chemically accessible and describe the computer-search strategy for finding pathways that maximize the product in Equation 14 for a set of specified decay factors. Many covalently coupled D-A model compounds that undergo photoinduced electron transfer have been constructed with both biological and nonbiological redox active chromophores. When one translates the reported decays of rate with bridge size to decay per bond factors of the tunneling matrix element, through-bond ε_C decay factors are calculated in the range ~ 0.7–0.4 (55). We have chosen a value of 0.6 because it is a reasonable average value for the decay per bond (see 64 for details). Although ratios of rates depend on the choice, if all ε_Cs are assumed to be the same, the qualitative results of the single pathway calculations are insensitive to the exact value chosen (because ε_C appears as a prefactor in all three terms). The key relationship is between ε_C and the through-space decay constant. Through-space interactions are treated as stretched bonds, with couplings that are weaker than the bonded couplings by an amount commensurate with the length of the interaction beyond the reference covalent-bond length. An additional factor, usually taken as 1/2, is added to account for the generally unfavorable orientation effects associated with through-space interactions. The decay length, 1.7 Å^{-1} for the through-space interaction, arises from the calculation of penetration through a one-dimensional square barrier, which drops with exponential decay constant $(2m_e E_B/\hbar^2)^{1/2}$, where m_e is the electron mass and E_B is the tunneling electron energy, about 10 eV (11). Tunneling energies chosen in the 5–10 eV range have been explored. Again, the results are insensitive to the specific value. The hydrogen-bond decay is treated as two covalent bonds from hetero-atom to heteroatom, allowing one to adjust the coupling if the bond length is longer or shorter than the reference length. Thus, we have arrived at the following parameter set (8, 9):

$$\varepsilon_C = 0.6 \qquad\qquad\qquad 16a.$$

$$\varepsilon_H = \varepsilon_C^2 \exp[-1.7(R-2.8)] \qquad\qquad 16b.$$

$$\varepsilon_S = (1/2)\varepsilon_C \exp[-1.7(R-1.4)]. \qquad\qquad 16c.$$

In these expressions, the distances, R, are in Å units and the decay factors, ε, are unitless. The reference covalent bond distance is chosen as 1.4 Å (2.8 Å for two bonds). These decay factors include the minimal amount of physical detail needed to understand the structural dependence of electronic coupling in a bridge. As such, they provide a starting point for the development of structure-function relationships that, if promising, will be elaborated to include numerous fascinating complications arising from quantum interference within and between pathways, bond energetic differences, and geometric fluctuations from assumed atomic positions, to name a few.

Finding the Best Path

How are the pathway searches actually performed? These parameters are consistent with typical binding energies for electron-transfer localized states as well as theoretical and experimental studies of model compounds (9). Each decay factor ε is associated with an effective distance d_{eff} where:

$$d_{eff}(i) = -\log \varepsilon(i). \qquad \qquad 17.$$

We refer both to decay factors and connection lengths throughout the paper. The strength of the coupling arising from a single (noninterfering) pathway is proportional to the product of decay factors for each step on the path: $\Pi_i \varepsilon_i$. The computational challenge is to analyze the highly interconnected network of bonded and nonbonded contacts in a protein and specify the bonds that maximize this product. This is precisely the well-known minimum-distance-in-a-graph problem. The minimum-distance problem addresses finding the shortest pathway between two points in an interconnected network. Because Equation 17 associates the decay factor with an effective distance, we can restate our search for the maximum pathway couplings as a search for the shortest effective distance between donor and acceptor in the corresponding network. Graph-theory strategies for solving the minimum-distance problem are discussed elsewhere (17).

The first step in using graph theory to find electron-transfer pathways in proteins is to construct a labeled graph (17) corresponding to the superset of all potential pathways. Covalent bonds (established as described below) are first mapped onto vertices. Establishing which vertices are to be joined by edges requires progressively more computation for adjacent covalent bonds, hydrogen bonds, and through-space contacts. The lengths of the edges (i.e. the decays) are determined by the distances between the atoms and the nature of the interaction (Equation 16). The covalent bonds are specified implicitly by the Brookhaven Protein Data Bank files. Covalent interactions, those between bonds anchored at a common atom, are easily identified. Commercial software is used to look up these connections for the known amino acids and other residues, which are then appended to the Protein Data Bank data. These amended Protein Data Bank files are used as input to the PATHWAYS software written by J. N. Betts. Directed by data in the parameter files, the program looks up the model-predicted decays (Equation 16) for the various bond types and stores them. Hydrogen bonds are identified as having acceptable: (a) hydrogen-donor and hydrogen-acceptor groups (donors: -NHx; acceptors: carbonyl oxygens; both: -OH), (b) donor-hydrogen-acceptor angle, and (c) donor-acceptor distance (Å). These values are specified in a parameter file. Edges representing the hydrogen bonds are added to the connection list, and lengths that represent these decays are added to the list of segment lengths. Next, potential through-space connections are sought within a limited radius of each atom, typically 6 Å. No through-space connections longer than 6 Å contribute to significant pathways, so they are ignored to shorten the data-processing time. The through-space connections are established for each atom, X, as follows. First, the investigator composes a list, L, containing all bonds/vertices within range of X and attempts to eliminate as many of the entries as possible. Through-space connections are eliminated between atoms that have a significantly stronger bond-mediated connection. The first through-space connections the program eliminates from L are those that are redundant with preexisting covalent and hydrogen bonds. The vertices remaining in L are sorted on the basis of their distances from X, shortest first. Next, a depth-first shortest-path search (17) is performed with X as the root, finding the shortest distance to atoms with potential through-space connections. The depth of the search is limited to a length that corresponds to the through-space decay from X to atoms within the through-space cutoff radius. If the search returns without having located the potential atom, the through-space contact is the shortest path to it, and the connection is thus added to the master connection (adjacency) list, and its corresponding length is added to the list of lengths. Otherwise, the through-space connection is discarded and the next vertex in L becomes the new target. In this way, shorter through-space contacts can disqualify longer ones, further decreasing the number of connections added to the graph.

Two standard search strategies are used to arrive at the minimum-distance path between two points in an interconnected network, referred to as depth-first and breadth-first searches. Depth-first searches begin at a specified point and step along allowed connections until no additional forward steps remain (a dead-end is reached) or the target site is found. If a dead-end occurs, the search backtracks by one step and then seeks alternative forward steps from that point, and so on until the target atom is found. Breadth-first searches simultaneously consider all paths radiating from the starting point by keeping track of each vertex and its distance. At each step of the search, a new vertex is added. The vertex chosen to be added is always the one that minimizes the effective distance to the donor at that stage. When the acceptor atom is the one that is added, the minimum-distance pathway has been found. We use a depth-first algorithm. The advantage of the depth-first search for our applications is its pathway orientation, i.e. each excursion represents a potentially acceptable pathway and the paths within a given factor of the best pathway are easily tabulated and accumulated.

RUTHENATED CYTOCHROMES

The molecules we have employed in experiments aimed at extracting T_{DA} values are ones in which ruthenium complexes are attached to surface histidines of structurally characterized proteins (2, 13, 22, 24, 30, 36, 40, 41, 44, 45, 49, 54, 61, 68, 73, 74, 74a, 75, 77–79). Surface modification of a protein is expected to be nonperturbative, so the structure of the modified protein is presumably the same as that of the native protein. Hence, the distance and the intervening medium involved in electron transfer between the native- and synthetic-protein redox sites are known. Altering the site of attachment allows one to vary both the distance and the intervening medium for electron transfer. Changing the ligands in the ruthenium modification reagent also permits one to study free-energy effects on the rate of the reaction.

Cytochrome c

HIS33 DERIVATIVES   The first experimental work on the electron-transfer reactions of Ru-modified proteins involved horse-heart cytochrome c modified by coordination of pentaammineruthenium to His33 (Figure 2) (75, 77). The rate of intramolecular electron transfer from $Rua_5(His33)^{2+}$ ($a = NH_3$) to the ferriheme ($T = 298$ K), measured using photochemical techniques, is $30(\pm 5)$ s^{-1} (Table 1). The reaction exhibits a rather small activation enthalpy (2 kcal mol^{-1}) and a large negative activation entropy (-43 eu). Measurements of the temperature dependences of the $Rua_5(His)^{3+/2+}$ and $Fe^{3+/2+}$ potentials in $Rua_5(His33)$-Fe-cyt c have provided estimates of $\Delta G°$ [$-4.3(\pm 2)$ kcal mol^{-1}, 298 K], $\Delta H°$ [$-11.5(\pm 10)$ kcal mol^{-1}], and $\Delta S°$ [$-25(\pm 3)$ eu] for the Ru(II)Fe(III) intramolecular electron-transfer reaction. Given these thermodynamic quantities, and the temperature dependence (2–40°C) of the electron-transfer rate in $Rua_5(His33)$-Fe-cyt c, one can extract values of λ and T_{DA} from Equation 2 using a classical expression for FC (51). Nonlinear least-square fits to the data suggest that $\lambda = 1.2$ eV and $T_{DA} = 0.03$ cm^{-1} (74a). This value of the reorganization energy is quite close to that predicted by the Marcus cross relation (59) [$\lambda_{12} = (\lambda_1 + \lambda_2)/2$] using the reorganization energies for the Fe-cyt c ($\lambda_{11} = 1.04$ eV) and $Rua_5(py)^{3+/2+}$ ($\lambda_{22} = 1.20$ eV) self-exchange reactions (15, 51).

A clear understanding of the electronic-coupling strengths in metalloprotein electron-transfer reactions depends upon reliable values of λ and T_{DA}. In addition to studies of temperature dependences, analysis of the driving-force dependence of electron transfer rates can also provide electron-transfer parameters. In the low-driving-force regime ($-\Delta G° \ll \lambda$), the variation of rate with free energy does not strongly depend upon λ, and it is difficult to obtain a good value for this parameter. Much better values of λ and T_{DA} can be obtained from high-driving-force measurements (i.e. $-\Delta G° \approx \lambda$). In this region, the driving-force curve flattens out and electron-transfer rates approach their maximum values.

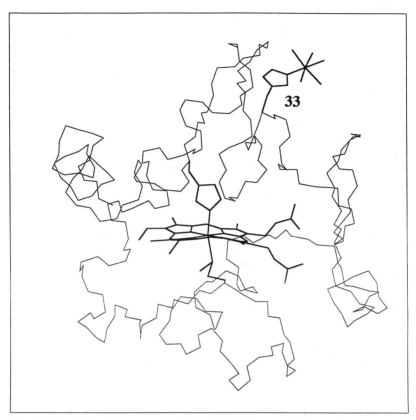

Figure 2 Peptide-backbone structure of Rua_5(His33)-Fe-cyt c. This complex was prepared by reaction of Rua_5(OH$_2$)$^{2+}$ with Fe(II)-cyt c for 24 h at room temperature. The pure singly modified derivative was isolated using ion-exchange chromatography and was extensively characterized by spectroscopic and chemical methods (77, 78).

It is difficult to prepare a Ru-ammine complex of Fe-cyt c in which the driving force for intramolecular electron transfer is much greater than 0.2 eV. Substitution of the native Fe center in cytochrome c with Zn, however, has led to high-driving-force intramolecular electron transfer. The lowest triplet-excited state of the Zn-porphyrin in Zn-cyt c has a 15-ms lifetime and is a potent reductant [$E° = -0.62$ V vs normal hydrogen electrode (NHE)]. The rates of direct photoinduced electron transfer and thermal recombination have been measured for three Rua_5L(His33)-Zn-cyt c proteins (L = NH$_3$, pyridine, isonicotinamide), spanning a 0.39-eV range in $\Delta G°$ (-0.66 to -1.05 eV; Table 1) (30, 54, 74). Fits of these data yield

Table 1 Rate constants and activation parameters for intramolecular electron-transfer reactions of Ru(His)-modified cytochrome c

Electron transfer	$-\Delta G^\circ$ (eV)	k_{ET} (s⁻¹)	$\Delta H^\ddagger$ (kcal mol⁻¹)	$\Delta S^\ddagger$ (eu)
His33 Derivatives ($d = 11.1$ Å)				
$Rua_5(His)^{2+} \rightarrow Fe(III)$[a]	0.18(2)	$3.0(5) \times 10^1$	2.0(5)	−43(5)
$Rua_4(isn)(His)^{2+} \rightarrow ZnP^+$ [b]	0.66(5)	$2.0(2) \times 10^5$	<0.5	−35(5)
$ZnP^* \rightarrow Rua_5(His)^{3+}$ [c]	0.70(5)	$7.7(8) \times 10^5$	1.7(4)	−27(5)
$Rua_4(py)(His)^{2+} \rightarrow ZnP^+$ [b]	0.74(5)	$3.5(4) \times 10^5$	<0.5	−34(5)
$ZnP^* \rightarrow Rua_4(py)(His)^{3+}$ [b]	0.97(5)	$3.3(3) \times 10^6$	2.2(4)	−22(5)
$Rua_5(His)^{2+} \rightarrow ZnP^+$ [c]	1.01(5)	$1.6(4) \times 10^6$	—	—
$ZnP^* \rightarrow Rua_4(isn)(His)^{3+}$ [b]	1.05(5)	$2.9(3) \times 10^6$	<0.5	−30(5)
His39 Derivatives ($d = 12.3$ Å)[d]				
$Rua_4(isn)(His)^{2+} \rightarrow ZnP^+$	0.66(5)	$6.5(7) \times 10^5$	−1.7(4)	−39(5)
$ZnP^* \rightarrow Rua_5(His)^{3+}$	0.70(5)	$1.5(2) \times 10^6$	1.3(3)	−27(5)
$Rua_4(py)(His)^{2+} \rightarrow ZnP^+$	0.74(5)	$1.5(2) \times 10^6$	−1.8(4)	−37(5)
$ZnP^* \rightarrow RuA_4(py)(His)^{3+}$	0.97(5)	$8.9(9) \times 10^6$	0.2(2)	−27(5)
$Rua_5(His)^{2+} \rightarrow ZnP^+$	1.01(5)	$5.7(6) \times 10^6$	−0.2(2)	−29(5)
$ZnP^* \rightarrow Rua_4(isn)(His)^{3+}$	1.05(5)	$1.0(1) \times 10^7$	0.2(2)	−27(5)
His62 Derivatives ($d = 14.8$ Å)[e]				
$ZnP^* \rightarrow Rua_5(His)^{3+}$	0.70(5)	$6.5(7) \times 10^3$	1.4(3)	−37(5)
$Rua_4(py)(His)^{2+} \rightarrow ZnP^+$	0.74(5)	$8.1(8) \times 10^3$	—	—
$ZnP^* \rightarrow Rua_4(py)(His)^{3+}$	0.97(5)	$3.6(4) \times 10^4$	—	—
$Rua_5(His)^{2+} \rightarrow ZnP^+$	1.01(5)	$2.0(2) \times 10^4$	0.7(7)	−37(5)

[a] References 61, 75.
[b] Reference 54.
[c] Reference 30.
[d] Reference 74.
[e] Reference 73.

$\lambda = 1.10$ eV and $T_{DA} = 0.12$ cm⁻¹ for the photoinduced reactions, and $\lambda = 1.19$ eV and $T_{DA} = 0.09$ cm⁻¹ for the recombinations. The electron-transfer parameters are not extremely sensitive to the nature of the reaction (photoinduced or recombination), and these reactions can be adequately described by a single pair of parameters: $\lambda = 1.15(10)$ eV and $T_{DA} = 0.1(2)$ cm⁻¹ (74a).

The similarity in reorganization energies for the Ru-Fe-cyt c and Ru-Zn-cyt c intramolecular electron-transfer reactions is to be expected. The total reorganization energy is a sum of inner-sphere (λ_i) and outer-sphere (λ_o) elements. Inner-sphere contributions arise from nuclear rearrangements in the Ru-ammine and metalloporphyrin complexes accompanying electron transfer. These rearrangements are rather small and have been estimated to contribute no more than 0.2 eV to λ for both Ru-Fe-cyt c and Ru-Zn-cyt c (54). The two sources of outer-sphere rearrangements are the solvent and the peptide matrix. Calculations based on a single-sphere dielectric continuum model (16) indicate a 0.6-eV contribution to λ_o from the solvent (54). From the structures of ferri- and ferrocytochrome cs, the peptide contribution to λ_o has been calculated to be about 0.2 eV (20). The sum of these individual components (1.0 eV) is in good agreement with the experimentally derived reorganization energy for the Ru-M-cyt c (M = Fe, Zn) systems.

HIS39 DERIVATIVES   Ru-ammine complexes have been bound to His39 of Zn-substituted cytochrome c from *Candida krusei* (68, 74). Intramolecular electron-transfer rates (Table 1) are approximately three times faster than those of corresponding reactions in His33 derivatives of horse-heart cytochrome c. The variation of rates with driving force in these derivatives suggests a 1.2(1) eV reorganization energy, indistinguishable from that found in the His33 complexes. The faster electron-transfer rates have been attributed to stronger donor-acceptor electronic coupling in the His39-modified protein (74).

The direct D-A distances in Ru(His33)-Zn-cyt c and Ru(His39)-Zn-cyt c are 11.1 and 12.3 Å, respectively; however, the T_{DA} is twofold larger for the His39 system. The pathway model is somewhat more consistent with the data: both the His33 and His39 pathways consist of 11 covalent bonds and 1 hydrogen bond (Figure 3). The n_{eff} values for His33 and His39 are 13.9 and 14.0 bonds, respectively (74a).

HIS62 DERIVATIVES   Site-directed mutagenesis creates many new opportunities for studying electron transfer in Ru-modified proteins. A yeast (*Saccharomyces cerevisiae*) cytochrome c variant has been characterized as having a surface histidine at position 62 (13). The Rua_5(His62) derivative of this mutant protein was prepared, and the rate of electron transfer from Ru(II) to Fe(III) was found to be 1.7 s^{-1} (Table 1) (13). Rua_5(His62) and Rua_4(His62) derivatives of Zn-substituted *S. cerevisiae* cytochrome c have also been examined. The rates of the photoinduced and thermal recombination reactions are more than two orders of magnitude slower than the rates of analogous reactions in His33 derivatives of horse-heart cytochrome c (73). The driving-force data are more limited than for the other His derivatives of cytochrome c, but again suggest that $\lambda \approx 1.2$ eV. The slower rates for the His62 derivatives are attributed to weaker electronic coupling. The direct D-A separation is 14.8 Å, while the effective number of bonds in the pathway is 20.6 (Figure 3) (74a). Both measures suggest that the His62 electron transfer reactions should be substantially slower than those found in His33 or His39 derivatives.

NATURE OF THE PATHWAYS   Qualitative differences can arise in the collection of best pathways found, depending on the protein structure. We have

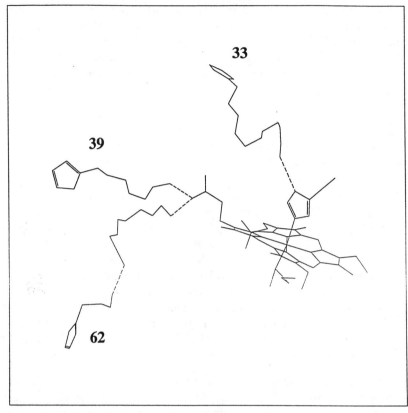

Figure 3 Predicted electronic-coupling pathways in Ru(His33)-, Ru(His39)-, and Ru(His62)-modified cytochrome *c*. Covalent bonds are depicted as solid lines and hydrogen bonds as dashed lines.

examined the paths within a factor of 10 of the best one in ruthenated His39 and His62 cytochrome *c*. In the His39 derivative, three routes feed into a single propionic acid side chain of the heme (Figure 4). The three pathways are more or less parallel and not highly interconnected. His62 has only two classes of pathways, but paths between and within each class have intertwined pathways near the His62 group, which are independent at intermediate distance and connect to independent parts of the heme. Pathway coupling calculations can be displayed in map form: Figure 5 is a coupling map showing the maximum pathway coupling to each α-carbon in cytochrome *c*.

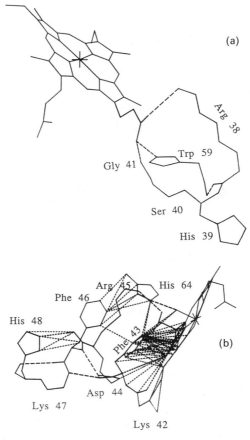

Figure 4 The best paths for (*a*) His39 cyt *c* and (*b*) His48 Mb are shown. Dotted lines are through-space contacts. Note that the best paths in cyt *c* are structurally related to one another, while several classes of pathways exist in Mb.

Cytochrome b$_5$

HIS26 DERIVATIVES   Three surface His residues of trypsin-solubilized bovine cytochrome b_5 (Tb_5) have been modified by coordination to Ru-penta-ammine complexes (His15, His80, His26) (40). Rates of intramolecular electron transfer from Fe(II) to Ru(III) have been measured in three His26 derivatives: Rua_5(His26)-Tb_5; mutant (Asn57 to Asp, Gln13 to Glu, Glu11 to Gln, His15 to Asn, His80 to Asn) lipase-solubilized cytochrome b_5 [Rua_5(His26)LMb_5]; and deuteroporphyrin-substituted (DP) Tb_5 [Rua_5(His26)DPb_5] (40, 41). Electron-transfer rates vary by more than an

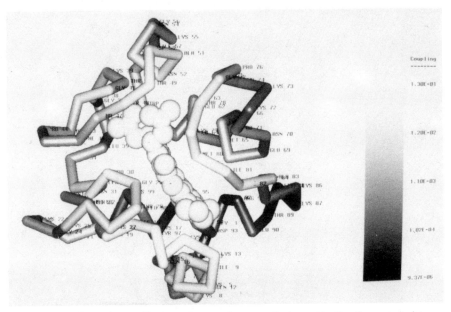

Figure 5 Electronic coupling map for cytochrome *c*. Amino acids directly connected to those coordinating the Fe or hydrogen-bonding to the heme are anomalously strongly coupled in reference to their through-space distance from the heme.

order of magnitude for the three proteins (Table 2). The small differences in driving force or estimated D-A separation cannot readily account for the variations in rate. Driving-force data are not available for this system, but changes in λ probably could not be responsible for the differences in electron-transfer rates. The pathway model has been invoked to account for the differences in rates. A critical through-space jump (from Leu25 to the heme) in the pathway from His26 to the heme is not constant in the three different proteins (Figure 6). The dramatic reduction in rate in $Rua_5(His26)DPb_5$ has been attributed to the absence of the heme 2-vinyl

Table 2 Electron-transfer rates in Ru(His26)-modified cytochrome b_5[a]

Electron transfer	$-\Delta G°$ (eV)	k_{ET} (s⁻¹)	d (Å)
Fe(II)-T$b_5 \to$ Rua_5(His26)$^{3+}$	0.08(2)	1.4(1)	12.1
Fe(II)-LM$b_5 \to$ Rua_5(His26)$^{3+}$	0.10(2)	5.9(5)	12.0
Fe(II)-DP$b_5 \to$ Rua_5(His26)$^{3+}$	0.13(2)	0.2(1)	12.9

[a] Reference 41.

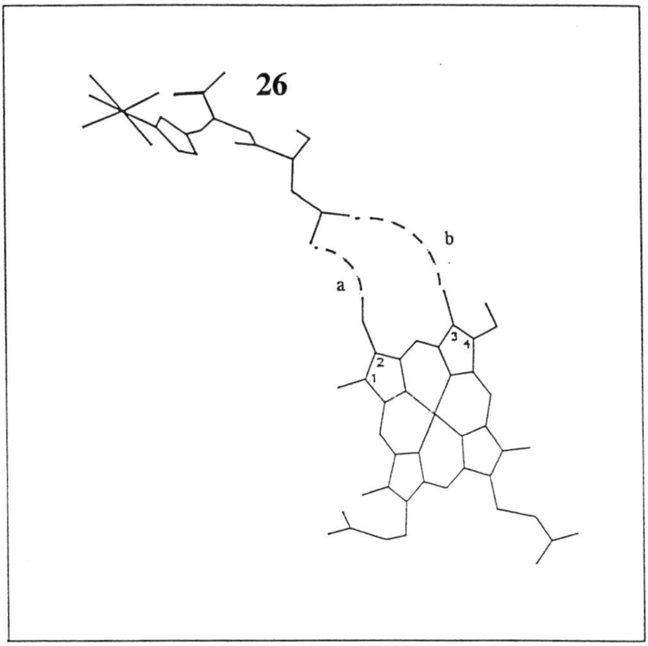

Figure 6   Best-pathway through-space jump from Leu25 to the heme in Ru(His26)-modified cytochrome Tb_5(a) and DPb_5 (b).

group, which is the terminus of the Leu25-to-heme through-space jump in the other two proteins (40, 41). A longer jump to the heme 3-methyl is predicted for Rua_5(His26)DPb_5, leading to a slower electron-transfer rate.

NATURE OF THE PATHWAYS   Pathways from His26 to the heme in cytochrome b_5 are somewhat less sparse than in cytochrome c. When the His63-Fe coupling (2.04-Å bond length) is treated as a through-space interaction, pathways through the vinyl group dominate as described above. Two other classes of pathways can be identified. Pathways arising from through-space interactions between the heme and residues His63 and Phe58 form a second tier of paths with weaker coupling than those described above.

Reorganization Energies and Electronic Couplings

Based on the few systems in which a reliable number has been extracted, $\lambda = 1.2$ eV appears to be a reasonable value for Ru-ammine-modified cytochromes (74a). Perhaps because of a lack of data and limited precision in the derived parameters, λ has not been found to be particularly sensitive to D-A separation or to the site of modification. In fact, the simple Marcus cross relation provides a reasonably good estimate of the reorganization energies in these reactions.

Unlike the reorganization energy, the electronic-coupling strengths in the Ru-modified cytochromes show a great deal of variability. Equation 15 expresses a simple distance dependence for T_{DA} that adequately describes electron transfer in model complexes with values of β between 0.8 and 1.2 Å^{-1}. This distance dependence, assuming a maximum electron-transfer rate of $10^{13}\ \text{s}^{-1}$ at close contact ($d = 3\ \text{Å}$), is represented by the solid ($\beta = 1.0\ \text{Å}^{-1}$) and dashed ($\beta = 0.8,\ 1.2\ \text{Å}^{-1}$) lines in Figure 7. Estimates of maximum electron-transfer rates (i.e. the rate at $-\Delta G^\circ = \lambda$) for Ru-modified cytochromes (Table 3) are plotted as a function of D-A separation (λ was assumed to be 1.2 eV for the cytochrome b_5 derivatives). Clearly all of the maximum rates lie below the values predicted by Equation 15; there is no simple correlation. The obvious conclusion is that, for a given D-A separation, the electronic coupling in the Ru-modified proteins is

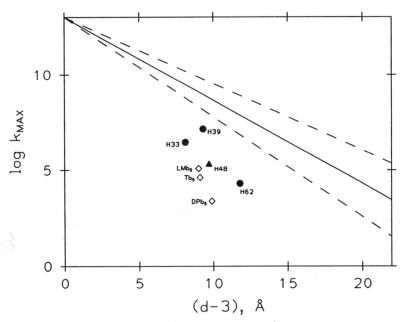

Figure 7 Plot of $\log k_{MAX}$ versus D-A distance (d) minus 3 Å (van der Waals contact) for Ru-modified proteins. Solid and dashed lines represent Equation 15 with $\beta = 0.8$, 1.0, and 1.2 Å^{-1}. Filled symbols indicate systems in which λ was estimated from a driving-force study. Open symbols indicate that an assumed value for λ (1.2 eV) was used to estimate k_{MAX}. ●, Cytochrome c; ▲, His48 derivative of Mb; ◇, His26 derivatives of cytochrome b_5.

Table 3 Maximum rates, D-A distances, coupling strengths, and effective bonds in pathways for Ru-modified proteins

	k_{max} (s^{-1})	$d(Å)$	T_{DA} (cm^{-1})	n_{eff} (bonds)
Ru(His39)cyt c^a	1.4×10^7	12.3	0.24	14.0
Ru(His33)cyt c^b	2.9×10^6	11.1	0.11	13.9
Ru(His62)cyt c^c	2.0×10^4	14.8	0.01	20.6
Ru(His26)Tb_5^d	4.1×10^4	12.1	0.01	19.0
Ru(His26)LMb_5^d	1.2×10^5	12.0	0.02	18.7
Ru(His26)DPb_5^d	2.4×10^3	12.9	0.003	20.3
Ru(His48)Mb^e	2.1×10^5	12.7	0.03	22.6

[a] Reference 74.
[b] Reference 54.
[c] Reference 73.
[d] Reference 41.
[e] Reference 74a.

substantially weaker than that predicted by a simple exponential decay with distance.

Our pathway model predicts the failure of exponential-decay correlations based on edge-edge distances. It also predicts that maximum electron-transfer rates correlate with the effective number of bonds in the pathway. [Multiplying n_{eff} by a canonical value of 1.4 Å/bond gives a tunneling length (σl) that replaces d in rate-distance correlations.] Maximum electron-transfer rates in the Ru-modified cytochromes are plotted against σl in Figure 8. A linear least-square fit yields the solid line with a slope of 0.7 Å^{-1}. Though the data are limited, the intercept at one bond (i.e. 1.4 Å) corresponds to a maximum electron-transfer rate of 3.4×10^{12} s^{-1}, which is in reasonable agreement with data from covalently coupled D-A complexes (33, 37, 76).

RUTHENATED MYOGLOBIN

His48 Derivatives

Myoglobin (Mb) is an oxygen-storage protein with 153 amino acids and a heme prosthetic group (1). Unlike cytochrome c, the heme is not covalently bound to the protein in Mb. This feature greatly facilitates metal substitution and has enabled the preparation of Ru(His48) proteins with six different metalloporphyrin active sites.

For cytochrome c, the evidence indicated that the reorganization energy for the electron-transfer reactions of the Zn-substituted protein would be nearly the same as that of the native-Fe protein. This, however, is not

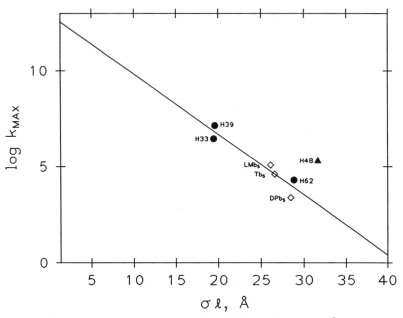

Figure 8 Plot of $\log k_{MAX}$ versus the tunneling length, σl ($= n_{eff} \times 1.4$ Å/bond), in the physical pathway between donor and acceptor for three Ru-modified derivatives of cytochrome c (●), three His26 derivatives of cytochrome b_5 (◇), and one Mb derivative (▲). The solid line is a linear least-square fit to the three cytochrome c points.

likely to be true in myoglobin: Fe(II)-Mb is a five-coordinate low-spin complex that, upon one-electron oxidation, binds a water molecule to form a six-coordinate species (1). This change in coordination number should be reflected in a greater reorganization energy in native Fe Mb, or even by electron-transfer rates limited by ligand binding or dissociation. The electron-transfer reactions of Ru-modified, metal-substituted Mb, however, are not accompanied by changes in metal coordination, and a single set of electron-transfer parameters should adequately describe these reactions. The rates of 18 different electron-transfer reactions in Ru(His48) Mb have been reported (Table 4) (2, 22, 24, 44, 45, 74a), spanning nearly 0.8 eV in driving force. Fitting the photoinduced and thermal recombination rates to a classical expression for FC yields $\lambda = 1.26$ eV and $T_{DA} = 0.03$ cm^{-1} (74a). The D-A separation in Ru(His48)Mb (12.7 Å) is quite similar to the distances in His33 and His39 derivatives of cytochrome c and does not readily explain the smaller value of T_{DA}. The best pathway in Ru(His48)Mb, however, is comprised of 22.6 effective bonds (eight more than found in the His33 and His39 pathways).

Table 4   Electron-transfer rates in Ru(His48)-modified myoglobin

Electron transfer	$-\Delta G^\circ$ (eV)	k_{ET} (s^{-1})
$H_2P^* \rightarrow Rua_5(His)^{3+}$ [a]	0.39($\pm$2)	7.6(8) $\times$ 10^2
$Rua_4(isn)(His)^{2+} \rightarrow ZnP^+$ [b]	0.61($\pm$2)	1.4(5) $\times$ 10^4
$PdP^* \rightarrow Rua_5(His)^{3+}$ [c]	0.64($\pm$2)	9.1(9) $\times$ 10^3
$Rua_4(py)(His)^{2+} \rightarrow ZnP^+$ [b]	0.69($\pm$2)	2.0(5) $\times$ 10^4
$CdP^* \rightarrow Rua_5(His)^{3+}$ [a,d]	0.79($\pm$2)	4.5(5) $\times$ 10^4
$MgP^* \rightarrow Rua_5(His)^{3+}$ [a,d]	0.81($\pm$2)	9.5(9) $\times$ 10^4
$ZnP^* \rightarrow Rua_5(His)^{3+}$ [b]	0.82($\pm$2)	7.0(7) $\times$ 10^4
$PdP^* \rightarrow Rua_4(py)(His)^{3+}$ [c]	0.91($\pm$2)	9.0(9) $\times$ 10^4
$Rua_5(His)^{2+} \rightarrow MgP^+$ [d]	0.91($\pm$2)	4.9(5) $\times$ 10^4
$Rua_5(His)^{2+} \rightarrow CdP^+$ [d]	0.92($\pm$2)	2.1(2) $\times$ 10^5
$Rua_5(His)^{2+} \rightarrow ZnP^+$ [b]	0.96($\pm$2)	1.5(5) $\times$ 10^5
$ZnP^* \rightarrow Rua_4(py)(His)^{3+}$ [b]	1.09($\pm$2)	2.0(2) $\times$ 10^5
$ZnP^* \rightarrow Rua_4(isn)(His)^{3+}$ [b]	1.17($\pm$2)	2.9(3) $\times$ 10^5
$Rua_5(His)^{2+} \rightarrow Fe(II)(CN-Br)$ [e]	0.09($\pm$2)	2.0(5)
$Fe(II)(CN-Br) \rightarrow Rua_4(isn)^{3+}(His)$ [e]	0.26($\pm$2)	5.5(5)
$Fe(II) \rightarrow Rua_5(His)^{3+}$ [f]	0.02($\pm$2)	4.0(5) $\times$ 10^{-2}
$Fe(II) \rightarrow Rua_4(py)(His)^{3+}$ [g]	0.28($\pm$2)	2.5(5)
$Fe(II) \rightarrow Rua_4(isn)(His)^{3+}$ [e]	0.35($\pm$2)	3.0(4)

[a] Reference 22.
[b] References 44, 74a.
[c] Reference 45.
[d] Reference 74a.
[e] Reference 79.
[f] Reference 24.
[g] Reference 49.

Cyanogen-bromide modification of His64 in the distal heme pocket of myoglobin inhibits coordination of a water ligand to the ferric heme (43, 56, 69). Therefore the reorganization energy for electron transfer in cyanogen-bromide-treated Ru(His48)-Fe-Mb will probably be nearly the same as that of the metal-substituted myoglobins. Fitting the two electron-transfer rates measured for this system (Table 4) to Equation 2, with λ equal to 1.26 eV, yields an electronic-coupling matrix element of 0.01 cm^{-1} (79). As in the case of Ru-modified cytochrome c, the apparent coupling strength in Ru-ammine–iron-heme reactions is somewhat smaller than that found for reactions involving Ru-ammines and metal-substituted porphyrins.

Three electron-transfer rates have been measured with Ru-ammines bound to His48 of native Fe myoglobin (Table 4) (24, 49). The reorganization energy for these reactions can be estimated by assuming that the coupling strength is the same as that found in the cyanogen bromide–treated systems (0.01 cm^{-1}) and by optimizing λ. The data suggest $\lambda = 1.48$

eV (74a), a 0.2-eV increase over the value found in systems that have no change in coordination number.

Nature of the Pathways

The pathways in cytochrome c are rather sparse and fairly independent compared to pathways in His48 Mb (Figure 4). This Mb derivative has two or three families of pathways, one connected to the heme by a hydrogen bond to Arg45, one connected through space to Phe43, and one connected through space to Lys42. In contrast to cytochrome c, loops interconnect these paths (by hydrogen-bond and through-space interactions) throughout the protein. The limitations of the single pathway approximation depend on the number of loops in the intervening medium, and it will be interesting to see (theoretically as well as experimentally) how well single-pathway models work for proteins of varied structural motifs.

Figure 8 also plots the maximum electron transfer rate for His48-modified Mb ($n_{eff} = 22.6$ bonds) (74a). This Mb point lies substantially above the line based on the cytochrome c and b_5 data, and clearly indicates a problem with the pathway model. In the simple form of this model, a single route is assumed to dominate the D-A coupling. The pathway-searching algorithm tends to support this assumption in the cytochromes, where single coupling paths stand out. In Mb, however, the pathway-searching algorithm identifies many nearly equivalent pathways: the one used for the point in Figure 8 represents the best route, but there are several close competitors. The problem is again the tunneling distance: with many nearly equivalent paths contributing to D-A coupling, n_{eff} will be substantially below 22.6 bonds for His48 Mb. Efforts are being made to refine the pathway model to accommodate multiple paths. If enough paths contribute to the overall electronic coupling in a given protein, the composition of any one path becomes relatively unimportant and tunneling lengths should closely parallel edge-edge distances.

CONCLUDING REMARKS

In addition to the utility of the pathway-mapping method in examining couplings between pairs of points in proteins, its simplicity allows the generation of global coupling maps from all atoms in a protein to the redox center. Such maps reveal important characteristic effects of primary, secondary, tertiary, and quaternary folded structure on the nature of the coupling to a specific patch of the protein. Regions anomalously strongly or weakly coupled to the redox center, given their distances, are easily identified (3), and evidence of these anomalous regions should appear in the experimental data. The simple pathway model appears to work relatively well for the cytochromes, which have few pathways. The His48 Mb data are not entirely consistent with the single-pathway analysis discussed here. Differences can arise from inadequacy of the single-path approximation, uncertainties in fitting of the experimental data, and inadequacies of using a simple classical expression for FC.

Our pathway technique is now being used to study other biological systems (19, 21, 29, 31, 32, 39, 57). New theoretical strategies are being implemented to further our understanding of tunneling pathways so that greater molecular detail can be included in the treatment of very large systems (see 66 for a description of the methods used). The long-term goal of this work is to obtain compact symbolic representations for proteins that include all the relevant pathways in the protein.

ACKNOWLEDGMENTS

Work in San Diego was funded by the National Science Foundation (Grant No. DMB-9018768) and a research contract from the Jet Propulsion Laboratory, supported by the Department of Energy's Catalysis/Biocatalysis Program. This work was performed in part at the Jet Propulsion Laboratory, California Institute of Technology, and was sponsored by the Department of Energy's Catalysis/Biocatalysis Program (Advanced Industrial Concepts Division), through an agreement with the National Aeronautics and Space Administration. Experimental work at the Beckman Institute was supported by the National Science Foundation and the National Institutes of Health.

Literature Cited

1. Antonini, E., Brunori, M. 1971. *Hemoglobin and Myoglobin in Their Reactions with Ligands.* Amsterdam: North Holland
2. Axup, A. W., Albin, M., Mayo, S. L., Crutchley, R. J., Gray, H. B. 1988. *J. Am. Chem. Soc.* 110: 435
3. Beratan, D. N., Betts, J. N., Onuchic, J. N. 1991. *Science* 252: 1285
4. Beratan, D. N., Hopfield, J. J. 1984. *J. Am. Chem. Soc.* 106: 1584
5. Beratan, D. N., Hopfield, J. J. 1984. *J. Chem. Phys.* 81: 5753
6. Beratan, D. N., Onuchic, J. N. 1989. *Photosynth. Res.* 22: 173
7. Beratan, D. N., Onuchic, J. N. 1991. *Adv. Chem. Ser.* 228: 71
8. Beratan, D. N., Onuchic, J. N., Betts, J. N., Bowler, B. E., Gray, H. B. 1990. *J. Am. Chem. Soc.* 112: 7915
9. Beratan, D. N., Onuchic, J. N., Gray, H. B. 1991. See Ref. 72, p. 97
10. Beratan, D. N., Onuchic, J. N., Hopfield, J. J. 1985. *J. Chem. Phys.* 83: 5325
11. Beratan, D. N., Onuchic, J. N., Hopfield, J. J. 1987. *J. Chem. Phys.* 86: 4488
12. Bialek, W., Bruno, W. J., Joseph, J., Onuchic, J. N. 1989. *Photosynth. Res.* 22: 15
13. Bowler, B. E., Meade, T. J., Mayo, S. L., Richards, J. H., Gray, H. B. 1989. *J. Am. Chem. Soc.* 111: 8757
14. Broo, S., Larsson, S. 1989. *J. Quant. Chem. Quant. Biol. Symp.* 16: 185
15. Brown, G. M., Sutin, N. 1979. *J. Am. Chem. Soc.* 101: 883
16. Brunschwig, B. S., Ehrenson, S., Sutin, N. 1986. *J. Phys. Chem.* 90: 3657
17. Buckley, F., Harary, F. 1990. *Distance in Graphs.* New York: Addison-Wesley

18. Caldeira, A. O., Leggett, A. J. 1983. *Ann. Phys.* 149: 374
19. Christensen, H. E. M., Conrad, L. S., Ulstrup, J., Mikkelsen, K. V. 1991. See Ref. 72, p. 57
20. Churg, A. K., Weiss, R. M., Warshel, A., Takano, T. 1983. *J. Phys. Chem.* 87: 1683
21. Conrad, D. W., Scott, R. A. 1989. *J. Am. Chem. Soc.* 111: 3461
22. Cowan, J. A., Upmacis, R. K., Beratan, D. N., Onuchic, J. N., Gray, H. B. 1988. *Ann. N.Y. Acad. Sci.* 550: 68
23. Cramer, W. A., Knaff, D. B. 1990. *Energy Transduction in Biological Membranes.* New York: Springer-Verlag
24. Crutchley, R. J., Ellis, W. R., Gray, H. B. 1985. *J. Am. Chem. Soc.* 107: 5002
25. da Gama, A. A. S. 1985. *Theor. Chim. Acta* 68: 159
26. da Gama, A. A. S. 1990. *J. Theor. Biol.* 142: 251
27. Davydov, A. S. 1987. *Phys. Status Solidi B* 90: 457
28. DeVault, D. 1984. *Quantum Mechanical Tunneling in Biological Systems.* New York: Cambridge Univ. Press. 2nd ed.
29. Durham, B., Pan, L. P., Long, J. E., Millett, F. 1989. *Biochemistry* 28: 8659
30. Elias, H., Chou, M. H., Winkler, J. R. 1988. *J. Am. Chem. Soc.* 110: 429
31. Farver, O., Pecht, I. 1989. *FEBS Lett.* 244: 379
32. Feher, G., Allen, J. P., Okamura, M. Y., Rees, D. C. 1989. *Nature* 339: 111
33. Fox, L. S., Kozik, M., Winkler, J. R., Gray, H. B. 1990. *Science* 247: 1069
34. Garg, A., Onuchic, J. N., Ambegaokar, V. 1985. *J. Chem. Phys.* 83: 4491
35. Goldman, C. 1991. *Phys. Rev. A* 43: 4500
36. Gray, H. B., Malmström, B. G. 1989. *Biochemistry* 28: 7499
37. Holten, D., Hoganson, C., Windsor, M. W., Schenck, C. C., Parson, W. W., et al. 1980. *Biochim. Biophys. Acta* 592: 461
38. Hopfield, J. J. 1974. *Proc. Natl. Acad. Sci. USA* 71: 3640
39. Jackman, M. P., McGinnis, J., Powls, R., Salmon, G. A., Sykes, A. G. 1988. *J. Am. Chem. Soc.* 110: 5880
40. Jacobs, B. A. 1991. *Preparation, characterization, and intramolecular electron transfer in pentaammineruthenium-modified derivatives of cytochrome b_5 and azurin.* PhD Thesis. Calif. Inst. Technol., Pasadena, Calif.
41. Jacobs, B. A., Mauk, M. R., Funk, W. D., MacGillivray, R. T. A., Mauk, A. G., Gray, H. B. 1991. *J. Am. Chem. Soc.* 113: 4390
42. Jortner, J. 1980. *Biochim. Biophys. Acta* 594: 139
43. Kamiya, N., Shiro, Y., Iwata, T., Iizuka, T., Iwasaki, H. 1991. *J. Am. Chem. Soc.* 113: 1826
44. Karas, J. L. 1989. *Long-range electron transfer in ruthenium-labelled myoglobin.* PhD Thesis. Calif. Inst. Technol., Pasadena, Calif.
45. Karas, J. L., Lieber, C. M., Gray, H. B. 1988. *J. Am. Chem. Soc.* 110: 599
46. Kuki, A., Wolynes, P. G. 1987. *Science* 236: 1647
47. Larsson, S. 1981. *J. Am. Chem. Soc.* 103: 4034
48. Larsson, S. 1983. *J. Chem. Soc. Faraday Trans.* 279: 1375
49. Lieber, C. M., Karas, J. L., Gray, H. B. 1987. *J. Am. Chem. Soc.* 109: 3779
50. Lin, S. H. 1989. *J. Chem. Phys.* 90: 7103
51. Marcus, R. A., Sutin, N. 1985. *Biochim. Biophys. Acta* 811: 265
52. Magarshak, Y., Malinsky, J., Joran, A. D. 1991. *J. Chem. Phys.* 95: 418
53. McConnell, H. M. 1961. *J. Chem. Phys.* 35: 508
54. Meade, T. J., Gray, H. B., Winkler, J. R. 1989. *J. Am. Chem. Soc.* 111: 4353
55. Mikkelsen, K. V., Ratner, M. A. 1988. *Chem. Rev.* 87: 113
56. Morishima, I., Shiro, J., Wakino, T. 1985. *J. Am. Chem. Soc.* 107: 1063
57. Natan, M. J., Baxter, W. W., Kuila, D., Gingrich, D. J., Martin, G. S., Hoffman, B. M. 1991. *Adv. Chem. Ser.* 228: 201
58. Newton, M. D. 1988. *J. Phys. Chem.* 92: 3049
59. Newton, M. D. 1991. *Chem. Rev.* 91: 767
60. Newton, M. D., Sutin, N. 1984. *Annu. Rev. Phys. Chem.* 35: 437
61. Nocera, D. G., Winkler, J. R., Yocom, K. M., Bordignon, E., Gray, H. B. 1984. *J. Am. Chem. Soc.* 106: 5145
62. Onuchic, J. N. 1987. *J. Chem. Phys.* 86: 3925
63. Onuchic, J. N., Beratan, D. N. 1987. *J. Am. Chem. Soc.* 109: 6771
64. Onuchic, J. N., Beratan, D. N. 1990. *J. Chem. Phys.* 92: 722
65. Onuchic, J. N., Beratan, D. N., Hopfield, J. J. 1986. *J. Phys. Chem.* 90: 3707
66. Onuchic, J. N., de Andrade, P. C. P., Beratan, D. N. 1991. *J. Chem. Phys.* 92: 1131
67. Onuchic, J. N., Wolynes, P. G. 1988. *J. Phys. Chem.* 92: 6495
67a. Ratner, M. A. 1990. *J. Phys. Chem.* 94: 4877
68. Selman, M. A. 1989. *Preparation and characterization and intramolecular electron transfer in a pentaammineruthenium derivative of* Candida krusei *cytochrome*

c. PhD Thesis. Calif. Inst. Technol., Pasadena, Calif.

69. Shiro, Y., Morishima, I. 1984. *Biochemistry* 23: 4879

70. Siddarth, P., Marcus, R. A. 1990. *J. Phys. Chem.* 94: 2985

71. Siddarth, P., Marcus, R. A. 1990. *J. Phys. Chem.* 94: 8430

72. Sigel, H., Sigel, A., eds. 1991. *Metal Ions in Biological Systems*, Vol. 27. New York: Marcel Dekker

73. Therien, M. J., Bowler, B. E., Selman, M. A., Gray, H. B., Chang, I.-J., Winkler, J. R. 1991. *Adv. Chem. Ser.* 228: 191

74. Therien, M. J., Selman, M. A., Gray, H. B., Chang, I.-J., Winkler, J. R. 1990. *J. Am. Chem. Soc.* 112: 2420

74a. Winkler, J. R., Gray, H. B. 1992. *Chem. Rev.* In press

75. Winkler, J. R., Nocera, D. G., Yocom, K. M., Bordignon, E., Gray, H. B. 1982. *J. Am. Chem. Soc.* 104: 5798

76. Wasielewski, M. R., Niemczyk, M. P., Svec, W. A., Pewitt, E. B. 1985. *J. Am. Chem. Soc.* 107: 5562

77. Yocom, K. M. 1981. *The synthesis and characterization of inorganic redox reagent-modified cytochrome* c. PhD Thesis. Calif. Inst. Technol., Pasadena, Calif.

78. Yocom, K. M., Shelton, J. B., Shelton, J. R., Schroeder, W. E., Worosila, G., et al. 1982. *Proc. Natl. Acad. Sci. USA* 79: 7052

79. Zewert, T. E. 1990. *Electron transfer in chemically and genetically modified myoglobins.* PhD Thesis. Calif. Inst. Technol., Pasadena, Calif.

Annu. Rev. Biophys. Biomol. Struct. 1992. 21:379–415

THE SINGLE-NUCLEOTIDE ADDITION CYCLE IN TRANSCRIPTION: a Biophysical and Biochemical Perspective

Dorothy A. Erie, Thomas D. Yager,[1] *and Peter H. von Hippel*

Institute of Molecular Biology and Department of Chemistry, University of Oregon, Eugene, Oregon 97403

KEY WORDS: DNA transcription, RNA polymerase, RNA synthesis, regulation of transcription, transcription complexes

CONTENTS

[1] Present Address: NSF Center for Molecular Biotechnology, Division of Biology (139–74), California Institute of Technology, Pasadena, California 91125.

379

1056–8700/92/0610–0379$02.00

PERSPECTIVES AND OVERVIEW

It is useful to view the mechanisms and regulation of RNA transcription at different levels of resolution. Each view stresses different aspects of the structure and behavior of the DNA-dependent RNA polymerase, which is the enzyme that catalyzes specific gene transcription. We review here the mechanism of transcription as catalyzed by the RNA polymerase of *Escherichia coli*, which is by far the best understood member of this class of enzymes.

Figure 1*A* shows the transcription process from the perspective of an

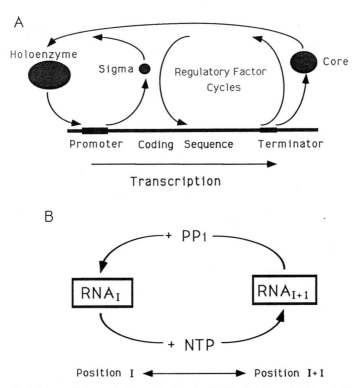

Figure 1 (*A*) Overall transcription cycle (see text). (*B*) Single nucleotide addition (or removal) cycle (see text).

operon. At this level, the operon (which may code for one or more genes or for one or more ribosomal or transfer RNA molecules) contains three important types of DNA sequences. (*a*) The promoter sequence signals the beginning of the operon and, as a consequence of its intrinsic and/or protein modulated affinity for polymerase holoenzyme, initiates specific transcript formation. The frequency of initiation at a particular promoter depends on its success in competing with the other promoters of the genome for free holoenzyme. (*b*) The coding sequence specifies the order of nucleotide residues in the mRNA, rRNA, or tRNA to be synthesized. (*c*) The terminator sequence marks the end of the transcribed region and brings about release of the nascent RNA transcript and of the polymerase. Termination may be controlled by the interaction of nucleotide sequences with the transcribing polymerase alone, or regulatory protein factors may be required as well.

These three sets of DNA sequences correspond functionally to the initiation, elongation, and termination phases of the overall transcription cycle, which begins and ends with polymerase free in solution. In addition to the main cycle representing the three phases of the transcription of an operon, Figure 1*A* also contains an upper regulatory loop that indicates that the successful transcription of an operon with this enzyme requires that the *E. coli* core RNA polymerase be augmented by a specificity subunit (σ) that enables it to recognize specific promoters and initiate transcription. At the end of the initiation phase, this σ factor is released, and the elongation and termination phases can be completed, in a minimal in vitro system, by core polymerase alone. Consequently, a minimal system capable of specific transcription (i.e. one that can initiate and terminate correctly) can be set up in a test tube using only a DNA fragment carrying appropriate promoter and terminator sequences, the *E. coli* polymerase holoenzyme, and the appropriate nucleotide triphosphates. The core polymerase (subunit composition $\alpha_2\beta\beta'$; see below), together with a σ subunit, comprise the RNA polymerase holoenzyme.

The overall cycle shown in Figure 1*A* is highly regulated in all three phases of transcription, both by extraneous protein factors that bind to the DNA template and/or to the transcription complex as it moves along the template, and by specific sequence elements (expressed either as DNA or RNA) that interact with the transcribing polymerase at each template position. The loop shown in Figure 1*A* marked *regulatory factor cycles* represents the large variety of regulatory proteins that bind to, and release from, the core polymerase in its passage through the elongation phase of transcription. These binding and release processes fine tune the stability and the rate of movement of the transcription complex along the template, and by so doing modulate the transcription of specific operons in accord with the requirements of the cell.

The molecular events involved in the transcription cycle, as portrayed schematically in Figure 1*A*, have (to the extent they are currently understood) been extensively reviewed in the past few years (50, 59, 97, 115, 141, 142, 148). We do not intend to reexamine this subject in any detail here.

Figure 1*B* schematically shows a higher resolution view of the transcription cycle. This cycle depicts the processive addition of a single nucleotide residue to the 3′-hydroxyl end of the nascent RNA chain located at template position I. At the end of this single nucleotide addition cycle, the chain is one nucleotide residue longer, and the transcription complex is poised to add another nucleotide at template position $I + 1$ or to remove the nucleotide residue at position I. This process is traditionally represented, in deceptively over-simplified form, by Equation 1, which represents the overall chemical reaction:

$$RNA_I + NTP \rightleftharpoons RNA_{I+1} + PP_i \qquad \qquad 1.$$

Recent progress in understanding the molecular-level details of the reaction portrayed in Equation 1 has come about largely because we can now isolate reasonably pure, homogeneous, and stable elongation complexes that are stalled (by NTP depletion) at specific DNA template positions (78, 91). Addition of the next (correct or incorrect) nucleotide triphosphate substrate and/or pyrophosphate allows one, in principle, to probe the rates and equilibria of individual steps (such as single-nucleotide incorporation, removal, or misincorporation) as a function of template sequence and solvent environment. Consequently, we can begin to examine the details of sequence- and factor-dependent transcriptional control at the chemical level. Only by investigating the transcription cycle at this highest level of resolution, and by understanding how its steps are perturbed by template sequence and/or interaction with protein regulatory factors, can we hope to uncover the molecular basis of the sequence-dependent events in transcription that are clearly crucial to the regulation of this central process of living cells.

Many questions need to be answered at this level of detail, as suggested by some examples. (*a*) Intrinsic (factor-independent) termination sites occur just after the transcribing polymerase has synthesized through a palindromic sequence that codes for the formation of a potentially stable stem-loop structure in the nascent RNA. How rapidly does this stem-loop structure form, and how does it interact with the moving transcription complex to drive the complex into the termination mode and thus cause transcript release? (*b*) The transcribing elongation complex pauses (for times several hundredfold longer than its dwell time at an average template position) at specific ρ-dependent termination sites, presumably to provide time for the RNA release protein, ρ, to move along the nascent RNA and detach the completed transcript. What signals this lengthy pause and how does the moving elongation complex respond to this signal? (*c*) On reading through the specific (*nut* or *qut*) site in transcription of the genome of phage λ, the N or Q antitermination proteins bind to the complex and the properties of the transcribing polymerase somehow change so that downstream termination signals are ignored. How does traversing the *nut* or *qut* site signal these changes, and how does the transcribing polymerase respond? These questions will not be definitively answered until we know, in molecular detail, what happens to the transcription complex at each of these loci.

This review focuses on transcription at this intimately mechanistic level, both by summarizing what (little) has so far been learned with stalled complexes, and by pulling together the substantial older literature at the level of the mechanistic enzymology that must now be reconsidered and reevaluated in light of new developments. This has been a rewarding exercise for us because it forms the underpinnings of the mechanistic investigations of transcription and transcriptional regulation in which we are currently engaged. We hope that some readers will also profit from this largely prospective review, the primary merit of which may be that it helps to illuminate (and to prepare a context for) studies that are yet to come.

THERMODYNAMICS OF RNA SYNTHESIS

Before considering the details of *E. coli* RNA polymerase structure and biochemistry, we analyze the free energy changes that drive the polymerase preferentially in one direction along the DNA template during RNA synthesis. This analysis is based on equilibrium thermodynamics and is thus largely independent of the mechanistic details of RNA transcript elongation that follow. One should remember in applying such a thermodynamic analysis, however, that the underlying assumption is that the complex reaches equilibrium at every template position.

The Gibbs Free Energy Function

We define a Gibbs free energy function (G_l) that has a unique and calculable value at each template position. The reference state for this function is defined as a transcription-elongation complex on a particular DNA template, located so that the 3'-hydroxyl terminus of the RNA transcript lies exactly 12 nucleotide positions downstream of the transcriptional start site.[2] Thus the putative 12-base pair (bp) RNA-DNA hybrid is complete, and the elongation complex has reached its mature state, but the RNA does not extend beyond the (double-stranded) hybrid. The concentrations of active polymerase molecules, of NTPs and PP_i, and of K^+, H^+, and Mg^{2+} are specified according to a set of initial reaction conditions.

G_I is then defined as the sum of three major terms[3] [further details will soon be available (T. D. Yager, J. Korte & P. H. von Hippel, in preparation)].

$$G_I = G_{chem,I} + \Delta G_{f,RNA,I} + \Delta G_{f,complex,I} \qquad 2.$$

The free energy terms of Equation 2 are defined as follows:

1. $G_{chem,I}$ is the Gibbs free energy of a purely chemical system corresponding to 1 mol of active elongation complexes located at position I on the template, with the associated free concentrations of NTP and PP_i. This is an extensive quantity and presumably could be calculated from absolute free energies of formation, according to the third law of thermodynamics.

2. $\Delta G_{f,RNA,I}$ is the free energy of formation of the folded structure of the RNA transcript that is located upstream of the end of the DNA-RNA hybrid at position I. This term is zero in the reference state, because no RNA exists outside of the transcription bubble. In general this free energy term consists of three components, corresponding to the following three elements of the tertiary structure of the nascent RNA: (a) the formation of duplex base-paired regions of the RNA (21, 44); (b) the stacking of adjacent nucleotide residues in single-stranded regions of the RNA (22); and (c) the specific chelation of divalent cations and small organic molecules to the RNA chain (64, 116, 119, 136).

3. $\Delta G_{f,complex,I}$, is the free energy of formation of the elongation complex at template position I, as defined by Yager & von Hippel (149). This term represents the free energy of formation of the ternary elongation complex at position I from pure double-stranded DNA, single-stranded (and

---

[2] This reference state is defined on the basis of the current consensus model of the ternary elongation complex of *E. coli*, as defined and justified extensively elsewhere (148, 149). If, for example, the DNA-RNA hybrid turns out to have a length different from the 12 bp of the consensus model (e.g. 120), then the reference state can, of course, be redefined appropriately. We note that initiation at different promoters, as well as other enviromental factors, will also lead to different reference states.

[3] In principle, a cratic (entropy of mixing) term should be added to the right side of Equation 2 to take into account the mixing of the RNA transcript with molecules of solvent. This term depends on the length and number of RNA transcripts synthesized from a fixed pool of NTPs; however, this term is small and generally can be ignored (T. D. Yager, J. Korte & P. H. von Hippel, in preparation).

unstructured) nascent RNA of length I, and core RNA polymerase in its free solution conformation.

The Gibbs Free Energy Difference Function

If the Gibbs free energy function, G_I, is constant from one position to the next along the DNA template, then no net thermodynamic driving force exists to move the elongation complex forward. The quantity $G_{I+1} - G_I$ must be nonzero to obtain a preferential movement in one direction. If this difference is less than zero, a net free energy decrease will accompany the forward movement of the elongation complex. On the other hand, if this difference is positive, then the elongation complex will be driven in the reverse direction, depolymerizing the RNA transcript as it proceeds. Thus, the thermodynamic free energy change that drives the elongation complex from position I to position $I+1$ is defined as:

$$\Delta G_{I \to I+1} = G_{I+1} - G_I \qquad\qquad 3.$$

The value of this function will vary signficantly with template position, as illustrated below.

The Chemical Free Energy Change

The chemical component of the free energy change can be calculated as follows:

$$\Delta G_{\text{chem},I \to I+1} = G_{\text{chem},I+1} - G_{\text{chem},I} = \Delta G^\circ_{\text{chem},I \to I+1} + RT \ln K \qquad 4.$$

where $\Delta G^\circ_{\text{chem},I \to I+1}$ is the chemical component of the standard free energy change of the reaction at template position I at standard state (1 M) concentrations of PP_i and NTP and K is the apparent equilibrium constant for the phosphoryl bond transfer reaction of Equation 1:

$$K = \frac{[PP_i]}{[NTP]} \qquad\qquad 5.$$

This equation is based on the assumption that the polymerase does not distinguish between RNA_I and RNA_{I+1}, which should be true (at least for homopolymers) once the transcription process has moved beyond the initiation phase, and that, therefore, the RNA can be simply considered (in terms of Equation 1) to act as a catalyst in the conversion of NTP to PP_i. Kato et al (72) have determined that $K \approx 100$ for the formation of poly (dA) from dATP monomers. The experimental approach in this study involved thin-layer chromatographic analysis of the products of a DNA polymerization reaction catalyzed by calf thymus terminal transferase at pH = 6.8, $[Mg^{2+}] = 8$ mM, and $T = 35°C$. We have carried out a similar study of the formation of poly (rA) from rATP, catalyzed by *E. coli* RNA polymerase (T. D. Yager & J. Korte, unpublished results), and have also obtained an experimental value of $K \approx 100$ under approximately the same conditions.

These two determinations may be checked for consistency with other data on the polymerization of homopolymers (112). The agreement is quite reasonable, given the somewhat different conditions under which the measurements were made. When all available data are averaged, we conclude that the standard free energy change for the synthesis of a RNA homopolymer, $\Delta G^\circ_{chem, l \to l+1}$, is -3.1 (± 0.8) kcal/mol of nucleotide polymerized. Thus, as expected, the synthetic process is favored under typical in vitro transcription conditions.

However, the above (experimental) determinations of the apparent equilibrium constant (K) measure factors besides the inherent chemical driving force. Monomers of rNTP, rNDP, or dNTP synthesize a homopolymer of RNA (or DNA), and it is well known that some homopolynucleotides— notably poly (rA)—spontaneously take on a helical structure in dilute (monovalent) salt solutions of neutral pH (8, 22, 40, 90, 112, 145). This helical structure is preserved upon the addition of 10 mM Mg^{2+} to such solutions (T. D. Yager & J. Korte, unpublished results). If we accept the determination that $\Delta G^\circ = -1$ kcal/mol (at $T = 37°C$) for the formation of helical structure between two adjacent adenine residues in a homopolymer (22), then to arrive at a true value for ΔG°_{chem} we must subtract this amount of free energy from the estimates of ΔG°_{chem} determined from the experimentally measured values of K cited above. Thus we obtain $\Delta G^\circ_{chem} \approx -2.1$ kcal/mol, which corresponds to an equilibrium constant of ~ 30 for the chemical component of the standard free-energy change for polymerization.

Under certain conditions, additional terms may be added to the right side of Equation 4 to take into account other chemical equilibria that may be linked to the chemical polymerization process. For example, the hydrolysis equilbrium, $PP_i + H_2O \rightleftharpoons 2P_i$, has been postulated to be important in vivo; however, recent estimates of the PP_i concentration in *E. coli* (82–84) suggest the contrary (see below).

One more term must be added to the right side of Equation 4 to account for linked ionic equilibria. Changes in the concentrations of H^+, Mg^{2+}, and K^+ ions away from their reference-state values can affect the equilibrium for RNA polymerization. This effect is mediated through linked ionic equilibria involving the differential binding of these cations to phosphate groups in NTP, PP_i, and the phosphodiester backbone of the growing RNA chain. These linked equilibria have been analyzed (T. D. Yager, J. Korte & P. H. von Hippel, in preparation) with the formalism of Alberty

(5, 6) and Phillips et al (113). The conclusion is that each step of RNA polymerization results in significant changes in the net binding of Mg^{2+} and H^+ during RNA polymerization.

RNA Folding

The quantity of importance in calculating the contribution of RNA folding to the thermodynamics of the reaction shown in Equation 1 is the difference in the free energies of formation of the folded RNA structures at positions I and $I+1$. We attempt to calculate this component of the energetics of the RNA synthesis reaction in three stages. (a) We subject the RNA sequence to an algorithm for secondary-structure prediction, using standard free-energy values for duplex base-pair formation in RNA (44). A reasonable prediction of secondary structure can be obtained if this structure is not too irregular (1). (b) We then analyze the RNA structure for any single-stranded regions that appear relatively unhindered in their conformation and that can form single-stranded helices. These regions are given an additional stabilization free energy of approximately -1 kcal/mol per pair of stacked nearest neighbors, in accord with experimental data (22). (c) Finally we ask whether the RNA structure might specifically chelate a Mg^{2+} ion or a small organic molecule, thereby gaining even greater thermodynamic stability. Based on the Mg^{2+} and spermidine binding behavior of yeast phenylalanyl tRNA, we expect such a binding event to contribute -5 to -10 kcal/mol of stabilization free energy to the entire RNA structure (64, 116, 119, 136).

A real calculation of the energetic contribution of RNA folding is limited by two problems. (a) Prediction of the tertiary structure of RNA is still very problematic, and the energetics of tertiary structure formation are poorly understood (e.g. 1). (b) We cannot yet predict the sites or free energies of chelation of divalent cations or other multicharged ligands on RNA sequences. These two problems are interrelated because tertiary structure in RNA is often cooperatively stabilized by the site-specific binding of small ligands.

Free Energy of Formation of the Transcription Complex

The difference between the free energy of formation of the transcription complex located at template positions I and $I+1$ $[\Delta(\Delta G_{f,complex,I \to I+1})]$ will also contribute to the total free energy change involved in a specific single nucleotide addition (or removal) reaction. The term $\Delta(\Delta G_{f,complex,I \to I+1})$ can be significantly positive or negative at specific template positions, depending on the identity of the base-pairs that open and close at the ends of the transcription bubble and at the ends of the DNA-RNA hybrid upon the I-to-$I+1$ translocation, and thus can have significant effects on the properties of the transcription complex as a function of template position (see discussion below). However, the average value of $\Delta(\Delta G_{f,complex,I \to I+1})$ will be close to zero.

PURIFICATION OF RNA POLYMERASE AND STALLED ELONGATION COMPLEXES

Purification Procedures and Assays

Work on this problem began over twenty years ago with the design of a purification procedure (25) that has been continually improved (56). However, the preparative procedure remains somewhat irreproducible for the following reasons. (*a*) The polymerase is easily damaged (in undefined ways); thus the fraction of polymerase that is active varies widely (30). (*b*) The polymerase undergoes a set of self-association reactions that complicate structural studies under conditions of high protein concentration (127, 139). (*c*) The polymerase core enzyme binds many different additional subunits at different points of the transcription cycle and under different physiological conditions, further complicating purification. (*d*) Finally, of course, one has to agree on what comprises an activity assay of the enzyme in its various forms, since polymerase preparations that seem identical in polymerizing activity can differ significantly in, for example, aspects of the kinetics of single-cycle misincorporation experiments on stalled complexes prepared in various ways (30; D. A. Erie, unpublished results).

Formation and Properties of Stalled Elongation Complexes

Investigation of the elongation phase of transcription has lagged behind that of initation and termination because it has been difficult to isolate sufficient quantities of purified homogeneous elongation complexes. This problem has been largely solved with procedures to isolate elongation complexes stalled at unique sites on the DNA template by specific NTP depletion (92). These complexes, however, are still slightly inhomogeneous. As described below, the details of the pathway by which a particular stalled complex is prepared can result in conformational and functional heterogeneity, and a preparation displaying homogeneity in one functional assay may be heterogeneous in another. Until a general procedure is devised for the preparation of complexes that are homogeneous in all functional assays, it will be necessary to characterize each new preparation thoroughly to allow comparison with other studies.

Early experiments (118) demonstrated that stable elongation complexes formed on poly d(AT) could be isolated using gel exclusion chromatography. These complexes were formed by allowing transcription to proceed for 1 min in the presence of UTP and ATP at 37°C. The reaction was then quenched with ethylenediaminetetraacetic acid (EDTA), chilled, and loaded onto a size-exclusion column. Stable elongation complexes were recovered that could support further template-directed elongation upon the addition of ATP and UTP. Such stalled complexes were stable at 4°C for up to a week and were used to investigate the kinetics of the elongation reaction on poly d(AT) without the complications of the initiation reaction.

In later studies, chain-terminating nucleotide analogs, such as 3'-O-Me-NTPs and 3'-dNTPs, were introduced in addition to the canonical NTPs to arrest elongation complexes on natural DNA templates at multiple defined positions (4, 16, 68, 70, 104, 105, 124). These chain-terminating NTPs can be removed via the pyrophosphorolysis reaction (3, 124), and the resulting shortened transcript (with a restored 3'-hydroxyl terminus) can be extended to full-length products (68, 70). Accordingly, chain-terminating NTP analogs incorporated into the 3'-end of the transcript can be used to make stable stalled elongation complexes. Although this method is an improvement over the quenching method described above, it still yields a distribution of complexes stalled at multiple sites. To permit a detailed exploration of the mechanism of RNA synthesis as well as the structure of a ternary elongation complex, one must obtain complexes that are stalled at unique template positions.

Stable elongation complexes stalled at specific template positions can be formed on natural templates using di- or trinucleotides as primers and only three of the four canonical NTPs. This procedure was used to form specific complexes on templates containing the T7A1, the λP_L, and the E. coli rrnB P1 promoters and their natural transcript sequences (92). Transcription from these promoters in the presence of the appropiate di- or trinucleotide initiator, ATP, CTP, and GTP resulted in the formation of stable elongation complexes stalled at positions just before the incorporation site of the first uridine residue. As previously observed with complexes stalled on poly d(AT) (118), these promoter-directed stalled complexes were also stable for more than a week at 4°C.

The ability to generate stable stalled elongation complexes at a single template position is a major breakthrough in the investigation of the elongation reaction. Use of stalled complexes at a single template base allows one to study the structure of an elongating ternary complex (79, 80, 102), the kinetics of addition of a single nucleotide residue (correct or incorrect) to an elongating RNA chain (41, 42), and the extent and type of misincorporation at a unique position (68). Stalling complexes at a unique position also allows the synchronization of RNA polymerase molecules, which is useful for measuring the lengths of specific transcriptional pauses (see below).

In addition to using the NTP depletion method, stalled complexes have been formed by inserting physical blocks to elongation on the DNA template. Blocking procedures that have been used include psoralen cross-links (128) and the binding of site-specific proteins to appropriate template sites (111). Stalled complexes made with psoralen cross-linked DNA have been used to investigate the structure of elongation complexes; however, because cross-linking is irreversible, elongation cannot proceed past the cross-linked position on the template. In contrast, stalled elongation complexes have been formed using a mutant of *Eco*RI that is defective in endonuclease activity but retains high specific binding affinity ($\sim 10^{13} \, \text{M}^{-1}$) under low salt conditions, thus functioning as a reversible block to transcript synthesis (111). Stalled complexes are formed in the presence of the *Eco*RI mutant at low salt; NTPs are removed by gel filtration; and the mutant *Eco*RI protein is dissociated from the DNA template by transferring the complexes to high salt. These specifically stalled complexes can then be further elongated by adding back NTPs.

The use of a reversible block of this type is particularly advantageous for making stalled complexes far from the promoter, because the only template sequence requirement is the presence of an *Eco*RI binding site. Accordingly, an *Eco*RI binding site can be cloned into the template at many different positions, and transcription can be performed in the presence of all four NTPs. One disadvantage of this method is that the transcription reactions must be run in high salt after stalled complex formation to prevent the rebinding of the *Eco*RI mutant enzyme. One probably could, however, use an excess of an oligonucleotide that contains the *Eco*RI binding site as a competitor to prevent rebinding of the mutant *Eco*RI to the transcription template or remove the *Eco*RI mutant protein by chromatography, thus allowing the stalled complexes to be chased in the presence of low salt.

The main difficulty with the above approaches is that any specific stalled elongation complex must be generated via initiation by σ factor–containing RNA polymerase holoenzyme at a specific promoter. This procedure can lead to conformational and sequence heterogeneity. Recent attempts to establish defined elongation complexes on natural templates directly with core polymerase, foregoing the initiation phase of transcription, are promising (S. Daube & P. H. von Hippel, unpublished results), but have not yet reached fruition. Most of the work described below has been done with stalled elongation complexes that have been naturally initiated, and is therefore subject to a caveat regarding possible heterogeneity.

STRUCTURE OF *E. COLI* RNA POLYMERASE

A high resolution structure would help elucidate the mechanism of RNA synthesis. Unfortunately, such information is not yet available for any DNA-dependent RNA polymerase. A variety of physical, chemical, and enzymatic methods, however, have been employed to probe the structure of *E. coli* RNA polymerase holoenzyme, core enzyme, and ternary elongation complexes as well as of the catalytic site.

The Holoenzyme

The RNA polymerase holoenzyme is required to initiate transcription specifically at the promoters that specify start sites for transcription. In addition to the functional $\alpha_2\beta\beta'$ core, the holoenzyme contains one molar equivalent of a σ subunit that is crucial for promoter recognition and the first steps of transcript initiation in vivo. Different σ factors that recognize different classes of promoters are synthesized in response to changes in environmental and developmental signals (58). In unstressed exponentially growing *E. coli* cells, the main ("housekeeping") sigma factor is σ^{70} (26),[4] and is the only σ factor that we consider here. This review is also not concerned with other transcription factors that regulate the properties and activity of the ternary (polymerase, DNA, and nascent RNA) transcription complex. Instead we restrict ourselves to a rigorous description of what is known about the mechanism and thermodynamics of the essential processes in the nucleotide addition cycle. Once this foundation is laid, information about additional protein factors that bind to and regulate the function of the elongation complex can be added more easily.

Core RNA Polymerase

Clearly, the core enzyme does far more than catalyze the (one-step) chemical reaction described in Equation 1. At the least, it facilitates the processive translocation of the enzyme along the DNA template as the nascent RNA chain is extended. It also carries helicase activities involved in opening the double-stranded DNA in front of the transcription complex to expose the single-stranded DNA template, and perhaps in closing the double-helix behind the transcription complex as well (45, 46). It is also involved in opening, closing, and otherwise manipulating the DNA-RNA hybrid at positions well removed from the actual catalytic site. In that it carries these properties as an inseparable part of the core polymerase, it differs from most DNA polymerase holoenzymes that must perform many of the same functions; in the DNA polymerases, the basic catalytic subunit can be

---

[4] The superscript refers to the approximate molecular weight (kDa) of the σ factor.

separated (and assayed) in the absence of the subunits that are primarily responsible for helicase and primase functions, for establishing processivity, and so forth (75).

The *E. coli* RNA polymerase core enzyme is well defined, with a subunit composition of $\alpha_2\beta\beta'$ (26). It also carries two mole equivalents of Zn(II) (34 and references therein). The genes for the core subunits have been cloned, sequenced, and mapped to the *E. coli* genome (27). Low resolution structural models of the core polymerase have been proposed, based on data from solution X-ray scattering (62, 98–100), solution neutron-scattering (61), and electron-diffraction investigations (36).

Because the $\alpha_2\beta\beta'$ complex is impossible to dissociate without denaturation, progress toward assigning specific functions to the subunits has been slow. Indeed, certain functions may depend specifically on the association of certain subunits. Clearly at least one of the zinc ions is bound to the β' subunit; however, it is not known if the second zinc ion is bound to the β' or the β subunit, or whether it is bound at the $\beta\beta'$ interface (34). Neither of the zinc ions can be removed from core or holoenzyme by treatment with EDTA or 1,10-phenanthroline without denaturating the enzyme. However, *E. coli* RNA polymerase containing Co(II) has been produced by growing *E. coli* on a Co(II)-supplemented, Zn(II)-depleted medium (132). This Co(II) enzyme has an activity identical to that of the Zn(II)-containing RNA polymerase. Genetic analysis and some protein cross-linking data have suggested that the β-subunit may carry the rNTP binding site of the enzyme. The α-subunits are known to be important for the correct assembly of core enzyme. In addition, the α-subunits are believed to be important for positive regulation in vivo (66).

THE ACTIVE SITE OF *E. COLI* RNA POLYMERASE

The Two-Site Model

It is generally accepted that *E. coli* RNA polymerase carries only a single active center that is involved in the catalysis of RNA polymerization (29, 76, 77). An early investigation (76) of the pyrophosphate-exchange reaction of *Azotobacter vinelandii* RNA polymerase led to the proposal of a two-site model for this catalytic process; it has been postulated that the 3′-hydroxyl terminus of the RNA resides in a product terminus site and that the NTP binds to a substrate site. (These features are shown schematically in Figure 2; position indices within the catalytic site, labeled $i+1$, i, and $i-1$, are also indicated in the figure.) A variety of subsequent studies on *E. coli* RNA polymerase (9, 14, 18, 31, 32, 39, 131, 152) support this model as well and suggest that it applies in general. Further structural and

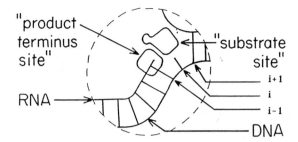

Figure 2   Two-site model of the catalytic site of DNA-dependent RNA polymerase (see text). The terms $i+1$, i, and $i-1$ represent position indices within the catalytic site.

mechanistic details of the substrate and product terminus sites have been provided by stereochemical studies of substrate binding and turnover.

Stereochemistry of RNA Synthesis

Ribonucleoside 5′-O-(1-thio-triphosphates) (α-thio-NTPs) are stereospecifically incorporated into RNA by *E. coli* RNA polymerase. In these reactions, the S_p diastereomer (A isomer) is greatly favored over the R_p diastereomer (B isomer) (14, 152). Figure 3*A* shows the structures and stereochemistry of these isomers. Investigations of the stereochemistry of RNA chain initiation and elongation using α-thio-NTPs (24, 39, 152) have revealed that inversion of configuration occurs at the α-phosphorous of the NTP in the synthesis reaction, while a retention of configuration is observed at the α-phosphorous in the pyrophosphate-exchange reaction. These results are consistent with a S_N^2 mechanism for the synthesis process and with the pyrophosphate exchange reaction being the reversal of the phosphodiester-bond formation. The S_N^2 mechanism requires that the 3′-hydroxyl group of the growing chain (at the product terminus site) and the PP_i group of the incoming NTP (at the substrate site) be located at apical positions of a trigonal bipyramid (152).

Structural Studies of the Polymerase Active Site

An early investigation of the kinetics of elongation on synthetic templates indicated that the triphosphate group dominates the binding affinity of the NTPs (118). In this study, the NTPs were found to be competitive inhibitors of one another in the synthesis process, with the inhibition constants (K_I) independent of the base moiety. This conclusion was strengthened by the observation that triphosphates inhibit synthesis to the same extent as the competing NTPs. Subsequent studies have employed a wide variety of nucleotide triphosphate and pyrophosphate analogs to probe the structure

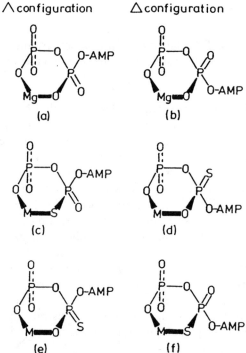

Figure 3 (*A*) Absolute configuration of the isomers of α-thio-ATP (ATPαS). Reproduced from Ref. 152. (*B*) Absolute configurations of the bidentate metal ion complexes of ATP (*a*, *b*) and of the A (*c*, *d*) and B isomers (*e*, *f*) of β-thio-ATP. Reproduced from Ref. 14.

and specificity of the NTP binding site (2, 9–14, 16, 24, 37, 39, 52, 53, 65, 67, 114, 126, 129, 130, 151–153). The pioneering work in this area was that of Eckstein and coworkers (10, 24, 39, 152), who extended their thio-NTP studies of the reaction to also probe the chemistry of the RNA polymerase active site. Examination of the substrate properties of the thio-NTPs with divalent metal ions that differ in their affinities for chelating sulfur and oxygen enabled these authors to propose a model for the structure of the NTP-containing substrate site (10).

α-THIO NTP DERIVATIVES   Investigation of the substrate properties of the α-thio derivatives revealed that only the A isomers (S_p configuration) of the α-thio NTP derivatives (Figure 3A) act as substrates. The K_m values of these A isomers were found to be approximately four times greater than those of the corresponding NTPs, while the V_{max} values were the same for the sulfur and oxygen derivatives. This result is consistent with a lower binding affinity for the α-thio species and indicates that the enzyme activity (calculated as substrate turnover rate) is unaffected by the substitution. In contrast, the B isomers (R configuration) do not serve as substrates; rather they appear to be weak inhibitors of the polymerization reaction (10, 152).

These results led to the proposal that a charged site on the enzyme interacts with the oxygens of the α-phosphate group. Because the α-thio-NTPs are chiral and because a positively charged group interacts more strongly with oxygen than with sulfur, the isomer in which the oxygen of the α-thio-phosphate group interacts with the charged group (in this case, the A isomer) should be the preferred substrate; thus explaining the lack of affinity of the enzyme for the B isomer. A similar explanation has been proposed for DNA polymerase I (14). In addition, replacement of Mg(II), which preferentially chelates oxygen, with ions such as Cd(II) that preferentially chelate sulfur over oxygen, did not affect the substrate properties of the α-S-NTPs. This result indicates that chelation of the metal ion with the α-phosphate group of the NTP is not required for enzyme activity.

β-THIO NTP DERIVATIVES   Investigation of the β-thio derivatives as a function of metal type have yielded further information about the structure of the NTP binding site as well as about the structure of the NTP-metal complex (14). In contrast to the α-thio NTPs, the substrate properties of the β-thio NTPs were sensitive to the metal ion present in the reaction buffer. Consequently, it was proposed that the divalent ion forms a bidentate complex with the NTP by chelating at the β- and γ-phosphate positions and that this metal-NTP complex is a substrate for RNA polymerase. For each diastereomer, two possible conformations of the bidentate complex can occur, depending on whether chelation is primarily through oxygen or primarily through sulfur. Figure 3B shows the possible conformations of the bidentate complexes of the β-thio-NTPs, as well as of the unmodified NTPs.

In the presence of Mg(II), the A and B isomers have approximately the same substrate properties; however, in the presence of Cd(II), which chelates sulfur more strongly than oxygen, the enzyme is essentially stereospecific for the B isomer. Because Cd(II) chelates primarily through sulfur, the data are consistent with the Δ configuration of the NTP being the active complex (Figure 3B). To account for the lack of selectivity between the A and B isomers in the presence of Mg(II), the authors propose an additional ion-pair interaction between the enzyme and the β-phosphate group. Because the ion-pair site prefers oxygen over sulfur and Mg(II) prefers oxygen over sulfur, and because the Δ configuration is the active bidentate complex, both isomers A and B only partially satisfy the binding specificity. These data, taken together with the results on the α-thio-NTPs and the stereospecificity of the polymerization reaction, led the authors to propose the stereochemical model of the NTP-bound substrate site shown in Figure 4A.

PYROPHOSPHATE ANALOGS   More recently, Rozovskaya and coworkers studied the effect of ten different pyrophosphate analogs on the pyro-phosphorolysis reaction catalyzed by RNA polymerase (126). Since pyro-phosphorolysis is the reverse reaction of synthesis (Equation 1), the ability of the various pyrophosphate analogs to support pyrophosphorolysis should also provide information about the specificity and structure of the NTP binding site. In this work, the authors combine data from a variety of studies on NTP analogs (references included in the list given at the beginning of this section) with their own data on pyrophosphate analogs to construct a detailed model of the configuration of the NTP substrate binding site. Inspection of their model shown in Figure 4B reveals that the oxygens of both the α- and β-phosphate groups can accommodate very few chemical substitutions and still remain active substrates while the γ-phosphate group can accommodate several bulky substituents in place of one of the nonbridging oxygens. Similarly, the 2'-OH group of the sugar has more stringent chemical substitution requirements than the 3'-OH group. In addition to providing insight into the structure of the NTP binding site, this chemical information is useful for designing new NTP analogs that are substrates for synthesis and that may be useful for probing the mechanism of synthesis.

MECHANISM OF RNA SYNTHESIS

To fully comprehend the mechanism by which RNA polymerase regulates gene expression, one must understand the details of the RNA poly-

---

Figure 4   (*A*) Model of the configuration of MgATP bound in the NTP binding site. Reproduced from Ref. 14. (*B*) Model of the configuration of MgATP and MgATP analogs that are substrates for RNA synthesis by *E. coli* RNA polymerase. Reproduced from Ref. 126.

(a)

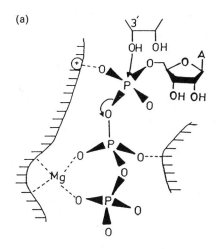

(b)

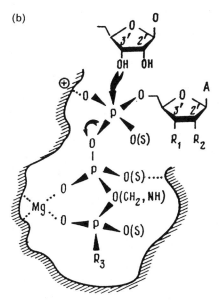

$R_1 = OCH_3, NH_2, N_3, H, NHCOCH_2Br, OH; R_2, R_3 = OH$

$R_2 = OH, OCH_3, N_3; R_1, R_3 = OH$

$R_3 = OH, F, OCH_3, OPhe,$ HN—⟨⟩, HN—⟨⟩—SO_3^-

$R_1, R_2 = OH$

$R_1 = NCS; R_2 = H; R_3 = OH$

merization reaction. That is, one should identify all of the steps in the kinetic pathway and determine which of the steps are rate limiting for both correct and incorrect nucleotide incorporation. In this section, we present a minimal mechanism for the addition (or removal) of a single nucleotide residue to (or from) an elongating RNA chain. As discussed in later sections, this minimal mechanism cannot explain all of the existing data on *E. coli* RNA polymerase transcription. The addition of one or more steps is required to account for conformational changes that occur in an elongating RNA polymerase complex. At present, however, the data are insufficient to allow the incorporation of these conformational changes into the overall kinetic scheme. Consequently, we present a mechanism that incorporates all of the steps for single nucleotide addition that are well defined. The minimal mechanism presented depends only on the well-accepted assumption that *E. coli* RNA polymerase has a single catalytic site (see above).

Minimal Kinetic Pathway for a Single Base Addition or Removal

The addition/removal of a single nucleotide to/from an elongating chain requires at least four steps: (*a*) NTP binding/release, (*b*) phosphodiester-bond formation/breakage, (*c*) pyrophosphate release/binding, and (*d*) translocation (forward/reverse) of the catalytic site relative to the terminus of the growing RNA chain. Each step is, in principle, reversible. A mechanistic scheme encompassing these steps is shown below:

$$EC + NTP \underset{1}{\overset{}{\rightleftharpoons}} EC{:}NTP \underset{2}{\overset{}{\rightleftharpoons}} EC{:}PP_i \underset{4a}{\overset{}{\rightleftharpoons}} EC_{+1}{:}PP_i$$

$$3a \updownarrow \qquad\qquad 3b \updownarrow$$

$$EC' + PP_i \underset{4b}{\overset{}{\rightleftharpoons}} EC_{+1} + PP_i$$

Scheme 1

where EC represents a ternary elongation complex stalled at a specific nucleotide residue, EC$'$ represents EC extended by a single nucleotide residue without movement of the active site, and EC$_{+1}$ represents a ternary complex in which EC is extended by a single nucleotide residue and the active site has moved forward such that it is poised to bind the next NTP. The following sections provide evidence for each step and discuss the kinetic importance of each step for both correct and incorrect incorporation.

NTP BINDING OR RELEASE   The interaction of NTPs with RNA polymerase has been extensively investigated. The apparent Michaelis constants (K_m)

for all four canonical NTPs (118), as well as the apparent K_m values of numerous NTP analogs, have been determined (references listed above). In general, these values range from approximately 20 μM to 100 μM for the canonical NTPs (118). The NTPs as well as pyrophosphate are competitive inhibitors of one another, with inhibition constants (K_I) on the order of 1 mM (118). This result is consistent with a single binding site for all of the NTPs (as opposed to a unique site for each of the four natural NTPs). These K_m and K_I values have been determined for the steady-state synthesis of long RNA chains and have not, in general, been determined as a function of template position. Significantly, the K_m value for a single NTP has been observed to vary greatly at different positions along the template (see section on pausing below) (91).

To what extent the apparent K_m values might reflect true NTP binding is not clear because of the very complex nature of the polymerization reaction. No data are available on the actual binding constants of the NTPs to an elongating (or stalled) RNA polymerase complex. Significantly, however, use of NTP concentrations sufficiently above the K_m yields pseudo–zero order kinetics of binding and allows one to probe the other steps in the kinetic pathway.

PHOSPHODIESTER-BOND FORMATION   Phosphodiester-bond formation proceeds via a S_N^2 mechanism in which the attack of the 3′-OH group and the release of pyrophosphate occur with in-line geometry (14). To test whether or not phosphodiester-bond formation is rate limiting, investigators have studied the effect of α-thio-NTPs on the kinetics. Solution studies have shown that the presence of the α-thio group reduces the rate of the chemical reaction at the α-phosphorous approximately 100-fold relative to the unmodified NTP (55). Consequently, if phosphodiester-bond formation is the rate-limiting step in the polymerization reaction, then the use of an A-isomer α-thio NTP (Figure 3A) in place of a NTP should result in an approximately 100-fold reduction in the rate of synthesis. Eckstein and coworkers (14) demonstrated that V_{max} for synthesis on poly d(AT) did not change when either oxygen-containing UTP or ATP was replaced with its α-thio equivalent. Consequently, the phosphodiester-bond formation does not appear to be rate limiting for correct incorporation of ATP and UTP using poly d(AT) as a template.

We have investigated the effect of α-thio-UTP on the misincorporation kinetics at a unique template position that requires CTP. In these studies, we did not observe a decrease in rate upon replacement of UTP with α-thio-UTP, thus suggesting that bond formation is also not the rate-limiting step for misincorporation at this position (41, 42; D. A. Erie, unpublished results). [This result contrasts with that obtained with *E. coli* and T7 DNA polymerase, in which phosphodiester-bond formation becomes partially rate limiting for misincorporation (81, 103, 146).] Without further kinetic studies, however, we cannot generalize this result to state that bond formation will not be rate limiting for all correct or incorrect nucleotide-incorporation reactions. [Note added in proof: Recent results (156) have shown that the effect of α-S-NTP substitution on V_{max} in systems such as this cannot always be used to determine whether bond formation is rate limiting.]

PYROPHOSPHATE EXCHANGE   As represented in Scheme 1, it is not known whether pyrophosphate release occurs before or after translocation. The order of translocation and pyrophosphate release will depend on the relative rate constants for the two processes, assuming that they can be treated as independent processes.

If translocation (step 4a) is rapid relative to pyrophosphate release from the untranslocated enzyme (step 3a), then pyrophosphate will be released after translocation (step 3b). In principle, pyrophosphate release after translocation should be fast because the translocated enzyme complex, EC_{+1}, should be ready to incorporate the next NTP. Pyrophosphate is a known inhibitor of synthesis, with a K_I of approximately 1 mM (4, 118).

If active-site translocation (step 4a) is slow relative to pyrophosphate release, then pyrophosphate release will occur prior to translocation (via step 3a). Although pyrophosphate exchange via step 4a is assumed to be rapid (68), the rate of release (and uptake) at this step remains undetermined. Significantly, pyrophosphate release is rate limiting for some phosphoryl-transfer reactions (74). In addition, pyrophosphate exchange via step 3a (prior to translocation) might have a K_m value as low as 1 μM (68, 70, 71). This proposed value stemmed from the observation that although the terminal nucleotide was sometimes removed at 1 μM PP_i, further pyrophosphorolysis required higher PP_i concentrations. It is important to note, however, that the same result would be observed if the K_m for PP_i of the enzyme complex before (via step 3a) or after (via step 3b) active-site translocation were lower than that for the penultimate nucleotide. Because the rate of pyrophosphorolysis varies greatly as a function of template sequence and position (68, 124–126), the latter explanation cannot be ruled out.

ACTIVE-SITE TRANSLOCATION   This step represents, at the least, the physical movement of the product terminus site and substrate site relative to a reference point on the DNA template. It does not necessarily involve a coordinate movement of the entire enzyme complex down the DNA. Very little direct experimental data have been obtained about the translocation event. To test whether translocation is rate limiting, one should investigate single- and double-nucleotide addition kinetics. Specifically, if translocation is rate limiting, then the rate of synthesis at active-site positions

i and $i+1$ (see Figure 2) should be slower than the sum of the single-base addition rates for adding a nucleotide at position i and then another at position $i+1$, because the latter event involves one less translocation event.

It has been suggested that translocation might constitute an error-checking step (i.e. a rate-limiting step for misincorporation) in elongation (68). However, this proposal is based on extents of reaction at 90 min as opposed to actual kinetic measurements. In experiments in which we measured rates of misincorporation at a single template position, we have not observed translocation to be rate limiting (41, 42; D. A. Erie, unpublished results). An investigation of these properties at several template positions will be necessary to determine if translocation is fast in general.

Pyrophosphorolysis

Pyrophosphorolysis of RNA by *E. coli* RNA polymerase was first observed by Maitra & Hurwitz in 1967 (95). Pyrophosphorolysis is the reverse reaction of RNA transcript synthesis; i.e. this process represents the processive removal of one or more ribonucleotides from the transcript in a ternary elongation complex. Pyrophosphorolysis is the only known mechanism by which a misincorporated nucleotide can be excised from an elongating transcript by the core enzyme.[5] This fact contrasts with the properties of most DNA polymerases, which have a separate exonuclease activity responsible for a large portion of error correction (75). Only a few studies have investigated the pyrophosphorolysis reaction and its role in maintaining fidelity (68, 70, 124–126).

Rozovskaya and coworkers investigated the effects of salt concentration, temperature, pyrophosphate concentration, and template position on the rate of pyrophosphorolysis. They formed a distribution of stalled complexes by quenching a transcription reaction with EDTA and removing the NTPs by using size exclusion chromatography. Pyrophosphate was added to the purified complexes and the rates of pyrophosphorolysis were measured by following the rate of formation of free labeled NTPs (rate averaged over all positions) and the rate of disappearance of specific transcripts (rates at unique positions). The average rate of pyrophosphorolysis (*a*) exhibits a linear dependence on temperature between 15°C and 37°C, (*b*) was independent of KCl concentration between 0.1 and 0.6 M, and (*c*) showed an apparent K_m of approximately 1 mM. Significantly, the rate of pyrophosphorolysis at different positions on the

---

[5] A NTPase activity that appears to preferentially hydrolyze incorrect NTPs prior to insertion has been observed in some RNA polymerase preparations. However, in at least two cases, the investigators were able to purify the NTPase activity away from the polymerase. Consequently, we believe that this NTPase activity is not an intrinsic property of the five-subunit holoenzyme. Further aspects of this putative activity are discussed in the section on fidelity, below.

template varied dramatically. At most positions, the half-life of this reaction ranged from < 1 s to 300 min. In general, the positions of the pauses in the pyrophosphorolysis reaction were different from those observed in the forward synthesis reaction. In a few cases, however, the RNA polymerase complex paused at the same positions (124, 125).

To investigate the properties of these paused complexes, the authors measured the stabilities of enzyme complexes that had been stalled at the same positions, but had arrived there either by synthesis or by pyrophosphorolysis. In a few cases, they found that the RNA polymerase dissociated 30–80% faster if it had arrived at the specific template position by pyrophosphorolysis rather than by synthesis. This result can be interpreted to mean that the enzyme can exist in two different conformational states, and that the distribution of the enzyme between these conformations depends either on the presence of NTPs or pyrophosphate or on the pathway of the enzymatic process. In either case, this result requires that the enzyme complex be able to assume at least two different conformations that are slow to interconvert (see below).

Fidelity

Many studies have examined misincorporation by *E. coli* RNA polymerase in vivo (20, 93, 121, 122) and in vitro (7, 17, 19, 23, 68, 94, 107–110, 133, 135, 140). In general, UTP is misincorporated in place of CTP, CTP in place of UTP, ATP in place of GTP, and GTP in place of ATP. Other misincorporations are significantly less frequent. Misincorporation probabilities ranging from 10^{-3} to 10^{-5} have been measured for *E. coli* RNA polymerase in vitro and in vivo (17, 19, 23, 68, 108, 109, 121, 122, 133). This wide range of error frequencies can probably be attributed to experimental differences (such as temperature, pH, salt concentration, NTP concentrations, RNA polymerase purification) as well as to sequence context. Many of these differences are considered in detail in a recent review (7); a few key experiments are discussed here.

FREQUENCY OF ERROR   In an early investigation (133), synthetic polydeoxyribonucleotides were used to study misincorporation of each NTP by *E. coli* RNA polymerase in vitro. The extent of misincorporation of CMP or GMP was measured using poly d(AT) as a template, and of AMP or UMP using poly d(CG) as a template. The observed frequencies of misincorporation in this study were: CTP (1 : 2400), ATP (1 : 9000), UTP (1 : 20,000), and GTP (1 : 42,000). Hence, CTP appeared to exhibit the highest rate of misincorporation of all NTPs tested, and was incorporated in place of UTP, but not in place of ATP. Significantly, of all possible point mutations, a single U-to-C mutation produces the smallest effect on the amino acid sequence or protein conformation (133). However, these studies were performed on synthetic templates, which may not be good models for natural DNA. Subsequent in vivo studies (121, 122) revealed that, although the observed error frequencies were similar to those listed above, the extent of misincorporation depended on template position as well as on sequence. Consequently the relative rates of misincorporation of the NTPs are likely to vary as a function of the position of the RNA polymerase on the DNA template.

EFFECT OF DIVALENT METAL IONS   Several investigations have measured the effect of divalent metal ions on the fidelity of transcription (23, 108, 110, 133). Because Mn(II) is known to have mutagenic effects in vivo, its effect on the fidelity of E. coli RNA polymerase has been of particular interest. Significantly, in all but one study (133), Mn(II) increased the rate of incorporation of an incorrect nucleotide. Specifically, upon replacement of Mg(II) with Mn(II), investigators observed a threefold increase in the synthesis of poly rG from poly d(TC)·poly d(AG) (110), a threefold increase in the incorporation of 8-hydroxy-GTP (in place of UTP) on poly d(AT) (23), and a threefold increase in the incorporation of CMP into poly r(AU) using poly d(AT) as a template (108). By contrast, in another study, a twofold decrease in misincorporation occurred for synthesis on poly d(AT) when Mg(II) was replaced with Mn(II) (133), which directly conflicts with the data from the other report (108).

There are two major differences between the two investigations: (a) One study used higher NTP concentrations with only ATP, UTP, and CTP present in the reaction mix (108), while the other investigation carried out transcription reactions with all four NTPs present at lower concentrations (133). (b) The two studies were carried out at different pH values: pH 7.1 (133) and pH 8.0 (108). Reduction of pH from 8.0 to 7.1 reduces the overall activity of E. coli RNA polymerase (118). Consequently, the observed differences in the effects of Mn(II) on RNA polymerase fidelity may result from differences in pH conditions. It is not clear whether these experimental differences can account for the contrasting effects of Mn(II) on the fidelity of transcription. The factors that determine E. coli RNA polymerase fidelity may be quite complex, and thus seemingly small differences in reaction conditions may result in significant differences in polymerase function.

Niyogi et al (108) investigated, in addition to Mn(II), the effect of several metal ions on the fidelity of transcription. They observed that only Mg(II), Mn(II), and Co(II) could support RNA synthesis. All other divalent ions investigated [i.e. Zn(II), Ca(II), Sr(II), Cu(II), Cd(II), and Ni(II)] required Mg(II) for activity and were inhibitory at low concentrations (<1 mM) even in the presence of Mg(II). Cd(II) increased the extent of mis-incorporation dramatically, and Ni(II) increased misincorporation slightly, while all the other ions did not affect the fidelity of transcription. These results, in conjunction with studies on chain initiation, led the authors to suggest that there may be a correlation between fidelity and the ability of a metal ion to increase chain initiation while inhibiting chain elongation (63, 108).

ROLE OF PYROPHOSPHOROLYSIS   Because RNA polymerase removes incor-porated bases in the presence of pyrophosphate, the pyrophosphorolysis reaction may be important for error correction in transcription (60, 68, 71). The intracellular concentration of pyrophosphate in *E. coli* cells was determined using a colorimetric assay (57) and was found to be ~ 0.5 mM (82, 84). This result is particularly interesting because the dogma of the transcription and replication fields has been that intracellular pyro-phosphate concentrations are kept low (< 10 μM) by cellular pyrophos-phatases and consequently make the synthesis of DNA or RNA effectively irreversible. Clearly this may not be the case, and thus, as suggested above, pyrophosphorolysis reactions could be important in maintaining the fidelity of transcription in vivo.

This measured pyrophosphate concentration is greater than that used in most in vitro investigations, in which the only pyrophosphate present is that produced from RNA synthesis, yielding in vitro pyrophosphate concentrations of 1–10 μM. An increase in pyrophosphate concentration from 10 μM to 1 mM results in a dramatic increase in the rate of the pyrophosphorolysis reaction (70, 71, 124, 125) and a large decrease in the overall rate of RNA synthesis (4, 68, 71, 118).

The effect of pyrophosphorolysis on the fidelity of *E. coli* RNA poly-merase in vitro has been investigated by measuring the effect of pyro-phosphate concentration on the extent of misincorporation at a single nucleotide position (68). These misincorporation studies were carried out on a synthetic 86-bp DNA fragment carrying a *tac18* promoter that coded for a transcript containing no cytosine residues prior to position +21. Stalled elongation complexes at position +20 were formed by carrying out transcription in the absence of CTP (see below). The identity of the misincorporated base and the extents of misincorporation at position +21 and of read-through past +21 were determined as a function of pyrophosphate and pyrophosphatase concentrations. At PP$_i$ con-centrations greater than 1 μM, U was preferentially misincorporated for C, but as the concentration of pyrophosphatase increased, the preference for U misincorporation disappeared. Unfortunately, interpreting the data at higher pyrophosphatase concentrations is difficult because many transcripts shorter than 21 nucleotides do not have the correct sequence, as well as posing other possible artifacts. It is not clear whether these abberations result from highly error-prone transcription (68) or if they represent an artifact due to the high pyrophosphatase concentrations used. The extent of read-through to position $+27$ (the position prior to the incorporation of the second C residue) increases slightly at high pyrophosphatase concentrations; however, the overall extent of misincorporation is apparently not affected by the presence of pyrophosphatase or pyrophosphate (Table I of 68).

Presently, the role of pyrophosphorolysis in transcription fidelity remains unclear. In principle, the importance of pyrophosphorolysis in error correction is determined by the rate of elongation of the transcript containing the misincorporated base, relative to the rate of removal of a misincorporated base by pyrophosphorolysis. Because the rates of pyrophosphorolysis, as well as the rates of elongation, depend strongly on template position, the significance of pyrophosphorolysis in regulating fidelity is probably a function of template position as well.

PROOFREADING MECHANISM?   It is generally believed that *E. coli* RNA polymerase does not proofread or correct errors by any mechanism other than pyrophosphorolysis. Several studies, however, suggest that RNA polymerase may carry a NTPase activity that could be involved in proofreading (93, 94, 107, 140; P. P. Chuknyisky, E. Tarien, J. J. Butzow & G. L. Eichhorn, submitted). In all of these investigations, a template-dependent NTPase activity in the *E. coli* RNA polymerase preparation that appears to act preferentially on the incorrect nucleotide triphosphate was observed. This NTPase activity may be associated with the β-subunit of RNA polymerase (93, 94); however, in two studies (140; P. P. Chuknyisky, E. Tarien, J. J. Butzow & G. L. Eichhorn, submitted), the authors were able to purify away the NTPase activity. Consequently, if indeed a NTPase proofreading mechanism is associated with *E. coli* RNA polymerase, it apparently is not covalently associated with any of the five subunits of the holoenzyme complex.

Multiple RNA Polymerase Conformations in Transcript Elongation

Both chemical and enzymatic methods have been used to probe the structures of stalled elongation complexes, to attempt to relate differences in these structures to differences in function. In principle, studies of stalled complexes at different template positions could also be used to ask more detailed structural and dynamic questions, such as whether the entire complex moves monotonically with the active site, or whether different

portions of the complex (as reflected in the overall footprint of the polymerase on the DNA), move asynchronously relative to the progress of
transcript polymerization. To approach questions such as these, extensive
footprinting studies with DNase I, exonuclease III, and λ exonuclease have
been carried out to establish the boundaries of the RNA polymerase
molecule on the DNA template (28, 79, 80, 88, 102, 128, 134). Hydroxyl-
radical footprinting has also been used to reveal protein-DNA contacts
within the region protected from enzyme digestion (102). The size and
position (relative to the 3′-OH terminus of the RNA) of the DNA footprints differed between templates, and also depended on template position.

In general, larger regions of DNA are protected in ternary complexes
that are stalled near the promoter (79, 80, 102, 134). Ternary complexes
(core polymerase, DNA, RNA) with transcripts less than approximately
20 nucleotides in length may exist in a strained conformation that is an
intermediate between an initiation complex that contains σ factor and a
mature elongation complex that no longer contacts the promoter region
(79, 80, 102, 134). This notion is supported by: (a) the result that the
lagging edge of the polymerase footprint is greatly reduced as the transcript
length increases while the leading edge is esentially unaffected (102), and (b)
the fact that the protection on the lagging edge can be partially destroyed in
the presence of heparin (80).

Only two systematic studies have examined the DNA protection patterns
of elongation complexes as a function of RNA transcript length (79, 102).
In one investigation, exonuclease III and hydroxyl-radical footprinting
were used to probe stalled complexes with transcript lengths ranging from
11 to 39 nucleotide residues (102). These complexes were formed on a
series of DNA templates that had been generated by cloning $d(AG)_n$
fragments of increasing length into a DNA template at a position 11
nucleotide residues downstream from the transcription start site. Consequently, the resulting ternary complexes all involved the same downstream
DNA sequences adjacent to different length tracts of $d(AG)_n$.

In a more recent investigation (79), stalled ternary complexes located at
several positions along two different transcription units were footprinted
with DNase I. These experiments differ in two ways from those of the
earlier study (102). First, DNase I was used to footprint the complexes in
the more recent study, while exonuclease III and hydroxyl radicals were
used to footprint the complexes in the earlier investigation. Second, the
RNA polymerase was "walked" down the two templates in the more
recent study, resulting in a series of complexes generated from a single
template, while each of the ternary complexes was formed on a different
DNA template in the earlier study.

In both investigations, the size of DNA footprint decreased as the transcript length increased up to ~ 20 nucleotide residues; however, the two investigations produced conflicting results for ternary complexes with transcripts longer than 20 residues. Very similar protection patterns for all the ternary complexes with transcripts greater than 20 nucleotides in length were observed in the study that employed multiple templates (102), while significantly different footprints were observed for each of the ternary complexes that were formed by walking the polymerase down the template (79). The earlier paper (102) proposed that after the synthesis of approximately 20 nucleotides, the RNA polymerase ternary complex reaches its mature state, at which point the DNA footprint becomes smaller and exhibits a monotonous change as it travels down the template. Significantly, these studies were performed on a template containing an alternating $d(AG)_n$ sequence, and the RNA polymerase contacts of complexes past position $+20$ remained the same on the leading edge and were all in the $d(AG)_n$ sequence on the lagging edge. The constancy of the footprint may not result from a mature complex but rather from the fact that both the upstream and downstream sequences contacted by the polymerase are essentially the same in all stalled complexes with transcript lengths exceeding 20 residues (79). Significantly, untranscribed downstream sequences affect pausing (89) and termination efficiency (137), which is consistent with the suggestion that downstream sequences affect the conformation of an elongating $E.\ coli$ RNA polymerase molecule (79).

An alternative view of an elongating complex is that the RNA polymerase adopts a multitude of conformations as it moves down the template and, furthermore, that the conformation of an elongating ternary complex may be perturbed by halting the polymerase because the enzyme conformation may be kinetically determined (79). This suggestion is supported by recent experiments (38) in which isolation of ternary complexes stalled at position $+20$ affected the pausing pattern 70 to 150 nucleotide residues downstream. Significantly, for a conformational change at position $+20$ to affect events such as pausing and termination downstream, the conformational change must either be irreversible or slow to interconvert relative to the rate of transcript synthesis. A wide variety of data support the notion that either slow or irreversible changes occur in an elongating ternary complex: (a) The stability of a stalled elongation complex depends upon whether the polymerase arrived at the stall site via synthesis or via pyrophosphorolysis (38, 124, 125) (see section on pyrophosphorolysis). (b) Termination efficiences are affected by transcribed upstream sequences as well as by untranscribed downstream sequences proximal to the terminator (51, 137, 138, 143). (c) The purification of stalled complexes perturbs pausing (38). (d) The rate of misincorporation at a single site for which the correct NTP is absent is significantly different before and after isolation of ternary complexes (D. A. Erie, unpublished results). Taken together, these results strongly support the hypothesis that *E. coli* RNA polymerase adopts several conformations as it moves down the template and that the conformations are kinetically determined.

Clearly, the path by which polymerase arrives at a site can affect its action at that site. If the polymerase has many intermediate states, then the conformation of the polymerase stalled at different positions may vary significantly (79). Furthermore, if stalling or ternary complex isolation modifies the polymerase conformation, the new conformation(s) is also likely to be affected by the conformation(s) prior to stalling or isolation. That is, each intermediate state may relax to a different ground-state conformation upon isolation. Thus, when transcription is resumed (by the addition of NTPs), the RNA polymerase may follow a different path with potentially different rate-limiting steps. This possibility significantly complicates the analysis of structural and kinetic data obtained using stalled elongation complexes. Consequently, one should know the history of the transcription complexes as well as the history of the holoenzyme when comparing studies. However, the connection, if any, between these events at the level of the overall conformation of the elongation complex and regulatory effects at the catalytic site of the enzyme remains to be elucidated.[6]

SPECIFIC PAUSING: SEQUENCE DEPENDENCE OF THE RATE OF TRANSCRIPT ELONGATION

Specific pausing in elongation is defined as the arrest of the elongation complex at a specific template position for a defined length of time, with or without the participation of a protein factor. This phenomenon is clearly a central feature in the regulation of transcription. The molecular basis of pausing at any template locus is still incompletely understood; thus a molecular understanding of the single-nucleotide addition cycle in transcription should aid in approaching this issue, by allowing one to determine at which step in the cycle the transcribing polymerase is actually arrested, what features of the template DNA (or the nascent RNA) are responsible for this arrest, how release from pausing occurs, and how the duration of

---

[6]If polymerase within elongation complexes stalled at specific template sites does indeed involve slowly relaxing (and perhaps pathway-dependent) conformations, then one must take this phenomenon into account in assessing the specific applicability in each case of the basic thermodynamic assumption made at the beginning of the thermodynamics section; i.e. that the elongation complex reaches equilibrium at each template position. Thus the validity of this assumption must be tested with kinetic experiments for each specific complex examined until general principles begin to emerge.

the pause is established. A formal definition of these events can be put forward in terms of activation energy barriers of the Eyring type (see 154, 155), but a detailed understanding must await kinetic and structural analysis of specifically stalled elongation complexes.

Thermodynamically Induced Pausing

With nucleoside triphosphates at a concentration of 1 mM and inorganic pyrophosphate at a concentration of 10 mM, in the absence of pyrophosphate hydrolysis, the synthesis of RNA is thermodynamically favorable at a value of $\Delta G_{I \rightarrow I+1} \approx -1$ to -4 kcal/mol of nucleotide polymerized. Although this driving force is not very large, it nonetheless is sufficient to ensure that, given certain boundary conditions, a RNA transcript of arbitrary sequence and length can be synthesized (see above). Such conditions are typical of in vitro transcription reactions. In vivo, the steady-state concentration of pyrophosphate will also influence the driving force for RNA synthesis (Equation 5).

We predict, based on the thermodynamic analysis leading to Equation 3, that the elongation complex will cease to move (but will remain stable) in the absence of a driving force. Elongation complexes on poly d(AT) or on natural DNA templates may be separated away from the NTP substrate and PP$_i$ products of transcription using a gel filtration column (15, 92, 118). Such isolated complexes remain stable for weeks at 4°C and may be restarted by simply adding back NTP.

The thermodynamic analysis leading to Equation 3 also predicts reverse movement of the elongation complex upon reversal of the thermodynamic driving force. Two relevant experiments are reported in the literature. (*a*) Experiments in which RNA polymerase is allowed to initiate transcription from the T7A1 promoter, and then is stalled by incorporation of 3'-O-Me-NTPs, have been carried out (3, 4, 123, 125, 126). When such stalled elongation complexes are exposed to inorganic pyrophosphate, the RNA transcript is pyrophosphorylized in a processive manner. Subsequent addition of regular NTPs causes the RNA transcripts to be reextended in a processive manner. (*b*) Similar observations have been made with *E. coli* RNA polymerase that contains regulatory subunits encoded by phage T4 (70). In this system, the modified polymerase initiates transcription from phage T4 late promoters.

The above discussion suggests that pausing should arise for thermodynamic reasons (i.e. because of the absence of a driving force) when one or more substrate concentrations is decreased below a threshold value. A series of pauses is generated on T7D111 DNA when the substrate concentration is made very low (3, 4, 92, 123, 125, 126). Our interpretation of this phenomenon is that, with a low thermodynamic driving force, the tendency for pausing to occur at certain positions in the transcript is high, and when the thermodynamic driving force is increased, nearly all of these pauses disappear. These types of pauses are often found one position before the incorporation of a uridine residue (4). Accordingly, we infer that, in the elongation complex, the free energy change for the addition of U residues to the transcript may be inherently low. Thus, pyrophosphorolysis should readily remove 3′-terminal U residues.

Physiological Pausing

Although we have argued that under typical in vivo and in vitro conditions a sufficient driving force ensures RNA synthesis, it does not necessarily follow that transcript elongation must always be rapid. In fact, much evidence points to a large variability in the transcriptional elongation rate, even under conditions of net favorable free energy change. Workers in several laboratories have experimentally observed pausing by RNA polymerase during transcript elongation (35, 43, 45, 49, 54, 69, 91, 96, 104–106, 117, 144). Transcriptional pausing interrupts the regular movement of the polymerase by presenting a higher-than-average activation energy barrier to elongation (see 154, 155). This is of interest from a molecular biological point of view for at least the following four reasons: (a) it may be the first step in certain simple termination events [e.g. at trp t_0 terminator (43)]; (b) it is the first step in many, if not all, ρ-dependent termination events; (c) it may be an important step in at least some antitermination events [e.g. in the antitermination system of phage λ (35, 54, 150)]; (d) it may help to synchronize the movement of RNA polymerase and ribosomes during transcriptional attenuation (85, 86, 88). Physiologically relevant pausing can be divided into two classes, on the basis of the mechanism by which it is induced.

SEQUENCE-DEPENDENT PAUSING   During the in vitro transcription of 6S RNA of phage λ (from the P'_R late promoter), the polymerase pauses at position 16 of the template. This pause is long enough to permit the isolation of a discrete RNA species (35, 54). This phenomenon occurs in the absence of any obvious capacity of the RNA (or DNA) sequence to form secondary structure(s). A similar lack of (obvious) secondary structure has been noted for pausing (or stalling) events in the $lacZ$ gene (transcribed from the $lacUV5$ promoter) (48, 49, 96), in the early region of phage T7, (69), in the $rrnB$ leader region of $E.$ $coli$ (73), and in form I SV40 DNA (46, 117). In the 6S RNA transcript of phage λ, the fact that the polymerase can be chased into the downstream sequence by adding λ antitermination protein Q suggests the physiological relevance of these observations (54). We note that, in the $lacUV5$ and $rrnB$ systems, pausing (or stalling) occurs during the early stages of the transcriptional event, i.e. at the point at which one would expect the polymerase to bind anti-termination protein(s). Pausing of this type may be caused by promoter-specific entry of the polymerase into an unusual conformational state (see above).

RNA HAIRPIN-INDUCED PAUSING   During transcription, the generation of a self-complementary sequence in the RNA can induce pausing of the polymerase. Such pausing is thought to occur at positions 90 and 92 in the attenuator region of the *trp* operon (87), and also at the t_0 terminator at the end of the *trp* operon (43). At the *trp* t_0 terminator, the pause constitutes a decision point; either elongation resumes (probability $\sim 80\%$) or termination occurs (probability $\sim 20\%$). Other possible cases of hairpin-induced pausing occur at six specific sites in SV40 form I DNA during transcription with *E. coli* RNA polymerase, (46, 117), at position 68 in the *trp* attenuator (87), and within the *thr* attenuator (47). In these cases, however, the evidence for RNA hairpin involvement is less direct.

Half-times for the release from this type of pausing range from 10 s to a few minutes (87, 117). Thus, the polymerase moves much more slowly through a pause site of this type than through an arbitrary DNA sequence, if we assume an average transcription rate of 30–50 base pairs per second (69, 118). The kinetics of read-through at the *trp*-attenuator pause site and at several of the SV40 pause sites appears to be first-order (87, 117), suggesting that a unimolecular (conformational) event is responsible for the release process.

Hairpin-induced pausing appears to be unique because the RNA hairpin may form within the transcription bubble (148, 149) and potentially disrupt the upstream portion of the RNA-DNA hybrid, rendering the proximal portion of the RNA-DNA hybrid unstable, as well as disrupting potentially important RNA-protein interactions. Thus, hairpin-induced pausing may represent an important physiological route out of the extremely stable elongation mode. However, at other types of terminators, routes out of the elongation mode that do not involve RNA hairpin formation must also exist. Defining these routes, and relating them to the temporary blockage of specific microscopic steps in the single nucleotide addition cycle, remains a problem for the future.

SUMMARY

This review has summarized the known features of the single-nucleotide addition reaction cycle in transcription. The reader will have noted that the information available is very incomplete, and that, in some cases, related experiments seem to lead to contradictory conclusions. We have tried to point out these discrepancies as they occur and to indicate areas where more experimentation is needed. We look forward to the day when all the microscopic steps of the single-nucleotide addition cycle can be identified and defined in thermodynamic, kinetic, and structural terms. At that point, we can begin to understand the principles that relate these parameters to template position and to the pathway of formation of a specific complex. It should be possible to provide specific molecular interpretations for observed effects on activation barrier heights to elongation and termination (154, 155) and to begin to understand the molecular bases of the regulation in these phases of transcription. Much work remains before this happy situation can be totally realized, but we feel that now the problem can at least be approached at this level. We hope that this review helps to illuminate the difficulties that remain.

ACKNOWLEDGMENTS

The experimental work from our laboratory on this topic, as well as the preparation of this review, has been supported, in part, by USPHS Research Grants GM-15792 and GM-29158 (to PHvH), by USPHS Individual Post-doctoral Fellowships GM-12915 (to DAE) and GM-10227 (to TDY), and by a grant to the Institute of Molecular Bioiogy from the Lucille P. Markey Charitable Trust. PHvH is an American Cancer Society Research Professor of Chemistry. We are grateful to many colleagues here and elsewhere for providing preprints of unpublished work and for many discussions that have helped us to define and clarify the ideas presented in this review.

Literature Cited

1. Abrahams, J. P., van de Berg, M., van Batenburgh, E., Pleij, C. 1990. *Nucleic Acids Res.* 18: 3035
2. Aivazashvili, V. A., Bibilashvili, R. S., Florent'ev, V. L. 1977. *Mol. Biol. (Moscow)* 11: 854
3. Aivazashvili, V. A., Bibilashvili, R. S., Vartikyan, R. M., Kutateladze, T. V. 1981. *Mol. Biol. (Moscow)* 15: 915
4. Aivazashvili, V. A., Bibilashvili, R. S., Vartikyan, R. M., Kutateladze, T. V. 1981. *Mol. Biol. (Moscow)* 15: 653
5. Alberty, R. A. 1968. *J. Biol. Chem.* 243: 1337
6. Alberty, R. A. 1969. *J. Biol. Chem.* 244: 3290
7. Anderson, R. P., Menninger, J. R. 1986. In *Accuracy in Molecular Processes*, ed. R. F. Rosenberger, D. J. Galas. p. 159. Chapman and Hall: New York
8. Applequist, J., Damle, V. 1966. *J. Am. Chem. Soc.* 88: 3895
9. Armstrong, V. W., Eckstein, F. 1976. *Eur. J. Biochem.* 70: 33
10. Armstrong, V. W., Eckstein, F. 1979. *Biochemistry* 18: 5117
11. Armstrong, V. W., Sternbach, H., Eckstein, F. 1974. *FEBS Lett.* 44: 157
12. Armstrong, V. W., Sternbach, H., Eckstein, F. 1976. *Biochemistry* 15: 2086

13. Armstrong, V. W., Sternbach, H., Eckstein, F. 1977. *Methods Enzymol.* 46: 346
14. Armstrong, V. W., Yee, D., Eckstein, F. 1979. *Biochemistry* 18: 4120
15. Arndt, K. M., Chamberlin, M. J. 1990. *J. Mol. Biol.* 213: 79
16. Axelrod, V. D., Vartikyan, R. M., Aivazashvili, V. A., Beabealashvili, R. S. 1978. *Nucleic Acids Res.* 5: 3549
17. Bass, I. A., Polonsky, Y. S. 1974. *FEBS Lett.* 48: 306
18. Beal, R. B., Pillai, R. P., Chuknyisky, P. P., Levy, A., Tarien, E., Eichhorn, G. L. 1990. *Biochemistry* 29: 5994
19. Bick, M. D. 1975. *Nucleic Acids Res.* 2: 1513
20. Blank, A., Gallant, J. A., Burgess, R. R., Loeb, L. A. 1986. *Biochemistry* 25: 5920
21. Borer, P. N., Dengler, B., Tinoco, I. Jr., Uhlenbeck, O. C. 1974. *J. Mol. Biol.* 86: 843
22. Brahms, J., Michelson, A. M., van Holde, K. E. 1966. *J. Mol. Biol.* 15: 467
23. Bruskov, V. I., Kuklina, O. V. 1988. *Mol. Biol. (Moscow)* 22: 580
24. Burgers, P. M. J., Eckstein, F. 1978. *Proc. Natl. Acad. Sci. USA* 75: 4798
25. Burgess, R. R. 1969. *J. Biol. Chem.* 244: 6160
26. Burgess, R. R. 1969. *J. Biol. Chem.* 244: 6168
27. Burgess, R. R., Erickson, B., Gentry, D., Gribskov, M., Hager, D., et al. 1987. See Ref. 117a, p. 3
28. Carpousis, A. J., Gralla, J. D. 1985. *J. Mol. Biol.* 183: 165
29. Chamberlin, M. J. 1974. *Annu. Rev. Biochem.* 43: 721
29a. Chamberlin, M. J., Losick, R., eds. 1976. *RNA Polymerase.* Cold Spring Harbor, NY: Cold Spring Harbor Lab.
30. Chamberlin, M. J., Nierman, W. C., Wiggs, J., Neff, N. 1979. *J. Biol. Chem.* 254: 10061
31. Chatterji, D., Wu, F. Y. H. 1982. *Biochemistry* 21: 4651
32. Chuknyisky, P. P., Rifkind, J. M., Tarien, E., Beal, R. B., Eichhorn, G. L. 1990. *Biochemistry* 29: 5987
33. Deleted in proof
34. Coleman, J. E. 1983. *Metal Ions Biology,* ed. T. G. Spiro, p. 219. New York: Wiley Interscience
35. Dahlberg, J. E., Blattner, F. R. 1973. In *Virus Research,* ed. C. F. Fox, W. S. Robinson, p. 533. New York: Academic
36. Darst, S. A., Kubalek, E. W., Kornberg, R. D. 1989. *Nature (London)* 340: 730

37. Dennis, D., Jurgensen, S., Sylvester, J. 1980. *Biochem. Biophys. Res. Commun.* 94: 205
38. Dissinger, S., Hanna, M. M. 1990. *J. Biol. Chem.* 265: 7662
39. Eckstein, F., Armstrong, V. W., Sternbach, H. 1976. *Proc. Natl. Acad. Sci. USA* 73: 2987
40. Eisenberg, H., Felsenfeld, G. 1967. *J. Mol. Biol.* 30: 17
41. Erie, D. A., von Hippel, P. H. 1991. *Biophys. J.* 59: 565
42. Erie, D. A., von Hippel, P. H. 1991. *J. Cell. Biochem. Suppl.* 15G: 241
43. Farnham, P. J., Platt, T. 1981. *Nucleic Acids Res.* 9: 563
44. Freier, S. M., Kierzek, R., Jaeger, J. A., Sugimoto, N., Caruthers, M. H., et al. 1986. *Proc. Natl. Acad. Sci. USA* 83: 9373
45. Gamper, H. B., Hearst, J. E. 1982. *Cold Spring Harbor Symp. Quant. Biol.* 47: 455
46. Gamper, H. B., Hearst, J. E. 1982. *Cell* 29: 81
47. Gardner, J. F. 1982. *J. Biol. Chem.* 257: 3896
48. Gilbert, W. 1976. See Ref. 29a, p. 193
49. Gilbert, W., Maizels, N., Maxam, A. 1974. *Cold Spring Harbor Symp. Quant. Biol.* 38: 845
50. Gill, S. C., Yager, T. D., von Hippel, P. H. 1990. *Biophys. Chem.* 37: 239
51. Goliger, J. A., Yang, X., Guo, H. C., Roberts, J. W. 1989. *J. Mol. Biol.* 205: 331
52. Grachev, M. A., Pletnev, A. G. 1980. *Bioorg. Khim.* 6: 1737
53. Grachev, M. A., Zaichikov, E. F. 1974. *FEBS Lett.* 49: 163
54. Grayhack, E. J., Yang, X., Lau, L. F., Roberts, J. W. 1985. *Cell* 42: 259
55. Gupta, A. P., Benkovic, P. A., Benkovic, S. J. 1984. *Nucleic Acids Res.* 12: 5897
56. Hager, D. A., Jin, D. J., Burgess, R. R. 1990. *Biochemistry* 29: 7890
57. Heinonen, J., Honkasalo, S. H., Kukko, E. I. 1981. *Anal. Biochem.* 117: 293
58. Helmann, J. D., Chamberlin, M. J. 1988. *Annu. Rev. Biochem.* 57: 839–72
59. Helmann, J. D., Masiarz, F. R., Chamberlin, M. J. 1988. *J. Bacteriol.* 170: 1560
60. Herbomel, P., Ninio, J. 1980. *C. R. Acad. Sci. Paris Ser. D* 291: 881
61. Heumann, H., Lederer, H., Baer, G., May, R. P., Kjems, J. K., Crespi, H. L. 1988. *J. Mol. Biol.* 201: 115
62. Heumann, H., Meisenberger, O., Pilz, I. 1982. *FEBS Lett.* 138: 273

414   ERIE, YAGER & VON HIPPEL

63. Hoffman, D. J., Niyogi, S. K. 1977. *Science* 194: 513
64. Holbrook, S. R., Sussman, J. L., Warrant, R. W., Church, G. M., Kim, S.-H. 1977. *Nucleic Acids Res.* 4: 2811
65. Hurwitz, J., Yarbrough, L., Wickner, S. 1972. *Biochem. Biophys. Res. Commun.* 48: 628
66. Igarashi, K., Fujita, N., Ishihama, A. 1991. *J. Mol. Biol.* 218: 1
67. Ishihama, A., Enami, M., Nishijima, Y., Fukui, T., Ohtsuka, E., Ikehara, M. 1980. *J. Biochem. (Tokyo)* 87: 825
68. Kahn, J. D., Hearst, J. E. 1989. *J. Mol. Biol.* 205: 291
69. Kassavetis, G. A., Chamberlin, M. J. 1981. *J. Biol. Chem.* 256: 2777
70. Kassavetis, G. A., Zentner, P. G., Geiduschek, E. P. 1986. *J. Biol. Chem.* 261: 14256
71. Kassavetis, G. A., Zentner, P. G., Geiduschek, E. P. 1987. See Ref. 117a, p. 471
72. Kato, K., Goncalves, J. M., Houts, G. E., Bollum, F. J. 1967. *J. Biol. Chem.* 242: 2780
73. Kingston, R. E., Chamberlin, M. J. 1981. *Cell* 27: 523
74. Knowles, J. R. 1980. *Annu. Rev. Biochem.* 49: 877
75. Kornberg, A., Baker, T. A. 1991. *DNA Replication.* San Francisco: Freeman. 2nd ed.
76. Krakow, J. S., Fronk, E. 1969. *J. Biol. Chem.* 244: 5988
77. Krakow, J. S., Rhodes, G., Jovin, T. M. 1976. See Ref. 29a, p. 216
78. Krummel, B., Chamberlin, M. 1992. *J. Mol. Biol.* In press
79. Krummel, B., Chamberlin, M. 1992. *J. Mol. Biol.* In press
80. Krummel, B., Chamberlin, M. J. 1989. *Biochemistry* 28: 7829
81. Kuchta, R. D., Benkovic, P., Benkovic, S. P. 1988. *Biochemistry* 27: 6716
82. Kukko, E., Heinonen, J. 1982. *Eur. J. Biochem.* 127: 347
83. Kukko, K. E., Lintunen, M., Inen, M. K., Lahti, R., Heinonen, J. 1989. *J. Bacteriol.* 171: 4498
84. Kukko-Kalske, E., Heinonen, J. 1985. *Int. J. Biochem.* 17: 575
85. Landick, R., Carey, J., Yanofsky, C. 1985. *Proc. Natl. Acad. Sci. USA* 82: 4663
86. Landick, R., Carey, J., Yanofsky, C. 1987. *Proc. Natl. Acad. Sci. USA* 84: 1507
87. Landick, R., Yanofsky, C. 1984. *J. Biol. Chem.* 259: 11550
88. Landick, R., Yanofsky, C. 1987. *J. Mol. Biol.* 196: 363
89. Lee, D. N., Phung, L. E., Stewart, J., Landick, R. 1990. *J. Biol. Chem.* 265: 15145
90. Leng, M., Felsenfeld, G. 1966. *J. Mol. Biol.* 15: 455
91. Levin, J. R., Chamberlin, M. J. 1987. *J. Mol. Biol.* 196: 61
92. Levin, J. R., Krummel, B., Chamberlin, M. J. 1987. *J. Mol. Biol.* 196: 85
93. Libby, R. T., Gallant, J. A. 1991. *Mol. Microbiol.* 5: 999
94. Libby, R. T., Nelson, J. L., Calvo, J. M., Gallant, J. A. 1989. *EMBO J.* 8: 3153
95. Maitra, U., Hurwitz, J. 1967. *J. Biol. Chem.* 242: 4897
96. Maizels, N. 1973. *Proc. Natl. Acad. Sci. USA* 70: 3585
97. McClure, W. R. 1985. *Annu. Rev. Biochem.* 54: 171
98. Meisenberger, O., Heumann, H., Pilz, I. 1980. *FEBS Lett.* 122: 117
99. Meisenberger, O., Heumann, H., Pilz, I. 1981. *FEBS Lett.* 123: 22
100. Meisenberger, O., Pilz, I., Heumann, H. 1980. *FEBS Lett.* 120: 57
101. Deleted in proof
102. Metzger, W., Schickor, P., Heumann, H. 1989. *EMBO J.* 8: 2745
103. Mizrahi, V., Henrie, R. N., Marlier, J. F., Johnson, K. A., Benkovic, S. P. 1985. *Biochemistry* 24: 4010
104. Morgan, W. D., Bear, D. G., von Hippel, P. H. 1983. *J. Biol. Chem.* 258: 9553
105. Morgan, W. D., Bear, D. G., von Hippel, P. H. 1983. *J. Biol. Chem.* 258: 9565
106. Morgan, W. D., Bear, D. G., von Hippel, P. H. 1984. *J. Biol. Chem.* 259: 8664
107. Ninio, J., Bernardi, F., Brun, G., Assairi, L., Lauber, M., Chapeville, F. 1975. *FEBS Lett.* 57: 139
108. Niyogi, S. K., Feldman, R. P. 1981. *Nucleic Acids Res.* 9: 2615
109. Ozolina, O. N., Oganesyan, M. G., Kamzolova, S. G. 1980. *FEBS Lett.* 110: 123
110. Paetkau, V., Coulter, M. B., Flintoff, W. F., Morgan, A. R. 1972. *J. Mol. Biol.* 71: 293
111. Pavco, P. A., Steege, D. A. 1990. *J. Biol. Chem.* 265: 9960
112. Peller, L. 1967. *Biochemistry* 15: 141
113. Phillips, R. C., George, P., Rutman, R. J. 1969. *J. Biol. Chem.* 244: 330
114. Pinto, D., Sarocchi, L. M. T., Guschlbauer, W. 1979. *Nucleic Acids Res.* 6: 1041
115. Platt, T. 1986. *Annu. Rev. Biochem.* 55: 339
116. Quigley, G. J., Teeter, M. M., Rich, A.

1978. *Proc. Natl. Acad. Sci. USA* 75: 64

117. Reisbig, R. R., Hearst, J. E. 1981. *Biochemistry* 20: 1907

117a. Reznikoff, W. S., Burgess, R. R., Dahlberg, J. E., Gross, C., Record, M. T. Jr., Wickens, M. P., eds. 1987. *RNA Polymerase Regulation and Transcription, Proc. Steenbock Symp. 16th.* New York: Elsevier

118. Rhodes, G., Chamberlin, M. J. 1974. *J. Biol. Chem.* 249: 6675

119. Rialdi, G., Levy, J., Biltonen, R. 1972. *Biochemistry* 11: 2473

120. Rice, G. A., Kane, C. M., Chamberlin, M. J. 1991. *Proc. Natl. Acad. Sci. USA* 88: 4245

121. Rosenberger, R. F., Foskett, G. 1981. *Mol. Gen. Genet.* 183: 561

122. Rosenberger, R. F., Hilton, J. 1983. *Mol. Gen. Genet.* 191: 207

123. Rozovskaya, T. A., Bibilashvili, R. S., Zarudnaya, M. I., Kosaganov, Y. N. 1981. *Mol. Biol. (Moscow)* 15: 79

124. Rozovskaya, T. A., Chenchik, A. A., Bibilashvili, R. S. 1981. *Mol. Biol. (Moscow)* 15: 636

125. Rozovskaya, T. A., Chenchik, A. A., Bibilashvilli, R. S. 1982. *FEBS Lett.* 137: 100

126. Rozovskaya, T. A., Chenchik, A. A., Tarusova, N. B., Bibilashvili, R. S., Khomutov, R. M. 1981. *Mol. Biol. (Moscow)* 15: 1205

127. Shaner, S. L., Piatt, D. M., Wensley, C. G., Yu, H., Burgess, R. R., Record, M. T. J. 1982. *Biochemistry* 21: 5539

128. Shi, Y., Gamper, H., Van Houten, B., Hearst, J. E. 1988. *J. Mol. Biol.* 199: 277

129. Simon, L., Meyers, T., Mednieks, M. 1965. *Biochem. Biophys. Acta* 103: 189

130. Slepneva, I. A., Vainer, L. M. 1982. *Mol. Biol. (Moscow)* 16: 763

131. Solaiman, D., Wu, F. Y. H. 1984. *Biochemistry* 23: 6369

132. Speckhard, D. C., Wu, F. Y.-H., Wu, C.-W. 1977. *Biochemistry* 16: 5228

133. Springgate, C. F., Loeb, L. A. 1975. *J. Mol. Biol.* 97: 577

134. Straney, D. C., Crothers, D. M. 1987. *J. Mol. Biol.* 193: 267

135. Strniste, G. F., Smith, D. A., Hayes, F. N. 1973. *Biochemistry* 12: 603

136. Teeter, M. M., Quigley, G. J., Rich, A. 1980. In *Nucleic Acid–Metal Inter-*

actions, ed. T. G. Spiro, p. 145. New York: Wiley-Interscience

137. Telesnitsky, A., Chamberlin, M. J. 1989. *Biochemistry* 28: 5210

138. Telesnitsky, A. P. W., Chamberlin, M. J. 1989. *J. Mol. Biol.* 205: 315

139. Travers, A. A., Lamond, A. I., Mace, H. A. F. 1982. In *Promoters: Structure and Function,* ed. R. L. Rodriguez, M. J. Chamberlin, p. 216. New York: Praeger

140. Volloch, V. Z., Rits, S., Tumerman, L. 1979. *Nucleic Acids Res.* 6: 1535

141. von Hippel, P. H., Bear, D. G., Morgan, W. D., McSwiggen, J. A. 1984. *Annu. Rev. Biochem.* 53: 389

142. von Hippel, P. H., Yager, T. D., Gill, S. C. 1992. In *Transcription Regulation,* ed. S. McKnight, K. Yamamoto. Cold Spring Harbor, NY: Cold Spring Harbor Lab. In press

143. Whalen, W., Ghosh, B., Das, A. 1988. *Proc. Natl. Acad. Sci. USA* 85: 2494

144. Winkler, M. E., Yanofsky, C. 1981. *Biochemistry* 20: 3738

145. Witz, H. G., Luzzati, V. 1965. *J. Mol. Biol.* 11: 620

146. Wong, I., Patel, S. S., Johnson, K. A. 1991. *Biochemistry* 30: 526

147. Deleted in proof

148. Yager, T. D., von Hippel, P. H. 1987. In *Escherichia coli and Salmonella typhimurium,* ed. F. C. Neidhardt, J. L. Ingraham, B. K. Law, B. Magasanik, M. Schechter, H. E. Umbarger, p. 1241. Washington, DC: Am. Soc. Microbiol.

149. Yager, T. D., von Hippel, P. H. 1991. *Biochemistry* 30: 1097

150. Yang, X., Roberts, J. W. 1989. *Proc. Natl. Acad. Sci. USA* 86: 5301

151. Yarbrough, L. R., Schlageck, J. G., Baughman, M. 1979. *J. Biol. Chem.* 254: 12069

152. Yee, D., Armstrong, V. W., Eckstein, F. 1979. *Biochemistry* 18: 4116

153. Yount, R. G. 1975. In *Advances in Enzymology and Related Areas of Molecular Biology,* ed. A. Meister, p. 1. New York: Cornell Univ. Med. College

154. von Hippel, P. H., Yager, T. D. 1991. *Proc. Natl. Acad. Sci. USA* 88: 2307

155. von Hippel, P. H., Yager, T. D. 1992. *Science* 255: 809

156. Herschlag, D., Piccirilli, J. A., Cech, T. R. 1991. *Biochemistry* 30: 4844

Annu. Rev. Biophys. Biomol. Struct. 1992. 21:417–39

PROTEIN INVOLVEMENT IN TRANSMEMBRANE LIPID ASYMMETRY

Philippe F. Devaux

Institut de Biologie Physico-Chimique, 13, rue Pierre et Marie Curie, F-75005 Paris, France

KEY WORDS: flippase, aminophospholipid translocase, phosphatidylserine, endocytosis, cell shape

CONTENTS

Introduction[1]

The evidence that phospholipids are asymmetrically distributed in biological membranes is compelling. This situation is possible because the transverse diffusion, or lipid flip-flop, is a slow process in phospholipid bilayers, as demonstrated for the first time in 1971 by Kornberg & McConnell (76). These authors found, with spin-labeled lipids in sonicated vesicles, a half-time of passage of several hours, a value since confirmed using many other techniques. An asymmetrical lipid synthesis could explain lipid asymmetry. However, in the past six years, the existence of several proteins specially involved in the control of transmembrane lipid asymmetry has

---

[1] Abbreviations used in this review are: PE, phoshpatidylethanolamine; PS, phosphatidylserine; PC, phosphatidylcholine; SM, sphingomyelin; PI, phosphatidylinositol; PIP, phosphatidylinositol 4-monophosphate; PIP$_2$, phosphatidylinositol 4,5-bisphosphate; PA, phosphatidic acid; PG, phosphatidylglycerol; CL, cardiolipin; TNBS 2,4,6-trinitrobenzene sulfonate; ER, endoplasmic reticulum.

417

1056–8700/92/0610–0417$02.00

been demonstrated. Several authors have also proposed various mechanisms apart from asymmetrical synthesis by which lipid asymmetry could be induced or modified in membranes. Finally, many researchers have speculated about the biological functions associated with lipid asymmetry and lipid transport through membranes. Several reviews have already examined the subject of lipid asymmetry in biological and model membranes (38, 46, 80, 101, 141). This chapter emphasizes protein involvement in transmembrane lipid asymmetry. I discuss particularly the putative role of the aminophospholipid translocase in generating lipid asymmetry in eukaryotes. Finally, I review the current hypothesis concerning biological functions associated with the membrane polarization resulting from lipid asymmetry and the shape changes triggered by transmembrane lipid transport.

Lipid Asymmetry in Biomembranes and Model Systems: a Critical Appraisal

Following the pioneering work of Bretscher in 1972 (14), many workers measured the transmembrane distribution of endogenous phospholipids in mammalian red cells using various techniques. These techniques comprise chemical labeling with nonpenetrating agents (for example with TNBS or fluorescamine), immunological methods, enzymatic assays with phosphatidylserine (PS)-dependent proteins, phospholipase digestion of membrane phospholipids, use of phospholipid exchange proteins, and physical methods such as X-ray diffraction and NMR. Previous reviews have discussed the validity of the various approaches (46, 101). None of these techniques is without drawbacks, particularly when quantitative statements are required. For example, attacking a membrane with exogenous phospholipases results in a progressive membrane degradation that can lead eventually to lipid scrambling. Thus, the determination of the lipids of the outer and inner leaflet, respectively, from the pattern of lipid degradation can be hazardous. Similarly, nonpenetrating probes, like fluorescamine, often in reality penetrate the membranes slowly. In brief, confirmation by several techniques is necessary; moreover, one should keep in mind that the limit of accuracy is generally of the order of $\pm 10\%$ of the lipids.

Figure 1 shows what is now a classic scheme corresponding to the outer and inner distribution of the main phospholipids of the human red cell membrane. Results from several laboratories appear on the same figure. Clearly there is total agreement concerning the preference of aminophospholipids [phosphatidylserine (PS) and phosphatidylethanolamine (PE)] for the inner monolayer, whereas the choline-containing lipids [phosphatidylcholine (PC) and sphingomyelin (SM)] reside essentially in the

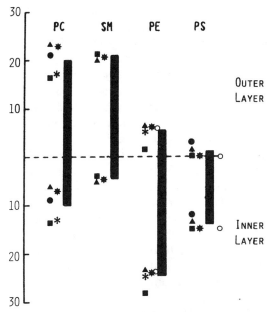

Figure 1 Transmembrane distribution of the four main phospholipid species in human erythrocytes. The results are indicated in percentage of total phospholipids. The data are gathered from six different publications and refer to nonpathological cells: (*star*) Verkleij et al (135); (*solid triangle*) Van Meer et al (134); (*asterisk*) Williamson et al (139); (*solid square*) Bergmann et al (5); (*solid circle*) Dressler et al (42); (*open circle*) Gordesky et al (55).

outer monolayer. However, after 20 years of investigation, we still do not know if 0 or 10% of PS is in the outer monolayer and conversely what fraction of the SM molecules can be found in the inner monolayer. Yet, this level of precision would be interesting, particularly when discussing the physiological role of lipid asymmetry. The data on red blood cells presented in Figure 1 should be completed by more recent information on the transmembrane distribution of plasmalogen PE, which, like the corresponding diacylglycerol phospholipid (71), is found preferentially in the inner monolayer as well as on phosphatidylinositol (PI) and its derivatives. Reportedly, 20% of PI, PIP$_2$, and phosphatidic acid (PA), but no PIP, are located in the outer monolayer (16, 52). In addition to the asymmetry of the head-group distribution, the average fatty acid composition of PS and PE shows more unsaturation than that of PC and SM (97); furthermore, within the same class of phospholipids (SM and PE), acyl chains from the outer monolayer differ from those of the inner mono-layer (11, 71). Finally, cholesterol transmembrane distribution in erythrocytes has been investigated by using cholesterol oxidase to selectively degrade cholesterol in the outer monolayer (13) and by using fluorescent analogs of cholesterol (58). Although Hale & Schroeder in 1982 (58) concluded that cholesterol is enriched in the outer monolayer of rat red blood cells, a recent article by Schroeder et al (113) suggests from two independent studies with fluorescent analogs that a larger fraction of cholesterol is located in the inner monolayer of erythrocytes. Definitive conclusions about the sterol distribution are certainly hampered by the rapid flip-flop of this noncharged molecule.

The compositional asymmetry in red cells is accompanied by the asymmetrical physical properties of this membrane (116, 126, 139). Several laboratories have shown that the viscosity of the outer monolayer is greater than that of the inner monolayer as determined with fluorescent or paramagnetic probes. In particular, we have shown that the rate of lateral diffusion of fluorescent phospholipids is approximately five times higher in the inner monolayer of erythrocytes than in the outer monolayer (94). This difference can be accounted for by the difference in phospholipid composition and does not require an asymmetrical distribution of cholesterol (29).

Erythrocytes from other mammals have yielded similar results in spite of the different proportions of the four main phospholipids in different species. The situation is more complex with other eukaryotic cells because the plasma membrane is only a small fraction of the total of cell membranes. Nevertheless, many laboratories have analyzed the lipid topology in purified plasma membranes and organelles. The main results are collected in Tables 1 and 2.

Table 1 clearly shows that, overall, the asymmetry of phospholipid distribution in human red cells is found in the plasma membrane of most eukaryotes. To what extent the quantitative variations reported for specific cell membranes are significant is a matter of debate. Indeed, purified plasma membrane may be contaminated by subcellular organelles. Moreover, the purification of the membranes is certainly responsible for a partial lipid scrambling. We recently showed that hypotonic lysis of red cells induces a partial scrambling of their lipids (S. L. Schrier, A. Zachowski & P. F. Devaux, unpublished data). This phenomenon is more pronounced if the lysis is carried out in the presence of Ca^{2+} (137). Also, as discussed later in this review, in certain cells such as platelets, a reorientation of a fraction of the lipids accompanies activation (6). Thus, the population of cells examined in some instances may have contained a fraction of activated cells with a nonrepresentative lipid asymmetry.

As is the case with erythrocytes, the phospholipid asymmetry of the plasma membrane of eukaryotes is accompanied by an asymmetrical trans-

Table 1 Quantitative results on the phospholipid asymmetry in the plasma membrane of eukaryotic cells

Cell type	Percent in outer layer					Reference
	PC	SM	PE	PS	PI	
Red blood cell (human)			see Figure 1		20	16, 52
Platelet (human)	62		54	6	34	136
	45	93	20	9	16	104
Platelet (pig)	40	91	34	6		20
Kidney brush border (rabbit)	34	80	23	15		133
Intestinal brush border (rabbit)	26		28			3
Intestinal brush border (trout)			50	32		103
Heart sarcolemna (rat)	43	93	25	0		105
Embryo fibroblast (chick)			34	17		117
Embryo myoblast (chick)			66	46		117
Brain synaptosomes (mouse)			10–15	20		49
LM fibroblast (mouse)			4–6	5		50
Hepatocytes (rat)						
Bile canalicular surface	85	63	50	0	0	65
Contiguous surface	82	0	0	14	0	65
Sinusoidal surface	85	66	55	0	0	65
Krebs II ascites (mouse)	51	46	45	20	30	110
Yeast			30–25	10–20	30–25	18

membrane viscosity. Such asymmetries were reported for platelets (74) and fibroblasts (125).

The labile character of the phospholipid transmembrane distribution and the difficulty of purifying homogeneous fractions are certainly also responsible for the discrepancies in the results obtained in cell organelles. Table 2 was in fact assembled from the literature to show the difficulty in obtaining definitive conclusions about lipid topology in organelles. In a living organism, lipids are continuously involved in the cellular traffic associated with exocytosis, endocytosis, lipid catabolism, and lipid synthesis. Thus, the lipid distribution is a dynamic process and the state of an isolated organelle such as the endoplasmic reticulum or a mitochondrion might depend drastically upon the conditions of isolation.

Only a few results have been collected from bacteria, generally with gram-positive organisms that possess a single plasma membrane. No general rules can be inferred (see 40, 54, 101, 119).

In conclusion, lipid asymmetry is probably a general feature in eukaryotic as well as in prokaryotic membranes. The model of the human red cell is probably representative of the topology of the plasma membrane

Table 2 Phospholipid asymmetry in organelles[a]

Membrane	Cell	Species	Cytoplasmic side	Random	Lumenal or matrix side	Reference
Retina disk	Rod outer segment	Cow	PS, PE	PS, PE		121
						41
						93
Synaptic vesicle	Electric organ	Torpedo	PE, PC	PC		89
		Ray	PE, PI			37
Chromaffin granule	Adrenal medulla	Cow	PE, PC	PS	PS	15
Gastric vesicle	Gastric mucosa	Pig	PS, PE, PC	SM	SM	100
Sarcoplasmic reticulum	Muscle	Rabbit	PS, PE, PC	PC	PS, PI, SM	60, 64, 131
Outer mitochondrial	Yeast	Saccharomyces cerevisiae	PE	PC, PI	PE	122
Inner mitochondrial	Liver	Rat	PE	PC	PE	87
				PE	PI, CL	99
						28
	Heart	Cow	PE		PE	81
Lysosome	Liver	Rat	PE	PC	SM, PI	99
Nucleus	Liver	Rat	PS, PE, PC	PS, PE, PC	SM, PI	99
Golgi	Liver	Rat	PS, PE	PC	SM, PI	99
				PC, PE, PI		123
Endoplasmic reticulum	Liver	Rat	PS, PE	PC	SM, PI	99
				PC, PE, PI		123
				PC	PE	132
	Brain	Chick	PC, SM	PS, PE		66, 72
						39

[a] This table contains a few contradictory results that reveal the difficulty in obtaining reliable data with purified organelles.

of eukaryotes. General rules are more difficult to infer in subcellular organelles.

In model systems, phospholipid asymmetry can be generated in liposomes with a mixed lipid composition. For example, NMR studies showed many years ago that sonicated vesicles composed of a mixture of phospholipids are generally asymmetrical. That is, in a mixture of PE and PC, PE is preferentially found inside, whereas in a mixture of PC and PG, PG is preferentially outside (4, 12, 83, 84, 90). This spontaneous segregation has been attributed to the packing problem arising in vesicles with a small diameter. Phospholipid with a small head group would be forced to the inner monolayer, while a larger head group would point to the outside. Such phenomena could cause a lipid asymmetry in organelles with a low radius of curvature, for example in mitochondrial cristae or in retinal discs.

Asymmetrical large unilamellar vesicles can be obtained through selective enzymatic or chemical modifications of external lipids (35, 76). Specific lipids, e.g. lyso derivatives or spin-labeled and fluorescent lipids with one relatively short chain, can also be added externally by spontaneous transfer (34, 48, 102). Alternatively, phospholipids from the external monolayer of a vesicle can be exchanged with the lipids of another membrane through the use of phospholipid exchange proteins (85).

Finally, workers in Cullis' laboratory have shown that certain classes of lipid corresponding to weak bases or weak acids such as free fatty acids, PA, and PG can be reoriented in a lipid bilayer by changing the pH. These investigators studied the kinetics of such reorientations and generated asymmetrical unilamellar vesicles. On the other hand, a change in pH (or $\Delta\Psi$) is not sufficient to force PS, CL, or PE to adopt an asymmetrical distribution (44, 69, 111).

Protein Involvement in Transmembrane Lipid Passage

The spontaneous passage of neutral lipids such as diacylglycerol (51) or fatty esters and probably cholesterol is rapid, with characteristic times on the order of seconds. On the contrary, phospholipid transverse diffusion in a bilayer is a slow process with characteristic times on the order of hours or days depending upon the chain length, degree of unsaturation, and the nature of the head groups (92) as well as upon the overall composition of the membrane. Cholesterol appears to increase the transverse stability of phospholipids (95), while detergent (79) and/or addition of membrane proteins can accelerate lipid flip-flop in reconstituted systems (36). Thus, the packing problem caused within the lipid lattice by the rough surface of any intrinsic protein inserted in the bilayer probably destabilizes the phospholipids at lipid-protein interfaces, and because the rate of lateral diffusion is fast (in-plane exchange rates on the order of 10^7–10^6 s^{-1}), a single protein can accelerate the flip-flop of a large population of lipids. For example, gramicidin enhances the transbilayer reorientation of lipids in erythrocyte membranes by inducing the locally hexagonal H_{II} phase (21, 129). Such extreme situations may exist at least temporarily in biological membranes.

Various proteins play specific roles in the establishment, maintenance, and cancellation of phospholipid asymmetry in eukaryotic and probably prokaryotic cells. Figure 2 is a scheme that attempts to summarize the

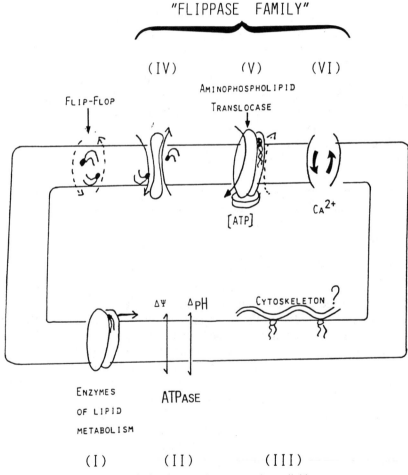

Figure 2 Protein involvement in transmembrane lipid passage.

various classes of proteins involved. Note that these proteins are in fact distributed in the plasma membrane and in subcellular organelles and may not coexist in the same membrane as schematically shown in this figure for the sake of simplicity. The first class of proteins, probably the most important in relation to lipid asymmetry, is constituted by membrane-bound enzymes that are responsible for phospholipid synthesis. At least the last stages of lipid synthesis and lipid remodeling are membranous and, hence, vectorial by nature. The orientation of the enzymes in the endoplasmic reticulum (ER), in mitochondria, and in the Golgi complex where most lipids are synthesized, therefore plays a crucial role in their subsequent orientation once shuttled to their target membranes, e.g. the plasma membrane (for a review, see 10, 68). Even erythrocytes that have a low metabolic activity contain enzymes that influence the transmembrane distribution. For example, Hirata & Axelrod (67) showed that the methyl-ation of PE is accompanied by its transmembrane reorientation. More recently, Andrick et al (1) demonstrated the fast translocation of PC to the outer membrane leaflet of human erythrocytes after its synthesis at the inner membrane surface by reacylation of lyso-PC. Thus, unlike model systems, biomembranes are made asymmetrically, and apparently fusion events, which take place during cell life and cell division, do not totally scramble lipid orientation.

A second class of proteins (II) that can be indirectly responsible for lipid asymmetry is composed of the ATPases that generate potential gradients and/or pH gradients. The strong pH gradient found in lysosomes polarizes the membrane of these organelles. But even the small acidic character of erythrocyte cytoplasm can explain the accumulation of exogenously added free fatty acids on the outer monolayer of erythrocyte (this is accompanied by the formation of echinocytes—see below). Changes in the com-positional asymmetry of phospholipids associated with the increment in the membrane surface potential have been reported in yeast (18). However, one should keep in mind that the potential or pH does not suffice to force most charged lipids to flip. As reported by Cullis' group, only the neutral form of the lipids can traverse the bilayer; the pH gradient traps a certain distribution but is not the driving force.

Hubbell (70) proposed an interesting model to explain the stable lipid asymmetry that supposedly exists in disc membranes. The model is based on the polarization through the membrane that results from fixed charges distributed asymmetrically on rhodopsin. This electric polarization would eventually segregate PS on the cytoplasmic side of the discs and indirectly influence PE distribution because of preferential interaction between PE and PS molecules. However, this model requires free passage of lipids between both monolayers in order to reach equilibrium. Such a rapid flip-flop is not excluded in disc membranes that contain very long unsaturated lipids, though this observation is yet to be verified.

A question mark indicates the class III proteins appearing in Figure 2. Several reports in the literature have suggested that cytoskeletal proteins, for example spectrin in red cells, could be responsible for maintaining lipid asymmetry (27, 57, 91, 138). However, as discussed in a previous review (38), the arguments are always indirect and may be erroneous. In fact, several recent articles devoted to erythrocyte lipid asymmetry concluded that cytoskeleton proteins play little or no role in the maintenance of phospholipid asymmetry (17, 56, 106). The latter articles are based on experiments in which the lipid asymmetry was monitored in the absence of cytoskeleton or after partial denaturation of spectrin and band 4.1.

Molecules of classes IV, V, and VI correspond to a protein family sometimes called *phospholipid flippases*, following the terminology invented by M. Bretscher. This family includes very different proteins. Molecule IV is a flippase whose existence was originally demonstrated in rat liver endoplasmic reticulum (ER) by Bishop & Bell in 1985 (9). Using a water-soluble short chain phospholipid (dibutyroyl-PC), these authors demonstrated the rapid passage through purified ER of the PC analog. The process was saturable and sensitive to proteases and chemical modifications and, according to these authors, specific for PC. A different transporter was postulated for lyso-PC (73). Using the same membrane preparation and spin-labeled lipids with one short chain and one long chain, we also found a rapid lipid flip-flop ($\tau_{1/2} \approx 10$ min at 37°C) but with very little specificity [see Figure 3 (bottom)]. Competition experiments demonstrated that lyso-PS and PC use the same pathway (63). Reconstitution experiments using a crude extract of microsomal proteins confirmed the existence of the flippase in ER (2). The same experiment using proteins from the red cell membrane failed. This process, which is a non-energy-requiring catalysis of phospholipid flip-flop, can be classified as a facilitated diffusion. Note that an appropriate name for this putative protein, yet to be purified, would be "flip-flop-ase" because both directions of transport, not just the flip, can be stimulated. Clearly this protein is indispensable in the membranes where lipids are being processed in that it allows a proper equilibration between lipids in both leaflets. One, therefore, may postulate the existence of similar protein(s) in bacterial membranes. Fast phospholipid translocations have indeed been measured in *Bacillus megaterium* (82).

Protein V represents the aminophospholipid translocase. This protein, originally discovered in the membrane of human erythrocytes (115) and later in the plasma membrane of many eukaryotic cells such as platelets (124), lymphocytes (143), fibroblasts (88), and synaptosomes (144), was

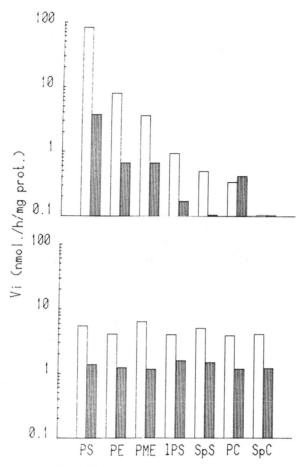

Figure 3 Comparison of the initial velocities of outside-inside translocation of spin-labeled phospholipids, at 37°C. (*Top*) Human red blood cells; (*bottom*) rat liver microsomes. The dashed bars correspond to experiments carried out after incubation with 1 mM N-ethyl-maleimide. Abbreviations are: PS, phosphatidylserine; PE, phosphatidylethanolamine; PC, phosphatidylcholine; PME, monomethyl-phosphatidylethanolamine; lPS, lyso-phos-phatidylserine; SpS, sphingosyl-phosphorylserine; SpC, sphingomyelin. Adapted from Herrmann et al (63) and Morrot et al (95).

also found in chromaffin granules, i.e. in a subcellular organelle (142). This protein selectively transports aminophospholipids (PS and PE) from the outer to the inner monolayer of the plasma membrane. Contrary to the flippase in endoplasmic reticulum (protein IV), the lipid selectivity is very high as indicated in Figure 3 (top) where the initial rates of outside-inside movements of different lipids are plotted. The movement is vectorial, requires cytosolic Mg-ATP ($K_m \approx 1$ mM), works against a chemical gradient and, thus, corresponds to an active transport. The mechanism is inhibited by N-ethyl maleimide ($K_i \approx 0.3$ mM), cytosolic vanadate (50 μM), AlF^{4-} ($\sim 50\ \mu$M) as well as by cytosolic Ca^{2+} ($\sim 1\ \mu$M).

The transmembrane equilibrium distribution of exogenously added lipids appears remarkably similar to that of endogenous lipids. For example, spin-labeled PS, PE, PC, and SM reach an equilibrium corresponding respectively to 95, 80, 30, and 5% of the lipid analogs in the inner monolayer. At 37°C, the plateau is attained in approximately 10 min with PS and in 1 h with PE. More than 10 h are necessary to estimate the final distribution of the other lipids (PC and SM) (95). Similar results were obtained in various laboratories with radioactive lipids (128), fluorescent lipids (25), and short-chain lipids (32, 33). Note that in all these experiments, the labeled lipids incorporated in the outer monolayer corresponded to a small fraction of the total lipids. To date, no studies have demonstrated that a totally scrambled membrane from red cells can recover its native lipid asymmetry by the action of the aminophospholipid translocase. This aspect is discussed later in the review.

The aminophospholipid translocase has not yet been unambiguously identified. Connor & Schroit have proposed, based on experiments with radioactive photoactivable PS, a 32-kilodalton (kDa) polypeptide as the putative protein (26, 27). We and other groups have selected a vanadate-sensitive 120-kDa Mg-ATPase (31, 96). Antibodies are currently being raised against the latter protein.

Protein VI is a very speculative protein of the flippase family. The evidence is strong that under physiological conditions, in some cells, the lipid asymmetry can be suddenly scrambled, thereby exposing PS on the outer layer of the plasma membrane. Platelets are the best-documented system in this regard (6, 7). Depending on the stimulus, phospholipid transbilayer asymmetry of the plasma membrane is more or less lost during platelet activation. Increase in cytosolic Ca^{2+} by addition of Ca^{2+} and ionophore strongly stimulates lipid scrambling, which is accompanied by vesicle shedding (22). Similar observations were made with erythrocytes, although the lipid scrambling triggered by cytosolic Ca^{2+} is less efficient (19, 22, 24, 59). Importantly, not only PS but PE also flops to the outer monolayer while PC flips inside. However, the efficiency of Ca^{2+}-induced reorientation of SM is weak (P. Williamson, A. Kulick, A. Zachowski, R. A. Schlegel & P. F. Devaux, submitted). The time scale of this lipid reorientation precludes a simple inhibition of the aminophospholipid translocase by Ca^{2+}. Indeed, when the translocase is inhibited, the randomization of lipid distribution normally takes hours or days to move through the spontaneous diffusion pathway. Ca^{2+} alone, although it interacts with PS or PA to form rigid domains, does not suffice to destroy the bilayer. Thus, a specific protein could be responsible for this Ca^{2+}-induced randomization in platelets and possibly in other cells. One mechanism that could account for the observed phenomenon would involve the formation of nonbilayer structures following the phospholipase induced production of diacylglycerol. Indeed, researchers have shown in model systems that physiological levels of diacylglycerol can destabilize lipid bilayers (120). Alternatively, partial disturbances of the bilayer structure could occur during fusion of the granules that accompanies in some instances platelet stimulation or during fusion of the plasma membrane that takes place upon shedding of membrane microvesicles (22). The Ca^{2+} pathway for lipid scrambling persists as long as cytosolic Ca^{2+} remains elevated, and disappears promptly when Ca^{2+} levels fail (P. Williamson, A. Kulick, A. Zachowski, R. A. Schlegel & P. F. Devaux, submitted). However, other laboratories have reported that flip sites were only transient during platelet or red cell stimulation by ionophore (8, 59). So, in conclusion, the mechanism of this fast lipid scrambling is far from being understood.

Generation and Maintenance of Lipid Asymmetry: Model Systems and Biomembranes

As already stated, biomembranes are not assembled de novo. A cell with its chemically polarized membranes gives rise to a second cell in which the membranes are identically polarized. Cell division involves breaking and fusion of membranes. But these processes do not appear to cause important lipid redistribution. To demonstrate the remarkable stability of the transmembrane asymmetry during the exchange of membranes within a cell, i.e. during vesicular traffic, fluorescent sphingomyelin (C_6-NBD-SM) can be inserted into the outer leaflet of fibroblast plasma membrane. At room temperature or above, the fluorescent lipid is endocytosed and, after passage through the Golgi complex, the labeled SM is recycled back to the plasma membrane where it is found exclusively again on the outer leaflet. This experiment shows not only that sphingomyelin remains on the same leaflet corresponding to the lumenal side of the Golgi stacks but also that most other phospholipids remain with the same orientation during this membrane traffic, in order to keep the necessary balance between the two monolayers. A small fraction of SM is degraded at each cycle but, under steady-state conditions, the same fraction is resynthesized at the Golgi complex (77, 78; J. M. El Hage Chahine, S. Cribier & P. F. Devaux, submitted). Newly synthesized SM is reinjected into the lipid circulation with a correct transmembrane orientation because of the sidedness of the enzymes involved in lipid metabolism. This process of subtle correction is probably representative of the mechanism of control of lipid asymmetry that undoubtedly involves a series of enzymes.

Could the aminophospholipid translocase alone generate the normal lipid asymmetry in a totally randomized erythrocyte membrane? This question pertains to the role of the aminophospholipid translocase on the transmembrane distribution of PC and SM. The experiment is not simple because most procedures of lipid randomization are partial. ATP depletion alone, on the other hand, would require days (or weeks!) to achieve a total lipid scrambling. Instead of total scrambling, one can achieve an out-of-equilibrium distribution by adding exogenous phospholipids to the outer monolayer. In several laboratories, labeled lipids, including PC and SM, were added in trace amounts to the outer monolayer of erythrocytes. With variable kinetics, the phospholipid analogs eventually reached a transmembrane distribution similar to that of the corresponding naturally occurring lipids. In fact, the similarity between the steady-state distribution of the labeled lipids and that of unlabeled lipids is striking. Thus, one may conclude that the activity of the amino-lipid pump suffices to sort aminolipids from choline-containing lipids. To explain the asymmetrical distribution of PC and SM, one would not need to postulate the existence of a PC (or SM) outward pump but simply that the occupancy of the inner lipid state by the aminophospholipids forces PC and SM to eventually accumulate in the outer monolayer. In case of scrambling, the mere passive diffusion of PC and SM concomitantly to the active inward transport of PS and PE would establish the segregation. But this view may in fact be erroneous. The model, as it is, is derived from the model explaining the formation of ion gradients through membranes, but it may not apply directly to lipids. Indeed, the inward movement of lipids without a simultaneously outward movement of another lipid (that is a flip without a flop) means that the two monolayers acquire progressively unequal surface areas and can no longer fit to each other. This process leads to membrane curvature and, if lipid transfer continues, to vesiculation and shedding. Thus, generating a lipid asymmetry from a totally scrambled lipid distribution appears to be impossible if the two mechanisms of flip and flop have very different kinetics, which would be the case in erythrocytes in which the aminophospholipid translocase activity is only counterbalanced by the very slow diffusion of PC and SM.

However, if only a small fraction of the lipids are involved in a transmembrane redistribution, as in the articles cited above, the difference in kinetics may be acceptable. For example, in the spin-label experiment carried out by Morrot and collaborators (95), the labeled lipids represented approximately 1% of the total phospholipid content. After several hours, the four phospholipid analogs tested were asymmetrically distributed as naturally occurring lipids in red blood cells. During these experiments, a shift from discocytes to echinocytes immediately after probe addition, and eventually from echinocytes back to discocytes and stomatocytes if the labeled lipids were aminophospholipids, considerably modified the cell morphology. In fact, Daleke & Huestis used similar shape changes to monitor the transmembrane passage of lipids in red cells (32, 33). Recent work showed that the reorientation of less than 1% of the phospholipids of a giant liposome, triggered by a change in pH, is accompanied by important shape changes (see Figure 4) (48).

In conclusion, the aminophospholipid translocase fulfills an important function in controlling the aminophospholipid asymmetry, particularly in sequestering PS from the outer leaflet of plasma membranes. Probably because of the lower affinity of the enzyme for PE, under steady-state conditions the equilibrium distribution of PE is only $\sim 70\text{--}80\%$. But the aminophospholipid translocase is just one of the several enzymes responsible for the lipid asymmetry. Thus, if scrambling of a large fraction of the phospholipids can be triggered physiologically by a Ca^{2+} burst in some cells (such as platelets) we infer that return to normal asymmetry, if it ever occurs, cannot be achieved without partial vesiculation of the membranes.

Biological Functions of Phospholipid Flippases

The three types of protein included here in the flippase family (IV, V, and VI in Figure 2) play very different roles in the lipid transmembrane traffic. As already mentioned, the nonspecific phospholipid flippase (class IV) probably does not coexist with classes V and VI in the plasma membrane of eukaryotes. This protein was discovered in ER membranes and most likely functions in the redistribution of newly synthesized lipids on both sides of the ER. A priori, a nonspecific flippase that catalyzes lipid translocation in both directions will not be associated with a specific pump that tends to accumulate a subpopulation of lipids on one side of a membrane. On the other hand, a PC-specific flippase, of the type postulated by Bishop & Bell (9), would be useful in the plasma membrane. Coupled with the aminophospholipid translocase, it would facilitate the establishment of the phospholipid asymmetry (see the preceding section). However, Backer & Dawidowicz (2) clearly showed that such a protein does not exist in red blood cells.

The association of the aminophospholipid translocase (protein V) with the putative Ca^{2+}-triggered flippase (protein VI) can be compared to the association of an ATP-dependent ion pump and an ionophore triggered by a specific ligand. However, as discussed above, the reversibility of lipid scrambling is questionable. So the real question is: what is the function of a transmembrane lipid segregation?

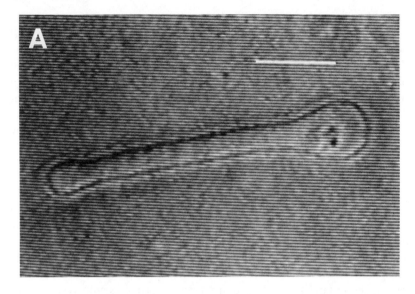

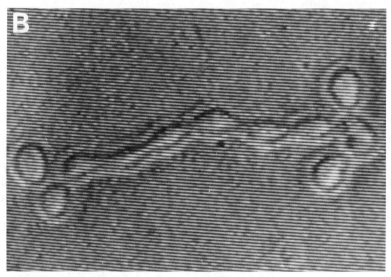

Figure 4 Shape change of a giant liposome induced by the reorientation of ~1% of the phospholipids. The liposome contains 99% PC and 1% PG. The latter lipids accumulate on the outer monolayer when the external pH is brought to 9.5. The bar corresponds to 20 μm (48).

I envision two types of functions. The first type deals with specific interactions of a subclass of lipids, particularly PS, that, if present, can be recognized on particular cell surface or can modulate enzyme activity. A fraction of the cell membranes are therefore tagged not only by proteins but also by the lipids. This may be important in cell sorting within the plasma as well as vesicle sorting within eukaryotic cells. The second type of function for lipid segregation deals with the bending imposed on a membrane by a transfer of phospholipids. I discuss the two aspects separately.

Phosphatidylserine interacts specifically with various membrane-bound enzymes. For example, protein kinase C activity depends strongly upon PS concentration (98, 109). Similarly, G proteins and annexins that correspond to a whole family of enzymes involved in many different cell functions are PS-dependent enzymes (53, 75). Thus, within a cell, these enzymes can select their target membranes if PS is asymmetrically distributed on an organelle's surface. However, the best example of a physiological modulation of enzyme activity controlled by flippases concerns a plasma membrane and is the conversion from prothrombin to thrombin induced by the sudden reorientation of PS at the outer surface of platelets. Platelet stimulation gives rise to a partial lipid scrambling with the appearance of PS on the outer monolayer of the plasma membrane as well as the release of shedded vesicles with a scrambled lipid distribution (see above for references). This phenomenon creates a PS interface on the external monolayer of the platelet membrane that stimulates the conversion of prothrombin to thrombin. This conversion is the first stage of the cascade of events involved in blood coagulation.

The progressive appearance of PS on the outer surface of aged erythrocytes may signal cell elimination. This postulation is based on experiments that showed that ghosts with an artificially scrambled lipid distribution are recognized preferentially by macrophages and endothelial cells (112, 114, 127). Recently, Fadok and collaborators provided evidence for macrophage recognition of PS on apoptotic lymphocytes and demonstrated the existence of PS receptors on macrophages (47). Progressive oxidation of the aminophospholipid translocase and the consecutive unpairing of the mechanism of maintenance of lipid asymmetry would be responsible for the lipid scrambling in aged erythrocytes. Up until now, however, it has not been possible to measure a significant variation of PS distribution in aged red cells, isolated on the grounds of their sedimentation characteristics (62). So the above mentioned theory is only valid if a very small fraction of PS on the outer layer is sufficient to tag old cells as such. Work is in progress to see if antibodies raised against PS can detect externally exposed PS on aged red cells with a better sensitivity than the phospholipase A_2 technique.

Aging may not be the only cell dysfunctioning accompanied by lipid reorientation. Sickled red blood cells have a measurable fraction of PS on their outer leaflet; simultaneously, these cells have a shorter life time in blood circulation than normal red cells (86). Also, tumorigenic, undifferentiated murine erythroleukemic cells express seven- to eightfold more PS in their outer leaflet than do their undifferentiated nontumorigenic counterparts. Increased expression of PS in the tumorigenic cells directly correlated with their ability to be recognized and bound by macrophages (23). Similarly, elevated expression of PS in the outer membrane leaflet of human tumor cells as well as recognition by activated human blood monocytes was reported recently (130).

Yet another hypothesis to explain the role of transmembrane lipid asymmetry is the different fusogenic properties of various lipid interfaces. PC and SM resist membrane fusion because of the stability of the corresponding bilayer (or monolayer) structure and also because of the long-range hydration shell of these lipids. On the contrary, PS (and PE) interfaces form smaller layers of bound water, thereby allowing closer contact between different membranes (108); secondly, they are more fusogenic, particularly in the presence of Ca^{2+}, because of their propensity to undergo phase transitions at physiological temperature from bilayer to nonbilayer phase (30).

Thus, the normal lipid polarization of plasma membranes prevents cell-cell fusion because their outer layer contains PC and SM. Interestingly, myoblasts are one of the few exceptions. These cells contain a large proportion of aminophospholipids on the outer monolayer of their plasma membrane. Myoblasts are, precisely, cells that fuse together (117). However, the actual physical principle that explains the capacity of cells to fuse has been questioned in recent work from Blumenthal's laboratory. Indeed, Herrmann et al (61) attempted to elucidate the role of phospholipid head-group specificity in modulating virus fusion to erythrocyte ghosts by using lipid scrambling or chemical modification of the outer leaflet. The results showed that fusion of influenza virus as well as vesicular stomatitis virus (VSV) was affected by the presence of unsaturated fatty acyl chains in the outer leaflet, but not by specific phospholipids. Moreover, in the case of myoblasts, the fluidity of the plasma membrane increases rapidly before the onset of fusion (107). Thus, lipid packing properties of the interacting membranes may be the important factor.

Within a cell, fusion of Golgi-derived vesicles with the plasma membrane is facilitated by the fluid PS-PE interface. Real fusion competence also requires that exocytic vesicles expose similar aminophospholipids on their outer cytosolic face. This seems to be the case for chromaffin granules and would involve the activity of an aminophospholipid translocase located in a subcellular organelle (142).

Cullis' group carried out very elegant experiments on model systems in which the fusion between large unilamellar vesicles was modulated in the presence of Ca^{2+} by the transmembrane reorientation of a small fraction of phosphatidic acid (PA) under the influence of a change in pH (43). Of course in real cells, specific proteins are certainly required for the targeting of the fusion events, but the lipid interface provides one form of recognition between membranes of the various organelles.

A different phenomenon may be the most important biological function associated with transmembrane phospholipid redistribution. This topic deals with shape changes caused by the transfer of lipids from one mono-layer to the other of a membrane. In 1974, Sheetz & Singer (118), on the basis of experiments with human erythrocytes, proposed the bilayer couple hypothesis. This theory accounts for red cell shape changes by the selective dilation of the outer or inner monolayer resulting from the intercalation of drugs on either side of the cell. The actual shape of erythrocytes results from the simultaneous action of the bilayer and the cytoskeleton. Platelets, which have different cytoskeleton proteins, undergo different shape changes when the same amphiphilic drugs are intercalated. But, for both systems, the addition of a small percentage of lipids on one leaflet ($\sim 1\%$) triggers the formation of membrane protrusions. We have already mentioned that shape changes have been triggered in large unilamellar vesicles devoid of proteins by the reorientation of a very small percentage of lipids. Thus, while in erythrocytes the activity of the aminophospholipid translocase seems limited to the maintenance of an overall discoid shape, in cells provided with a higher translocase activity that transports amino-phospholipids (PS and PE) from the outer to the inner leaflet, the inva-ginations could lead to endocytic vesicles (for more details on such a model, see 38). The proteins considered to provide the driving force for membrane pitching off (clathrin) could in fact be present in order to localize the regions of the membrane where the invaginations start. Extra-polation of such an idea leads one to suggest that Golgi membranes should contain an aminophospholipid translocase, which could participate in the formation of Golgi vesicles, oriented towards the cytosol. As for vesicles formed from the ER, they could be generated by a mismatch between rates of lipid synthesis on one side of the membrane and rates of lipid flip-flop by a type IV phospholipid flippase.

Summary and Conclusions

Transmembrane asymmetry has been extensively studied in eukaryotic cells. It is as yet only clearly demonstrated in the plasma membrane of a few cells. Subcellular organelles have evidence of lipid asymmetry, but very little consistent quantitative data exist. Proteins involved in transmembrane passage of lipids comprise enzymes of lipid metabolism and also the so-called phospholipid flippases that are either passive or active putative lipid transporters. The aminophospholipid translocase that pumps amino-phospholipids from the outer to the inner monolayer of the plasma membrane of eukaryotes is a Mg^{2+}-ATP dependent protein with a high lipid selectivity. Lipid asymmetry provides an asymmetrical environment for membrane enzymes. Thus, PS (and PE) reorientation could be a way of controlling or triggering specific enzymes. Also, the asymmetrical distribution of phospholipids most likely determines the fusion-competent membranes and/or which sides of membranes should fuse. Finally, the lipid pump as well as all enzymes responsible for the net transmembrane flux of phospholipids may provide the driving force for membrane bending, notably during the formation of endocytic vesicles.

Clearly, real progress in this area will be made only if the proteins of the flippase family are purified and antibodies obtained that will permit the recognition and localization of these proteins in various cells. Also, specific inhibitors as well as mutants would allow one to infer more directly what are the real functions of these proteins. At a late stage, the protein purification will eventually permit speculation on the mechanism of action of a pump that must transport simultaneously hydrophilic and hydrophobic groups through a membrane.

ACKNOWLEDGMENTS

The author thanks Drs. A. Zachowski and S. Sweeney for critically reading this manuscript. Work is supported by grants from the Centre National de la Recherche Scientifique (URA 526), the Institut National de la Santé et de la Recherche Médicale (N° 900104) and the Université Paris VII.

Literature Cited

1. Andrick, C., Bröring, K., Deuticke, B., Haest, C. W. M. 1991. *Biochim. Biophys. Acta* 1064: 235–41
2. Backer, J. M., Dawidowicz, E. A. 1987. *Nature* 327: 341–43
3. Barsukov, L. I., Bergelson, L. D., Spiers, M., Hauser, J., Semenza, G. 1986. *Biochim. Biophys. Acta* 882: 87–99
4. Berden, J. A., Barker, R. W., Radda, G. K. 1975. *Biochim. Biophys. Acta* 375: 186–208
5. Bergmann, W. L., Dressler, V., Haest, C. W. M., Deuticke, B. 1984. *Biochim. Biophys. Acta* 772: 328–36
6. Bevers, E. M., Comfurius, P., Zwaal, R. F. A. 1983. *Biochim. Biophys. Acta* 736: 57–66

7. Bevers, E. M., Tilly, R. H. J., Senden, J. M. G., Comfurius, P., Zwaal, R. F. A. 1989. *Biochemistry* 28: 2382–87
8. Bevers, E. M., Verhallen, P. F. J., Visser, J. W. G., Comfurius, P., Zwaal, R. F. A. 1990. *Biochemistry* 29: 5132–37
9. Bishop, W. R., Bell, R. M. 1985. *Cell* 42: 51–60
10. Bishop, W. R., Bell, R. M. 1988. *Annu. Rev. Cell Biol.* 4: 579–610
11. Boeghein, J. P. J., van Linde, M., Op den Kamp, J. A. F., Roelofsen, B. 1983. *Biochim. Biophys. Acta* 735: 438–42
12. Bramhall, J. 1986. *Biochemistry* 25: 3479–86
13. Brasaemble, D. L., Robertson, A. D., Ahle, A. D. 1988. *J. Lipid Res.* 29: 481–89
14. Bretscher, M. S. 1972. *Nature New Biol.* 236: 11–12
15. Buckland, R. M., Radda, G. K., Shennan, C. D. 1978. *Biochim. Biophys. Acta* 513: 321–37
16. Bütikofer, P., Lin, Z. W., Chiu, D. T.-Y., Lubin, B., Kuypers, F. A. 1990. *J. Biol. Chem.* 265: 16035–38
17. Calvez, J. Y., Zachowski, A., Herrmann, A., Morrot, G., Devaux, P. F. 1988. *Biochemistry* 27: 5666–70
18. Cerbon, J., Calderon, V. 1991. *Biochim. Biophys. Acta* 1067: 139–44
19. Chandra, R., Joshi, P. C., Bajpai, V. K., Gupta, C. M. 1987. *Biochim. Biophys. Acta* 902: 253–62
20. Chap, H. J., Zwaal, R. F. A., van Deenen, L. L. M. 1977. *Biochim. Biophys. Acta* 467: 146–64
21. Classen, J., Haest, C. M. W., Tournois, H., Deuticke, B. 1987. *Biochemistry* 26: 6604–12
22. Comfurius, P., Senden, J. M. G., Tilly, R. H. J., Schroit, A. J., Bevers, E. M., Zwaal, R. F. A. 1990. *Biochim. Biophys. Acta* 1026: 153–60
23. Connor, J., Bucana, C., Fidler, I. J., Schroit, A. J. 1989. *Proc. Natl. Acad. Sci. USA* 86: 3184–88
24. Connor, J., Gillum, K., Schroit, A. J. 1990. *Biochim. Biophys. Acta* 1025: 82–86
25. Connor, J., Schroit, A. J. 1987. *Biochemistry* 26: 5099–5105
26. Connor, J., Schroit, A. J. 1988. *Biochemistry* 27: 848–51
27. Connor, J., Schroit, A. J. 1990. *Biochemistry* 29: 37–43
28. Crain, R. C., Marinetti, G. V. 1979. *Biochemistry* 18: 2407–14
29. Cribier, S., Morrot, G., Neumann, J.-M., Devaux, P. F. 1990. *Eur. Biophys. J.* 18: 33–41
30. Cullis, P. R., de Kruijff, B. 1979. *Biochim. Biophys. Acta* 559: 399–420
31. Daleke, D. L., Cornely-Moss, K. A., Smith, C. M. 1991. *Biophys. J.* 59: 381a
32. Daleke, D. L., Huestis, W. H. 1985. *Biochemistry* 24: 5406–16
33. Daleke, D. L., Huestis, W. H. 1989. *J. Cell. Biol.* 108: 1375–85
34. Dao, H. N. T., McIntyre, J. C., Sleight, R. G. 1991. *Anal. Biochem.* 196: 46–53
35. de Kruijff, B., Baken, P. 1978. *Biochim. Biophys. Acta* 507: 38–47
36. de Kruijff, B., van Zoelen, E. J. J., van Deenen, L. L. M. 1978. *Biochim. Biophys. Acta* 509: 537–42
37. Deutsch, J. W., Kelly, R. B. 1981. *Biochemistry* 20: 378–85
38. Devaux, P. F. 1991. *Biochemistry* 30: 1163–73
39. Dominski, J., Binaglia, L., Dreyfus, H., Massarelli, R., Mersel, M., Freysz, L. 1983. *Biochim. Biophys. Acta* 734: 257–66
40. Donohue-Rolfe, A. M., Schaechter, M. 1980. *Proc. Natl. Acad. Sci. USA* 77: 1867–71
41. Drenthe, E. H. S., Klompmakers, A. A., Bonting, S. L., Daemen, F. J. M. 1980. *Biochim. Biophys. Acta* 603: 130–41
42. Dressler, V., Haest, C. W. M., Plasa, G., Deuticke, B., Erusalimsky, J. D. 1984. *Biochim. Biophys. Acta* 775: 189–96
43. Eastman, S. J. 1991. *Studies of the generation and function of phopholipid asymmetry.* PhD thesis. University of Vancouver, Vancouver, British Columbia
44. Eastman, S. J., Hope, M. J., Cullis, P. R. 1991. *Biochemistry* 30: 1740–45
45. Deleted in proof
46. Etemadi, A.-H. 1980. *Biochim. Biophys. Acta* 604: 423–75
47. Fadok, V. A., Voelker, D. R., Campbell, P. A., Cohen, J. J., Bratton, D. L., Henson, P. M. 1991. *J. Exp. Med.* Submitted
48. Fadok, E., Devaux, P. F. 1992. *Biophys. J.* In press
49. Fontaine, R. N., Harris, R. A., Schroeder, F. 1990. *Neurochemistry* 34: 269–77
50. Fontaine, R. N., Schroeder, F. 1979. *Biochim. Biophys. Acta* 558: 1–12
51. Ganong, B. R., Bell, R. M. 1984. *Biochemistry* 23: 4977–83
52. Gascard, P., Tran, D., Sauvage, M., Sulpice, J.-C., Fukami, K., et al. 1991. *Biochim. Biophys. Acta* 1069: 27–36
53. Geisow, M. J., Walker, J. H. 1986. *TIBS* 11: 420–23
54. Goldfine, H., Johnson, N. C., Bishop,

438   DEVAUX

D. G. 1982. *Biochem. Biophys. Res. Commun.* 108: 1502–7
55. Gordesky, S. E., Marinetti, G. V., Love, R. 1975. *J. Membr. Biol.* 20: 111–32
56. Gudi, S. R. P., Kumar, A., Bhakuni, V., Ghodale, S. M., Gupta, C. M. 1990. *Biochim. Biophys. Acta* 1023: 63–72
57. Haest, C. W. M., Plasa, G., Kamp, D., Deuticke, B. 1978. *Biochim. Biophys. Acta* 509: 21–32
58. Hale, J. E., Schroeder, F. 1982. *Eur. J. Biochem.* 122: 649–61
59. Henseleit, U., Plasa, G., Haest, C. 1990. *Biochim. Biophys. Acta* 1029: 1217–27
60. Herbette, L., Blaisie, J. K., Defoor, P., Fleischer, S., Bick, R. J., et al. 1984. *Arch. Biochem. Biophys.* 234: 235–42
61. Herrmann, A., Clague, M. J., Purl, A., Morris, S. J., Blumenthal, R., Grimaldi, S. 1990. *Biochemistry* 29: 4054–58
62. Herrmann, A., Devaux, P. F. 1990. *Biochim. Biophys. Acta* 1027: 41–46
63. Herrmann, A., Zachowski, A., Devaux, P. F. 1990. *Biochemistry* 29: 2023–27
64. Hidalgo, C., Ikemoto, N. 1977. *J. Biol. Chem.* 252: 8446–54
65. Higgins, J. A., Evans, W. H. 1978. *Biochem. J.* 174: 563–67
66. Higgins, J. A., Piggot, C. A. 1982. *Biochem. Biophys. Acta* 693: 151–58
67. Hirata, F., Axelrod, J. 1978. *Proc. Natl. Acad. Sci. USA* 75: 2348–52
68. Hjelmstad, R. H., Bell, R. M. 1991. *Biochemistry* 30: 1731–40
69. Hope, M. J., Cullis, P. R. 1987. *J. Biol. Chem.* 262: 4360–66
70. Hubbell, W. L. 1990. *Biophys. J.* 57: 99–108
71. Hullin, F., Bosant, M.-J., Salem, N. Jr. 1991. *Biochim. Biophys. Acta* 1061: 15–25
72. Hutson, J. L., Higgins, J. A. 1982. *Biochim. Biophys. Acta* 687: 247–56
73. Kawashima, Y., Bell, R. M. 1987. *J. Biol. Chem.* 262: 16495–16502
74. Kitagawa, S., Matsubayashi, M., Kotani, K., Usui, K., Kametani, F. 1991. *J. Membr. Biol.* 119: 221–27
75. Klee, C. 1988. *Biochemistry* 27: 6645–53
76. Kornberg, R. D., McConnell, H. M. 1971. *Biochemistry* 10: 1111–20
77. Koval, M., Pagano, R. E. 1989. *J. Cell. Biol.* 108: 2169–81
78. Koval, M., Pagano, R. E. 1990. *J. Cell. Biol.* 111: 429–42
79. Kramer, R. M., Hasselbach, H.-J., Semenza, G. 1981. *Biochim. Biophys. Acta* 643: 233–42

80. Krebs, J. J. R. 1982. *J. Bioenerg. Biomembr.* 14: 141–57
81. Krebs, J. J. R., Hauser, H., Carafoli, E. 1979. *J. Biol. Chem.* 254: 5308–16
82. Langley, K. E., Kennedy, E. P. 1979. *Proc. Natl. Acad. Sci. USA* 76: 6245–49
83. Lentz, B. R., Alford, D. R., Dombrose, F. A. 1980. *Biochemistry* 19: 2555–59
84. Litman, B. J. 1974. *Biochemistry* 13: 2844–48
85. Low, M. G., Zilversmit, D. B. 1980. *Biochim. Biophys. Acta* 596: 223–34
86. Lubin, B., Chiu, D., Bastacky, J., Roelofsen, B., van Deenen, L. L. M. 1981. *J. Clin. Invest.* 67: 1643–49
87. Marinetti, G. V., Senior, A. E., Love, R., Broadhurst, C. I. 1976. *Chem. Phys. Lipids* 17: 353–62
88. Martin, O. C., Pagano, R. E. 1987. *J. Biol. Chem.* 262: 5890–98
89. Michaelson, D. M., Barkai, G., Barenholz, Y. 1983. *Biochem. J.* 211: 1155–62
90. Michaelson, D. M., Horwitz, A. F., Klein, M. P. 1973. *Biochemistry* 12: 2637–43
91. Middelkoop, E., Lubin, B. H., Bevers, E. M., Op den Kamp, J. A. F., Comfurius, P., et al. 1988. *Biochim. Biophys. Acta* 937: 281–88
92. Middelkoop, E., Lubin, B. H., Op den Kamp, J. A. F., Roelofsen, B. 1986. *Biochim. Biophys. Acta* 855: 421–24
93. Miljanich, G. P., Nemes, P. P., White, D. L., Dratz, E. A. 1981. *J. Membr. Biol.* 60: 249–55
94. Morrot, G., Cribier, S., Devaux, P. F., Geldwerth, D., Davoust, J., et al. 1986. *Proc. Natl. Acad. Sci. USA* 83: 6863–67
95. Morrot, G., Herve, P., Zachowski, A., Fellmann, P., Devaux, P. F. 1989. *Biochemistry* 28: 3456–62
96. Morrot, G., Zachowski, A., Devaux, P. F. 1990. *FEBS Lett.* 266: 29–32
97. Myher, J. J., Kuksis, A., Pind, S. 1989. *Lipids* 24: 396–407
98. Newton, A. C., Koshland, D. E. 1990. *Biochemistry* 29: 6656–61
99. Nilsson, O. S., Dallner, G. 1977. *Biochim. Biophys. Acta* 464: 453–58
100. Olaisson, H., Mardh, S., Arvisson, G. 1985. *J. Biol. Chem.* 260: 11262–67
101. Op den Kamp, J. A. F. 1979. *Annu. Rev. Biochem.* 48: 47–71
102. Pagano, R. E., Martin, O. C., Schroit, A. J., Struck, D. K. 1981. *Biochemistry* 20: 4920–27
103. Pelletier, X., Mersel, M., Freysz, L., Leray, C. 1987. *Biochim. Biophys. Acta* 902: 223–28
104. Perret, B., Chap, H. J., Douste-Blazy,

L. 1979. *Biochim. Biophys. Acta* 556: 434–46
105. Post, J. A., Langer, G. A., Op den Kamp, J. A. F., Verkleij, A. J. 1988. *Biochim. Biophys. Acta* 943: 256–66
106. Pradhan, D., Williamson, P., Schlegel, R. A. 1991. *Biochemistry* 30: 7754–58
107. Prives, J., Shinitzky, M. 1977. *Nature* 268: 761–63
108. Rand, R. P., Parsegian, V. A. 1989. *Biochim. Biophys. Acta* 988: 351–76
109. Rando, R. R. 1988. *FASEB J.* 2: 2348–55
110. Record, M., El Tamer, A., Chap, H., Douste-Blazy, L. 1984. *Biochim. Biophys. Acta* 778: 449–56
111. Redelmeier, T. E., Hope, M. J, Cullis, P. R. 1990. *Biochemistry* 29: 3046–53
112. Schlegel, R. A., Prendergast, T. W., Williamson, P. 1985. *J. Cell Physiol.* 123: 215–18
113. Schroeder, F., Nemecz, G., Wood, W. G., Joiner, C., Morrot, G., et al. 1991. *Biochim. Biophys. Acta* 1066: 183–92
114. Schroit, A. J., Madsen, J. W., Tanaka, Y. 1985. *J. Biol. Chem.* 260: 5131–38
115. Seigneuret, M., Devaux, P. F. 1984. *Proc. Natl. Acad. Sci. USA.* 81: 3751–55
116. Seigneuret, M., Zachowski, A., Herrmann, A., Devaux, P. F. 1984. *Biochemistry* 23: 4271–75
117. Sessions, A., Horwitz, A. F. 1983. *Biochim. Biophys. Acta* 728: 103–11
118. Sheetz, M. P., Singer, S. J. 1974. *Proc. Natl. Acad. Sci. USA* 71: 4457–61
119. Shukla, S. D., Green, C., Turner, J. M. 1980. *Biochem. J.* 188: 131–35
120. Siegel, D. P., Banschbach, J., Yeagle, P. L. 1989. *Biochemistry* 28: 5010–19
121. Smith, H. G. Jr., Fager, R. S., Litman, B. J. 1977. *Biochemistry* 16: 1399–1405
122. Sperka-Gottlieb, C. D. M., Hermetter, A., Paltauf, F., Daum, G. 1988. *Biochim. Biophys. Acta* 946: 227–34
123. Sundler, R., Sarcione, S. L., Alberts, A. W., Vagelos, P. R. 1977. *Proc. Natl. Acad. Sci. USA* 74: 3350–54
124. Sune, A., Bette-Bobillo, P., Bienvenüe, A., Fellmann, P., Devaux, P. F. 1987. *Biochemistry* 26: 2972–78
125. Sweet, W. D., Wood, W. G., Schroeder, F. 1987. *Biochemistry* 26: 2828–35
126. Tanaka, K. I., Ohnishi, S.-I. 1976. *Biochim. Biophys. Acta* 426: 218–31
127. Tanaka, Y., Schroit, A. J. 1983. *J. Biol. Chem.* 258: 11335–43
128. Tilley, L., Cribier, S., Roelofsen, B., Op den Kamp, J. A. F., van Deenen, L. L. M. 1986. *FEBS Lett.* 194: 21–27
129. Tournois, H., Leunissen-Bijvelt, J., Haest, C. W. M., de Gier, J., de Kruijff, B. 1987. *Biochemistry* 26: 6613–21
130. Utsugi, T., Schroit, A. J., Connor, J., Bucana, C. D., Fidler, I. J. 1991. *Cancer Res.* 51: 3062–66
131. Vale, M. G. P. 1977. *Biochim. Biophys. Acta* 471: 39–48
132. van den Besselaar, A. M. H. P., de Kruijff, B., van den Bosch, H., van Deenen, L. L. M. 1978. *Biochim. Biophys. Acta* 510: 242–55
133. Venien, C., Le Grimellec, C. 1988. *Biochim. Biophys. Acta* 942: 159–68
134. Van Meer, G., Gahmberg, C. G., Op den Kamp, J. A. F., van Deenen, L. L. M. 1981. *FEBS Lett.* 135: 53–55
135. Verkleij, A. J., Zwaal, R. F. A., Roelofsen, B., Comfurius, P., Kastelijn, D., van Deenen, L. L. M. 1973. *Biochim. Biophys. Acta* 323: 178–93
136. Wang, C. T., Shia, Y. I., Chen, J. C., Tsai, W.-J., Yang, C. C. 1986. *Biochim. Biophys. Acta* 856: 244–58
137. Williamson, P., Algarin, L., Bateman, J., Choe, H.-R., Schlegel, R. A. 1985. *J. Cell. Physiol.* 123: 209–14
138. Williamson, P., Antia, R., Schlegel, R. A. 1987. *FEBS Lett.* 219: 316–20
139. Williamson, P., Bateman, J., Kozarsky, K., Mattocks, K., Hermanowicz, N., et al. 1982. *Cell* 30: 725–35
140. Deleted in proof
141. Zachowski, A., Devaux, P. F. 1990. *Experientia* 46: 644–56
142. Zachowski, A., Henry, J.-P., Devaux, P. F. 1989. *Nature* 340: 75–76
143. Zachowski, A., Herrmann, A., Paraf, A., Devaux, P. F. 1987. *Biochim. Biophys. Acta* 897: 197–200
144. Zachowski, A., Morot Gaudry-Talarmain, Y. 1990. *J. Neurochem.* 55: 1352–56

Annu. Rev. Biophys. Biomol. Struct. 1992. 21:441–83

STRUCTURE AND MECHANISM OF ALKALINE PHOSPHATASE

Joseph E. Coleman

Department of Molecular Biophysics and Biochemistry, Yale University, New Haven, Connecticut 06510

KEY WORDS: zinc enzymes, enzyme mechanisms (alkaline phosphatase), crystal structure (alkaline phosphatase), ^{31}P NMR (alkaline phosphatase), ^{113}Cd NMR (alkaline phosphatase)

CONTENTS

441

1056–8700/92/0610–0441$02.00

INTRODUCTION

Alkaline phosphatase is often cited as the most frequently referenced enzyme (55). This fact relates more to the widespread use of alkaline phosphatase activity in human serum as an enzymatic signal for a variety of disease states involving particularly the liver and bone, than to a greater number of investigations directed at the molecular properties of the enzyme. The emergence in the literature of the enzyme alkaline phosphatase began around 1907 when Suzuki et al first suggested that phosphatases constituted a separate class of eukaryotic enzymes (70). By 1912, the enzyme we now know as alkaline phosphatase was defined by the work of Grosser & Husler (40) and von Euler (75), who showed that while it was present in a variety of tissues, the enzyme, which could hydrolyze glycerophosphate and fructose 1–6 diphosphate, was present in highest amount in intestinal mucosa. von Euler & Funke (76) used the word phosphatase for the first time in 1912. The enzyme from intestinal mucosa, particularly calf intestine, became the prototype for investigators exploring the properties of the enzyme itself.

Not until 1961 did Engstrom discover that the intestinal enzyme formed a phosphoseryl residue when incubated with phosphate esters at low pH (27, 28). The enzyme's catalysis of ^{18}O exchange into inorganic phosphate strongly supported the notion that the phosphoserine is a significant intermediate on the catalytic pathway (3, 65, 69). The demonstration that transfer of phosphate by the enzyme from an ester to a second alcohol leads to retention rather than inversion of configuration around the phosphorous (46) supported the conclusion derived from much previous evidence that the mechanism involves two sequential in-line nucleophilic attacks at phosphorous, the first by the hydroxyl of Ser102 on the incoming phosphomonoester and the second on the phosphoseryl intermediate by solvent water or an alcohol acceptor (32–34, 38).

In the late 1950s and early 1960s, investigators discovered that *Escherichia coli* possessed an alkaline phosphatase that was derepressible by phosphate starvation (21, 31, 42, 72). Its gene, *phoA*, was part of the *pho* regulon consisting of the group of genes in *E. coli* whose products are involved in phosphate transport and metabolism (4, 22, 38, 53) (for bibliography, see 22, 38). The *E. coli* enzyme had similar catalytic properties, similar pH-rate profile, and formed the same phosphoseryl intermediate as the intestinal enzyme (66, 67). The amino acid sequences of the mammalian enzymes, derived from their cDNA sequences, can be fit into the primary structure of the bacterial enzyme, with the proper adjustments for some insertions and deletions (47). With such adjustments, most of the critical active-site residues described below are conserved between the eukaryotic and bacterial enzymes.

In 1962, the *E. coli* alkaline phosphatase joined the class of zinc metallo-enzymes with the demonstration by Plocke et al (62) that the enzyme contained stoichiometric amounts of zinc, a finding also confirmed in later studies of the calf intestinal enzyme (30). These early studies showed that Zn(II) is required for activity, and many subsequent studies have confirmed this observation, including the demonstration that the metal is required for initial phosphate binding and thus for the formation of the phosphoseryl intermediate (3). The great stability over a wide range of pH of the metal-free apophosphoryl enzyme, which can be formed by removal of the metal ion from the Cd(II) enzyme, demonstrates that the metal ion is required for dephosphorylation of the phosphoseryl intermediate as well (18).

The most detailed information on the structure and function of the enzyme is available for the *E. coli* enzyme. This review is a synthesis of the solution data and the recently completed crystal structures of the *E. coli* alkaline phosphatase and its two phosphoenzyme intermediates at 2.0-Å and 2.5-Å resolution, respectively (48). The phosphoenzymes are E·P, the noncovalent complex formed between inorganic phosphate and the enzyme, and E-P, the covalent or phosphoseryl intermediate, formed by the phosphorylation of Ser102.

GENERAL STRUCTURE OF *E. COLI* ALKALINE PHOSPHATASE

Alkaline phosphatase exists in the periplasmic space of *E. coli* as a dimer of identical subunits each containing 429 amino acids (11). The four Cys residues are present as two intrachain disulfides. The monomers are synthesized as a preenzyme containing a Leu-rich signal peptide of 22 residues (7, 45, 56, 57). Processing occurs via a signal peptidase after secretion through the membrane (17). Recent data suggest that formation of active enzyme upon dimerization may be a complex process involving some modulator molecules (J. F. Chlebowski, personal communication). A comparison of the amino acid sequences of the phosphorylated peptides isolated from the enzyme with the complete amino acid sequence showed that the phosphorylated residue was Ser102. Figure 1*a* shows the overall shape and polypeptide conformation found in the crystal structure of the dimer. Figure 1*b* shows a ribbon diagram of the secondary structure of the monomer.

SUMMARY OF SUBSTRATE SPECIFICITY AND KINETICS OF ALKALINE PHOSPHATASE

Alkaline phosphatase is thought to be strictly a phosphomonoesterase, although one recent investigation found a low phosphodiesterase activity

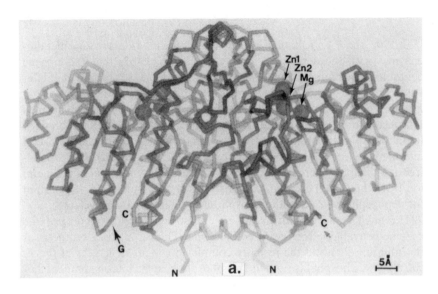

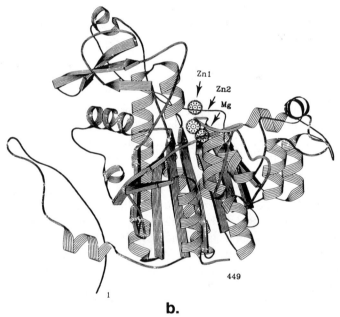

Figure 1 (*a*) Alpha-carbon trace of the dimer of *E. coli* alkaline phosphatase. The non-crystallographic two-fold axis is vertical and the maximum dimension of the dimer is horizontal. The three metal ions at each active center are shown as spheres and the two active sites of the dimer are 30 Å apart. (*b*) Ribbon drawing of the monomer of *E. coli* alkaline phosphatase. The three metal ions are shown as stippled spheres, Zn1, Zn2, and Mg as indicated. The center of the monomer consists of a 10-stranded β-sheet flanked by 15 helices of varying lengths. A second 3-stranded β-sheet and an α-helix form the top of the molecule in this view. Reprinted from Ref. 48.

(J. F. Chlebowski, personal communication). The enzyme hydrolyzes not only oxyphosphate monoesters (23, 29, 41, 63), but also a variety of O- (58, 59) and S-phosphorothioates (19), phosphoramidates (63), thiophosphate, and phosphate (3, 19, 65, 69); hydrolysis of the latter group is reflected by the catalysis of the exchange of ^{18}O from $H_2^{18}O$ into inorganic phosphate (3, 65, 69) or the release of H_2S from thiophosphate (19). The enzyme has an alkaline pH maximum, and the rate follows an approximately sigmoid pH-rate profile with an apparent pK_a of ~ 7.5 (19, 34, 50, 63). Table 1 summarizes substrate structure, reaction products, and k_{cat} values. In the case of oxyphosphate monoesters, the k_{cat} is apparently independent of the R group, which can vary from a large protein molecule to a methyl group (63). This finding reflects the fact that either the dephosphorylation of E-P or the dissociation of the product, P_i, is the rate-controlling step depending on pH. A variety of NMR methods have demonstrated that the latter step is rate limiting at alkaline pH (38, 44). In hydrolysis of P_i (^{18}O exchange) or release of H_2S, however, the phosphorylation of Ser102 by the substrate appears to be so slow as to be rate controlling (9, 19, 63).

Alkaline phosphatase reactions can be fit to the general kinetic formulation given in Scheme 1,

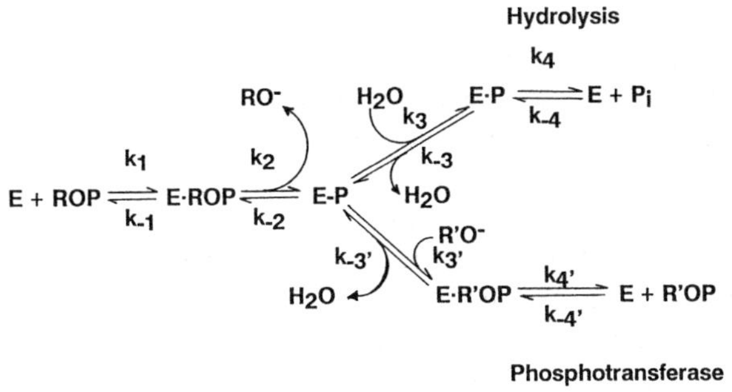

Scheme 1

which includes the covalent phosphoseryl intermediate, E-P, formed when Ser102 is phosphorylated, and the noncovalent complex, $E \cdot P$, which is formed with the product, P_i. At pH 5.5 and below, the $E\text{-}P \rightleftharpoons E \cdot P$ equilibrium favors E-P such that P_i can phosphorylate Ser102 to form high equilibrium concentrations of E-P (for summary, see 63). Scheme 1 also includes the finding that solvent, H_2O, is not the only acceptor for the phosphate from E-P. Almost any alcohol will serve as an acceptor at pH values above 9 and acceptor concentrations near 1 M as shown by recent ^{31}P NMR assays (38). Traditionally, amino alcohols with the amino group

Table 1 Values of k_{cat} for phosphate monoesters hydrolyzed by alkaline phosphatase

Substrate (conditions)		k_{cat}, pH 8.0 (s^{-1})
$ROPO_3^{2-}$	(0.1 M Tris)	8.5^a
$ROPO_3^{2-}$	(1.0 M Tris)	13–45
$ROPO_3^{2-}$	(1.0 M Tris), Co(II)	≈ 2
$RSPO_3^{2-}$	(1.0 M Tris)	30
$RNHPO_3^{2-}$	(1.0 M Tris)	28
$ROPSO_2^{2-}$	(0.1 M Tris)	0.005
$ROPSO_{2-}$	(1.0 M Tris)	0.09
$ROPSO_2^{2-}$	(1.0 M Tris), Co(II)	0.17
$HSPO_3^{2-}$		0.26
$HOPO_3^{2-}$		0.15–0.2

^{a} When a single k_{cat} is given, it stands for a representative value
for substrates that have been the subject of relatively few studies.
If a range is given, it reflects a substrate for which a great many
values of V_{max} are available in the literature.

on the carbon adjacent to that carrying the accepting OH, e.g. Tris and
ethanolamine, have been used to demonstrate this phosphotransferase
activity (63). These acceptors not only have enhanced acceptor activity,
but show maximum transferase activity around pH 8 (63). The rate rapidly
falls off at higher pH values, pH 8–11 (38). Analysis of the high-resolution
crystal structure does not as yet suggest the reason for this special reactivity
of amino alcohols. The mechanism of the phosphotransferase activity
based on a variety of NMR evidence is postulated to involve the coordination of the alcoxide ion to one of the zinc ions at the active site
instead of a water molecule (38).

Since the original isolation of a phosphorylated serine from alkaline
phosphatase by Engström's laboratory (27, 28), kinetic analyses of the
enzyme reaction have included steps for the formation and dephosphorylation of the serylphosphate. Rapid-flow kinetic methods applied to
examine the initial phases of the hydrolysis of nitrophenyl phosphates by
the enzyme revealed that the enzyme produced a relatively rapid burst of
phenolate product followed by a steady-state rate at acid pH, but no burst
was observed at alkaline pH, where the enzyme was maximally active. The
acid burst was readily explained by the finding that dephosphorylation of
E-P was very slow, 0.1 s^{-1}, and rate limiting. The possible rate-limiting
step at alkaline pH was less clear. The rate of phosphorylation of the serine
hydroxyl at pH 5.5, calculated from the burst rate, ranged from 17 to 30
s^{-1} as assembled from numerous studies. In 1973, Bloch & Schlessinger

(8) demonstrated that the rapid-flow kinetics were badly distorted by phosphate that was bound to the native enzyme and carried along through most standard isolation procedures. When phosphate-free enzyme was employed for rapid-flow measurements, they observed instantaneous bursts of RO^- (within the 3-ms dead time of the instrument) at both pH 5.5 and 8.0. The readdition of phosphate abolished the burst at alkaline pH and slowed down the burst rate at acid pH. Thus, contaminating phosphate can abolish the burst at alkaline pH by the prior formation of $E \cdot P$, but in general cannot completely abolish the burst at pH 5.5, because E-P is not 100% formed. Even more importantly, most stock enzymes were diluted from neutral pH where no E-P was present at the time of mixing. Thus, $HOPO_4^{2-}$ simply competed with $ROPO_4^{2-}$ binding at acid pH. Because phosphorylation from the monoester is so much more rapid than from phosphate, the rate of release of RO^- slowed during the transient phase, despite the fact that the ester still carried out most of the phosphorylation of the enzyme. An important fact emerging from these studies is that phosphorylation from $ROPO_4^{2-}$, even at acid pH, is a much more rapid process than previously believed. Since the bursts at both pH 5.5 and pH 8.0 are instantaneous, k_2, the phosphorylation rate in Scheme 1, must be at least 300 s^{-1} throughout the pH range from pH 5.5 to 8.0 and may be even faster.

The values of many of the kinetic and equilibrium constants describing the alkaline phosphatase reaction (Scheme 1) are plotted in Figure 2 as a function of pH. The pH-rate profile, expressed as k_{cat}, is presented as a sigmoid function corresponding to a single pK_a of 7.5 (Figure 2a). After collection of most of the published data on pH-rate profiles for the E. coli enzyme, this curve was chosen to represent k_{cat} (see 19, 50, 58, 65). Although not all pH-rate profiles fit the theoretical curve for a single ionization, the most extensive analyses of pH-rate profile data using Dixon plots (log V_{max} vs pH) show that the pH-rate profile can be adequately fit by a single pK_a (50). This finding suggests, but does not prove, that a single proton dissociation is involved. Under conditions usually employed for alkaline phosphatase assays, the pK_a for V_{max} is ~7.5; however, depending on whether neutral buffers, cationic buffers or added organic solvents are present, the apparent pK_a has been observed to vary from 6.58 to 7.55 (50). K_m values for phosphate monoesters remain constant as a function of pH until above pH 8, where an increase in the magnitude of K_m can be fit with an apparent pK_a near 9 (Figure 2b) (50). Thus, V_{max}/K_m plots are bell-shaped if high pH values are included. The increase in K_m at high pH may be connected with a phenomenon of phosphate dissociation at high pH observed using ^{31}P NMR and discussed further below.

Direct measurements of k_3, the rate for dephosphorylation of the phos-

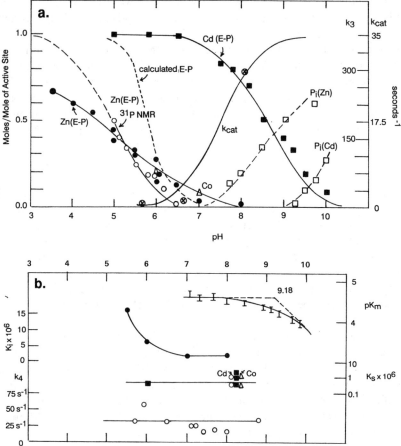

Figure 2 Summary of kinetic constants, equilibrium constants, and concentration of phosphoenzyme intermediates describing the interaction of phosphate monoesters and phosphate with *E. coli* alkaline phosphatase as functions of pH. (*a*) (*Solid circle*) Moles of E-^{32}P formed per mole of active site by the native zinc enzyme. (*Open circle*) E-P per mole of active site as determined using ^{31}P NMR. (*Dashed line*) Expected moles of E-P formed per mole of active site calculated from kinetic constants (52). (*Solid square*) E-P formed by Cd$_6$AP per mole of active site as determined by labeling with H^{32}PO$_4^{2-}$ and using ^{31}P NMR. (*Open triangle*) E-^{32}P formed by CoAP. (*Solid line*) The central sigmoid curve labeled k_{cat} represents the pH-profile of k_{cat} (see text). (*Circled X*) k_3, value for the desphosphorylation rate of E-P determined as described in the text. (*Open square*) P$_i$ (moles per mole of active site) dissociating from the Zn$_4$Mg$_2^-$ and Cd$_6$ alkaline phosphatase; at acid pH, both enzymes bind 2 mol of phosphate per mole of dimer. (*b*) (I) K_m for hydrolysis of ROPO$_4^{2-}$. (*Solid circle*) K_i for inhibition of ROPO$_4^{2-}$ hydrolysis by phosphate. K_s represents equilibrium constants for ^{32}P$_i$ binding to AP as determined by equilibrium dialysis for the Zn (*solid sqaure*), Cd (*open circle*) and Co (*open triangle*) enzymes. (*Open circle*) k_4, dissociation rate of phosphate from E·P as determined using ^{31}P NMR in version transfer.

phoseryl residue (E-P), are difficult to obtain. The relatively few values in the literature are those calculated in order to fit reaction profiles observed in rapid flow kinetics. Because $k_{-3}/k_3 = $ E-P/E·P, many reasonably accurate values of this ratio are available. Estimates of k_3 vs pH taken from kinetic analyses of the alkaline phosphatase reaction are plotted in Figure 2a. Because most rapid-flow kinetics studied prior to 1973 were distorted by the presence of contaminating inorganic phosphate bound to the enzyme (8), some modification of the estimates of the magnitude of k_3 are required, especially at alkaline pH. One can determine a lower limit for k_3 from the dead time of the stopped-flow instrument because an instantaneous burst of ~ 1 mol of RO$^-$ per mole of active site is observed at alkaline pH for the phosphate-free enzyme and because this burst results from the slow, 35 s^{-1}, rate-limiting dissociation of E·P. Therefore, as noted above, k_3 must be $\geqslant 300$ s^{-1} at pH 8.0; the scale for k_3 in Figure 2a has been adjusted to reflect this.

The equilibrium concentration of E-P (1.0 represents maximum possible formation of phosphoserine) for the Zn, Co, and Cd enzymes has been plotted from data obtained by ^{32}P labeling of the enzyme by incubation with $H^{32}PO_4^{2-} \rightleftharpoons H_2{}^{32}PO_4^-$, followed by manual quenching (3, 65). The curve marked "calculated" is the equilibrium concentration of E-P formed as a function of pH predicted by Wilson and his colleagues from the kinetic constants for the $E\text{-}P \rightleftharpoons E\cdot P \rightleftharpoons E + P_i$ reaction as assembled from the extensive kinetic data (52). These investigators suggested that the reason the predicted curve is steeper than the observed values obtained from several laboratories using ^{32}P labeling is the difficulty of quenching the enzyme rapidly enough to trap all the phosphoserine.

The $E\text{-}P \rightleftharpoons E\cdot P$ equilibrium vs pH also has been determined using ^{31}P NMR to avoid perturbing the equilibrium by the method of detection. The ^{31}P NMR of the enzyme-bound phosphate can quantitate these two intermediates from pH 10 to 5. Between pH 7 and 10, no detectable E-P is present at equilibrium. Between pH 7 and 5, the ratio of E-P/E·P rises along a sigmoid curve and reaches a value of 1 at pH 5. Below pH 5, the zinc enzyme is unstable. Because the ratio is determined accurately by ^{31}P NMR at close intervals over half the pH function, one can extrapolate a sigmoid function for the E-P/E·P ratio with a midpoint at pH 5 as shown in Figure 2a. Values of k_4 for dissociation of P_i remain relatively constant from pH 5.7 to 8.8 as determined using ^{31}P NMR inversion transfer (Figure 2b) (Table 2) (38). Values of the equilibrium constant for phosphate binding, K_s, as determined by equilibrium dialysis using $H^{32}PO_4^{2-}$ are shown for pH 6 and pH 8.8, the latter for the Zn, Co, and Cd enzymes (3). For the Zn enzyme, K_i values for phosphate kinetically determined by Wilson's laboratory are shown for pH values of 5.5, 6.0, 7.0, and 8.0 (52).

Table 2 Dissociation rates of the product, inorganic phosphate, from the active site of alkaline phosphatase as a function of the metal ion composition of the enzyme[a]

Enzyme	k_{off} (s^{-1})
$Zn(II)_4AP$ (pH 8.8)	35
$Zn(II)_4AP$ (pH 5.7)	33
$Zn(II)_4AP + 1.0$ M Cl^- (pH 8.0)	60–260[b]
$[Zn(II)_A Mg(II)_B]_2AP$ (pH 8.0)	≈ 1
$[Zn(II)_A Mg(II)_B]_2AP + 0.1$ M Cl^- (pH 9.0)	1.8
$[Zn(II)_A Mg(II)_B]_2AP + 1$ M Cl^- (pH 9.0)	≈ 15
$[Zn(II)_A Cd(II)_B]_2AP$ (pH 9.0)	≈ 2
$Cd(II)_6AP$ (pH 9.0)	< 1
$Cd(II)_6AP + 1$ M Cl^- (pH 9.0)	≈ 10

[a] All samples were in 0.01 M Tris-acetate (38).
[b] Too fast to measure directly by ^{31}P NMR inversion transfer; limits given are based on the inversion transfer measurement at 162 MHz.

The value of k_3, the dephosphorylation rate of E-P, falls rapidly from pH 8.0 ($\geqslant 300$ s^{-1}) to pH 6.3 (~ 1.3 s^{-1}), over the same pH range in which k_{cat} falls by $\sim 90\%$ (Figure 2a). Thus, the pH-rate profile (from alkaline to acid pH) is coincident with a change in the rate-limiting step from phosphate dissociation to dephosphorylation of the phosphoserine. At pH 8, k_3 exceeds the rate of dissociation of the product phosphate, k_4, by ~ 10-fold. At pH 6.3, however, the relationship is reversed; k_4 is 26-fold faster than k_3 and is no longer rate limiting. On the other hand, k_3 is not yet as slow as k_{-3}, the rate of phosphorylation of Ser102 from E·P, and thus significant equilibrium concentrations of E-P are not observed at pH 6.3. At pH 5, k_3 has decreased further such that $k_3 = k_{-3}$ and [E-P] = [E·P] at equilibrium (Figure 2a). Judging by ^{18}O exchange experiments, both constants must be on the order of 0.1 s^{-1}. The possible identity of the $AH \rightleftharpoons A^- + H^+$ equilibria governing k_3 and the pH-rate profile are discussed in the section on structure and mechanism.

Phosphate is both a substrate and competitive inhibitor of the enzyme. Phosphate binding appears to be essentially pH independent between pH 5.5 and 8.0 if the values for K_i and K_s are taken as a guide (Figure 2b) (3, 52, 63). In support of this conclusion is the fact that the dissociation rate of inorganic phosphate from the enzyme, k_4, is also pH independent from pH 5.5 to 8.8 (38). A pH independence of phosphate binding to alkaline phosphatase is surprising because two proton dissociations of phosphoric acid may fall in the pH range 5 to 10, $H_2PO_4^- \rightleftharpoons HPO_4^{2-} + H^+$ (pK$_a$ = 6.8) and $HPO_4^{2-} \rightleftharpoons PO_4^{3-} + H^+$ (normal pK$_a \approx 12$). The latter could affect the

AP-phosphate equilibrium if $E \cdot P$ forces formation of the trianion as some reasoning suggests (see below). An enzyme active center, which excludes all but specific water molecules, may limit proton access from the bulk solvent as well. Even in the apophosphoryl enzyme, which is formed by removing Cd from the E-P form of the enzyme, the ^{31}P chemical shift shows that the dianion form of the phosphoseryl group is not titrated to become the monoanion until below pH 4.0 after the enzyme unfolds (34).

At variance with the kinetic constants that suggest that phosphate binding is pH independent is the observation, made using ^{31}P NMR, that while Zn_4AP remains saturated with phosphate to pH 7.0, above pH 7.0 bound phosphate significantly decreases such that $[E \cdot P] = [P_i]$ at pH 10 (Figure 2a) when enzyme is 2 mM and phosphate 4 mM (33). The latter finding appears paradoxical, since the measurement of k_4 by NMR inversion transfer shows that the dissociation rate remains constant at ~ 35 s^{-1} under the same conditions and over the same pH range (Figure 2b). While one could postulate that the "on" constant for phosphate binding changes at high pH, this seems unlikely. If a water molecule on Zn_A becomes $Zn-^-OH$ at alkaline pH, phosphate binding will compete with hydroxide binding to Zn_A. In support of this postulate is the observation that phosphate does not begin to dissociate from the cadmium enzyme until well above pH 9.0 (Figure 2a) (33). However, if both bound phosphates on the enzyme were competing equally with ^-OH, then k_4 should increase as it does in the case of Cl^- competition (Table 2). One possible explanation of this paradox is negative cooperativity of phosphate binding, i.e. phosphate at one active site is bound less tightly than at the other at pH values above 7.0. Then most of the remaining $E \cdot P$ will be at the tight binding site and the inversion transfer will be weighted in favor of this site.

Negative cooperativity has not been discussed thus far in this review. The phenomenon formed a significant part of earlier discussions of the alkaline phosphatase reaction because many early experiments measuring $H^{32}PO_4^{2-}$ binding or burst magnitude showed that only a single bound phosphate per dimer or a single active site was phosphorylated. When sample-preparation techniques were changed such that samples with a full complement of metal ions were prepared, two E-P or two $E \cdot P$ complexes per dimer were easily formed under most conditions, especially at pH values below 7. Note that the Cd_6AP retains 1 mol of E-P per active site or 2 mol/dimer until the pH rises above 7.0 (Figure 2a). From pH 7 to 9, the sum of $E-P + E \cdot P$ also remains 2/dimer for the Cd_6 enzyme (32). Likewise, when enzymes uncontaminated with phosphate were employed in rapid-flow experiments, most burst stoichiometries approached 2/dimer (8).

Before we discard negative cooperativity in alkaline phosphatase as an artifact, however, I must point out that in the alkaline pH range several sensitive NMR techniques can detect unequal binding constants for the two enzyme-bound phosphates. Detailed ^{31}P NMR titrations of the Zn_4AP and the Cd_6AP with P_i show that at pH 6 both enzymes titrate linearly the formation of 2 mol of enzyme-bound phosphate per mole of dimer. The Cd_6AP does the same at pH 8, but the Zn_4AP titrates the formation of only 1 mol of $E \cdot P$ under the NMR conditions employed (33). The same phenomenon is apparent when phosphate binding to the enzyme is evidenced by ^{35}Cl line broadening resulting from the binding of two $^{35}Cl^-$ ions to each Zn_A. At pH 6, the phosphate ions displace one chloride from each Zn_A site, i.e. half the Cl^-. In contrast, at pH 8 one phosphate displaces only one quarter of this Cl^- in a stoichiometric fashion; displacement of the other quarter requires up to six phosphates per dimer (37). Thus, inequivalent phosphate binding affinities may be involved in product release.

The rate-limiting phosphate product dissociation accounts for burst kinetics observed at alkaline pH by stopped-flow methods when a phosphate-free enzyme is employed (5, 20). Because the enzyme does not appear to recognize the R group of a phosphomonoester, researchers have often assumed that phosphate ester binding affinity was similar to that of phosphate. Indeed, the best measurement of K_m values have been $\sim 10^{-6}$ M for $ROPO_3^{2-}$, although they increase to almost 10^{-4} M for an O-phosphorothioate, $ROPSO_2^{2-}$ (19, 58). When an acceptor alcohol is present, the rate of the phosphotransferase activity is always additive to that of the initial phosphohydrolase as has been confirmed using accurate ^{31}P-NMR measurement techniques (38). Because the dissociation of P_i is rate limiting for the hydrolysis reaction under these conditions, the dissociation of the new product ester in the transferase reaction is clearly considerably more rapid than phosphate dissociation. K_m varies as a function of the metal-ion species, Zn or Co, at the active center (19), but the K_i for phosphate is rather similar for the Zn, Co, and Cd enzymes [$(0.75 \pm 0.25) \times 10^{-6}$ M] (3). If the dissociation rate constant for $ROPO_3^{2-}$ were ~ 35 s^{-1} as it is for phosphate, then K_m would not represent k_{-1}/k_1, since the phosphorylation rate at pH 8 is at least 10^2 s^{-1} and probably even faster.

In comparing the kinetic pattern observed for phosphate esters as substrates and the information derived from using phosphate as substrate to form E-P, one should keep in mind that phosphorylation of the enzyme by $HOPO_3^{2-}$ has become rate-limiting, as concluded from the fact that the ^{18}O exchange rate, 0.1 to 0.2 s^{-1}, is slower than the dephosphorylation of E-P over most of the pH range and is always slower than the dissociation of P_i. The ^{18}O exchange reaction is pH independent, evidence that the apparent pK_a reflected in the normal pH-rate profile is that of a group

primarily affecting a step following formation of the phosphoseryl intermediate (see below). This pH independence, presumably controlled by a
slow phosphorylation, is confirmed by the hydrolysis of thiophosphate,
which releases H_2S (19). The rate of release of H_2S from thiophosphate is
the same at pH 5.5 and 8.0 and is only slightly more rapid than the rate
of ^{18}O exchange into phosphate catalyzed by the enyzme (Table 1).

The above background is useful in considerations of the nature of the
transition state in the alkaline phosphatase mechanism and whether the
reaction is primarily associative via the initial attack of the Ser-O$^-$ on
the phosphorous or whether the enzyme mechanism involves significant
dissociative features via activation of the leaving group as in non-enzyme-
catalyzed phosphomonoester hydrolysis (6, 49, 78). Recent investigations
have probed this question and confirmed that k_{cat}/K_m values for a variety
of substrates as functions of the pK_a of the leaving group show β values
of ~ 0.1 rather than the value of ~ 1 expected for a dissociative reaction
(51, 78). Although these newer findings and earlier, less rigorous kinetics
have been interpreted to mean that the enzyme mechanism is purely nucleophilic in character, forming a five-coordinate intermediate, the high resolution crystal structure of E·P reveals interesting structural arrangements
of metal and phosphate that bear on this view of the mechanism, as
discussed in the next section of this perspective.

Using the phosphotransferase reaction to capture as a second chiral
phosphate ester the phosphate from E-P initially formed by a chiral phosphomonoester containing ^{16}O, ^{17}O, and ^{18}O, Jones et al (46) demonstrated
that the alkaline phosphatase reaction proceeds with retention of configuration around phosphorus. This result suggested that the reaction path
consists of two in-line nucleophilic attacks; the first by the Ser-OH (or Ser-
O$^-$) and the second by solvent H_2O (or ^-OH).

THE METALLOENZYME NATURE OF ALKALINE PHOSPHATASE

The original analytical data reporting that alkaline phosphatase was a Zn
metalloenzyme showed two Zn ions per dimer (62). Subsequent determinations of the zinc content by the original laboratory and other investigators showed that with different preparation techniques the Zn:protein
dimer ratio was generally 4 and under some circumstances could reach 6
(1, 10, 25, 60). Numerous studies contribute to these conclusions; it is now
certain that a fully active native alkaline phosphatase contains four Zn
and two Mg ions, the Zn occupying sites designated A and B, while Mg
occupies sites designated as C. The A, B, and C sites were first unequivocally demonstrated using ^{113}Cd NMR. The $^{113}Cd_6$ enzyme shows three

454   COLEMAN

NMR signals at 153, 70, and 0 ppm relative to $Cd(ClO_4)_2$, each of which integrates into two Cd ions per dimer (Figure 3) (32, 35). Solution studies suggested that two sites, believed to be the A and B sites as defined from the ^{113}Cd NMR (Figure 3), were filled by Zn in the native protein (1, 10, 25). The crystal structure of the native zinc enzyme confirms the occupancy of sites A and B by Zn and of site C by Mg (48). The signal at 153 ppm is sensitive to conditions resulting from the exposure of this site to the addition of ligands from solution, H_2O, or anions. Thus, the chemical shift, δ, has been observed to vary from 150 to 170 ppm (see below).

Based on what is now known of ^{113}Cd NMR chemical shifts as a function of ligand donor atoms, the shift of 153 ppm, assigned to A-site ^{113}Cd, is compatible with a site containing two His N atoms serving as donors with oxygen atoms as the remaining donors (see crystal structure below). The ^{113}Cd NMR signal at 70 ppm is compatible with assignment to the B site containing one His N, where the rest of the donors are oxygen; while the ^{113}Cd chemical shift of 0 ppm is expected from a site such as the C site, which is composed of all oxygen donors. The variable metal stoichiometry displayed by alkaline phosphatase preparations is readily accounted for because the ammonium sulfate used in practically all preparative pro-

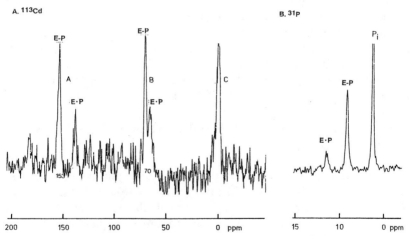

Figure 3 ^{113}Cd NMR (*A*) and ^{31}P NMR (*B*) of $^{113}Cd_6AP$ (3 mM) in 0.01 M Tris HCl, pH 8.3, containing 2 mol of bound phosphate in the presence of equimolar free P_i (^{31}P $\delta = 3$ ppm). At pH 8.0, $\sim 80\%$ of the enzyme is present as E-P (^{31}P $\delta = 8.7$ ppm), and $\sim 20\%$ is present as E·P (^{31}P $\delta = 13.0$ ppm). The ^{113}Cd signals at 153 and 70 ppm reflect the ^{113}Cd ions in sites A and B for an enzyme in the E-P form, while the small peaks, 20 and 8 ppm upfield respectively, are the signals from the A- and B-site ^{113}Cd of an enzyme in the E·P form. Data are from Ref. 32.

cedures can easily remove Zn from the B site as well as from the A site at high pH. In fact, the best way to prepare the apoenzyme is to dialyze the enzyme at pH 9 against buffered 2 M ammonium sulfate (33).

The relationship between occupancy of the three metal-ion binding sites, A, B, and C, on each monomer and phosphatase activity was not an easy one to define, but required enzymes with known metal:protein stoichiometry as well as knowledge of which sites were occupied (33, 34, 38). Mixed-site occupancy occurs easily when metal ions are present at less than full stoichiometry. While a $(Zn_A Zn_B Mg_C)_2$ enzyme has maximal activity, an enzyme containing only two Zn ions, one at each A site, is not inactive. Such a two-Zn enzyme binds phosphate and catalyzes phosphorylation of Ser102 (2). In fact, if Mg occupies both the B and C sites, the activity of the $(Zn_A Mg_B Mg_C)_2$AP is near normal in the phosphotransferase reaction (Table 3) (21). In contrast, the normal hydrolysis reaction is much depressed in the $(Zn_A Mg_B Mg_C)_2$AP (Table 3) (21, 38). Because standard

Table 3   Effect of metal-ion species on the E-P $\rightleftharpoons$ E·P equilibrium at the active center of alkaline phosphatase (AP) and the k_{cat} values

Metal site occupancy at active center	k_{cat} s^{-1}	pH at which [E-P] = [E·P][a]	^{31}P chemical shift, ppm	
			E-P	E·P
$[Zn(II)_A Zn(II)_B]_2$AP	35	5.0	8.6	4.3
$[Zn(II)_A Zn(II)_B Mg(II)_C]_2$AP	35	5.0	8.6	3.4
$[Zn(II)_A Mg(II)_B]_2$AP (0.01 M Tris)	1	4.0	8.5	1.8
$[Zn(II)_A Mg(II)_B]_2$AP (1 M Tris)	30	—	—	—
$[Zn(II)_A Cd(II)_B]_2$AP	2	6	8.0	12.6
$[Cd(II)_A Cd(II)_B]_2$AP	0.001[b]	10	8.4	13.4
$[Cd(II)_A Cd(II)_B Cd(II)_C]_2$AP	<0.1[c]	8.7	8.7	13.0
$[Cd(II)_A Zn(II)_B]_2$AP (unstable)	—	7	9.3	
ApoPhosphorylAP	—	—	5.8	
$[Co(II)_A Co(II)_B]_2$AP	2	≈5[d]	ND[e]	
$[Mn(II)_A Mn(II)_B]_2$AP	0.2[c]	≈6.5[d]	ND	

[a] These values were determined from ^{31}P-NMR of the enzyme vs pH unless otherwise indicated.

[b] This is the rate of phosphorylation from E·P taken from the NMR experiment shown in Figure 7. Since the major intermediate accumulating at pH 8 is E-P, dephosphorylation of E-P, k_3, cannot be faster. Thus the turnover, k_{cat}, cannot be faster than 0.001 s^{-1}.

[c] The lower limit for turnover determined by the standard colorimetric assay; i.e. it represents the background from zinc contamination of the best apoenzyme preparations assayed in metal-free buffers and substrates. The value 0.2 s^{-1} is readily detected above the apoenzyme background under metal-free assay conditions (64).

[d] Taken from ^{32}P labeling data (3).

[e] Not detected due to line broadening by the paramagnetic metal ions. Data are from Ref. 16 and 66. Assays were at pH 8, 0.01 M Tris unless otherwise stated.

assays employ 1 M Tris buffer, this difference is not routinely detected. Surprisingly, a large activation of the hydrolysis + transferase reaction by Mg is only observed for the two-Zn species; Mg occupancy of the C site in a 4-Zn enzyme, $(Zn_A Zn_{B-C})_2 AP$, enhances total activity relatively little if at all. In all the studies of *E. coli* alkaline phosphatases of defined metal-ion stoichiometry, detecting significant effects of the C-site metal ion on structure or function has proved difficult. This statement may not apply to the mammalian enzymes, which undergo much more dramatic activation by Mg even when maximum Zn ions are present (22).

The above brief introduction to the properties of alkaline phosphatase is intended only to set the background for the main purpose of this perspective, which is an attempt to synthesize the findings of the recent 2.0-Å crystal structure of the enzyme and its two phosphoenzyme intermediates with the extensive solution data bearing on the catalytic mechanism of alkaline phosphatase. The resultant synthesis gives the clearest picture yet of the active center and the intermediates on the reaction path of alkaline phosphatase. For detailed descriptions of the earlier kinetic, spectroscopic, and other physicochemical studies of the enzyme, earlier reviews should be consulted (23, 34, 63).

COORDINATION CHEMISTRY AT THE ACTIVE CENTER OF ALKALINE PHOSPHATASE

The coordination chemistry at the active center of alkaline phosphatase is best presented by a detailed description of the structure around each of the three metal ions at the active center of the native enzyme that has the metal composition $Zn_A Zn_B Mg_C$. Multinuclear NMR investigations of the enzyme done in the past have used the designations A, B, and C for the three sites; the crystal structure uses the designations 1, 2, and 3. Figure 4a presents the general structure of the active center by a stereo view of the immediate region of the active center including the three metals (48). Figure 4b shows a computer-graphics representation of the E · P complex of the native $Zn_4 Mg_2$ enzyme that includes the metal-ligand bonds, the slowly exchanging water molecules, the hydrogen bonds, and the amino acid side chains located within the immediate region of the active center (48). Both representations are taken from the structure of the E · P complex, i.e. with phosphate bound noncovalently at the active center by soaking crystals of the $(Zn1Zn2Mg3)_2 AP$ in phosphate at neutral pH. This structure has been determined at 2-Å resolution and all information suggests it should represent the authentic E · P intermediate. The three metal ions form a cluster in which the metal-to-metal distances trace a triangle of $3.94 \times 4.88 \times 7.09$ Å. Table 4 lists the metal-metal distances, the ligands

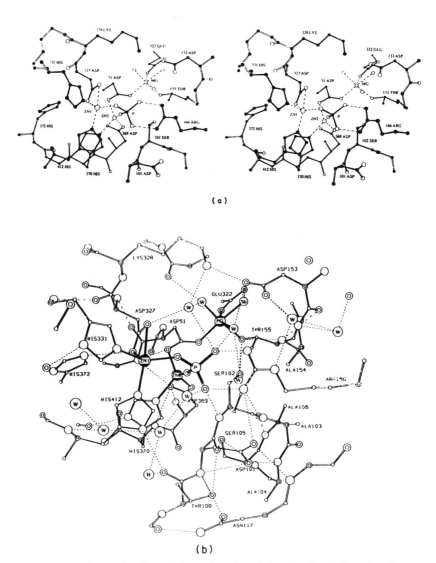

Figure 4 (*a*) Stereo drawing of the active site of the *E. coli* alkaline phosphatase, $(Zn1Zn2Mg3)_2AP$ plus 2 mM HPO_4^{2-}, pH 7.5. Atoms are shaded by atom type. Some residues and water molecules are omitted for clarity. (*b*) The active-site region of the E·P complex (2-Å resolution) including all the atoms within 10 Å of the phosphorus atom. Water molecules are labeled *W*. Hydrogen bonds are shown as broken lines.

Table 4 Summary of the metal-metal and metal-ligand distances (Å) for the dimer of $(Zn1,Zn2,Mg3)_2$alkaline phosphatase[a]

Metal to metal	Atom	Distances (Å)	
		Subunit A	Subunit B
Zn1–Zn2		3.94	4.81
Zn2–Mg		4.88	4.66
Zn1–Mg		7.09	7.03
Metal-ligand			
	Zn1 coordination		
Asp327	OD1	2.00	2.26
	OD2	2.30	2.53
His331	ND1	1.96	2.07
His412	NE2	2.04	2.04
PO_4	O1	1.97	2.12
	Zn2 coordination		
Asp51	OD1	2.13	2.03
Asp369	OD1	1.79	1.80
His370	ND1	2.05	2.01
PO_4	O2	1.97	2.23
	Mg coordination		
Asp51	OD2	2.07	1.96
Thr155	OG1	2.15	2.05
Glu322	OE1	2.26	1.93
Water	O	2.03	1.92
Water	O	1.90	2.00
Water	O	2.32	2.03

[a] The data are taken from Ref. 48.

for each site, and the metal-ligand bond lengths. These distances vary slightly, as observed in the separate monomers, A and B, related by the two-fold axis of the dimer, but the significance of these differences is not clear at present.

The active center is located at the carboxyl end of the central β-sheet, and one monomer provides all the ligands to the three metal ions. The electron-density map of $E \cdot P$ is well defined except for the disordered hydroxyl group of Ser102 (see below). Despite the close packing of the metal centers, there is only one bridging ligand, the carboxyl of Asp51, which bridges between Zn2 and Mg3 or Cd2 and Cd3 in the Cd_6 enzyme. Figure 5 diagrams the coordination around Zn1, Zn2, and Mg3 as it exists in the $E \cdot P$ complex.

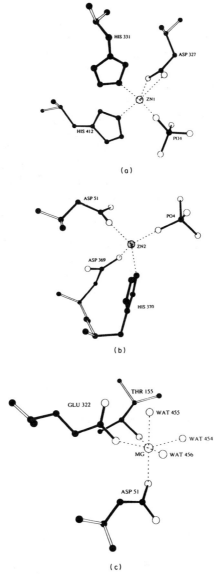

Figure 5 Coordination spheres of the three metals in the E · P complex of $(Zn1Zn2Mg3)_2AP$: (*a*) Zn1, (*b*) Zn2, and (*c*) Mg. Conditions as in Figure 4. The figure is reproduced from Ref. 48.

Zn1 (A) Coordination

The A site or Zn1, which upon substitution with first-transition metal ions shows spectroscopic properties of a typical Zn(II) metalloenzyme (2, 34), has four ligands from the protein, which include both carboxyl oxygens of Asp327, the N3 of His331, and the N3 of His412. In the absence of HPO_4^{2-}, water relaxation data (64) and $^{35}Cl^-$ NMR data (37) suggest that the coordination sphere of the A site is completed by two H_2O molecules. In the E·P complex, one of the phosphate oxygens forms a typical co-ordinate bond with Zn1, with a Zn1-O bond length of 1.97 Å and a Zn-O-P bond angle of 120° (Figure 5a). Water-relaxation data using the Mn enzyme show that one of the water molecules coordinated to the A-site metal is displaced by phosphate (64). ^{35}Cl NMR reveals a similar displacement of a monodentate ligand at A-site, i.e. Cl^-, by phosphate binding to the Zn enzyme (37). The Zn1 coordination in E·P can best be described as pseudotetrahedral, where both carboxyl oxygens of Asp327 occupy one of the apices. His372, which was originally thought to co-ordinate Zn1, is not a direct ligand; it is 3.8 Å away from Zn1, and the N3 of the imidazole ring forms a hydrogen bond with one of the coordinated carboxyl oxygens of Asp327 (Figure 4b).

Zn2 (B) Coordination

In the E·P complex, Zn2 is coordinated tetrahedrally by the N3 of His370, one of the carboxyl oxygens of the bridging Asp51, and one of the carboxyl oxygens of Asp369 (Figure 5b). The tetrahedral coordination is completed by one of the phosphate oxygens. While the Zn2-O bond length is 1.97 Å, identical to that for the Zn1-O bond, the Zn2-O-P bond angle is nearly linear (175°). The OH of Ser102 is disordered in the E·P complex but appears to form a coordinate bond with Zn2 in the phosphate-free enzyme (see below).

Mg3 (C) Coordination

The Mg site can be described best as a slightly distorted octahedron consisting of the second carboxyl oxygen of the bridging Asp51, one of the carboxyl oxygens of Glu322, and the hydroxyl of Thr155, while the rest of the coordination sites are filled by three slowly exchanging water molecules (numbered 454 to 456) (Figure 5c). Asp153 is not a direct ligand as orginally believed (68, 80), but is an indirect ligand in that the carboxyl group forms hydrogen bonds with two coordinated water molecules (454 and 455) that are the direct ligands to Mg (Figure 4b). The Mg site does not appear close enough to participate directly in the hydrolysis mechanism, but could of course contribute to the shape of the electrostatic potential around the active center (see below).

Enzyme-Bound Phosphate in the E·P Intermediate

Because the relationship between the amino acid side chains and the phosphate in the E·P intermediate forms the basis for the initial discussion of the relationship of the crystal structure to solution studies of the mechanism, additional details of the structure are outlined here. In addition to oxygen-metal bonds to Zn1 and Zn2 made by two of the oxygen atoms of phosphate, the other two phosphate oxygens in E·P hydrogen bond to the guanidinium group of Arg166 (Figure 4a). Figure 6a shows the electron density map on which this structure is based. The guanidinium group is involved in an additional hydrogen-bond network that includes hydrogen bonds to Asp101 and a water molecule (Wat459), the latter held by Asp153 and possibly also by Tyr169. Of the two phosphate oxygens involved with the guanidino group, one is further hydrogen bonded to the amide of Ser102, and the second seems to be involved with two of the slowly exchanging water molecules. One of these molecules (Wat454) is coordinated to Mg, while the second (Wat457) forms a bridge between the phosphate oxygen and Lys328 (Figure 4b). Zn1, O1, P, O2, and Zn2 are nearly coplanar.

Enzyme-Bound Phosphate in the E-P Intermediate

As shown in Figure 2, the substitution of Cd for Zn shifts the pH stability of the covalent phosphoryl enzyme well into the alkaline pH range. Ser102 of the Cd_6 enzyme remains 90% phosphorylated at pH 7.5; hence, crystals of the Cd_6 enzyme when soaked in phosphate can be used to determine a structure of the E-P intermediate. The electron density map at 2.5-Å resolution of the E-P intermediate formed by Cd_6AP is shown in Figure 6b and should be compared to the electron density map of the E·P complex of the Zn_4Mg_2 enzyme at 2-Å resolution shown in Figure 6a. An ester bond between the phosphate and the hydroxyl of Ser102 is clearly present. Cd2 also appears to form a coordinate bond with the ester oxygen. The phosphate group has moved slightly deeper into the active-center cavity, and whether an oxygen of the phosphate remains close enough to Cd1 to retain a coordinate bond is difficult to determine from the electron density alone (see discussion of mechanism below). The two hydrogen bonds between phosphate oxygens and the guanidino group of Arg166 are maintained in the E-P complex.

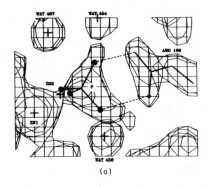

(a)

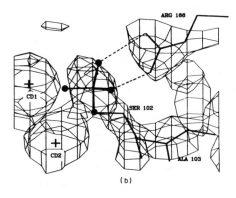

(b)

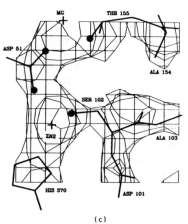

(c)

Figure 6 (a) $2F_o\text{-}F_c$ electron-density map of the active-site region of $(\text{Zn1Zn2Mg2})_2\text{AP}$ as the E·P phosphoenzyme intermediate. (b) Electron-density map of Cd_6AP plus 2 mM HPO_4^{2-}, pH 7.5; atoms within 8.0 Å of Ser102 are omitted from the structure factor and phase calculations. The final refined model is superimposed on the density map. (c) Electron-density map of $(\text{Zn1Zn2Mg3})_2\text{AP}$, pH 7.5, in the absence of phosphate; atoms within 8.0 Å of Ser102 are omitted in the calculation of the structure factor and phases. The final refined model is superimposed on the density map. The figure is reproduced from Ref. 48.

CHANGES IN ACTIVITY OF ALKALINE PHOSPHATASE ON SUBSITUTING CADMIUM, COBALT, OR MANGANESE FOR THE NATIVE ZINC ION

The substitution of the native Zn ions in sites A(1) and B(2) with other first transition or IIB metal ions significantly changes k_{cat} as well as the rate constants for individual steps. While the structural reasons for all these changes are not immediately obvious, the results have been helpful in understanding specific aspects of the mechanism.

The most dramatic change is the fall in k_{cat} upon Cd substitution from ~ 35 s^{-1} to a rate impossible to detect using standard assay techniques. Both ^{32}P labeling at low pH and NMR detection of E-P and E·P, however, show that the Cd enzyme forms both of these phosphoenzyme intermediates. Inversion transfer from ^{31}P$_i$ to the E·^{31}P complex on the Cd$_6$ enzyme show that k_4, the dissociation of the product phosphate, has slowed to less than 1 s^{-1} as a result of the Cd substitution (Table 2). The dissociation of phosphate, however, is no longer the rate-limiting step for the Cd enzyme. By following the formation of E-P via observation of its ^{31}P NMR resonance, the phosphorylation rate of the cadmium enzyme from HOPO$_3^{2-}$, k_{-3}, is $\sim 10^{-3}$ s^{-1} at pH 9.0 (see Figure 7 below). Over much of the pH range, however, k_3, the dephosphorylation of E-P, must be even slower because the major equilibrium species of intermediate is E-P until the pH is above 9 (Figure 2a). One of the possible explanations for the latter remarkable fall in k_3 is that the solvent nucleophile required for the dephosphorylation step is coordinated to the A-site metal, and its pK$_a$ has been shifted far to alkaline pH by the Cd substitution. Although the NMR studies show the Cd enzyme following all the steps of the native enzyme, it is essentially an enzyme in slow motion.

Substitution of Co, on the other hand, causes far less drastic changes. While k_{cat} falls significantly, 2–10 s^{-1} depending on preparation (Table 3) (19), the pH-rate profile for V_{max} remains nearly the same as that for the zinc enzyme, with an apparent pK$_a$ of ~ 7.5 (19). Compatible with this finding is the observation that significant equilibrium concentrations of E-^{32}P form only below pH 7. The acid instability of the Co enzyme prevents determination of the complete pH dependence of the E-P/E·P ratio (3). The Co substitution, however, is accompanied by a dramatic switch in the relative magnitudes of phosphate dissociation, k_4, vs the rephosphorylation rate of Ser102 from E·P, k_{-3}. ^{31}P NMR can be used to accurately measure the exchange of ^{18}O out of HP^{18}O$_4^{2-}$ as catalyzed by alkaline phosphatase, since an isotope shift in the ^{31}P signal is induced proportional to the number of ^{18}O oxygens in the phosphate (9). The exchange catalyzed by the native

Zn(II) enzyme is compatible with a kinetic scheme in which E·P dissociates at least 10 times more rapidly than E-P is reformed, in agreement with the rate constants given above, i.e. $k_4 = \sim 35$ s^{-1} (Table 2), while the rephosphorylation rate, k_{-3}, is ~ 0.2 s^{-1} for Zn. On the other hand, Co(II) catalyzes the exchange of approximately three phosphate oxygens per turnover, showing that several rephosphorylations of the Ser102 occur before E·P can dissociate. The multiple ^{18}O exchanges from E·P catalyzed by the Co enzyme allow the conclusion that E·P is a dynamic complex in which the phosphate oxygens interchange their positions on a reasonably fast time scale, probably between 10 and 100 times per second to accommodate both the ^{18}O exchange data and the k_{cat} observed for the Co enzyme. Although paramagnetic broadening of the bound phosphate by Co(II) prevents the measurement of k_4 for the Co enzyme by the accurate NMR methods, similar equilibrium dissociation constants measured for phosphate binding to the Co and Zn enzymes (3) suggest that the phosphate dissociation rates may be similar. Thus Co appears to catalyze phosphorylation of Ser102 from E·P more rapidly than Zn. While precise explanations of the above phenomena are not possible, even with the 2-Å map of the E·P complex, they do emphasize the close interactions between the phosphate and the metal ions.

Substitution of Mn for Zn produces an enzyme with far less activity, but one that is nevertheless detectable by the standard assays with p-nitrophenyl phosphate and estimated to be 0.2 s^{-1} (64). Although very low, the latter is significantly greater than the turnover number for the Cd enzyme. While the kinetics of the Mn enzyme have not been investigated in detail, part of the fall in k_{cat} must reflect a fall in k_3, the dephosphorylation rate of E-P, because significant equilibrium concentrations of E-P are formed by the Mn enzyme at pH 8 and above (3).

CONCLUSIONS ON STRUCTURE AND MECHANISM OF ALKALINE PHOSPHATASE DERIVED FROM MULTINUCLEAR NMR

Investigators used ^{113}Cd NMR of the ^{113}Cd$_6$AP to originally identify the presence of three separate metal-ion binding sites, A, B, and C, on each monomer of alkaline phosphatase (32). The chemical shifts of two of these sites, A and B, depend on which phosphoenzyme intermediate, E·P or E-P, is present (Figure 3), suggesting originally that both Cd$_A$ and Cd$_B$ were near the phosphate binding site as the structure now shows. ^{31}P NMR signals can be detected from both E·P and E-P intermediates and have been valuable probes of the mechanism. The ^{31}P NMR signal of E·P has provided the demonstration by saturation and inversion transfer that the dissociation of inorganic phosphate, $k_d \approx 35$ s^{-1}, is the slowest, and therefore the rate-limiting, step in the mechanism (38). The chemical shifts of the ^{31}P NMR resonances of the two alkaline phosphatase intermediates as well as the pH at which [E·P] = [E-P] for each metalloderivative of the enzyme are summarized in Table 3 and suggest several general conclusions.

For the native $(Zn_A Zn_B Mg_C)_2$ enzyme, E·P has a resonance at 4 ppm, while E-P resonates 8 ppm downfield of phosphoric acid. The chemical shift of the E-P signal is relatively insensitive to the substitution of the various metal-ion species at sites A or B. In marked contrast, the chemical shift of the E·P signal is highly sensitive to the nature of the metal ion in both sites, shifting from the most upfield position of 1.8 ppm in the $(Zn_A Mg_B Mg_C)_2$AP to 13 ppm in the $(Cd_A Cd_B Cd_C)_2$AP. This great sensitivity of the δ of E·P to the nature of the metal ion suggested that the phosphate of E·P was coordinated to one or both metal ions. In the case of the $(Cd_A Cd_B Cd_C)_2$AP, the phosphate of E·P appeared to be coordinated to only one of the active-center ^{113}Cd ions based on the observation that the ^{31}P signal for E·P is a doublet showing a single 30-Hz ^{31}P-^{113}Cd coupling (Figure 7a) (33). Heteronuclear decoupling shows that this coupling comes from the A-site ^{113}Cd, a conclusion supported by the disappearance of this coupling in the $(Zn_A Cd_B)_2$AP hybrid enzyme (Figure 7d) (36). Although the coupling disappears, upon Zn substitution for the A-site ^{113}Cd, the unusual downfield chemical shift of 12.6 ppm is maintained in a $(Zn_A Cd_B)_2$ hybrid (Table 3, Figure 7d), which leads to the unexpected conclusion that Cd in the B site rather than the A site induces the unusual downfield shift of the E·^{31}P signal. This observation became less surprising when the crystal structure of E·P showed that a second phosphate oxygen is as close to $Zn_B(2)$ as the more normally coordinated oxygen is to $Zn_A(1)$ (Figure 4b).

In contrast to the changes in chemical shift of the E·^{31}P signal, the resonance of the phosphoserine, E-^{31}P, remains between 8.6 and 8.4 ppm no matter what metal ions are in the A, B, and C sites (Table 3). Likewise, in heteronuclear-decoupling experiments, no change in the linewidth of the E-^{31}P singlet is observed on irradiation of either the ^{113}Cd$_A$ or ^{113}Cd$_B$ signals. These characteristics of the phosphorous nucleus in the E-P complex led to the suggestion that at least on the appropriate NMR time average, the phosphate of E-P is not coordinated to either A-site or B-site metal ions. However, if the $Cd_B(2)$ is coordinated to the ester oxygen as the electron density map suggests, a ^{113}Cd-O-^{31}P coupling may not be resolved. The structure in the immediate vicinity of the phosphoseryl-102 is significantly influenced by the metal ions, since removal of the Cd ions from the E-P form of the Cd_6 enzyme results in an apophosphoseryl

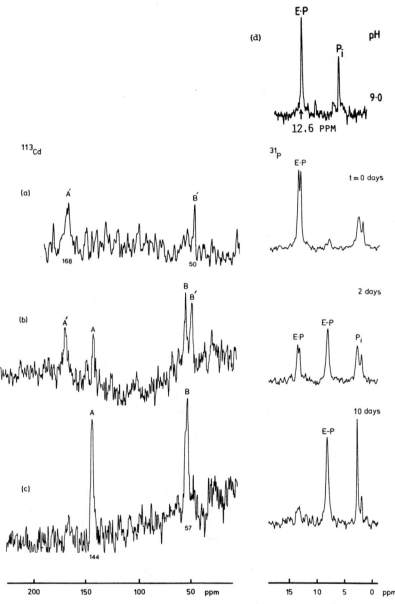

Figure 7 Time course of the slow phosphorylation of ($^{113}Cd_A{}^{113}Cd_{B-C})_2AP$ (2.76 mM) containing two equivalents of P_i at pH 9.0. The spectra on the right are ^{31}P NMR (80.9 MHz) and on the left are ^{113}Cd NMR (*a*, 44.3 MHz; *b,c*, 19.96 MHz). (*d*) ^{31}P spectrum of the phospho-$Zn(II)_ACd(II)_B$ alkaline phosphatase hybrid at pH 9.0. The data are from Ref. 32 and 36.

enzyme that has a ^{31}P chemical shift that moves upfield to 5.8 ppm from 8.7 ppm (Table 3).

The above NMR characterizations are graphically illustrated by both ^{113}Cd and ^{31}P NMR signals during the phosphorylation of (^{113}Cd$_A$ ^{113}Cd$_{B-C}$)$_2$AP by inorganic phosphate. The E·P species (^{31}P doublet at 13 ppm) forms rapidly (Figure 7a). This species slowly phosphorylates the enzyme over a period of days (Figures 7b,c). At two days, half of the enzyme has become E-P (^{31}P singlet at 8.7 ppm). Simultaneously, the ^{113}Cd signals have each split into two, reflecting the different values for Cd$_A$ and Cd$_B$ in the E·P and E-P forms of the enzyme, respectively. Perhaps reflecting the release of the coordinate bond between the phosphate and ^{113}Cd$_A$ in E·P, the shift of the ^{113}Cd signal from site A on formation of E-P is 20 ppm, while that from ^{113}Cd$_B$ is only 8 ppm (Figure 7b). The metal-ion species at site A largely determines the pH at which [E·P] = [E-P] or the pH at which $k_3 = k_{-3}$ (21, 24, 33). This pH shifts from 5 for Zn$_4$AP to 8.7 for Cd$_6$AP, while remaining at pH 6 for the (Zn$_A$Cd$_B$)$_2$AP hybrid (Table 3). Because k_{-3} appears to be pH independent, based on the ^{18}O exchange out of HP^{18}O$_4^{2-}$ catalyzed by the enzyme, this extreme change in the pH dependence of k_3 must relate to an effect of Cd$_A$ on the dephosphorylation of E-P.

Dephosphorylation of E-P is absolutely metal-ion dependent, and Cd is a "softer" metal than Zn and therefore is expected to affect lowering the pK$_a$ of a coordinated water less. If the nucleophile required for the dephosphorylation of E-P were a metal-hydroxide formed from a solvent H$_2$O coordinated to Zn$_A$, then k_3 would vary with the Zn·OH$_2 \rightleftharpoons$ Zn·$^-$OH + H$^+$ dissociation. The titration data in Figure 2 indicate that the pK$_a$ of a water coordinated to Zn$_A$ would have to be ~ 7.5 in order to match both the pH dependence of k_3 and the pH dependence of k_{cat}. Because below the pK$_a$ of the Zn·OH$_2$, the concentration of the Zn·$^-$OH nucleophile would continue to fall by 10-fold for each 1-unit further drop in pH, k_3 would fall as well. Thus, when the pH reaches a value where k_3 matches k_{-3}, E-P will build up along a sigmoid curve whose midpoint is the pH at which $k_3 = k_{-3}$ (Scheme 1). Because Cd$_A$ moves the pH at which $k_3 = k_{-3}$ toward the alkaline by ~ 3.7 pH units, the postulate of a metal$_A$-hydroxide as the nucleophile in the dephosphorylation of Ser102 requires that the pK$_a$ of the Cd·OH$_2 \rightleftharpoons$ Cd·$^-$OH + H$^+$ equilibrium be at least 3.7 pH units higher than that for the corresponding zinc equilibrium. How much above pH 8.7 the pK$_a$ of the Cd·OH$_2$ is depends on the value of k_{-3}, which we do not know for the Cd enzyme.

The nucleophile in both the hydration and esterase reactions catalyzed by carbonic anhydrase is a Zn-hydroxide at the active center of the enzyme, and the Zn·OH$_2 \rightleftharpoons$ Zn·$^-$OH + H$^+$ equilibrium is described by a pK$_a$ of

6.8 (71). The substitution of Cd for the native Zn ion shifts this pK_a to 9.3, and the apparent pK_a of the sigmoid pH profile of k_{cat} for esterase activity shifts from 6.8 to 9.3 (71). Thus, a shift in the pK_a of a coordinated solvent molecule has a precedent in another zinc metalloenzyme and is one of the few changes expected of a Cd substitution that could account for such a dramatic shift in the pH dependence of a rate constant for an enzyme reaction.

CORRELATION OF STRUCTURE AND MECHANISM

Michaelis Complex with a Phosphate Monoester

The electron density map of the active center in the absence of phosphate indicates a bond between the oxygen of Ser102 and Zn2 (Figure 6c), supporting the notion that one of the functions of Zn2(A) is to activate the Ser hydroxyl to Ser-O$^-$. However, the 2-Å map of the E·P complex from which nucleophilic attack of the Ser O$^-$ would occur shows that this coordination position is occupied by one of the phosphate oxygens, leaving the serine side chain free in the cavity (disordered). Nevertheless, some activation may be conferred by the positive charge density, and in the E·P complex, protons may not have access to the Ser-O$^-$. The structure of the E·P complex with the $(Zn_AZn_BMg_C)_2AP$ indicates that the four oxygens of the phosphate are each in contact with a positively charged center, one with Zn_A, two in a hydrogen bond network with the guanidino group of Arg166, and the fourth with Zn_B through the unusual P-O-Zn bond angle of almost 180° described earlier. Perhaps this unusual bond, rather than the lack of a bond, in the E·P complex of the cadmium enzyme accounts for the inability to observe detectable ^{113}Cd-^{31}P coupling to the ^{113}Cd at the B site.

The Zn1-O-P-O-Zn2 bridge and the two hydrogen bonds between the two other phosphate oxygens places the oxygen of Ser102 in the expected position for nucleophilic attack on the phosphorous nucleus, a position that would become one of the apical positions if a five-coordinate intermediate were formed. The oxygen coordinated to Zn1 would occupy the opposite apical position. These relationships are best seen in Figure 4a. If the E·P structure is extrapolated to that of E·ROP (with which E·P must share at least some features in common), then the oxygen coordinated to Zn_A must be the ester oxygen. None of the other positions would allow space for the attachment of an R group, which can range in size from CH_3 to a macromolecule. This observation suggests that in the normal hydrolysis reaction, Zn_A is an electrophile activating the leaving group, much as protonation of the ester oxygen does in the model systems. Thus, the alkaline phosphatase mechanism may have as significant a dissociative component provided by activation of the leaving group by Zn_A as it does an associative component provided by the attack of Ser102, the latter activated by the second Zn ion. An electrophilic activation by the Zn would explain why the β values for k_{cat}/K_m observed for substrates that cannot protonate the leaving group (phosphopyridines) do not differ significantly compared with those that can (oxyesters) (51); both β values are equally small (51). A dissociative character of the alkaline phosphatase reaction has been suggested by the low magnitude of secondary isotope effects when the nonbridging oxygens of the substrate are labeled with ^{18}O (77). This is compatible with the observation that an alkoxide, RO^-, appears to be the species coordinated to $Zn_A(1)$ in the phosphotransferase mechanism (38). Thus a Zn_A-coordinated alkoxide as the immediate leaving group in normal hydrolysis is entirely possible.

The Phosphoseryl Intermediate

As noted above, the very large alkaline shift in the pH at which [E-P] = [E·P], induced by Cd at the A site (Table 3), provides a means for visualizing the E-P complex in the crystal structure. A normal-appearing ester bond has formed with Ser102 and the phosphate is slightly deeper in the active center cavity than in the case of the E·P complex (Figure 6b). The electron-density map of the E-P complex shows that Cd2 forms a coordinate bond with the ester oxygen of the seryl phosphate (Figure 6b). The latter would suggest that the metal in site B(2) has the same function in the second half of the mechanism as the metal in site A(1) has in the first half, i.e. activation of the leaving group. The possibility of a phosphate oxygen remaining in contact with Cd1 in the E-P complex is not clear from the electron-density map (Figure 6b). Mechanistic considerations suggest that if the nucleophile in the final hydrolysis reaction is a solvent coordinated to metal A(1), then the coordination of an electron-donating group of the substrate to the same metal ion as the nucleophile would not facilitate this step.

Hydrolysis of the Phosphoseryl Intermediate

The crystal structure of the E-P complex indicates that a solvent molecule in position to be a nucleophile adding to the phosphate nucleus from the apical position opposite to that occupied by the seryl ester would clearly be placed in the vicinity of Zn(1). An obvious choice is to place the solvent as one coordinated to Zn1 in the approximate position originally occupied by the coordinated phosphate ester oxygen in the E·P complex (Figure 4). For the reasons described in the previous section, the ionization of a coordinated solvent molecule on metal A is the simplest explanation for the pH-rate profile and for the behavior of the pH-dependent $E\text{-}P \rightleftharpoons E \cdot P$ equilibrium upon the Cd for Zn substitution.

Dissociation of the Product, Inorganic Phosphate, the Rate-Limiting Step

As discussed above, at alkaline pH (8 to 9) where alkaline phosphatase is maximally active, dissociation of the product, P_i, is rate limiting for the native $(Zn_A Zn_B Mg_C)_2$ enzyme, as most easily demonstrated by NMR methods. For the native enzyme, the reported values for k_4 (Scheme 1) have ranged from 20 to 50 s^{-1} (19, 44). This value is approximately the range reported in the literature for k_{cat}, 13–70 s^{-1}, under a variety of conditions (19, 29, 41, 63). At acid pH, the rate-limiting step changes to dephosphorylation of the phosphoseryl intermediate, primarily because of a dramatic fall in the rate constant, k_3, for this reaction from $\geqslant 300$ s^{-1} (pH 8) to ~ 0.5 s^{-1} (pH 5.5) (19). This fall in k_3 is compatible with the notion that the nucleophile for this dephosphorylation is a Zn-hydroxide at the A site that becomes protonated in the acid form of the enzyme, thus markedly reducing the concentration of active nucleophile present (21).

As outlined in the earlier section on kinetics, both the rate of phosphate dissociation, k_4, and the rate of phosphorylation of Ser102 by $E \cdot P$, k_{-3}, depend on the species of metal ion present at both A and B sites. Both metal sites seem to be involved in the regulation of the phosphate dissociation because the rate for the $Zn_A Cd_B$ hybrid enzyme shows a less dramatic fall in k_4 to ~ 2 s^{-1}, compared with the $Cd_A Cd_B$ enzyme in which k_4 is < 1 s^{-1} (Table 2) (38). The structure of the $E \cdot P$ complex as revealed by the crystal structure does not directly suggest a reason for this metal-ion dependence of k_4. Because metal-phosphate bonds to both A- and B-site metal ions are required for phosphate binding, dissociation probably depends critically on the detailed charge distribution at the sites as well as on subtle aspects of the coordination geometry. The latter may be somewhat different for the larger Cd(II) ion, i.e. 0.97 Å compared with 0.74 Å for Zn(II). It is not clear, however, why the larger Cd(II) ion results in slower dissociation of phosphate.

Early kinetic studies called attention to the fact that an activation of alkaline phosphatase caused by increasing ionic strength should be distinguished from the "apparent" activation caused by the additive transferase activity (61). Because 1 M concentrations of Tris usually carry significant Cl$^-$ concentrations as well, these separate effects can be confusing. The ionic strength effect (activation), e.g. from the addition of NaCl, can be accounted for by the fact that the anion, Cl$^-$, enhances the dissociation rate for phosphate as shown in Table 2. Even the relatively slow phosphate dissociation from the $(Zn_A Mg_B Mg_C)_2 AP$ can be enhanced ~ 15-

fold by 1 M Cl$^-$ (Table 2). The molecular mechanism of this effect appears adequately explained by the ^{35}Cl NMR (Zn_4Mg_2 enzyme) and ^{113}Cd NMR (Cd_6 enzyme) observations that Cl$^-$ can occupy two coordination sites at the A-site metal ion (37). Thus, Cl$^-$ is in competition with one of the phosphate-oxygen-metal bonds and can thus labilize the bound phosphate of E·P.

Because of the apparent lack of effect of pH on phosphate binding to the enzyme through the range of the second pK_a of phosphate, investigators have always argued that the phosphate is forced to bind to the enzyme active center as the dianion (63). The phosphate-dissociation rate is independent of pH from pH 8.8 to pH 5.5 as has been shown directly with ^{31}P NMR inversion transfer for Zn_4AP (38) (Figure 2). All forms of E-P show ^{31}P chemical shifts more downfield than the dianion of free phosphoserine, for which the $\delta = 4$ ppm (Table 3). The ^{31}P chemical shifts of all forms of E·P, with the exception of that for $(Zn_AMg_BMg_C)_2AP$, are downfield of that for the dianion forms of free P_i, $\delta = 3$ ppm. The $(Zn_AMg_BMg_C)_2AP$ enzyme has an unusually far upfield ^{31}P resonance for E·P (Table 3) and a very slow off rate for phosphate, $k_4 = 1.0$–1.8 s^{-1} (Table 2). This slowing of the rate-limiting step in the hydrolysis reaction is an adequate explanation for the fact that in the presence of an acceptor like Tris, where the majority of the reaction is phosphotransferase rather than hydrolysis, k_{cat} does not decrease for the $(Zn_AMg_BMg_C)_2AP$, while if no acceptor is present, k_{cat} is 10% of that for the native enzyme. This assertion follows because the dissociation of an ester, e.g. R′OP as the transferase product, is much faster than HOP as discussed in more detail below.

The Phosphotransferase Reaction

The transfer of the phosphate from E-P to an acceptor alcohol by alkaline phosphatase was discovered early in kinetic studies of the enzyme (26, 63). The fact that a two- to fourfold enhancement in the rate of RO$^-$ release could be observed by adding an acceptor like Tris(tris-hydroxymethyl aminomethane) (Table 1) led to the routine inclusion of 1 M Tris in the standard assay of alkaline phosphatase. The enhanced rate of release of p-nitrophenolate made the assay significantly more sensitive. Product analysis showed that the enhanced activity resulted almost entirely from the formation of a new phosphate monoester, Tris-phosphate. The rate of formation of the original hydrolysis product, phosphate, remained relatively unaffected (63, 79).

Isolation of nonchromophoric phosphate esters is difficult, and relatively little quantitative data on the phosphotransferase reaction have accumulated over the years. Recently, ^{31}P NMR proved to be a convenient method of simultaneously following the phosphotransferase and hydrolysis reactions (38). Most phosphate monoesters, even those with relatively similar R groups, have sufficiently different ^{31}P chemical shifts to be distinguished. The separate signals for *p*-nitrophenylphosphate, P_i, and phospho-Tris are shown in Figure 8*a* illustrating a ^{31}P NMR spectrum of a standard assay mix (20 mM *p*-nitrophenylphosphate-1 M Tris) a few minutes after adding assay concentrations of alkaline phosphatase.

Figure 8*b* shows examples of the pH-dependencies of phosphotransferase reactions as followed by ^{31}P NMR, employing two rather different acceptors, Tris and glycerol. The data are presented as the ratio of new ester product to the hydrolysis product, phosphate, as a function of time, which is also the ratio of the rates of the two separate reactions,

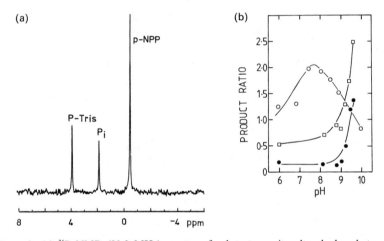

Figure 8 (*a*) ^{31}P NMR (80.9 MHz) spectra of substrate, *p*-nitrophenyl phosphate and products, inorganic phosphate, and O-Tris phosphate during hydrolysis and phosphotransfer as catalyzed by alkaline phosphatase. The composition at the start of reaction was 20 mM *p*-nitrophenyl phosphate in 1 M Tris or 3 M glycerol, pH 8, 293 K. To this was added alkaline phosphatase (5×10^{-8} M). The spectra were collected after about 50% hydrolysis and represent 80 scans. (*b*) pH Dependence of transferase and hydrolase products in the presence of 1 M Tris and 3 M glycerol. (*Open circle*) Ratio of initial rates of formation of Tris phosphate to inorganic phosphate; (*open square*) ratio of initial rates of formation of glycerol C1, C3, and C2 monophosphate to inorganic phosphate; (*solid circle*) ratio of initial rates of formation of glycerol C2 monophosphate to glycerol C1,C3 monophosphate. Note that at pH 9.5 the C2 transferase product exceeds the C1+C3 product by the ratio 1.3 : 1.0. The reaction mixture in the case of glycerol contained initially 3 M glycerol in 50 mM Tris (the latter solely as buffer and not at high enough concentration to result in competition with 3 M glycerol). Enzyme (10^{-7}–10^{-8} M) was used depending on pH. The substrate concentration was 20 mM. The figure is reproduced from Ref. 38.

phosphotransferase/phosphohydrolyase. The two curves for glycerol represent the formation of the equivalent C1 + C3 monophosphates and the C2 monophosphate. All three hydroxyl groups of glycerol are approximately equally phosphorylated by the enzyme. Tris is a much more effective acceptor in the neutral pH range than glycerol. The phosphotransferase reaction also increases in rate as the pH approaches the pK_a of the amino group, ~ 8 for Tris (63). This observation led to the suggestion that the neutral species of the amino alcohols were the most effective acceptors (63). The transferase activity of Tris, however, peaks at pH 8, falling rapidly to higher pH values (Figure 8b). At pH 9 and above, nonamino alcohols like glycerol, ethanol, and propanol are substantially more efficient acceptors than Tris (Figure 8b).

The rapid increase in the phosphate transfer to aliphatic alcohols above pH 9 is compatible with an arrangement in which the accepting alcohol is in the alcoxide form when bound at the active center and accepts the phosphoryl group from the seryl phosphate intermediate (38). If the oxygen of the acceptor coordinates Zn_A, as seems likely (38), then the apparent pK_a of the -C-OH will be lowered. An alcoxide has also been postulated to be the form of ethanol bound to alcohol dehydrogenase (82), another zinc enzyme in which an open coordination position on a zinc ion is the driving force for the formation of the alcoxide below its pK_a. At concentrations 0.5 M or greater, Tris and glycerol shift the ^{113}Cd resonance from the A site upfield by 14 and 6 ppm, respectively, at pH 9 (38). These ^{113}Cd chemical shift changes may represent the displacement of a water ligand by the alcoxide of the acceptor (38). Both the enhanced acceptor efficiency of the amino alcohols below the pK_a of the amino group and the rapid decline upon deprotonation of the amino group (Figure 8b) could result from the lowering of the pK_a of the -CH_2-OH group caused by the adjacent -C-NH_3^+ group such that the alcoxide of the amino alcohols is formed more readily (has a lower pK_a) below the pK_a of the amino group than when the neutral form of the amino group is present.

SUMMARY OF THE MECHANISM OF ALKALINE PHOSPHATASE AS BASED ON SOLUTION DATA AND THE CRYSTAL STRUCTURE

Figure 9 shows the Michaelis complex of the dianion of a phosphate monoester bound to the active center of Ser102 along with the steps leading to the phosphorylation of Ser102 and its subsequent dephosphorylation. The probable structural relationships are taken from the crystal structure of the E·P complex of the native zinc enzyme (Figure 4b) and the E-P complex of the cadmium enzyme (Figure 6b). Zn_A coordinates the ester

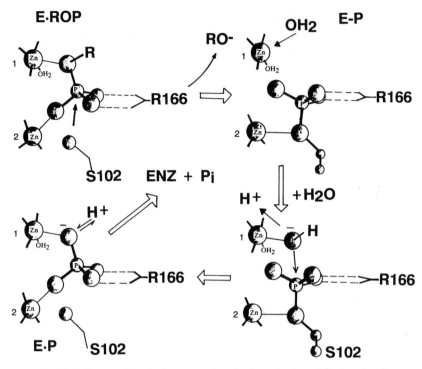

Figure 9   Major intermediates in the proposed mechanism of action of alkaline phosphatase. The dianion of a phosphate monoester, ROPO$_4^{2-}$, forms E·ROP in which the ester oxygen coordinates Zn1; a second oxygen coordinates Zn2, forming a phosphate bridge between the Zn1 and Zn2; while the other two phosphate oxygens form hydrogen bonds (*dashed lines*) with the guanidium group of R166. Ser102 is the nucleophile in the first half of the reaction and would occupy the position opposite to the leaving group, RO$^-$, in a five-coordinate intermediate. Upon formation of E-P, the phosphate (as the dianion of a phosphoseryl residue) moves slightly into the cavity of the active center, but maintains a coordinate bond between Zn2 and the ester oxygen as well as the two hydrogen bonds with R166. A water molecule coordinates Zn1 in the position occupied originally by the ester oxygen of the substrate. At alkaline pH, the water dissociates a proton to become Zn-$^-$OH in position to be the nucleophile for the hydrolysis of the phosphoseryl ester. E·P forms as the phosphate moves away from the serine and as one of the phosphate oxygens again coordinates Zn1 to reestablish a phosphate bridge. E·P is pictured as a phosphate trianion for the reasons discussed in the text. Dissociation of phosphate from E·P is the slowest, 35 s^{-1}, and therefore the rate-limiting, step.

oxygen, activating the leaving group. Zn$_B$, 3.9 Å away, coordinates a second phosphate oxygen, while the other two phosphate oxygens form hydrogen bonds with the guanidino group of Arg166. The leaving group is pictured as the alcoxide, RO$^-$. Activation of this leaving group by the

A-site metal ion via a bond with the ester oxygen appears to be one of the functions of this ion in the first stage of the alkaline phosphatase reaction. The oxygen of Ser102 is in the other apical position to form the new ester bond with the phosphorous. Dissociation of RO^- and formation of the phosphoseryl intermediate is associated with movement of the phosphate farther into the cavity (Figure 6b). Hence, when the alcoxide leaves, its coordination site on Zn_A can be occupied by a water molecule that must dissociate a proton and become a $Zn-^-OH$. The strongest evidence for this metal-induced proton dissociation is the large alkaline shift (3.7 pH units) in the pH dependence of the $E \cdot P \rightleftharpoons E-P$ equilibrium when the much softer metal ion, Cd(II), is substituted for Zn(II). The $Zn-^-OH$, placed in the apical postion opposite to the seryl ester, occupies the place of the original leaving group and thus is ideally positioned to be the nucleophile in the second stage of the hydrolysis reaction (Figure 9).

The second stage of the reaction is nearly a mirror image of the first stage. Zn_B now activates the leaving group by forming a coordinate bond with the ester oxygen of the phosphoseryl residue (Figure 9). The hydroxyl coordinated to Zn_A attacks the phosphorous from the other apical position, and the transition state will decay into $E \cdot P$. The issue of whether the new phosphate oxygen remains negatively charged is discussed below, but the dissociation of phosphate anion in the $E \cdot P$ intermediate is remarkably slow, $35\ s^{-1}$.

As discussed in connection with the phosphotransferase reaction, why the dissociation of $R_2OPO_3^{2-}$ is more rapid than that of $HOPO_3^{2-}$ if the latter is bound as the dianion is unclear. One possibility is that coordination of phosphate to both Zn ions as well as hydrogen bonding of the other two oxygens to the guanidino group of Arg166 forces the formation of the trianion, OPO_3^{3-}. On the other hand, the bound $ROPO_3^{2-}$ can only be a dianion. Zn_A does seem to be capable of lowering the pK_a of bound water by several pH units as well as inducing the alcoxide in the phosphotransferase reaction. Thus, lowering the third pK_a of phosphate may not be so unexpected as it might at first appear. Such a postulate would provide an explanation as to why dissociation of phosphate from the active center is so much slower than that for the dianion of a phosphate ester. The higher negative-charge density would also explain why phosphorylation of Ser102 by both phosphate and thiophosphate is so slow compared to phosphorylation by any phosphate ester. The pK_a of the leaving group for thiophosphate, H_2S, is 6.9 compared to a pK_a of 15.7 for HOH, the leaving group in phosphorylation from phosphate. Yet in the presence of rate-controlling phosphorylation, the difference in the phosphorylation of Ser102 by these two agents is at most only twofold (Table 1), despite the large ΔpK_a between the leaving groups. If both substrates were bound as trianions, poor leaving groups (probably requiring protonation first) and high charge density around the phosphorous could account for the very slow phosphorylation step as well as slow dissociation of the noncovalently bound species.

In the case of most enzyme-catalyzed phosphorylation or phospho-transferase reactions, investigators have tended to assume that such biological reactions were nucleophilic and associative and formed classic five-coordinate intermediates, the leaving group departing from the opposite apical position. This assumption was made despite the fact that in model systems most phosphate mono- and diester hydrolyses apparently proceed by a dissociative mechanism with the transient production of the highly electrophilic metaphosphate, $[PO_3^-]$ (6, 49, 78). Only phosphate triester hydrolysis follows a nucleophilic path in model systems (6, 49, 78). Enzymes could presumably make the nucleophilic path more favorable by creating protein-binding sites that successfully reduced the negative charge around phosphate, a significant inhibitory factor in mono- and diester hydrolysis in model systems. Determination of the predicted chirality changes around phosphate during enzyme-catalyzed phosphate incor-porations, i.e. inversion if no covalent enzyme intermediate was formed and retention if a covalent enzyme intermediate was formed as in alkaline phosphatase, tended to solidify the nucleophilic point of view. However, the finding that the Zn ions activate the leaving group in both the initial phosphorylation of the active-center serine and its dephosphorylation suggests that there may be significant dissociative character to both reactions. While the enzyme might hold a metaphosphate rigid enough to prevent scrambling of chirality, the evidence that the phosphate oxygens exchange positions relatively rapidly in the Co(II) enzyme does not favor the existence of free PO_3^- at the active site. Whether a classic five-coordinate intermediate is a true transition state in the alkaline phosphatase reaction remains an open question.

SITE-DIRECTED MUTANTS OF *E. COLI* ALKALINE PHOSPHATASE

Cloning of the *phoA* gene has allowed researchers to employ site-directed mutagenesis to change several of the amino acid side chains at the active center of alkaline phosphatase. The results of mutations at Ser102 and Arg166 have been most informative relative to mechanism, while mutations of several surrounding residues have revealed subtle influences on the rate. The results of these mutations are summarized below.

Ser102 → Cys102, Ala102, Leu102

The Ser102 → Cys102 mutant shows between 30 and 90% of normal activity against p-nitrophenyl phosphate and 2,4-dinitrophenyl phosphate depending on conditions. The range of turnover values results both from the fact that the phosphotransferase/phosphohydrolase ratio is increased and that k_{cat} depends on the nature of the leaving group. The Cys102 enzyme has a k_{cat} of 4.6 s^{-1} with 4-nitrophenyl phosphate and a k_{cat} of 15 s^{-1} with 2,4-dinitrophenyl phosphate under conditions where k_{cat} for the wild-type enzyme is 18 s^{-1} (39). In addition, the pH profile of the Cys102 enzyme shows no clearly apparent pK_a of activity. Lastly, a covalent S-phosphorothioate cannot be isolated from the enzyme by quenching at low pH (39). Most of the above findings on the Cys102 mutant can be explained if the rate-limiting step has changed to phosphorylation throughout the pH range. Throughout the pH range, phosphorylation of the native enzyme by ROPO$_4^{2-}$ occurs at the rate of 10^2 to 10^3 s^{-1}; thus, the phosphorylation rate can fall by 10- or even 100-fold without significantly lowering k_{cat}. These findings also suggest that dephosphorylation of the S-phosphorothioate formed with Cys102 is occuring more rapidly than for the normal covalent intermediate. A detailed kinetic study is required to sort out the rate constants of the Cys102 mutant. Phosphotransfer from a ^{16}O-, ^{17}O-, and ^{18}O-labeled phosphate ester to an acceptor catalyzed by the Cys102 mutant revealed retention of configuration around the phosphorous, proving that the reaction pathway has not been substantially changed (12).

The Ser102 → Ala102 or Leu102 mutants are not completely devoid of activity. The k_{cat} values are reported to be $\sim 1/1000$ and $\sim 1/500$ of those for the wild-type enzyme (14). K_m values for ROPO$_4^{2-}$ and K_i values for P$_i$ are reported to be normal as is the pH-rate profile. Because residue 102 is not directly involved in the structure of E·P, the lack of alteration in substrate and phosphate binding is not surprising. Since Zn$_A$ carries two coordinated H$_2$O molecules, as shown using NMR relaxation methods (37, 64), a water remaining on Zn$_A$ may be in a position to directly attack the ester of E·ROP at a low rate. An alkoxide, R$_2$O$^-$, could do the same and account for the detection of some phospho-Tris formed by these mutants (14).

Arg166 → Lys166, Glu166, Ser166, Ala166

All four mutations of Arg166 result in enzymes that remain active but demonstrate an increase in K_m and a decrease in phosphate affinity (13, 15). Although a decrease in phosphate binding affinity might increase the rate of phosphate dissociation, k_4, and therefore k_{cat}, the fact that the opposite occurs suggests that the loss of a positively charged center, helping to reduce the negative charge density at phosphorous, is the more important function. This fact also suggests that despite a significant dissociative aspect to the mechanism, the alkaline phosphatase reaction must retain significant aspects of a nucleophilic hydrolysis mechanism. This conclusion is supported by the finding for these mutants that when the nucleophile is water (hydrolysis), a relatively poor nucleophile, k_{cat} is reduced more by the mutation than when RO^- (phosphotransfer), a better nucleophile, is the nucleophile in the second half of the reaction. Likewise, the leaving group in the first half of the mechanism, phosphorylation of Ser102, has a more pronounced effect on the observed k_{cat} of the Arg166 mutants, e.g. k_{cat} decreases 10-fold on shifting from p-nitrophenolate as the leaving group to phenolate for both the Lys and Glu mutants. The effect of the Lys mutant must result from the different topological placement of the positive charge by the shorter lysyl side chain.

The fact that changes related to the bond-making and -breaking steps are now reflected in k_{cat} suggest that these mutations may have changed the relative values of the rate constants such that phosphate departure is no longer the slowest and therefore exclusively rate-limiting step. Further investigation is needed. While reduced in affinity, the phosphate binding is nevertheless adequately maintained in the Arg166 mutants by the interactions with the metal ions and the further hydrogen bonds with bridging water molecules to Mg_C and Lys328 (Figure 4b). E. E. Kim & H. W. Wyckoff (in preparation) have determined the crystal structure of the Arg166 → Ala166 mutant, which shows no changes in the active center except for the truncation of the density at the β-carbon of residue 166. Thus, the changes in the reaction parameters described above can be attributed exclusively to the functions of the Arg166 side chain.

Lys328 → His328, Ala328

Despite the conservation of many of the active-site residues found at the active center of the E. coli enzyme in several mammalian alkaline phosphatase isozymes, it has been puzzling why the mammalian enzymes uniformly show k_{cat} values at least an order of magnitude larger than that of the bacterial enzyme (for review, see 22). One intriguing structural finding at the active center of the bacterial enzyme is that Lys328, replaced by a His in all mammalian alkaline phosphatases, is bridged to the bound phosphate in E·P through a water molecule (Figure 4b). The latter water molecule is also hydrogen bonded to one carboxyl oxygen of Asp327, the bidentate ligand to Zn_A. The other oxygen of Asp327 makes a hydrogen bond with the N3 of His372 as discussed in the section on structure.

Because of the difference in the nature of residue 328 between the mammalian and bacterial enzymes and the close association of the Lys328 side chain with the A-site metal ligands as well as with phosphate via hydrogen bonds, two single site mutations of this residue have been examined, Lys328 → His328 and Lys328 → Ala328 (54, 81).

At pH 10.3, the Lys328 → Ala328 mutant shows a 14-fold increase in k_{cat} in the presence of Tris as an acceptor and a 6-fold increase in k_{cat} in the absence of the acceptor (15). At pH 8.0 in 1 M Tris, k_{cat} for the mutant enzyme was 81 s^{-1} and for the wild-type enzyme was 16 s^{-1}. The Lys328 → His328 is similar, but the enhancement of k_{cat} is not as large. Both mutant enzymes show reduced affinity for phosphate. K_m for ROPO$_4^{2-}$ is increased from 21 μM for the wild-type enzyme to 159 μM for the Ala328 mutant and 58 μM for the His328 mutant. Some significant changes are observed in the alkaline pH-rate profile of the mutant enzymes both in the presence and absence of a phosphate acceptor as well as in the magnitude and rate of the burst observed at both acid and alkaline pH, suggesting that the relative values of k_3 (dephosphorylation of E-P) and k_4 (phosphate dissociation) may have been changed by the mutation. Xu & Kantrowitz (81) suggest these changes might result from a change in the pH dependence of k_3, reflecting a change in the pK_a of the solvent H$_2$O coordinated to Zn$_A$. We lack sufficient detail on the pH dependence of the individual rate constants to be certain of the precise origin of the observed changes in pH-dependent functions. In another zinc enzyme, carbonic anhydrase, a series of detailed studies of rate-constant changes vs pH for several site mutations and a crystal structure of an isozyme carrying three of the side-chain changes show that changes in residues near the active center that alter the hydrogen-bonding patterns of the ordered water molecules near the Zn-coordinated solvent are far more effective in altering the pK_a of the co-ordinated solvent than are mutations of charged residues in the active site cavity that do not alter the hydrogen bond structure (73).

Several other site mutations of residues near the active center increase k_{cat}. These include Asp101 → Ala101, which increases k_{cat} 4.2-fold (80), as well as several mutations in the polypeptide chain region from residue 99 to 109. Mandecki et al (54) screened for "up" mutants in this region and found that V99A, T100V, A103D, A103C, and T107V all increase k_{cat} two- to fourfold. Residues 101 to 112 form a helical stem that holds Ser102 in place at the active center. Thus, alterations in k_{cat} are not surprising. What is perhaps unexpected is that most changes enhance k_{cat}. The assays are in 50 mM Tris; thus, the increases in k_{cat} primarily relate to the hydrolysis reaction. In the case of the *E. coli* enzyme, in which the dissociation of the phosphate is a very slow and rate-limiting step at alkaline pH, several slight perturbations of the topology at the active center can enhance this step. What evolutionary advantage prevented such mutations from evolving naturally is unclear. Perhaps phosphotransferase (not inhibited by phosphate departure) is a much more important reaction to *E. coli* than we currently appreciate because the natural acceptor has not been identified.

SUMMARY

Alkaline phosphatase was the first zinc enzyme to be discovered in which three closely spaced metal ions (two Zn ions and one Mg ion) are present at the active center. Zn ions at all three sites also produce a maximally active enzyme. These metal ions have center-to-center distances of 3.9 Å (Zn1-Zn2), 4.9 Å (Zn2-Mg3), and 7.1 Å (Zn1-Mg3). Despite the close packing of these metal centers, only one bridging ligand, the carboxyl of Asp51, bridges Zn2 and Mg3. A crystal structure at 2.0-Å resolution of the noncovalent phosphate complex, E·P, formed with the active center shows that two phosphate oxygens form a phosphate bridge between Zn1 and Zn2, while the two other phosphate oxygens form hydrogen bonds with the guanidium group of Arg166. This places Ser102, the residue known to be phosphorylated during phosphate hydrolysis, in the required apical position to initiate a nucleophilic attack on the phosphorous. Extrapolation of the E·P structure to the enzyme-substrate complex, $E \cdot ROPO_4^{2-}$, leads to the conclusion that Zn1 must coordinate the ester oxygen, thus activating the leaving group in the phosphorylation of Ser102. Likewise, Zn2 appears to coordinate the ester oxygen of the seryl phosphate and activate the leaving group during the hydrolysis of the phosphoseryl intermediate. Both of these findings suggest that there may be a significant dissociative character to each of the two displacements at phosphorous catalyzed by alkaline phosphatase. A water molecule (or hydroxide) coordinated to Zn1 following formation of the phosphoseryl intermediate appears to be the nucleophile in the second step of the mechanism. Dissociation of the product phosphate from the E·P intermediate is the slowest, $35 \, s^{-1}$, and therefore the rate-limiting, step of the mechanism at alkaline pH.

Since the determination of the initial crystal structure of alkaline phosphatase, two other crystal structures of enzymes involved in phosphate ester hydrolysis have been completed that show a triad of closely spaced zinc ions present at their active centers. These enzymes are phospholipase C from *Bacillus cereus* (structure at 1.5-Å resolution) (43) and P1 nuclease from *Penicillium citrinum* (structure at 2.8-Å resolution) (74). Both enzymes hydrolyze phosphodiesters. Substrates for phospholipase C are phosphatidylinositol and phosphatidylcholine, while P1 nuclease is an endonuclease hydrolyzing single stranded ribo- and deoxyribonucleotides. P1 nuclease also has activity as a phosphomonoesterase against 3'-terminal phosphates of nucleotides. The Zn ions in both enzymes form almost identical trinuclear sites. Zn1 and Zn3 are ~ 3.2 Å apart and are linked by a bridging carboxylate of an Asp residue as well as a bridging H_2O or ^-OH ion. Zn2 is an isolated site ~ 5.8 Å from Zn1 and ~ 4.7 Å from Zn3.

Are the three enzymes with trinuclear Zn sites at their active centers related? The general arrangement of the zinc ions is similar, but alkaline phosphatase and the other two enzymes are significantly different. All three metal sites in P1 nuclease and phospholipase C are typical Zn binding sites with mixed oxygen and nitrogen donors, while the third site in alkaline phosphatase is made up of all oxygen donors, which may explain its preference for Mg. The aspartate carboxylate bridging two of the Zn ions appears to define a binuclear zinc site in the two diesterases. In contrast, the bridging aspartate carboxylate defines the Zn-Mg pair in native alkaline phosphatase. As discussed in this review, the two nonbridged Zn ions, 3.9 Å apart in alkaline phosphatase, appear to form the major functional pair forming the phosphate bridge. In contrast, the few substrate analog binding studies done on the diesterases suggest that the isolated Zn2 site interacts with the phosphate diester (43). On the other hand, difference maps for phosphate bound to both P1 nuclease and phospholipase C show that an interaction with inorganic phosphate can take place involving coordination to all three zinc ions and raises the possibility that all three Zn ions could be catalytically involved at some stage of a complete mechanism.

Alkaline phosphatase is not closely related structurally to the other two enzymes. Alkaline phosphatase has a relatively small amount of α-helical structure on both faces of a large core of parallel and antiparallel β-sheets. The secondary structure of the two diesterases is composed almost entirely of α-helices, and their structures are closely related (43, 74). In addition, alkaline phosphatase forms a phosphoseryl intermediate, while both P1 nuclease and phospholipase C catalyze single-step hydrolyses, inverting the chirality around phosphate. While it is too early to state whether the trinuclear zinc sites found in the three phosphohydrolases reflect related functions, the data available at present suggest that the presence of multiple Zn ions located at a single enzyme active center add many alternatives to the reaction pathways available to zinc metalloenzymes.

ACKNOWLEDGMENT

I thank Harold W. Wyckoff and Eunice Kim for many helpful discussions and suggestions. The crystallography of alkaline phosphatase was supported by Grant GM22778. Original work in the author's laboratory was supported by NIH Grant DK09070.

Literature Cited

1. Anderson, R. A., Bosron, W. F., Kennedy, F. S., Vallee, B. L. 1975. *Proc. Natl. Acad. Sci. USA* 72: 2989–93
2. Applebury, M. L., Coleman, J. E. 1969. *J. Biol. Chem.* 244: 709–18
3. Applebury, M. L., Johnson, B. P., Coleman, J. E. 1970. *J. Biol. Chem.* 245: 4968–76
4. Bachman, B. J., Low, K. B., Taylor, A. L. 1976. *Bacteriol. Rev.* 40: 116–67
5. Bale, J. R. 1978. *Fed. Proc.* 37: 1287
6. Benkovic, S. J., Schray, K. J. 1973. *Enzymes* 8: 201–38
7. Benson, S. A., Hall, M. N., Silhavy, T. J. 1985. *Biochemistry* 54: 101–34
7a. Bertini, I., Luchinat, C., Maret, W., Zeppezaur, M., eds. 1986. *Zinc Enzymes.* Basel: Birkhäuser
8. Bloch, W. A., Schlessinger, M. J. 1973. *J. Biol. Chem.* 248: 5794–5805
9. Bock, J. L., Cohn, M. 1978. *J. Biol. Chem.* 253: 4082–85
10. Bosron, W. F., Anderson, R. A., Falk, M. C., Kennedy, F. S., Vallee, B. L. 1977. *Biochemistry* 16: 610–14
11. Bradshaw, R. A., Cancedda, F., Ericsson, L. H., Neuman, P. A., Piccoli, S. P., et al. 1981. *Proc. Natl. Acad. Sci. USA* 78: 3473–77
12. Butler-Ransohoff, J. E., Kendall, D. A., Freeman, S., Knowles, J. R., Kaiser, E. T. 1988. *Biochemistry* 27: 4777–80
13. Butler-Ransohoff, J. E., Kendall, D. A., Kaiser, E. T. 1988. *Proc. Natl. Acad. Sci. USA* 85: 4276–78
14. Butler-Ransohoff, J. E., Rokita, S. E., Kendall, D. A., Banzon, J. A., Carano, K. S., Kaiser, E. T., Matlin, A. R. 1992. *J. Org. Chem.* 57: 142–45
15. Chaidaroglou, A., Brezinski, J. D., Middleton, S. A., Kantrowitz, E. R. 1988. *Biochemistry* 27: 8338–43
16. Chaidaroglou, A., Kantrowitz, E. R. 1989. *Protein Eng.* 3: 127–32
17. Chang, C. N., Inouye, H., Model, P., Beckwith, J. 1980. *J. Bacteriol.* 142: 726
18. Chlebowski, J. F., Armitage, I. M., Tusa, P. P., Coleman, J. E. 1976. *J. Biol. Chem.* 251: 1207–16
19. Chlebowski, J. F., Coleman, J. E. 1974. *J. Biol. Chem.* 249: 7192–7202
20. Chlebowski, J. F., Coleman, J. E. 1976. *J. Biol. Chem.* 251: 1202–6
21. Coleman, J. E. 1987. In *Phosphate Metabolism and Cellular Regulation in Microorganisms,* ed. A. Torriani-Gorini, F. G. Rothman, S. Silver, A. Wright, E. Yagil, pp. 127–38. Washington, DC: Am. Soc. Microbiol.
22. Coleman, J. E., Besman, M. J. A. 1987. In *Hydrolytic Enzymes,* ed. A. Neuberger, K. Brocklehurst, pp. 377–406. New York: Elsevier
23. Coleman, J. E., Chlebowski, J. F. 1979. *Adv. Inorg. Biochem.* 1: 1–66
24. Coleman, J. E., Gettins, P. 1986. See Ref. 7a, pp. 77–99
25. Coleman, J. E., Nakamura, K., Chlebowski, J. F. 1983. *J. Biol. Chem.* 258: 386–95
26. Dayan, J., Wilson, I. B. 1964. *Biochim. Biophys. Acta* 81: 620–28
27. Engström, L. 1961. *Biochim. Biophys. Acta* 52: 49–59
28. Engström, L., Agren, G. 1962. *Biochim. Biophys. Acta* 56: 606–7
29. Fernley, H. N., Walker, P. G. 1969. *Biochem. J.* 111: 187–94
30. Fossett, M., Chappelet-Tordo, D., Lazdunski, M. 1974. *Biochemistry* 13: 1783–88
31. Garen, A., Levinthal, C. 1960. *Biochim. Biophys. Acta* 38: 470–83
32. Gettins, P., Coleman, J. E. 1983. *J. Biol. Chem.* 258: 396–407
33. Gettins, P., Coleman, J. E. 1983. *J. Biol. Chem.* 258: 408–16
34. Gettins, P., Coleman, J. E. 1983. *Adv. Enzymol.* 55: 381–452
35. Gettins, P., Coleman, J. E. 1982. *Fed. Proc.* 41: 2966–73
36. Gettins, P., Coleman, J. E. 1984. *J. Biol. Chem.* 259: 4991–97
37. Gettins, P., Coleman, J. E. 1984. *J. Biol. Chem.* 259: 11036–40
38. Gettins, P., Metzler, M., Coleman, J. E. 1985. *J. Biol. Chem.* 260: 2875–83
39. Ghosh, S. S., Back, S. C., Rokita, S. E., Kaiser, E. T. 1986. *Science* 231: 145–48
40. Grosser, P., Husler, J. 1912. *Biochem. Z.* 39: 1
41. Halford, S. E., Bennett, N. G., Trentham, D. R., Gutfreund, H. 1969. *Biochem. J.* 114: 243–51
42. Horiuchi, T., Horiuchi, S., Mizuno, D. 1959. *Nature (London)* 183: 1529–30
43. Hough, E., Hansen, L. K., Birknes, B., Jynge, K., Hansen, S., et al. 1989. *Nature (London)* 338: 357–60
44. Hull, W. E., Halford, S. E., Gutfreund, H., Sykes, B. D. 1976. *Biochemistry* 15: 1547–61
45. Inouye, H., Barnes, W., Beckwith, J. 1982. *J. Bacteriol.* 149: 434–39
46. Jones, S. R., Kindman, L. A., Knowles, J. R. 1978. *Nature (London)* 257: 564–65
47. Kim, E. E., Wyckoff, H. W. 1989. *Clin. Chim. Acta* 186: 175–88
48. Kim, E. E., Wyckoff, H. W. 1991. *J. Mol. Biol.* 218: 449–64

49. Knowles, J. R. 1980. *Annu. Rev. Biochem.* 49: 877–919
50. Krishnaswamy, M., Kenkare, U. W. 1970. *J. Biol. Chem.* 245: 3956–63
51. Labow, B. I. 1989. *Mechanisms of phosphoryl transfer by alkaline phosphatase from E. coli.* MS thesis. Brandeis Univ.
52. Levine, D., Reid, T. W., Wilson, I. B. 1969. *Biochemistry* 8: 2374–80
53. Ludke, D., Bernstein, J., Hamilton, C., Torriani, A. 1984. *J. Bacteriol.* 159: 19–25
54. Mandecki, W., Shallcross, M. A., Sowadski, J., Tomazic-Allen, S. 1991. *Protein Eng.* 4: 801–4
55. McComb, R. B., Bowers, G. N., Posen, S. 1979. *Alkaline Phosphatase.* New York: Plenum
56. Michaelis, A., Beckwith, J. 1982. *Annu. Rev. Microbiol.* 36: 435–65
57. Muller, M., Blobel, G. 1984. *Proc. Natl. Acad. Sci. USA* 81: 7737–41
58. Mushak, P., Coleman, J. E. 1972. *Biochemistry* 11: 201–5
59. Neumann, H. 1968. *J. Biol. Chem.* 243: 4671–76
60. Petitclerc, C., Lazdunski, C., Chappelet, D., Moulin, A., Lazdunski, M. 1970. *Eur. J. Biochem.* 14: 301–8
61. Plocke, D. J., Vallee, B. L. 1962. *Biochemistry* 1: 1039–43
62. Plocke, D. J., Levinthal, C., Vallee, B. L. 1962. *Biochemistry* 1: 373–78
63. Ried, T. W., Wilson, I. B. 1971. *Enzymes* 4: 373–415
64. Schulz, C., Bertini, I., Viezzoli, M. S., Brown, R. D., Koenig, S. H., Coleman, J. E. 1989. *Inorganic Chem.* 28: 1490–96
65. Schwartz, J. H. 1963. *Proc. Natl. Acad. Sci. USA* 49: 871–78
66. Schwartz, J. H., Lipmann, F. 1961. *Proc. Natl. Acad. Sci. USA* 47: 1996–2005
67. Schwartz, J. H., Crestfield, A. M., Lipmann, F. 1963. *Proc. Natl. Acad. Sci. USA* 49: 722–29
68. Sowadski, J. M., Handschumacher, M. D., Murthy, H. M. K., Foster, B. A., Wyckoff, H. W. 1985. *J. Mol. Biol.* 186: 417–33
69. Stein, S. S., Koshland, D. E. 1952. *Arch. Biochem. Biophys.* 39: 229–30
70. Suzuki, U., Yoshimura, K., Takaishi, M. 1907. *Bull. Coll. Argric. Tok. Imp. Univ.* 7: 503
71. Tashian, R. E., Hewett-Emmett, D. *Ann. New York Acad. Sci.* 429: 1–640
72. Torriani, A. 1960. *Biochim. Biophys. Acta* 38: 460–69
73. Tu, C., Paranawithana, S. R., Jewell, D. A., Tanhauser, S. M., LoGrasso, P. V., et al. 1990. *Biochemistry* 29: 6400–5
74. Volbeda, A., Lahm, A., Sakiyama, F., Suck, D. 1991. *EMBO J.* 10: 1607–18
75. Von Euler, H. 1912. *Z. Physiol. Chem.* 79: 375
76. Von Euler, H., Funke, Y. 1912. *Z. Physiol. Chem.* 77: 488
77. Weiss, P. M., Cleland, W. W. 1989. *J. Am. Chem. Soc.* 111: 1928–29
78. Westheimer, F. H. 1968. *Acc. Chem. Res.* 1: 70–78
79. Wilson, I. B., Dayan, J., Cyr, K. 1964. *J. Biol. Chem.* 239: 4182–85
80. Wyckoff, H. W., Handschumacher, M. D., Murthy, H. M. K., Sowadski, J. M. 1983. *Adv. Enzymol. Relat. Areas Mol. Biol.* 55: 453–80
81. Xu, X., Kantrowitz, E. R. 1991. *Biochemistry* 30: 7789–96
82. Zeppezauer, M. 1986. See Ref. 7a, pp. 417–34

SUBJECT INDEX

A

Acanthamoeba castellanii
  actin-profilin complex of, 68–69
Acetone-water exchange
  in vapor phase, 6–7
Acetylcholine
  anion channels gated by, 267
  cation channels gated by, 267
Acetylcholine receptor
  cation channels of
    blockade at, 282–83
    noncompetitive inhibitors of, 284–85
    single-channel conductance of, 271
  subunit composition of, 268
Acid hydrolysis
  bond rupture in, 12
Actin, 49–73
  adenosine triphosphate binding domain of, 305
  complexed with deoxyribonuclease I
    crystal structure of, 52–57
  function of, 63–71
  isoforms of, 62–63
  nucleotide hydrolysis and, 149
  polymerization of, 50
  structure of, 51–63
Actin-binding proteins, 50
Actin-depolymerizing factor, 68
Actin filament
  structure of, 59–62
α-Actinin
  function of, 69–70
Actophorin, 68
Adenosine diphosphate
  resonances of
    pH dependence of, 16
Adenosine triphosphatase
  clathrin-uncoating, 298
  lipid asymmetry and, 425
Adenosine triphosphate
  in actin, 56–57
  cation channels gated by, 267
  hydrolysis of
    heat-shock protein 70 and, 305–6
  protein folding and, 314
  reactions involving adenyl group, 13
  resonances of
    pH dependence of, 16

Adenyl-transfer reactions
  similarity to phosphoryl-transfer reactions, 13
Adenyl-transferring enzymes, 14
Adseverin
  homology to gelsolin, 70
Affinity labeling
  active site of Rubisco and, 130
Alamethicin peptide-dipalmitoylphosphatidylcholine complexes
  magnetization transfer curves for, 43
Alamethicin undecapeptides
  nuclear magnetic resonance spectroscopy of, 40–43
Alanine
  helix-forming tendency of, 96, 108
Alcaligenes eutrophus
  Rubisco of
    crystallography of, 126
Alkaline phosphatase, 441–81
  active center of
    coordination chemistry at, 456–61
  changes in activity of, 463–64
  dimer of
    alpha-carbon trace of, 444
  kinetics of, 443–53
  mechanism of, 473–76
  metalloenzyme nature of, 453–56
  site-directed mutants of, 476–80
  structure and mechanism of
    correlation of, 468–73
  multinuclear nuclear magnetic resonance and, 464–68
  structure of, 443
  substrate specificity of, 443–53
Alkyl N-methylglucamides
  precipitates formed by, 325
Alkylsulfates
  precipitates formed by, 325
Aluminum fluoride
  microtubule assembly and, 163
Alzheimer's disease
  amyloid precursor protein in, 236

Amino acids
  helix-forming propensities of, 96, 109–11
  helix-propagation parameters for, 101
Aminophospholipids
  in red cell membrane, 418–19
Aminophospholipid translocase, 426–28
Amphiphiles
  micelle formation by, 325
  solubilizing
    interactions with membrane proteins, 331–33
α-Amylase inhibitor
  structure of, 184–85
Amyloid precursor protein
  Alzheimer's disease and, 236
Anabena eutrophus
  Rubisco of
    subunit interactions in, 128
Anesthetics
  local
    neurotransmitter-gated ion channels and, 277–84
Anisotropy
  chemical-shift, 26–27
Apomyoglobin
  hydrogen-exchange labeling with, 252–53
Arabidopsis thaliana
  Rubisco of, 121
Archaebacteria
  ribosomes of
    crystallization of, 80
    thermoprotection factor of, 317
Arginine
  neurotransmitter-gated ion channels and, 279
Asialoglycoprotein receptor
  transmembrane domain of, 235
Aspartate receptor
  signal transduction by, 232
Atomic probes, 1–22
Azotobacter vinelandii
  RNA polymerase of
    pyrophosphate-exchange reaction of, 392

B

Bacillus cereus
  phospholipase C of, 481

494   SUBJECT INDEX

transcript elongation and,
405–8
RNA polymerase holoenzyme,
391
RNA synthesis
fidelity of, 402–5
mechanism of, 396–408
pyrophosphorolysis in, 401–2
single-base addition/removal
in, 398–401
stereochemistry of, 393
thermodynamics of, 383–88
Rubisco, 119–40
activation of, 122–23, 136–37
active site of, 130–32
carboxylation reaction of,
123, 138–40
conformational changes during
catalysis, 135–36
enolization of, 137–38
homooligomeric assembly of,
311
L$_2$ dimer of, 127–28
L$_8$S$_8$ molecule of, 128–29
L subunit of, 126–27
phosphorylated compounds
binding to, 132–35
photosynthesis/
photorespiration and,
120–21
protein crystallography and,
126–29
reactions/reaction in-
termediates of, 124–25
small subunits of, 129–30
S subunit of, 128
structure and function of,
136–40
synthesis and assembly of,
121–22
three-dimensional structure of,
126–36
Rubisco-binding protein, 122
Rubisco subunit-binding protein,
294, 306–8
Ruthenated cytochromes
electron-transfer reactions of,
361–71
Ruthenated myoglobin
electron-transfer reactions of,
371–74

S

Saccharomyces cerevisiae
cytochrome c variant of
surface histidine of, 365
heat-shock protein genes of,
300
Sarcoplasmic reticulum
solubilization of, 330

Schneider, G., 119–43
Scholtz, J. M., 95–118
Scintillation counting
structure change in hemoglobin and, 250
Sequential assignment method
nuclear magnetic resonance
spectroscopy and, 170–
71
Serine proteinase inhibitor
nuclear magnetic resonance
structure of, 184
Serotonin
cation channels gated by,
267
Severin
homology to gelsolin, 70
Signal transduction
monomolecular models for,
228–30
oligomerization and, 231–33
oligomerization models for,
230
tyrosine kinase receptor and,
232–33
Silvius, J. R., 323–48
Single-helix proteins
topology of, 227
two-stage folding and, 226–
27
Site-directed mutagenesis, 21
active site of Rubisco and,
130
alkaline phosphatase and,
476–80
neurotransmitter-gated ion
channels and, 269
QX-222 binding site and,
281–82
Smith, S. O., 25–47
Spectrin, 69–70
lipid asymmetry and, 426
Spectroscopy
coherent anti-Stokes Raman,
205
femtosecond, 199–220
experimental techniques in,
201–5
heme protein dynamics
and, 205–10
nuclear Overhauser enhancement, 170–74
photon echo, 205
total correlation, 170
transient absorption, 203–4
transient infrared absorption,
204–5
transient Raman, 204
See also Nuclear magnetic resonance spectroscopy
S-peptide
helix stop in, 103

Sphingomyelin
transmembrane distribution of,
429–30
Spinach
Rubisco of
crystallography of, 126
Staphylococcal nuclease
peptides of
helix formation in, 102
Statistical mechanics
helix formation in, 98–99
Stereocilia
actin bundles in, 52
Stress fibers, 52
Sulfolobus shibatae
thermoprotection factor of,
317
Sulfur-amino acid metabolism
isotopic tracers and, 7
Synaptosomes
aminophospholipid translocase
of, 426
Synchrotron radiation
crystallography of ribosomal
particles and, 89
Synecococcus
Rubisco of
crystallography of, 126

T

T-cell receptor
dimeric, 232
single-helix
transmembrane segments
of, 227
transmembrane domain of,
235
Temperature
hydrogen-exchange rates and,
247
micelle-forming properties of
detergents and, 325
photosynthetic reaction centers
and, 216–17
Tendamistat
structure of, 184–85
Tetrahymena thermophila
actin of
deoxyribonuclease I and,
57–58
mitochondria of
heat-shock protein 60 of,
308
Thermodynamics
helix formation in, 97–98
of RNA synthesis, 383–
88
Thermophiles
ribosomes of
crystallization of, 79–80

CUMULATIVE INDEXES

CONTRIBUTING AUTHORS, VOLUMES 17–21

496

CHAPTER TITLES, VOLUMES 17–21

INDEXED BY KEYWORD

Rubisco

Scanning Microscopy

Secondary Structure

Selective Deuteration

Sensory Rhodopsin

Sequence

β-Sheet

Signal Transduction

Signaling

Thermodynamic

Three-Dimensional Structures

Thick Filament

Time-Resolved

ANNUAL REVIEWS INC.

a nonprofit scientific publisher
4139 El Camino Way
P. O. Box 10139
Palo Alto, CA 94303-0897 • USA

ORDER FORM
ORDER TOLL FREE
1-800-523-8635
(except California)
FAX: 415-855-9815

Annual Reviews Inc. publications may be ordered directly from our office; through booksellers and subscription agents, worldwide; and through participating professional societies.

Prices are subject to change without notice.   ARI Federal I.D. #94-1156476

- **Individuals:** Prepayment required on new accounts by check or money order (in U.S. dollars, check drawn on U.S. bank) or charge to MasterCard, VISA, or American Express.

- **Institutional Buyers:** Please include purchase order.

- **Students:** $10.00 discount from retail price, per volume. Prepayment required. Proof of student status must be provided. (Photocopy of Student I.D. is acceptable.) Student must be a degree candidate at an accredited institution. Order direct from Annual Reviews. Orders received through bookstores and institutions requesting student rates will be returned.

- **Professional Society Members:** Societies who have a contractual arrangement with Annual Reviews offer our books at reduced rates to members. Contact your society for information.

- **California orders** must add applicable sales tax.

- **CANADIAN ORDERS:** We must now collect 7% General Sales Tax on orders shipped to Canada. Canadian orders will not be accepted unless this tax has been added. Tax Registration # R 121 449-029. Note: Effective 1-1-92 Canadian prices increase from USA level to "other countries" level. See below.

- **Telephone orders,** paid by credit card, welcomed. Call Toll Free **1-800-523-8635** (except in California). California customers use 1-415-493-4400 (not toll free). M-F, 8:00 am - 4:00 pm, Pacific Time. Students ordering by telephone must supply (by FAX or mail) proof of student status if proof from current academic year is not on file at Annual Reviews. Purchase orders from universities require written confirmation before shipment.

- **FAX: 415-855-9815   Telex: 910-290-0275**

- **Postage paid by Annual Reviews** (4th class bookrate). UPS domestic ground service (except to AK and HI) available at $2.00 extra per book. UPS air service or Airmail also available at cost. UPS requires street address. P.O. Box, APO, FPO, not acceptable.

- **Regular Orders:** Please list below the volumes you wish to order by volume number.

- **Standing Orders:** New volume in the series will be sent to you automatically each year upon publication. Cancellation may be made at any time. Please indicate volume number to begin standing order.

- **Prepublication Orders:** Volumes not yet published will be shipped in month and year indicated.

- **We do not ship on approval.**

ANNUAL REVIEWS SERIES *Volumes not listed are no longer in print*		Prices, postpaid, per volume		Regular Order Please send Volume(s):	Standing Order Begin with Volume:
		Until 12-31-91 USA & Canada / elsewhere	After 1-1-92 USA / other countries (incl. Canada)		
Annual Review of ANTHROPOLOGY					
Vols. 1-16	(1972-1987)....................	$33.00/$38.00			
Vols. 17-18	(1988-1989)....................	$37.00/$42.00 ⎫ $41.00/$46.00			
Vols. 19-20	(1990-1991)....................	$41.00/$46.00 ⎭			
Vol. 21	(avail. Oct. 1992).................	$44.00/$49.00	$44.00/$49.00	Vol(s)._____	Vol._____
Annual Review of ASTRONOMY AND ASTROPHYSICS					
Vols. 1, 5-14,	(1963, 1967-1976)				
16-20	(1978-1982)....................	$33.00/$38.00			
Vols. 21-27	(1983-1989)....................	$49.00/$54.00 ⎫ $53.00/$58.00			
Vols. 28-29	(1990-1991)....................	$53.00/$58.00 ⎭			
Vol. 30	(avail. Sept. 1992).............	$57.00/$62.00	$57.00/$62.00	Vol(s)._____	Vol._____
Annual Review of BIOCHEMISTRY					
Vols. 30-34, 36-56	(1961-1965, 1967-1987) ...	$35.00/$40.00			
Vols. 57-58	(1988-1989)....................	$37.00/$42.00 ⎫ $41.00/$47.00			
Vols. 59-60	(1990-1991)....................	$41.00/$47.00 ⎭			
Vol. 61	(avail. July 1992)	$46.00/$52.00	$46.00/$52.00	Vol(s)._____	Vol._____

ANNUAL REVIEWS SERIES	Prices, postpaid, per volume			
	Until 12-31-91 USA & Canada / elsewhere	After 1-1-92 USA / other countries (incl. Canada)	Regular Order Please send Volume(s):	Standing Order Begin with Volume:
Volumes not listed are no longer in print				

Annual Review of **BIOPHYSICS AND BIOMOLECULAR STRUCTURE**

Vols. 1-11	(1972-1982)	$33.00/$38.00			
Vols. 12-18	(1983-1989)	$51.00/$56.00	$55.00/$60.00		
Vols. 19-20	(1990-1991)	$55.00/$60.00			
Vol. 21	(avail. June 1992)	$59.00/$64.00	$59.00/$64.00	Vol(s)._____	Vol.____

Annual Review of **CELL BIOLOGY**

Vols. 1-3	(1985-1987)	$33.00/$38.00			
Vols. 4-5	(1988-1989)	$37.00/$42.00	$41.00/$46.00		
Vols. 6-7	(1990-1991)	$41.00/$46.00			
Vol. 8	(avail. Nov. 1992)	$46.00/$51.00	$46.00/$51.00	Vol(s)._____	Vol.____

Annual Review of **COMPUTER SCIENCE**

Vols. 1-2	(1986-1987)	$41.00/$46.00	$41.00/$46.00		
Vols. 3-4	(1988, 1989-1990)	$47.00/$52.00	$47.00/$52.00	Vol(s)._____	Vol.____

Series suspended until further notice. Volumes 1-4 are still available at the special promotional price of $100.00 USA /$115.00 other countries, when all 4 volumes are purchased at one time. Orders at the special price must be prepaid.

Annual Review of **EARTH AND PLANETARY SCIENCES**

Vols. 1-10	(1973-1982)	$33.00/$38.00			
Vols. 11-17	(1983-1989)	$51.00/$56.00	$55.00/$60.00		
Vols. 18-19	(1990-1991)	$55.00/$60.00			
Vol. 20	(avail. May 1992)	$59.00/$64.00	$59.00/$64.00	Vol(s)._____	Vol.____

Annual Review of **ECOLOGY AND SYSTEMATICS**

Vols. 2-18	(1971-1987)	$33.00/$38.00			
Vols. 19-20	(1988-1989)	$36.00/$41.00	$40.00/$45.00		
Vols. 21-22	(1990-1991)	$40.00/$45.00			
Vol. 23	(avail. Nov. 1992)	$44.00/$49.00	$44.00/$49.00	Vol(s)._____	Vol.____

Annual Review of **ENERGY AND THE ENVIRONMENT**

Vols. 1-7	(1976-1982)	$33.00/$38.00			
Vols. 8-14	(1983-1989)	$60.00/$65.00	$64.00/$69.00		
Vols. 15-16	(1990-1991)	$64.00/$69.00			
Vol. 17	(avail. Oct. 1992)	$68.00/$73.00	$68.00/$73.00	Vol(s)._____	Vol.____

Annual Review of **ENTOMOLOGY**

Vols. 10-16, 18	(1965-1971, 1973)				
20-32	(1975-1987)	$33.00/$38.00			
Vols. 33-34	(1988-1989)	$36.00/$41.00	$40.00/$45.00		
Vols. 35-36	(1990-1991)	$40.00/$45.00			
Vol. 37	(avail. Jan. 1992)	$44.00/$49.00	$44.00/$49.00	Vol(s)._____	Vol.____

Annual Review of **FLUID MECHANICS**

Vols. 2-4, 7	(1970-1972, 1975)				
9-19	(1977-1987)	$34.00/$39.00			
Vols. 20-21	(1988-1989)	$36.00/$41.00	$40.00/$45.00		
Vols. 22-23	(1990-1991)	$40.00/$45.00			
Vol. 24	(avail. Jan. 1992)	$44.00/$49.00	$44.00/$49.00	Vol(s)._____	Vol.____

Annual Review of **GENETICS**

Vols. 1-12, 14-21	(1967-1978, 1980-1987)	$33.00/$38.00			
Vols. 22-23	(1988-1989)	$36.00/$41.00	$40.00/$45.00		
Vols. 24-25	(1990-1991)	$40.00/$45.00			
Vol. 26	(avail. Dec. 1992)	$44.00/$49.00	$44.00/$49.00	Vol(s)._____	Vol.____

Annual Review of **IMMUNOLOGY**

Vols. 1-5	(1983-1987)	$33.00/$38.00			
Vols. 6-7	(1988-1989)	$36.00/$41.00	$41.00/$46.00		
Vol. 8	(1990)	$40.00/$45.00			
Vol. 9	(1991)	$41.00/$46.00	$41.00/$46.00		
Vol. 10	(avail. April 1992)	$45.00/$50.00	$45.00/$50.00	Vol(s)._____	Vol.____